LIBRARY-LRC
TEXAS HEART INSTITUTE

The Ventricular Arrhythmias of Ischemia and Infarction

Electrophysiological Mechanisms

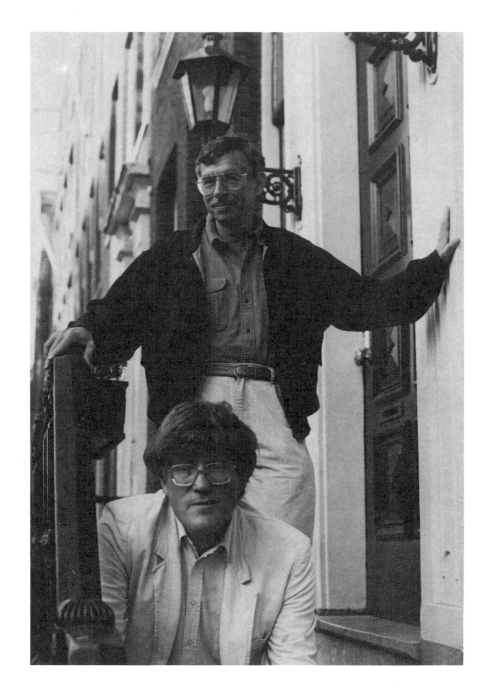

The Authors in Amsterdam

The Ventricular Arrhythmias of Ischemia and Infarction

Electrophysiological Mechanisms

By

Andrew L. Wit, PhD
Professor of Pharmacology, Department of Pharmacology,
College of Physicians and Surgeons of Columbia University
New York, NY

and

Michiel J. Janse, MD
Professor of Experimental Cardiology, Department of Clinical and
Experimental Cardiology,
University of Amsterdam and the
Interuniversity Cardiology Institute
Amsterdam, The Netherlands

**Futura Publishing
Company, Inc.**
Mount Kisco, NY

Library of Congress Cataloging-in-Publication Data

Wit, Andrew L.
    The ventricular arrhythmias of ischemia and infarction :
electrophysiological mechanisms / by Andrew L. Wit and Michiel
J. Janse.
        p. cm.
    Includes bibliographical references and index.
    ISBN: 0-87993-376-3
    1. Arrhythmia. 2. Ventricular fibrillation. 3. Myocardial
infarction—Complications and sequelae. 4. Coronary heart
diseases—Complications and sequelae. I. Janse, Michiel
Johannes. II. Title
    [DNLM: 1. Arrhythmia—physiopathology. 2. Electrophysiology.
3. Heart Ventricle—physiopathology. 4. Myocardial Infarction—
physiopathology. WG 330 W891v]
RC685.A65W58   1992
616.1′28—dc20
DNLN/DLC   91-46933
for Library of Congress   CIP

Copyright © 1993

Published by
Futura Publishing Company, Inc.
2 Bedford Ridge Road
Mount Kisco, New York 10549

LC #: 91-46933
ISBN #: 0-87993-376-3

Every effort has been made to ensure that the information in this book is as up to date and accurate as possible at the time of publication. However, due to the constant developments in medicine, neither the author, nor the editor, nor the publisher can accept any legal or any other responsibility for any errors or omissions that may occur.

All rights reserved.

No part of this book may be translated or reproduced in any form without written permission of the publisher.

Printed in the United States of America.

Printed on acid-free paper.

Acknowledgments

Kind Hearts and Coronaries

We assume that the reader will associate the title of this dedication with the film *Kind Heart and Coronets,* in which Sir Alec Guinness played almost every part. On the other hand, readers may recognize the original source, the poem "Lady Clara Vere de Vere" by Tennyson, containing the phase "Kind hearts are more than coronets". Our variation reflects to a certain extent our feelings about the subject of this book. No matter how often observed, a heart that suddenly goes into ventricular fibrillation is an awesome sight. The kind heart, one that has been beating faithfully and uncomplainingly for millions and millions of beats, is suddenly betrayed by the hand that feeds it, its coronary arteries. Since both of us (A.L.W. and M.J.J) have worked for many years on the electrophysiological changes that result from disturbances of coronary blood flow and have done so together with many colleagues and friends, our dedication is twofold. First to the kind hearts that were the subject of our research and second to the kind hearts that worked with us:

Maurits A. Allessie
Arlene Albala
J. Desmond Allen
Jacques M.T. de Bakker
Charly N.W. Belterman
Felix Bonke
Penelope A. Boyden
F. James Brennan
Frans J.L. van Capelle
Alessandro Capucci
René Cardinal
Juan Cinca
James Coromilas
Ruben Coronel
Kenneth H. Dangman
Jesse Davis*
Stephen M. Dillon
Eugene Downar
Karl P. Dresdner

John J. Fenoglio, Jr.*
Jan W.T. Fiolet
Peter L. Friedman
Phyllis I. Gardner
Leonard S. Gettes
Robert Glassman
Michael S. Hanna
Richard N.W. Hauer
Norbert M. van Hemel
Jaap van Hulst
Josje Janse
Ronald W. Joyner
Harayr S. Karagueuzian
André G. Kléber
Richard P. Kline
Karel Koch
Itsuo Kodama
Marijke Kraayenhof
Wim Lammers

*deceased

vi // Acknowledgments

Herve Moréna*
Christoph Naumann d'Alnoncourt
Tobias Opthof
Ron J.G. Peters
Tuan Duc Pham
Anand R. Ramdat Misier
Shira Rohde
Gerald Nassif
Adam E. Saltman
Aart Schene
Peter J. Schwartz
Wim L. ter Smitte

James Stewart
Sara J.A. Tasseron
Jorgen Tranum-Jensen
Gea-Ny Tseng
Philip C. Ursell
Jessica T. Vermeulen
Bernd Waldecker
Hsueh Hwa Wang
Melvin B. Weiss
Arthur A.M. Wilde
Robert L. Wilensky
Francien J.G. Wilms-Schopman

Preface

On the Origin of Ischemic Heart Disease, Ventricular Fibrillation, and Sudden Death

From our viewpoint today, it seems remarkable that it took such a long period of time before it was widely recognized in the 1960s that sudden death in patients with coronary artery disease is often caused by ventricular arrhythmias, notably ventricular fibrillation. We say this because it had been known for more than a century that sudden death in humans was associated with coronary artery obstruction and that coronary artery obstruction in experimental animals caused ventricular fibrillation. In the 18th century, Heberden first described the clinical syndrome of angina pectoris as "a sort of undescribable anguish across the breast", syncope, and eventually sudden death, but did not relate this syndrome to abnormalities of the coronary arteries (Snellen 1984). In 1779, both John Hunter, an English surgeon and anatomist, and Edward Jenner, famous for the cow-pox vaccine, almost simultaneously reported for the first time extensive ossification and calcification of the coronary arteries in patients with angina who died suddenly (Snellen 1984). At that time, Charles Parry also published a book (*An Inquiry into the Symptoms and Causes of the Syncope Anginosa Commonly Called Angina Pectoris*) in which he described in detail autopsies on patients who suffered from angina with sudden death, some of whom also probably had infarcts: ". . . after having examined the more important parts of the heart, without finding any thing by means of which I could account either for his sudden death, or the symptoms preceding it, I was making a transverse section of the heart pretty near to its base, when my knife struck against something so hard and gritty, as to notch it. I well remember looking up to the ceiling, which was old and crumbling, conceiving that some plaister had fallen down. But on further scrutiny the real cause appeared: the coronaries were becoming bony canals" (Parry 1799). After investigating several cases of sudden death, Parry wrote that ". . . the coronaries may be so obstructed as to intercept the blood, which should be the proper support of the muscular fibers of the heart". He considered this condition to result in "diminishing the energy of the heart" and added in a footnote: "By the energy of the heart I mean not merely the readiness, but also the degree of irritability or excitability" (Parry 1799). Subsequently, Quain (1850) demonstrated the damage to the heart (infarction) resulting from the coronary obstruction. Therefore, at the time Erichsen in 1840 ligated a coronary artery of a dog in the experimental laboratory, the link between coronary obstruction, ischemia, and sudden death had been established. Erichsen's experiments showed that coronary artery occlusion caused the action of the ventricles to cease, with "a slight tremulous motion alone continuing", providing the connection between coronary occlusion and ventricular fibrillation (Erichsen 1841–1842). Later experiments around the turn of the century confirmed and expanded these findings (Begold 1867; Porter 1894; 1896; Cohnheim and Von Schulthess-Rechberg 1881; Lewis 1909).

The clinical importance of the experimental results showing that coronary occlusion causes ventricular fibrillation was not at all recognized, except by a few individuals such as McWilliam. In 1889, based on his own experimental studies, he suggested that: ". . . sudden syncope from plugging or obstructing some portion of the coronary system (in patients) is very probably determined or ensured by the occurrence of fibrillar contractions in the ventricles. The cardiac pump is thrown out of gear, and the last of its vital energy is dissipated in a violent and prolonged turmoil of fruitless activity in the ventricular walls". However, in widely distributed textbooks, such as *Diseases of the Heart* by Sir James Mackenzie (1918) these ideas were ignored and only three lines were devoted to ventricular fibrillation in the 76 pages on cardiac arrhythmias. Wenckebach's monograph on arrhythmias of the heart (1904) does not mention ventricular fibrillation at all. A Dutch textbook of 1935 states: ". . . from that time on (i.e., since the electrocardiograph became widely used in both the clinic and in the experimental laboratory), fibrillation, and especially atrial fibrillation, became important in the clinic. Since ventricular fibrillation usually results in sudden cardiac death, it is, of course, of much less importance. Besides, ventricular fibrillation occurs much less frequently than atrial fibrillation" (De Boer 1935, our translation). Ventricular fibrillation was clearly considered to be of no clinical importance.

Indeed, in a paper written in 1923 entitled: *Some Applications of Physiology to Medicine*, MacWilliam (his name is now spelled MacWilliam instead of McWilliam, as in the 1889 paper) writes: "It may be permissible to recall that in the pages of this journal thirty-four years ago I brought forward a new view as to the causation of sudden death by a previously unrecognized form of failure of the heart's action in man (e.g., ventricular fibrillation)—a view fundamentally different from those entertained up to that time. Little attention was given to the new view for many years . . . At that time the current conception of the relations of the experimental physiology of the heart to practical medicine was widely removed from what it now is . . . it was not then recognized that most of the disturbances that have been experimentally induced in the mammalian heart (for example, fibrillation, flutter, heart-block, extra-systoles of various types, rhythms of abnormal origin, alternation of the heart beat, etc.) have their clinical counterparts in the manifold derangements of function in diseased conditions in man . . . In more recent times the view that ventricular fibrillation is a cause of sudden death in man has been accepted by numerous observers." It was not, however, universally accepted. MacWilliam's lament could with equal poignancy have been written many decades later.

The reasons why ventricular fibrillation was so neglected probably were that it was difficult to document its occurrence in man, and that it could not be treated (Lown 1979a). Sporadically, case reports documenting ventricular fibrillation in man appeared (Hoffman 1911; Halsey 1915). However, it was not until the advent of the coronary care unit in the late 1960s, where electrocardiograms were recorded from patients in the early phase of myocardial infarction, that the frequent occurrence of ventricular fibrillation in man with acute myocardial ischemia was appreciated (Julian et al. 1964; Lown et al. 1967a). At that time, mobile coronary care units recording cardiograms from individuals suffering cardiac arrest outside the hospital provided further evidence that ventricular fibrillation was present in many cases (Pantridge et al. 1967; Cobb et al. 1975). The fact that by this time electrical defibrillation was made not only possible but easy as well (Lown et al. 1962) undoubtedly contributed to the interest in sudden death and its underlying mechanisms generated in the past 20 years. (Lown 1979a; 1979b).

Although the history of mechanisms of disorders of cardiac rhythm is long, MacWilliam being the dominant figure in the 19th century, and with important contributions of Mines, Garrey, and Lewis in the period between 1910 and 1924, the study of arrhythmia mechanisms caused by ischemia and infarction is of more recent origin. Some of the first important studies came from the laboratory of Wiggers, where it was shown that the threshold for fibrillation induced by electrical current was much reduced after coronary artery occlusion (Wiggers et al. 1940). Wiggers postulated that ectopic impulses would be able to initiate ventricular fibrillation because of this reduction. Shortly thereafter, Harris and Rojas (1943) proposed a mechanism in which current flow across the boundary between ischemic and nonischemic myocardium caused these ectopic beats. The first investigations in which attempts were made to study the effect of acute ischemia on transmembrane potentials of single myocardial cells date from the late 1950s and early 1960s (Kardesh et al. 1958; Samson and Scher 1960; Prinzmetal et al. 1961). Our story begins at this point. Both of us began working in the late 1960s, one (A.L.W.) with Hoffman and Cranefield on electrophysiological mechanisms of arrhythmias, the other (M.J.J.) in Durrer's laboratory where, among other studies, experiments on arrhythmias caused by ischemia and infarction had been undertaken. This book is based to a large part on experimental studies performed in our own laboratories. We follow the axiom of MacWilliam stated above in ascribing an important relation of "the experimental physiology of the heart to practical medicine", a concept that was also ingrained in us by our own teachers Dirk Durrer, Brian Hoffman, and Paul Cranefield. We owe them a special debt of gratitude. Therefore, much of the text describes experimental studies. We do not mean this book to be a complete review on all the literature dealing with arrhythmias, ischemia, and infarction. This would be an impossible task anyway: in a period of two-and-a-half years, from January 1980 to June 1982,

6,027 papers were published carrying the word "arrhythmia" in either title or key words. For "ischemia" the number was 6,484, and for "infarction" 11,268 (Dialog Database, Los Angeles). We did not relish the prospect of reading some 150,000 papers in order to have a complete picture of everything published in about 20 years on these subjects. Undoubtedly we have overlooked important contributions.

A.L.W.
M.J.J.

Contents

Chapter I

Basic Mechanisms of Arrhythmias

Before examining the electrophysiological consequences of ischemia and infarction, we will describe the different electrophysiological mechanisms that cause arrhythmias. The recording of transmembrane electrical events of individual myocardial cells with microelectrodes has provided much of the information necessary for understanding these mechanisms. The importance of this approach was recognized and emphasized in the 1960s by Hoffman and Cranefield (Hoffman and Cranefield 1964). They proposed that although arrhythmias may have many different pathological causes, in the final analysis they are the result of critical alterations in cellular electrophysiology. During the subsequent decades many scientists investigating arrhythmias followed their lead and the literature is replete with publications on cellular mechanisms. (For some reviews see Hoffman and Cranefield 1964; Cranefield 1975; Moe 1975; Wit and Bigger 1975; Wit and Cranefield 1978; Wit et al. 1980; Hoffman and Rosen 1981; Spear and Moore 1982; Wit and Rosen 1984; Gilmour and Zipes 1986; Janse 1986a; Wit and Rosen 1986; Cranefield and Aronson 1988; Wit and Rosen 1989). From this vast literature a general schema on classifications of mechanisms has been formulated (Hoffman and Rosen 1981), which is shown in Table 1. This schema subdivides the general causes of arrhythmias into two: abnormalities in impulse initiation and abnormalities in impulse conduction. Both abnormalities may also occur simultaneously. Each has subclassifications. All these mechanisms come into play at one time or another to cause the arrhythmias of cardiac ischemia and infarction.

Arrhythmias Caused by Abnormal Impulse Initiation

Abnormalities of impulse initiation are one cause of arrhythmias. The term "impulse initiation" is used to indicate that an electrical impulse can arise in a single cell or group of closely coupled cells through depolarization of the cell membrane, and once initiated spread through the rest of the heart. Impulse initiation occurs because of localized changes in ionic currents that flow across the membranes of single cells. There are two major causes for the impulse initiation that may result in arrhythmias: automaticity and triggered activity. Each has its own unique cellular mechanism resulting in membrane

---

Table 1*

I. Abnormal Impulse Initiation
   A. Automaticity
      1. Normal automaticity
      2. Abnormal automaticity
   B. Triggered Activity
      1. Early afterdepolarizations
      2. Delayed afterdepolarizations
II. Abnormal Impulse Conduction
   A. Conduction block leading to ectopic pacemaker "escape"
   B. Unidirectional block and reentry
      1. Ordered reentry
      2. Random reentry
   C. Reflection
III. Simultaneous Abnormalities of Impulse Initiation and Conduction
   A. Impaired conduction caused by phase 4 depolarization
   B. Parasystole

---

* (Modified from Hoffman and Rosen 1981.)

depolarization. Automaticity is the result of spontaneous (diastolic) depolarization (see Figure 1.1), whereas triggered activity is caused by afterdepolarizations (see Figure 1.12 later in this chapter). These different cellular mechanisms result in arrhythmias that have very different electrocardiographic characteristics, including their mode of onset, their rate, their mode of termination, and their response to interventions such as external pacemakers and drugs.

Automaticity

It is convenient to subdivide automaticity into two kinds, normal and abnormal, although sometimes the subdivision may be somewhat artificial. Normal automaticity is found in the primary pacemaker of the heart—the sinus node—as well as in certain subsidiary or latent pacemakers that can become the pacemaker under conditions that are described later. Impulse initiation is a normal property of these latent pacemakers. On the other hand, abnormal automaticity, whether the result of experimental interventions or pathology, only occurs in cardiac cells when major (abnormal) changes occur in their transmembrane potentials, in particular, steady state depolarization of the resting potential. This property of abnormal automaticity is not confined to any specific latent pacemaker cell type, but may occur almost anywhere in the heart. Arrhythmias characterized by abnormalities in the rate, regularity, or site of origin of the cardiac impulse can result from either normal or abnormal automaticity.

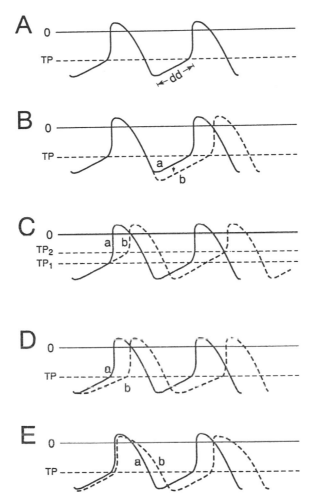

Figure 1.1: Diagrams of sinus node action potentials illustrating normal automaticity caused by spontaneous diastolic depolarization and the factors that change the rate of impulse initiation. Panel A shows a typical sinus node action potential with spontaneous diastolic depolarization, "dd". Panel B shows change in rate that occurs when the maximum diastolic potential is shifted to a more negative level (from a to b). Panel C shows change in rate caused by change in threshold potential to a less negative level (from TP_1 to TP_2). Panel D shows change in rate that occurs when the slope of phase 4 depolarization is decreased (from a to b). Panel E shows change in rate that occurs when the action potential duration is increased (from a to b).

Normal Automaticity

Normal Pacemaker Mechanisms   The normal site of impulse initiation is the sinus node. The cause of normal automaticity in the sinus node is a spontaneous decline in the transmembrane potential during diastole, referred to as the pacemaker potential or phase 4 or diastolic depolarization (we use the terms interchangeably) first recorded in isolated, superfused preparations from the mammalian heart with a microelectrode by West in 1955. Diastolic depolarization can also be recorded from the sinus node in the *in situ* animal or human heart with an extracellular electrode. During *in situ* recordings, the amplification must be high because the extracellular currents that flow during the pacemaker potential are very small (Cramer et al. 1977; Hariman et al. 1980). Diastolic depolarization is that part of the sinus node membrane potential labeled "dd" in the top panel (A) of Figure 1.1. (Baumgarten and Fozzard (1986) point out that care should be taken not to confuse electrical diastole with mechanical diastole because the two are not temporally coincident.) When the depolarization reaches threshold potential (dashed line "TP"), the upstroke of the spontaneous action potential is initiated. This fall in membrane potential during phase 4 reflects a gradual shift in the balance between inward and outward membrane currents in the direction of net inward (depolarizing) current. Studies have been done to elucidate and characterize the membrane currents that cause diastolic (phase 4) depolarization in the sinus node using voltage-clamp techniques in small tissue preparations and in single dissociated sinus node cells. At this time (1991) the cause of the pacemaker potential is still controversial. There is some evidence that diastolic depolarization results from the turning on of an inward current called "i_f", that is activated after repolarization of the sinus node action potential (Brown and DiFrancesco 1980; DiFrancesco and Ojeda 1980; DiFrancesco 1990). The i_f current is carried by Na^+ and K^+ as shown by ion substitution experiments; the reversal potential of the current is intermediate between the Na^+ and K^+ equilibrium potentials (DiFrancesco 1990). From the voltage-clamp studies, it is known that the i_f channels are inactivated at positive membrane potentials, begin to activate after hyperpolarization to around -40 mV, and are fully activated after hyperpolarization to around -100 mV (Yanagihara and Irisawa 1980; DiFrancesco 1986; DiFrancesco et al. 1986). Because the maximum diastolic potential of the sinus node pacemaker cells is between -60 and -70 mV, the i_f current is turned on during repolarization to this level although it is not fully activated at the maximum diastolic potential. Activation of the i_f conductance also has a time dependency, and therefore the inward current continues to increase after complete repolarization, causing the progressive fall in the membrane potential during phase 4. Despite the fact that i_f is not fully activated in sinus node cells at the maximum diastolic potential, DiFrancesco (1990) has stated that it generates sufficient current density to be the primary cause of spontaneous diastolic depolarization. However, an important role for a time-dependent decrease in a potassium conductance, i_K, in causing spontaneous diastolic depolarization has also been proposed (Brown 1982; Brown et al. 1982). Activation of this outward potassium current after the upstroke of the action potential plays a major role in causing repolarization in sinus node cells (Nakayama et al. 1984; Shibasaki 1987) and determines the most negative level of the membrane potential upon complete repolarization (Irisawa and Giles 1990). After complete repolarization, this potassium conductance decreases with time, resulting in membrane depolarization during diastole. In addition, activation of both T- and L-type inward calcium currents (Reuter 1984; Bean 1985) during the diastolic depolarization contributes to further phase 4 depolarization (Hagiwara et al. 1988; Doerr et al. 1989). The L-type calcium current also causes the upstroke of the sinus node action potential (Noma et al. 1977; Brown et al. 1984). Brown et al. (1984) have also provided evidence for a secondary component of slow inward current possibly mediated by intracellular calcium release that may contribute to the last part of diastolic depolarization. Current i_f may contribute to diastolic depolarization in this model, but is not the primary cause. Therefore, there may be no single pacemaker current in the sinus node but rather, a number of currents may contribute to the occurrence of automaticity (Irisawa and Giles 1990).

The intrinsic rate at which sinus node pacemaker cells initiate impulses is determined by the interplay of three factors (Hoffman and Cranefield 1960):

(a) the maximum diastolic potential;
(b) the threshold potential; and
(c) the rate or slope of phase 4 depolarization.

The third factor (c) is related to the properties of the pacemaker current(s). A change in any one of these factors will alter the time required for phase 4 depolarization to carry the membrane potential from its maximum diastolic level to threshold, and thereby alter the rate of impulse initiation. For example, if the maximum diastolic potential increases (becomes more negative) going from solid trace "a" to dashed trace "b" in Figure 1.1B, spontaneous depolarization to threshold potential will take longer and the rate of impulse initiation will fall. Conversely, a decrease in the maximum diastolic potential will tend to increase the rate of impulse initiation (going from trace b to trace a). Similarly, changes in threshold potential or changes in the slope of phase 4 depolarization will alter the rate of impulse initiation. In Figure 1.1C, a change in threshold potential from TP_1 to the less negative TP_2 causes spontaneous diastolic depolarization to proceed for a longer time (dashed action potential trace) before an impulse is initiated, slowing the rate. In Figure 1.1D, a decrease in the slope of spontaneous diastolic depolarization from a to b also results in a longer interval between action potentials (dashed trace) because of the longer time required for membrane potential to reach the threshold potential. In both Figures 1.1C and 1.1D, changes of threshold potential or slope of diastolic depolarization in the opposite direction would speed up the rate.

The alterations in the rate of impulse initiation in the sinus node resulting from the factors discussed above may lead to arrhythmias. They are often the result of the actions of the autonomic nervous system on the sinus node. Parasympathetic stimulation and the resultant release of acetylcholine hyperpolarizes the membrane potential through stimulation of muscarinic receptors and activation of a K current (Figure 1.1B) (Trautwein 1982; Soejima and Noma 1984). Acetylcholine also decreases inward calcium current and the i_f pacemaker current. The i_f current activation curve is shifted to more negative potentials so that less current is activated upon repolarization of the sinus node cells (DiFrancesco and Tromba 1988). A combination of these effects slows the rate. Sympathetic stimulation and norepinephrine release increases the slope of diastolic depolarization and therefore sinus rate by increasing L-type calcium current (Noma et al. 1980) and by shifting the activation threshold of i_f to more positive levels, so that there is increased activation of the inward current at the completion of action potential repolarization (DiFrancesco 1985; DiFrancesco 1986; DiFrancesco et al. 1986). These effects are mediated through β_1-receptor stimulation.

Another alteration in the transmembrane potentials of sinus node cells, a change in the duration of the action potential, may also influence their rate of firing. A prolongation of the action potential duration in the face of a constant diastolic period increases the time between successive action potential upstrokes and slows the rate. In Figure 1.1E, the dashed action potentials have a prolonged duration compared to the action potentials indicated by the solid trace. Shortening of the action potential duration has an opposite effect, speeding the rate if there are no offsetting changes in the diastolic interval. While a change in the sinus node action potential duration alone is not the primary mechanism for physiological or pathophysiological changes in sinus rate, it can be an important cause of rate changes that result from administration of some pharmacological agents (Opthof et al. 1986).

In addition to the sinus node, cells with pacemaking capability in the normal heart are located in some parts of the atria and ventricles, although they are not pacemakers while the sinus node is functioning normally. These are latent or subsidiary pacemakers. Because spontaneous diastolic depolarization is a normal property, the automaticity generated by these cells is classified as normal. In the atria, cells with well polarized membrane potentials (resting potentials of around -80 mV) and action potentials characterized by fast upstrokes, a plateau phase of repolarization and spontaneous diastolic depolarization, are located along the crista terminalis (Figure 1.2A) (Hogan and Davis 1968). Subsidiary atrial pacemakers with somewhat lower maximum diastolic potentials (-75 to -70 mV) and prominent phase 4 depolarization are located at the junction of the inferior right atrium and inferior vena cava, near or on the eustachian ridge (a remnant of the eustachian valve of the inferior vena cava) (Figure 1.2B) (Sealy et al. 1973; Jones et al. 1978; Randall et al. 1980; Rozanski et al. 1983; Rozanski and Lipsius 1985). Other potential atrial pacemakers are at the orifice of the coronary sinus (Figure 1.2C) (Wit and Cranefield 1977) and in the atrial muscle that extends into the tricuspid and mitral valves (Figure 1.2D) (Wit et al. 1973; Bassett et al. 1976; Rozanski 1987). Action potentials of cells in the valves have slow upstrokes that are depressed by verapamil and that are probably caused to a significant extent by L-type calcium current. In the atrioventricular (AV) junction, AV nodal cells possess the intrinsic property of automaticity (Figure 1.2E) (Kokubun et al. 1980) although there is still some uncertainty as to the exact location of these pacemakers in the node (James et al. 1979). The intrinsic rate of the atrial pacemakers is greater than that of AV junctional pacemakers (Randall et al. 1980). Both atrial and junctional subsidiary pacemakers are under autonomic

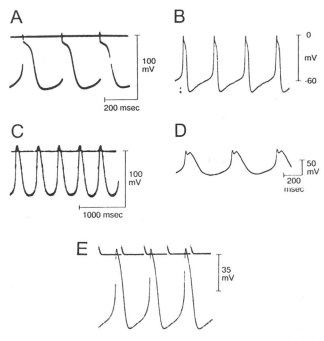

Figure 1.2: Transmembrane potentials recorded in isolated superfused preparations from some subsidiary pacemaker cells with the property of normal automaticity. Spontaneous diastolic depolarization that developed in the absence of overdrive suppression is shown in each panel. **A**: Atrial fiber in crista terminalis in the presence of isoproterenol. (Reproduced from Hogan and Davis (1968) with permission.) **B**: Atrial fiber in the inferior right atrium. (Reproduced from Rozanski and Lipsius (1985) with permission.) **C**: Atrial fiber in ostium of coronary sinus in the presence of norepinephrine. (Reproduced from Wit and Cranefield (1977) with permission.) **D**: Atrial fiber in stretched mitral valve leaflet. (Reproduced from Wit et al. (1973) with permission.) **E**: Atrioventricular (AV) nodal fiber of the rabbit heart after the AV node was separated from the atrium. (Reproduced from Wit and Rosen (1984) with permission.)

control with the sympathetics enhancing pacemaker activity through β_1-adrenergic stimulation and the parasympathetics inhibiting pacemaker activity through muscarinic receptor stimulation (Spear and Moore 1973; Randall et al. 1978; Wallick et al. 1979; Rozanski and Jalife 1986). In the ventricles, latent or subsidiary pacemakers are found in the His-Purkinje system where Purkinje fibers have the property of spontaneous diastolic depolarization (Figure 1.3) (Weidmann 1956; Hoffman and Cranefield 1960). In general, the intrinsic Purkinje fiber pacemaker rate is less than the rate of atrial and junctional pacemakers, and decreases from the His bundle to the distal Purkinje branches (Hope et al. 1976). The spontaneous diastolic depolarization in this region is also under similar autonomic control. As in the atria, sympathetic activation enhances automaticity (Vassalle et al. 1968), while parasympathetic activation can reduce it, mostly through inhibition of sympathetic influences (Levy 1971; Levy and Blattberg 1976) although acetylcholine does have a small direct de-

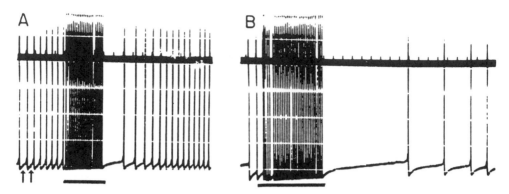

Figure 1.3: Overdrive suppression of normal automaticity in a canine Purkinje fiber. The action potentials are displayed at a slow oscilloscopic sweep speed so the time course of repolarization cannot be seen. The period of overdrive is indicated by the horizontal bar below the recordings. (Reproduced from Cranefield (1975) with permission.)

pressant effect on spontaneous diastolic depolarization of Purkinje fibers (Danilo et al. 1978; Gadsby et al. 1978).

The membrane currents causing the normal spontaneous diastolic depolarization at ectopic sites have also been studied. The most thorough analyses have been done on the pacemaker current in Purkinje cells using voltage-clamp techniques. These studies have shown the presence of an i_f pacemaker current, as in the sinus node, that is activated with hyperpolarizing voltage-clamp pulses in the range of potentials between -60 mV and -100 mV (DiFrancesco 1981a; 1981b; 1985). Thus, i_f channels are deactivated during the action potential upstroke and initial plateau phase of repolarization, but begin to activate as repolarization brings the membrane potential to levels more negative than about -60 mV. Because the activation kinetics are slow, the channels continue to activate throughout diastole, leading to an increasing net inward current (carried by Na^+) and diastolic depolarization (DiFrancesco 1981a; 1981b). Other currents are also likely to contribute to the pacemaker potential in Purkinje cells (Noble 1984; DiFrancesco 1985; DiFrancesco and Noble 1985; Gintant and Cohen 1988). These currents include the i_{K1} potassium current that is the major potassium conductance during diastole (Gintant and Cohen 1988). Two properties of this current are instrumental in its proposed role in the generation of the pacemaker potential. One is that the i_{K1} conductance shows inward rectification; that is, the conductance is large at negative membrane potentials near E_K and negligible at potentials more than 40 mV positive to E_K (Shah et al. 1987). The second is that i_{K1} conductance is influenced by the K^+ concentration outside the cell and increases in proportion to the square root of this concentration $[K^+]_o$ (Sakmann and Trube 1984). Because of these properties, the i_{K1} conductance is high immediately after repolarization because of the negative level of the membrane potential and an elevated level of K^+ outside the cell membrane, resulting from accumulation of K^+ leaving the cell during the action potential in restricted spaces or clefts between Purkinje cells (Kline and Kupersmith 1982). Cleft K^+ then decreases during diastole because K^+ is moved into the cells by the Na/K pump (called "deaccumulation" by Cranefield and Aronson 1988). The decrease in $[K^+]_o$ causes the K^+ conductance to decrease and the membrane to depolarize, contributing to phase 4 depolarization. The importance of this decrease in K^+ conductance is suggested by the failure of some investigators to observe spontaneous diastolic depolarization in single isolated disaggregated Purkinje cells (Robinson et al. 1987), a preparation in which there are no restricted extracellular spaces (clefts) and presumably little or no K^+ accumulation and deaccumulation. Another potassium current, the delayed rectifier (i_K) may also contribute to spontaneous diastolic depolarization in Purkinje fibers as has been proposed for the sinus node. This current is activated during the action potential and is a major factor in causing repolarization (Cohen et al. 1986). Decay of the i_K current after repolarization because the conductance is inactivated at the negative level of membrane potential, then contributes to the fall of K^+ conductance during diastole and diastolic depolarization. The steady state Na^+ window current is also expected to contribute to the inward pacemaker current during diastole (Gintant and Cohen 1988). Therefore, it is likely that the net increase in inward current during diastole causing spontaneous diastolic depolarization in Purkinje fibers is a result of an increase in an inward current (i_f) and a decrease in outward currents (i_{K1} and i_K). In the coming years the relative contributions of each of these currents are sure to be elucidated.

A membrane current similar to the i_f pacemaker current in Purkinje fibers may also be involved in the pacemaker activity in atrial and AV junctional pacemakers (Kokubun et al. 1980; 1982; Earm et al. 1983; Carmeliet 1984). Other membrane currents may also contribute to pacemaker activity in these cells. In atrial subsidiary pacemakers near the eustachian ridge and the AV valves, diastolic depolarization consists of two phases, an early rapid and short-lasting depolarization and a later slower and longer lasting depolarization (See Figure 1.2B). It has been suggested that the early rapid depolarization may be the result of the i_f pacemaker current while the longer lasting slower depolarization is a calcium-dependent process (Rubenstein and Lipsius 1989). This calcium-dependent process may not be entirely inward current through a calcium channel; a membrane current mediated by intracellular release of calcium from the sarcoplasmic reticulum (SR) may contribute. It has been proposed that calcium released from the SR acts on the sarcolemma to facilitate the inward movement of Na^+ during diastole that causes slow depolarization, a mechanism similar to the transient inward current that causes delayed afterdepolarizations (see section on Triggered Activity) (Rubenstein and Lipsius 1989). The inward current might result from Na/Ca exchange. The primary evidence for such a process is the depression of spontaneous firing rate of subsidiary atrial pacemakers caused by ryanodine (Rubenstein and Lipsius 1989), a chemical that inhibits calcium release from the sarcoplasmic reticulum (Sutko and Kenyon 1983; Marban and Wier 1985). Changes in the rate of firing of the subsidiary pacemakers is primarily dependent on changes in slope of the second phase of diastolic depolarization and not the first. A similar pacemaker mechanism also occurs in the atrial fibers of the AV valves (Rozanski 1987).

Suppression of Subsidiary Pacemakers In the normal heart in sinus rhythm, the intrinsic rate of impulse initiation owing to automaticity of cells in the sinus node is higher than that of the other potentially automatic cells, and the latent pacemakers are excited by propagated impulses from the sinus node before they can spontaneously depolarize to threshold potential. The function of the subsidiary pacemakers during normal rhythm is only to participate in conduction of the sinus impulse through the heart. Not only are latent pacemakers prevented from initiating an impulse because they are depolarized before they have a chance to fire, but also the diastolic (phase 4) depolarization of the latent pacemaker cells is actually inhibited because the cells are repeatedly depolarized by the impulses from the sinus node (Vassalle 1970; Vassalle 1977). This inhibition can be demonstrated by suddenly stopping the sinus node by, for example, vagal stimulation (vagal stimulation also inhibits subsidiary pacemakers in the atria and AV junction). Impulses then usually arise from a subsidiary pacemaker in the ventricular Purkinje system, but that impulse initiation is generally preceded by a long period of quiescence (Vassalle et al. 1967). Impulse initiation by the Purkinje fiber pacemaker then begins at a low rate and only gradually speeds up to a final steady rate that is, however, still slower than the original sinus rhythm. The quiescent period following abolition of the sinus rhythm reflects the inhibitory influence exerted on the subsidiary pacemaker by the dominant sinus node pacemaker. This inhibition is called overdrive suppression. Similarly, the sinus node also overdrive-suppresses subsidiary atrial pacemakers (Randall et al. 1982a).

The phenomenon of overdrive suppression can also be demonstrated in isolated, superfused cardiac pacemaker fibers as shown in Figure 1.3. At the left of panel A, action potentials recorded from an automatic Purkinje fiber, spontaneously firing at a rate of about 1 per second are shown. There is prominent phase 4 depolarization preceding the upstroke of each action potential (small arrow). The fiber bundle was stimulated rapidly at a rate of 3 per second for 25 seconds, during the period indicated by the horizontal line below the trace. After stimulation was stopped, there was a period of quiescence before the spontaneous rhythm began again at a slow rate that gradually increased to the rate that existed prior to stimulation. In panel B the overdrive was repeated for a longer time period, indicated by the horizontal bar, resulting in a longer period of postoverdrive quiescence before the spontaneous rhythm returned.

The mechanism of overdrive suppression has been characterized in microelectrode studies on isolated Purkinje fiber bundles exhibiting pacemaker activity such as the one shown in Figure 1.3 (Vassalle 1970). It is mostly mediated by enhanced activity of the Na^+-K^+ exchange pump that results from driving a pacemaker cell faster than its intrinsic spontaneous rate. During normal cardiac rhythm, the sinus node (or in the example in Figure 1.3, the electrical stimulus) drives the latent pacemakers at a faster rate than their normal (intrinsic) automatic rate. As a result, the intracellular Na^+ of the latent pacemakers is increased to a higher level than would be the case were the pacemakers firing at their own intrinsic rate. This is the result of Na^+ ions entering the cells during each action potential upstroke. The rate of activity of the sodium pump is largely determined by the level of intracellular Na^+ concentration (Glitsch 1979), so that pump activity is enhanced during high rates of stimulation (Vassalle 1970). The increased pump activity prevents intracellular Na^+ from rising to very high levels although, as mentioned before, there is an increase in the steady state Na^+ concentration at high rates of firing. Because the sodium pump moves more Na^+ outward than K^+ inward, it generates a net outward (hyperpolarizing) current across the cell membrane (Gadsby and Cranefield 1979a). When subsidiary pacemaker cells are driven faster than their intrinsic rate (such as by the sinus node), the enhanced outward pump current hyperpolarizes the membrane potential and suppresses spontaneous impulse initiation in these cells, which as described before, is dependent on the net inward current. When the dominant (overdrive) pacemaker is stopped, this suppression continues because the Na^+ pump continues to generate the outward current as it reduces the intracellular Na^+ levels towards normal. The continued sodium pump-generated outward current is responsible for the period of quiescence that lasts until the intracellular Na^+ concentration, and hence the pump current, becomes small enough to allow subsidiary pacemaker cells to depolarize spontaneously to threshold. Intracellular Na^+ concentration decreases during the quiescent period, because Na^+ is constantly being pumped out of the cell and little is entering (January and Fozzard 1984). Intracellular Na^+ and pump current continue to decline even after spontaneous firing begins because of the slow rate, causing a gradual increase in the discharge rate of the subsidiary pacemaker. The higher the overdrive rate, or the longer the duration of overdrive, the greater is the enhancement of pump activity (until a maximum effect is reached when the pump is saturated), so that the period of quiescence following the cessation of overdrive is directly related to the rate and duration of overdrive (see Figure 1.3) (Vassalle 1970).

Some suppression of subsidiary pacemakers may also occur after short periods of overdrive, even before the pump current significantly increases. This suppression is a result of an initial transient increase in extracellular K^+ caused by K^+ loss from the cells during the initial period of rapid activity. The increase in extracellular K^+ causes some membrane depolarization (prior to the hyperpolarization caused by the pump current) and increases membrane conductance, an effect that decreases spontaneous diastolic depolarization (Vassalle 1970). During overdrive, intracellular Ca^{2+} may also increase because of the increased frequency of action potentials (Lado et al. 1982). An increased intracellular Ca^{2+} contributes to overdrive suppression (Musso and Vassalle 1982) because Ca^{2+} increases membrane K^+ conductance that hyperpolarizes and opposes spontaneous diastolic depolarization (Isenberg 1977). The influences of elevated extracellular K^+ concentration and intracellular Ca^{2+} concentration are not nearly as important as that of the increased Na pump current during longer periods of overdrive.

The sinus node itself can also be overdrive-suppressed if it is driven at a rate more rapid than its intrinsic rate (Jordan et al. 1977; Kodama et al. 1980; Greenberg and Vassalle 1990). Thus, there may be a quiescent period after termination of a rapid ectopic arrhythmia before the sinus rhythm resumes (Gang et al. 1983). However, when overdrive suppression of the normal sinus node occurs, it is of lesser magnitude than that of subsidiary pacemakers overdriven at comparable rates (Jordan et al. 1977; Jones at al. 1978). The sinus node action potential upstroke is largely dependent on slow inward current carried by calcium through the L-type calcium channels, and far less sodium enters the fiber during the upstroke than in latent pacemaker cells such as Purkinje fibers. As a result, the activity of the sodium pump is probably not increased to the same extent in sinus node cells after a period of overdrive and, therefore, there is less overdrive suppression caused by enhanced sodium pump current. An increase in intracellular Ca^{2+} may contribute to the overdrive suppression of the sinus node because overdrive suppression of the node is markedly enhanced when extracellular Ca^{2+} is increased experimentally (Greenberg and Vassalle 1990). The relative resistance of the normal sinus node to overdrive suppression may be important in enabling it to remain as the dominant pacemaker even when its rhythm is transiently perturbed by external influences (such as transient shifts of the pacemaker to an ectopic site). The diseased sinus node, however, may be much more easily overdrive-suppressed (Breithardt et al. 1977).

In addition to its intrinsic resistance to overdrive suppression, the pacemaker cells of the sinus node are also protected from overdrive suppression during rapid atrial arrhythmias by the perinodal fibers that form the border between the sinus node and atrium (Strauss and Bigger 1972). During rapid irregular rhythms, such as atrial fibrillation, the center of the sinus node is protected because ectopic impulses block both in the perinodal region and the periphery of the node. Microelectrode recordings from the sinus node region of rabbits during atrial fibrillation showed that the average cycle length in the center of the sinus node was nearly the same as during normal sinus rhythm (Kirchhof 1989).

In addition to overdrive suppression being of paramount importance for maintenance of normal rhythm, the characteristic response of normally automatic pacemakers to overdrive, as discussed in the previous paragraphs, is often useful for identifying mechanisms of arrhythmias in the *in situ* heart where arrhythmia mechanisms cannot usually be identified by recording transmembrane potentials because of the technical difficulties. Not all mechanisms of arrhythmogenesis respond in the same way to overdrive as normally automatic pacemakers and the differences in response can sometimes be used to distinguish among mechanisms. We describe these differences in detail later in this chapter.

For the sake of completeness, we will at this time also describe the effects of single stimuli arising outside the pacemaker region on normal automaticity although it is a digression from the theme of our discussion on how the dominant pacemaker suppresses subsidiary pacemakers to maintain a normal rhythm. We will return to that theme shortly. The effects of single stimuli can also be used in the *in situ* heart to distinguish among arrhythmogenic mechanisms. A single premature impulse, either resulting from an electrical stimulus or arising spontaneously at an ectopic pacemaker site, might propagate into the sinus node and disturb the sinus rhythm or a single sinus or stimulated impulse during an ectopic rhythm might propagate into that pacemaker site and disturb that rhythm. The characteristic way in which the rhythm is disturbed might be of help in identifying arrhythmias caused by normal automaticity in the *in situ* heart. The effects of premature impulses on automatic rhythms have been studied on isolated, superfused preparations of the sinus node and Purkinje fiber bundles (Bonke et al. 1969; Klein et al. 1972; Klein et al. 1973a; 1973b; Dangman and Hoffman 1985). During sinus rhythm or the slow rhythm characteristic of a normally automatic Purkinje fiber, the cycle length following a prematurely stimulated impulse occurring late in diastole, and that succeeds in depolarizing the pacemaker (resetting it), is often prolonged compared to the regular spontaneous cycle length (Bonke et al. 1969; Klein et al. 1972; Dangman and Hoffman 1985). This effect is illustrated in Figure 1.4. In each trace (A-C) action potentials are shown recorded from a spontaneously active Purkinje fiber (cycle length 1570 msec). The record in trace A shows a prematurely stimulated impulse at the arrow with a coupling interval of 870 msec. The postextrasystolic cycle length of 1590 msec is longer than the unperturbed spontaneous cycle length. The prolongation resulted from depression of spontaneous diastolic depolarization of the premature action potential. The mechanism for the depression is uncertain. Occasionally some hyperpolarization following the premature action potential has also been noted, accounting for an increase in the time required for spontaneous diastolic depolarization to carry the membrane potential to threshold. In the sinus node

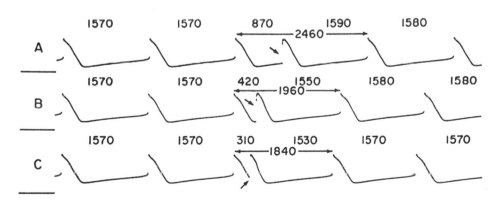

Figure 1.4: Effects of stimulated premature impulses on normal automaticity of a canine Purkinje fiber. The cycle lengths are indicated above the traces in each panel. The spontaneous cycle length is 1570 msec. The prematurely stimulated impulse is indicated by the arrow in each panel. The horizontal arrows above each trace indicate the sum of the premature cycle and the return (postextrasystolic) cycle that follows it. For example, in **A** the premature cycle is 870 msec, the postextrasystolic cycle is 1590 msec, and the sum of the two is 2460 msec. This is less than compensatory since twice the unperturbed spontaneous cycle is 3140 (see text for explanation). (Reproduced from Klein et al. (1972) with permission.)

the depression of the pacemaker potential following a single premature impulse is sometimes accompanied by a shift of the pacemaker site (Bonke et al. 1969; Klein et al. 1973b). Conceivably, this might also happen at ectopic pacemaker sites. Despite the prolonged extrasystolic cycle length, the cycle length following premature impulses occurring late in diastole is generally less than compensatory.

The meaning of the term compensatory is diagrammed in Figure 1.5. Trace A shows the cycle length of a spontaneous rhythm (S_1-S_1) that is 1000 msec. Trace B shows the time of occurrence of a premature impulse (S_2) that was stimulated during the spontaneous cycle length at a coupling interval of 750 msec. The impulse following the prematurely stimulated impulse (S_3) occurs at the time expected for the next impulse if there had been no stimulation, because the lengthening of the post-stimulus cycle length to 1250 msec exactly counterbalances the shortening of the premature cycle length. Thus, the S_1-S_2 interval plus the S_2-S_3 interval is equal to two S_1-S_1 intervals and the S_2-S_3

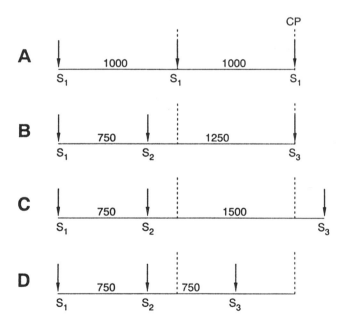

Figure 1.5: A diagram illustrating some possible effects of single premature impulses on normal automaticity. The arrows in panel A, labeled S_1, indicate the time of occurrence of spontaneous impulses at a cycle length of 1000 msec. Panel B shows a premature impulse stimulated at S_2 with a coupling interval of 750 msec to the spontaneous impulse S_1 (the dashed line in the middle is where the next spontaneous impulse would have occurred if there had been no premature impulse). The time of occurrence of the next spontaneous impulse 1250 msec after the premature impulse is indicated by S_3, on the dashed line indicating a compensatory pause (CP). In panel C, the time of occurrence of the spontaneous impulse S_3, following the premature impulse S_2, is 1500 msec, which is longer than compensatory. In panel D, the time of occurrence of the spontaneous impulse S_3, following the premature impulse, S_2, is 750 msec, which is less than compensatory.

interval is said to be compensatory. If the impulse following the premature depolarization comes later than expected, e.g., the sum of S_1-S_2 plus S_2-S_3 is greater than 2 times S_1-S_1, the postextrasystolic cycle length is said to be more than compensatory (Trace C), and if the impulse following the premature depolarization comes earlier than expected, e.g., the sum of S_1-S_2 plus S_2-S_3 is less than 2 times S_1-S_1, the postextrasystolic cycle length is said to be less than compensatory (Trace D).

After premature impulses delivered in midcycle, the postextrasystolic cycle is generally about the same as the basic cycle and also less than compensatory. After premature impulses delivered early in the basic spontaneous cycle the postextrasystolic cycle has been found to be shorter than the basic cycle (and still less than compensatory) in the studies on both the sinus node and Purkinje fibers, particularly when the rate of spontaneously firing is slow. The decrease in the postextrasystolic cycle length of spontaneously beating Purkinje fibers when the premature impulse was delivered during phase 3 of repolarization was mainly a result of the decrease in the duration of the premature action potential, the rate of spontaneous diastolic depolarization being either unchanged or slightly depressed (Klein et al. 1973b). This is also illustrated in Figure 1.4 where in traces B and C the stimulated premature impulse at the arrows is occurring earlier and earlier in the cycle length, and the postextrasystolic cycle length decreases as the coupling interval of the stimulated impulse decreases. For example, in trace C, the premature coupling interval is 310 msec and the cycle length following the premature impulse in 1530 msec compared to the cycle length of 1570 msec prior to stimulation. In the sinus node, the mechanism for the shortening of the postextrasystolic cycle is not obvious (Bonke et al. 1969; Klein et al. 1973b). Conduction delay from the sinus node to the atrium might sometimes mask the decrease in the sinus node cycle length, causing it not to be apparent in recordings from the atrium. In the experiments of Dangman and Hoffman (1985) on spontaneously firing Purkinje fibers, this shortening of the cycle following early premature impulses was not usually evident and the return cycle length remained unchanged from the spontaneous cycle length over a wide range of premature coupling intervals in most preparations. Figure 1.6 from their publication shows the relationship of the corrected return cycle (return cycle as a percent of the cycle prior to stimulation) to the premature cycle. Return cycles remain equal to the spontaneous cycle (corrected return cycle of 1) and are less than compensatory in this figure, throughout the range of premature coupling intervals. Shortening of the return cycle in Purkinje fibers following an early premature stimulus is probably dependent on the spontaneous rate being very slow and the action potential duration being very long. At faster rates at which the action potential duration during the basic rhythm is short, the duration of the action potential of the premature impulse compared to the basic impulse is not much different and therefore, the reason for the shortening of the cycle length is removed. Thus, shortening of the postextrasystolic cycle would not be expected after early premature impulses applied during an automatic tachycardia.

Now we return to our discussion on how subsidiary pacemakers in the

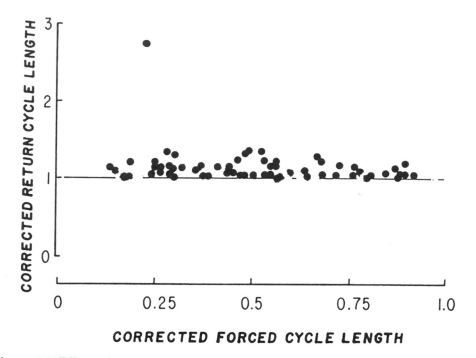

CORRECTED FORCED CYCLE LENGTH

Figure 1.6: Effects of premature stimuli on normal automatic rhythms in canine Purkinje fibers. Filled circles show the corrected return cycle (return cycle as a percent of the cycle prior to stimulation) following single stimulated premature impulses over a wide range of cycle lengths (expressed as corrected forced cycle length that is a fraction of the basic spontaneous cycle length). The return cycle, which is less than compensatory, did not change over a wide range of premature coupling intervals. (Reproduced from Dangman and Hoffman (1985) with permission.)

heart are normally suppressed and prevented from becoming the dominant pacemaker. Another mechanism that may suppress subsidiary pacemakers, in addition to overdrive suppression, is the electrotonic interaction between the pacemaker cells and nonpacemaker cells in the surrounding myocardium (Van Capelle and Durrer 1980). This mechanism may be particularly important in preventing AV nodal automaticity (Wit and Cranefield 1982; Kirchhof et al. 1988). Atrioventricular nodal cells have intrinsic pacemaker activity that may sometimes be nearly as rapid as that in the sinus node. This can be demonstrated in small pieces of the AV node superfused in a tissue chamber (Kokubun et al. 1980). Such pacemaker activity is not easily overdrive-suppressed, probably for the same reasons discussed above for the sinus node. However, the pacemaker activity of the AV node may be suppressed by axial (intracellular) current flowing through the connections between the node and surrounding atrial cells. The proposed mechanism is shown schematically in Figure 1.7A, where an AV nodal action potential with a low membrane potential and spontaneous diastolic depolarization is indicated by the solid trace (a), and the high level of transmembrane potential of an adjacent atrial cell without pacemaker

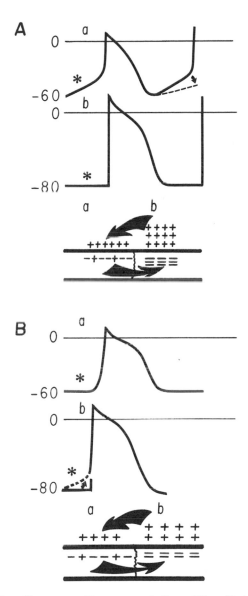

Figure 1.7: Panel A is a diagrammatic representation of the effects of current flow from a cell with a high resting potential of −80 mV (cell b) on the spontaneous diastolic depolarization of a cell with a lower resting potential of −60 mV (cell a). Panel B shows a diagrammatic representation of the effects of a cell with a steady low membrane potential of −60 mV (cell a) on diastolic depolarization in a cell with a higher membrane potential (cell b). (Reproduced from Wit and Rosen (1989) with permission.)

activity is shown by the solid trace (b). As a result of the more negative potentials of the atrial cells during diastole, current flow between them and the nodal cells should be in a direction that prevents spontaneous phase 4 depolarization of the nodal cells. The current flow is diagrammed below the action potential traces in a schematic representation of the membrane during the diastolic period. Because (a) has a lower potential than (b), there is a flow of positive charge from (b) to (a) in extracellular space and from (a) to (b) in intracellular space (axial current), opposing the decrease in membrane potential during spontaneous diastolic depolarization. The small arrow in action potential trace (a) points to the suppressed phase 4 depolarization. This current flow is apparently sufficient to prevent nodal automaticity despite the paucity of intercellular junctions in the nodal region. The same mechanism might also be operative in other regions of the atria where latent pacemaker cells are surrounded by nonpacemaker cells, or in the distal Purkinje system where the pacemaking Purkinje fibers are in contact with nonpacemaking working ventricular muscle (Van Capelle and Durrer 1980; Janse and Van Capelle 1982a; Opthof et al. 1987). In Figure 1.8, the effects of decreasing the coupling resistance and, therefore, increasing intercellular current flow between a pacemaker and a nonpacemaker cell, on automaticity in a computer simulation of Van Capelle and Durrer (1980) is shown. The bottom trace is the simulated transmembrane potential of a pacemaker cell and the top trace is the transmembrane potential of an adjacent nonpacemaker cell. In (A), when the two cells were not coupled (coupling resistance infinitely high) rapid firing of the pacemaker cell which did not conduct to the nonpacemaker cell is evident. In (B), (C), and (D) the coupling between the two cells was increased (coupling resistance was reduced thereby increasing intercellular current flow between

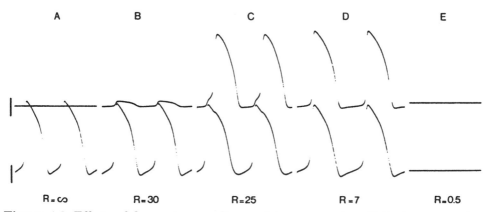

Figure 1.8: Effects of decreasing coupling resistance on automaticity in a computer simulation. The top trace shows membrane potential of the simulated nonpacemaker cell; the bottom trace shows membrane potential of the simulated pacemaker cell. Each panel (A-E) shows events that occurred at different coupling resistances between the cells (indicated below the bottom trace). (Reproduced from Van Capelle and Durrer (1980) with permission.)

the two cells) until in (E), the two cells were very tightly coupled. As coupling increased, the pacemaker impulse conducted to the nonpacemaker cell (C, D) but the electrotonic current flow during diastole (described above) slowed the pacemaker firing rate. Finally in (E), with tight coupling, pacemaker firing was prevented by the flow of current from the nonpacemaker cell to the pacemaker cell.

Arrhythmias Caused by Normal Automaticity   Arrhythmias caused by the normal automaticity of cardiac fibers may occur for several different reasons. Such arrhythmias might result simply from an alteration in the rate of impulse initiation by the normal sinus node pacemaker without a shift of impulse origin to a subsidiary pacemaker at an ectopic site; sinus bradycardia and tachycardia are such arrhythmias. The cellular mechanisms that can change the rate of impulse initiation in the sinus node have been described above and in Figure 1.1. During alterations in sinus rate there may be shifts of the pacemaker site within the sinus node (Hoffman and Cranefield 1960; Boineau et al. 1978; Gomes and Winters 1987).

A shift in the site of impulse initiation to one of the regions where subsidiary pacemakers are located is another factor that results in arrhythmias caused by a normal automatic mechanism. This would be expected to happen when any of the following occurs:

(a) The rate at which the sinus node activates subsidiary pacemakers falls considerably below the intrinsic rate of the subsidiary pacemakers;
(b) inhibitory electrotonic influences between nonpacemaker and pacemaker cells are interrupted; or
(c) impulse initiation in subsidiary pacemakers is enhanced.

The rate at which the sinus node activates subsidiary pacemakers may be decreased in a number of situations. Impulse initiation by the sinus node may be slowed or inhibited altogether by heightened activity in the parasympathetic nervous system (Toda and West 1965) or as a result of sinus node disease (Ferrer 1974). Alternatively, there may be block of impulse conduction from the sinus node to the atria or block of conduction from the atria to the ventricles. A latent pacemaker might also be protected from being overdriven by the sinus node if it is surrounded by a region in which impulses of sinus origin block (entrance block), prior to reaching the pacemaker cells. Such block, however, must be unidirectional so that activity from the pacemaker can propagate into surrounding myocardium whenever the surrounding regions are excitable. Some possible mechanisms for unidirectional block are discussed later in this chapter. The protected pacemaker is said to be a parasystolic focus (Katz and Pick 1956). In general, under these conditions such a protected focus of automaticity can fire at its own intrinsic frequency. Electrotonic current flow from surrounding regions may also influence the cycle length of a protected focus, either prolonging or abbreviating it, depending on whether the surrounding activity occurs during the early or late stage of diastolic depolarization (Jalife and Moe 1976; Moe et al. 1977; Jalife and Moe 1979). Under any of the above conditions (sinus slowing, sinoatrial (SA) or AV block, parasystolic focus) there may be "escape" of a subsidiary pacemaker as a result of the removal of overdrive suppression by the sinus pacemaker.

There is a natural hierarchy of intrinsic rates of subsidiary pacemakers, with atrial pacemakers having faster intrinsic rates than AV junctional pacemakers and AV junctional pacemakers having faster rates than ventricular pacemakers (Erlanger and Hirschfelder 1906; Erlanger and Blackman 1907; Eyster and Meek 1922; Hope et al. 1976; Vassalle 1977; Randall et al. 1980). Once overdrive suppression is removed by sinus node inhibition, the pacemaker with the fastest rate becomes the site of impulse origin (Vassalle 1977). As a result, there is a tendency for ectopic rhythms to arise in the atria when the sinus node impulse initiation is impaired or when there is sinus exit block. The most prevalent atrial pacemaker site in experimental studies is at the junction of the inferior vena cava and posterior wall of the right atrium (Randall et al. 1978; Euler et al. 1979; Loeb et al. 1980; Randall et al. 1982a; 1982b). Although these atrial pacemakers are highly sensitive to the overdrive-suppressive effects of the sinus node during sinus rhythm (Randall et al. 1982a), the ability to overdrive-suppress them diminishes with time after they gain control of the cardiac rhythm (Rozanski et al. 1984b). The mechanism for this change is not known. Initially after sinus node suppression, these pacemakers are highly dependent on sympathetic drive for continued activity although this dependence diminishes with time (Rozanski et al. 1984b). Atrial rhythms controlled by these subsidiary pacemakers can increase their rate in response to increased sympathetic activity and decrease their rate in response to increased parasympathetic activity (Randall et al. 1978; Loeb et al. 1980; Rozanski et al. 1984b). These atrial pacemakers may cause atrial arrhythmias if the sinus node or its arterial supply is damaged (El-Said et al. 1972; Gillette et al. 1980). Sinus node dysfunction during the sick sinus syndrome may also result in a pacemaker shift to an atrial ectopic site.

Sometimes, however, mechanisms that are responsible for the suppression of impulse initiation in the sinus node also suppress pacemaker activity in the atria so that ectopic impulse initiation may occur in the AV junction. Atrioventricular junctional pacemakers may be located either in the AV node or His bundle. These different sites have somewhat different properties including their intrinsic rate (faster in the node than in the His bundle), and response to autonomic nerve activity (parasympathetic activity suppresses AV nodal pacemakers to a greater extent than His bundle pacemakers). Atrioventricular junctional rhythms may occur during AV block because the site of block is often proximal to the junctional pacemaker location (James et al. 1979). If junctional pacemakers are also suppressed or if the site of disease causing AV block is in the His bundle or bundle branches, subsidiary pacemaker location is in the His-Purkinje system. The His bundle at the proximal end of the conducting system has a faster intrinsic rate than the more distally located Purkinje fibers (Hope et al. 1976). During the sick sinus syndrome there may be suppression of AV junctional automaticity because the disease extends to the

AV node and His bundle and ectopic ventricular beats rather than junctional beats sometimes occur during the period of sinus bradycardia or arrest. Idioventricular rhythm in patients with complete heart block is often characterized by a wide, aberrant QRS complex, indicating impulse initiation in the distal Purkinje system (Wolferth 1930; Klein et al. 1973a). In acute myocardial ischemia, particularly when occurring in the inferior wall, parasympathetic activity may be enhanced depressing sinus rate or AV conduction (Webb et al. 1972), and ectopic impulse initiation may arise in the ventricular specialized conducting system (Lie et al. 1974).

Any event that decreases intercellular coupling between latent, subsidiary, pacemaker cells and surrounding nonpacemaker cells may remove the inhibitory influence of electrotonic current flow on the latent pacemakers that was described in Figures 1.7 and 1.8 and allow them to fire at their intrinsic rate (Van Capelle and Durrer 1980). Coupling might be reduced by fibrosis that can separate myocardial fibers. For example, fibrosis in the atrial aspect of the AV junctional region that results in heart block might release nodal pacemakers from electrotonic suppression by surrounding atrial cells and permit them to become the dominant pacemakers driving the ventricles. Uncoupling might also be caused by factors that increase the intracellular Ca^{2+} (Dahl and Isenberg 1980) because elevated intracellular calcium levels increase coupling resistance between myocardial cells. This might result, for example, from treatment with digitalis (Weingart 1977) that inhibits sodium extrusion and thus increases calcium levels in the cell (Ellis 1977). In myocardial infarction, Purkinje fiber pacemakers may be uncoupled from damaged ventricular muscle cells, allowing the Purkinje fibers to fire at their normal intrinsic rates. Some inhibition of the sinus node is still necessary for the site of impulse initiation to shift to an ectopic site that is no longer inhibited because of uncoupling from surrounding cells, since as explained above, the intrinsic firing rate of subsidiary pacemakers is still slower than the sinus node.

Subsidiary pacemaker activity also may be enhanced causing impulse initiation to shift to ectopic sites even when sinus node function is normal. One cause may be enhanced sympathetic nerve activity. Norepinephrine released locally from sympathetic nerves steepens the slope of diastolic depolarization of latent pacemaker cells (Hoffman and Cranefield 1960; Wit et al. 1973; Tsien 1974; Davis 1975; Wit and Cranefield 1977) and diminishes the inhibitory effects of overdrive (Pliam et al. 1975). The increase in slope of spontaneous diastolic depolarization may result from effects of norepinephrine on the current i_f as described before, as well as from an increase in inward calcium current in those cells in which this current participates in pacemaker activity. Localized effects on subsidiary pacemakers may occur in the absence of sinus node stimulation (Armour et al. 1972). Therefore, sympathetic stimulation may enable membrane potential of ectopic pacemakers to reach threshold before they are activated by an impulse from the sinus node, resulting in ectopic premature impulses or automatic rhythms. There is evidence that in the subacute phase of myocardial ischemia increased activity of the sympathetic nervous system may enhance automaticity of Purkinje fibers, enabling them to escape from sinus node domination (see Chapter III). From studies on isolated tissues superfused with catecholamines and from studies on sympathetic stimulation in dogs, it appears that the limit for automatic rates generated by subsidiary pacemakers in the atria is close to 200/min (Randall 1977) and in the Purkinje fibers of the ventricles is around 120/min (Vassalle et al. 1968). Normal automaticity enhanced by sympathetic stimulation, therefore, probably does not cause very rapid ventricular rhythms although it might cause atrial tachycardia.

Enhanced subsidiary pacemaker activity also may not require sympathetic stimulation. The flow of current between partially depolarized myocardium and normally polarized latent pacemaker cells might enhance automaticity (Katzung et al. 1975). This mechanism has been proposed to be a cause of some of the ectopic beats that arise at the borders of ischemic areas in the ventricle (see Chapter II) (Janse and Van Capelle 1982a) and is diagrammed in Figure 1.7B. Ischemia causes a reduction in membrane potential of the affected cells. Thus, at the border of an ischemic area there is a transition between depolarized and normal tissue. In Figure 1.7B, cell a, (top trace) has a depolarized membrane potential of -60 mV while adjacent cell b has a higher membrane potential of -80 mV and the capability of spontaneous diastolic depolarization. As a result of the differences in membrane potential, current flow during diastole in extracellular space is from cell b to cell a, while in intracellular space it is from cell a to cell b as shown by the direction of the arrows in the diagram below the action potentials. The flow of current during diastole, therefore, is in the depolarizing direction for cell b, enhancing or causing spontaneous diastolic depolarization (dashed part of action potential (b)), possibly to an extent sufficient to cause spontaneous impulse initiation.

Inhibition of the electrogenic sodium-potassium pump results in a net increase in inward current during diastole because of the decrease in outward current normally generated by the pump and, therefore, may increase automaticity in subsidiary pacemakers sufficiently to cause arrhythmias. This might occur after adenosine triphosphate (ATP) is depleted during prolonged hypoxia or ischemia (Chapter II) or in the presence of toxic amounts of digitalis (Rosen et al. 1973a; 1973b). A decrease in the extracellular potassium level also enhances normal automaticity (Vassalle 1965), as does acute stretch (Deck 1964). Stretch can induce rapid automatic rates in Purkinje fibers with normal maximum diastolic potentials (Dudel and Trautwein 1954; Kaufmann and Theophile 1967). In experiments designed to stretch Purkinje fibers *in vitro*, spontaneous rate increased from values of around 30 beats/min to 85 beats/min when fibers were stretched to 138% of their initial length. Stretch of the ventricles can also induce arrhythmias in the intact heart (Hansen et al. 1990) although the site of origin of the ectopic impulses has not yet been localized. Stretch of the Purkinje system might occur in akinetic areas after acute ischemia or in ventricular aneurysms in hearts with healed infarcts. It has been proposed that stretch-induced automaticity results from the activation of special stretch-activated channels with a reversal potential of around -30 to -40 mV (Hansen et al. 1990). Activation of the channels normally occurs during systole and results in an outward current that accelerates repolarization. However, under abnormal conditions such as diastolic bulging, the channels may be activated during diastole. Because diastolic potential is more negative than the reversal potential, this would produce an inward current that causes spontaneous diastolic depolarization or an afterdepolarization (Hansen et al. 1990). Validation of this hypothesis requires additional experimental studies.

Abnormal Automaticity

Abnormal Pacemaker Mechanisms   Working atrial and ventricular myocardial cells do not normally have spontaneous diastolic depolarization and do not initiate spontaneous impulses even when they are not excited for long periods of time by propagating impulses. However, when the resting potentials of working atrial or ventricular myocardial cells are reduced sufficiently, spontaneous diastolic depolarization may occur and cause repetitive impulse initiation, a phenomenon called depolarization-induced automaticity or abnormal automaticity. (We use the two terms interchangeably.) The level of membrane potential at which abnormal automaticity occurs has varied in different studies but is often in a range between   70 and -90 mV (Brown and Noble 1969; Hauswirth et al. 1969; Imanishi and Surawicz 1976; Katzung and Morgenstern 1977). Depolarization of the membrane potential can be accomplished experimentally by the application of constant depolarizing current as shown in Figure 1.9. In panel A at the left, is an action potential recorded from a ventricular muscle cell in a guinea pig papillary muscle. Two superimposed traces, recorded while depolarizing current was passed through the preparation are shown. At membrane potential (a) there was no spontaneous activity, but when the current pulse depolarized the membrane potential to level (b) (about -60 mV), slow, rhythmic abnormal automatic activity occurred. Panels B, C, and D show that the rate of the abnormal automatic activity increased as membrane potential was depolarized to more positive levels. Depolarization to near 0 mV in E only elicited low-amplitude oscillations while there was no abnormal automaticity upon further depolarization (F). Experimentally applied stretch can also result in depolarization of papillary muscle cells and induce similar abnormal automaticity in muscle fibers (Kaufmann and Theophile 1967). Likewise, cells such as those in the Purkinje system which are normally automatic at high levels of membrane potential also show abnormal automaticity when the membrane potential is reduced (Imanishi 1971; Cranefield 1975). As we discussed before, the i_f channels that participate in normal pacemaker activity in Purkinje fibers have a gating mechanism controlling channel opening and closing that is dependent on the transmembrane voltage. At membrane potentials that are positive to about -60 mV, such as after the upstroke and during the early phases of repolarization, the channels are closed. In response to the negative potentials that occur after complete repolarization, the channels reopen generating the inward pacemaker current (DiFrancesco 1981a; 1981b). For this reason, when

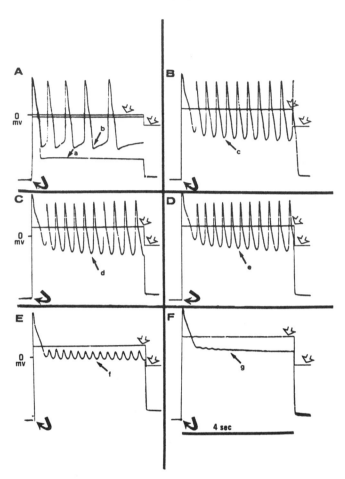

Figure 1.9: Effects of depolarizing membrane current on the membrane potential and automatic firing of a guinea pig papillary muscle. In each panel the current pulse is indicated by the unfilled arrows. In panel A, two superimposed traces are shown. Trace a shows a single action potential at the left induced by a stimulus in a normally polarized cell. The arrow (a) shows a level of depolarization insufficient to cause automaticity. Trace b shows abnormal automaticity in the same cell after membrane potential was depolarized by 20 mV with a current pulse. Panels B-F show the effects of further depolarization on the abnormal automaticity. In each panel the maximum diastolic potential during depolarization is indicated by the small arrows (c, d, e, f, g). (Modified from Imanishi and Surawicz (1976) with permission).

the steady state membrane potential of Purkinje fibers is reduced to around −60 mV or less as may sometimes occur in ischemic regions of the heart (see Chapter III), these normal pacemaker channels are not functional, and automaticity is not caused by the normal pacemaker mechanism. However, it can be caused by an "abnormal" mechanism (described below). In Figure 1.10, the transmembrane potential recorded from a spontaneously firing Purkinje fiber with normal automaticity is shown in panel A, and abnormal automatic activ-

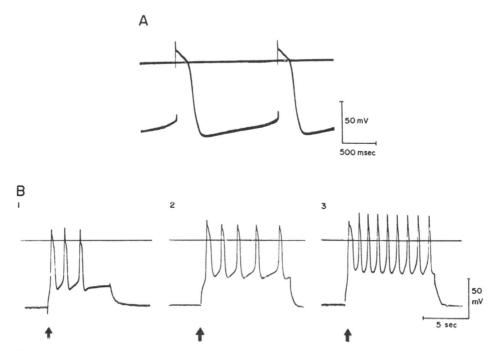

Figure 1.10: Normal and abnormal automaticity in a canine Purkinje fiber. Panel A shows transmembrane potential recording from a Purkinje fiber with a normal maximum diastolic potential of 85 mV and spontaneous diastolic depolarization. Panel B shows the abnormal automaticity that occurred when membrane potential was decreased. In 1 the fiber was depolarized (at the arrow) to a membrane potential of −45 mV by injecting a long-lasting current pulse through a microelectrode; in 2 the membrane potential was reduced to −40 mV (at arrow), and in 3 it was reduced to −30 mV (at arrow). (Reproduced from Wit and Friedman (1975) with permission.)

ity occurring while the membrane potential was depolarized to progressively lower membrane potentials is shown in panel B; 1, 2, and 3. As in the ventricular muscle, the abnormal automatic rate increased as membrane potential became more positive.

In Purkinje fibers, enhanced automaticity may also occur over the range of membrane potentials between the normal high level (around −90 mV) and the low level at which abnormal automaticity occurs (around −60 mV). At these intermediate levels of membrane potential there is no sharp distinction between normal and abnormal automaticity. Such a distinction is not a problem in atrial or ventricular cells in which normal automaticity does not occur.

A low level of membrane potential is not the only criterion for defining abnormal automaticity. If this was so, the automaticity of the sinus node would have to be considered abnormal. Therefore, an important distinction between abnormal and normal automaticity is that the membrane potentials of fibers showing the abnormal type of activity are reduced from their own normal level. For this reason, we do not classify automaticity in the AV node or valves, where membrane potential is normally low, to be abnormal automaticity.

On the basis of the results of voltage-clamp studies in guinea pig and cat ventricular muscle, Katzung and Morgenstern (1977) proposed a mechanism for the pacemaker activity that occurs at depolarized membrane potentials. A likely cause of automaticity at depolarized membrane potentials in muscle is activation and deactivation of the delayed rectifier K^+ current (i_K) (Noble and Tsien 1968). The conductance of this K^+ channel is activated during the normal action potential plateau and the outward current that flows through it contributes to repolarization. The channel then deactivates during diastole. No significant outward current flows through this channel at normal diastolic potentials because the resting potential lies near the reversal potential and the driving force is negligible (Katzung and Morgenstern 1977). However, when the membrane potential is depolarized (as by the current shown in the experiment described in Figure 1.9), an outward current flows through this channel that is activated at the depolarized membrane potentials. This current hyperpolarizes the membrane potential. As the channel then deactivates at the hyperpolarized potentials, spontaneous diastolic depolarization occurs. If either Na^+ or Ca^{2+} channels have been reactivated since the preceding action potential, the spontaneous depolarization caused by K^+ channel deactivation may lead to an upstroke caused by current flowing through one of these channels (depending on the level of the membrane potential) (Katzung and Morgenstern 1977). A similar mechanism might cause abnormal automaticity in partially depolarized Purkinje fibers. In another experimental model of abnormal automaticity, exposure of ventricular muscle cells to barium-containing solution depolarizes the resting potential by blocking i_{K1}. Under these conditions, cyclical increases and decreases in this K^+ current has been shown to play a role in spontaneous diastolic depolarization (Imoto et al. 1987).

It is uncertain how the data obtained in the experimental models described above apply to the abnormal automaticity observed in diseased cardiac fibers in which it is caused by depolarization that results from the effects of pathology on resting membrane conductances. Experiments on depolarized human atrial myocardium from dilated atria indicate that calcium-dependent processes may contribute to abnormal pacemaker activity at low membrane potentials (Escande et al. 1987; Kimura et al. 1988). Diastolic depolarization in depolarized atrial cells occurs in two phases, with an initial fast rate of depolarization followed by a slower rate of depolarization as we described for some subsidiary atrial pacemakers in normal atria. In experimental studies, the initial fast rate of depolarization was inhibited by cesium (an inhibitor of the i_f current), which reduced spontaneous firing rate slightly, suggesting that i_f makes a small contribution to pacemaking, even at these low membrane potentials (Escande et al. 1987). The second phase of diastolic depolarization was decreased when internal calcium was experimentally decreased, and increased when internal calcium was increased, causing marked changes in the firing rate. Ryanodine, which inhibits sarcoplasmic reticulum calcium release (Sutko and Kenyon 1983), also depressed the second phase of spontaneous diastolic depolarization (Escande et al. 1987; Kimura et al. 1988). On the basis of these properties, it was proposed that intracellular calcium controls membrane permeability to an inward current during diastole that leads to spontaneous diastolic depolarization and abnormal automaticity. It is also possible that Na/Ca exchange is involved in generating the inward current. The mechanism may be similar to the one causing the transient inward current responsible for delayed afterdepolarizations (see the section on Triggered Activity) except that in diseased human atria, an abnormal prolongation of the intracellular calcium transient occurs during the action potential to cause spontaneous diastolic depolarization, rather than an oscillatory change in intracellular calcium and membrane potential (an afterdepolarization) (Morgan and Morgan 1984; Escande et al. 1987). Previously Cranefield (1975), and later Cranefield and Aronson (1988) also suggested that there may be some similarities between abnormal automaticity and triggered activity occurring at depolarized levels of membrane potential. An inward calcium current may also contribute to abnormal automaticity in diseased and depolarized cardiac fibers (Kimura et al. 1988).

In summary, therefore, several different mechanisms probably cause abnormal automaticity including activation and deactivation of K^+ currents, calcium-dependent activation of an inward current, inward calcium currents, and even some contribution by the pacemaker current i_f. It has not yet been determined which of the above mechanisms are operative in the different pathological conditions in which abnormal automaticity may occur. We will discuss this problem further when we discuss abnormal automaticity caused by ischemia and infarction.

The upstrokes of the spontaneously occurring action potentials generated by abnormal automaticity may be caused by either Na^+ or Ca^{2+} inward currents or possibly, a mixture of the two. In the range of diastolic potentials between approximately -70 mV and -50 mV repetitive activity is dependent on extracellular Na^+ concentration and can be decreased or abolished by the Na^+ channel blockers lidocaine and tetrodotoxin, indicating that the Na^+ inward current is involved. In a diastolic potential range of approximately -50 mV to -30 mV, repetitive activity depends on extracellular Ca^{2+} concentration and is reduced by the Ca^{2+} channel blockers, Mn^{2+} and verapamil, indicating a role for the L-type Ca inward current (Cranefield 1975; Grant and Katzung 1976; Imanishi et al. 1978; January and Fozzard 1984).

The decrease in membrane potential of cardiac cells required for abnormal automaticity to occur may be induced by a variety of factors related to cardiac disease. Some of the causes of a low resting potential can be considered in terms of the Goldman-Hodgkin-Katz equation (Hodgkin and Katz 1949) which approximates the resting potential, V_r, of working myocardial cells over a wide range of extracellular K^+ concentrations.

$$V_r = \frac{RT}{F} \ln \frac{[K^+]_o + P_{Na}/P_K[Na^+]_o}{[K^+]_i + P_{Na}/P_K[Na^+]_i}$$

In this equation R is the gas constant, F is Faraday's constant, T is the absolute temperature, $[K]_o$ and $[K]_i$ are the extracellular and intracellular free K^+ concentrations or activity, respectively; P_{Na}/P_K is the ratio of the permeability coefficients for Na^+ and K^+ and $[Na]_o$ and $[Na]_i$ are the extracellular and intracellular free Na^+ concentrations or activity, respectively. The equation does not show the direct contribution of the electrogenic Na/K exchange pump to the resting potential although a single modification will (Cranefield and Aronson 1988). The several ways in which the resting potential can be made less negative according to this equation are that (1) $[K]_o$ might be increased, (2) $[K]_i$ might be decreased, or (3) the ratio of P_{Na}/P_K might be increased following either an increase in P_{Na} (sodium permeability of the sarcolemma) or a decrease in P_K (potassium permeability of the sarcolemma). Any one of these changes would by itself cause the resting potential to decline although a change in one (decrease in $[K]_i$ for example) would lead to a change in another (a decrease in P_K caused by the depolarization). (For a discussion of how the components in the equation interact, we refer the reader to the excellent discussion in Cranefield and Aronson (1988).) It is likely that more than one change occurs simultaneously in diseased cells (Gadsby and Wit 1981). As we discuss in subsequent chapters, some of these changes have been shown to occur during cardiac ischemia.

Although an increase in extracellular potassium concentration can reduce membrane potential, normal or abnormal automaticity in working atrial, ventricular, and Purkinje fibers usually does not occur when $[K]_o$ is elevated because of the increase in K^+ conductance (and, hence, net outward current) that results from an increase in $[K]_o$ (Gadsby and Cranefield 1977). This argues against abnormal automaticity being responsible for arrhythmias arising in acutely ischemic myocardium, where cells are partially depolarized by increased extracellular K^+ (Hill and Gettes 1980; Hirche et al. 1980; Kléber 1983). However, atrial fibers in the mitral valve (Wit and Cranefield 1976) and fibers in the AV node may have automatic activity even when extracellular K^+ is markedly elevated presumably because there is much less of an effect of elevated $[K]_o$ on K^+ conductance in these cells. A decrease in intracellular K^+ has been shown to occur in the Purkinje fibers that survive on the endocardial surface of infarcts and this decrease persists for at least 24 hours after the coronary occlusion (Dresdner et al. 1985; 1987) (see Chapter III). The reduction in $[K]_i$ contributes to the low membrane potential (Dresdner et al. 1987) and the accompanying abnormal automaticity (Friedman et al. 1973b; Lazzara et al. 1973). Isolated preparations of diseased atrial and ventricular myocardium from human hearts, superfused with Tyrode's solution, show phase 4 depolarization and abnormal automaticity at membrane potentials in the range of -50 to -60 mV (Hordof et al. 1976; Ten Eick and Singer 1979; Singer et al. 1981). It has been proposed that a decrease in membrane potassium conductance, P_K, is an important cause of the low membrane potentials in the atrial fibers (Ten Eick and Singer 1979).

Myocardial cells might also be partially depolarized by the flow of electrotonic current from an adjacent depolarized region. After placing papillary muscles in a three-compartment bath, and depolarizing the central compartment with a solution containing 145 mM K^+, Katzung et al. (1975) observed spontaneous activity in the adjacent normal test compartment where fibers became partially depolarized by the flow of current from the depolarized central compartment. This experiment was intended to mimic conditions that might exist in regional ischemia, where depolarized cells are found adjacent to polarized cells. (Extracellular K^+ in ischemic myocardium is, however, much lower than 145 mM.)

Suppression of Abnormal Subsidiary Pacemakers   In the heart, myocardial fibers with low resting potentials and a propensity for abnormal automaticity, should not fire automatically if the sinus node drives them faster than their intrinsic abnormal, automatic rate. An abnormal automatic focus should manifest itself and cause an arrhythmia when the sinus rate decreases below the intrinsic rate of the focus or when the rate of the focus increases above that of the sinus node, as was discussed for latent pacemakers with normal automaticity. A similar interplay between maximum diastolic potential, threshold potential and rate of phase 4 depolarization, as discussed for a normally automatic focus (see Figure 1.1), determines the rate of impulse initiation by the abnormal pacemaker. However, there is an important distinction between the effects of the dominant sinus pacemaker on the two kinds of automaticity, that is, abnormal automaticity is not overdrive-suppressed to the same extent as the normal automaticity that occurs at high levels of membrane potential (Carmeliet 1980; Hoffman and Dangman 1982; Dangman and Hoffman 1983). Figure 1.11 shows the failure of overdrive to suppress abnormal automaticity in an experiment on a Purkinje fiber in which abnormal automaticity was caused by adding $BaCl_2$ to the Tyrode's superfusate, resulting in a reduction of maximum diastolic potential to around -50 mV. The first five action potentials at the left occurred at a cycle length of 810 msec during the spontaneous rhythm. A period of overdrive was then begun at a cycle length of 500 msec, denoted by the

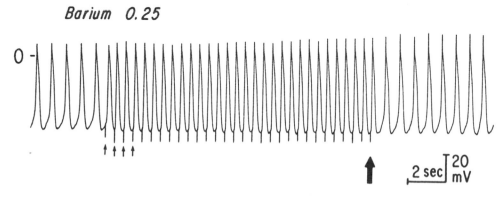

Barium 0.25

Figure 1.11: Transmembrane potential recording from canine Purkinje fiber showing effect of overdrive stimulation on abnormal automaticity. Small arrows indicate stimulus artifacts. Large arrow indicates the end of the overdrive period. (Reproduced from Dangman and Hoffman (1983) with permission).

stimulus artifacts (small arrows) and was terminated at the large arrow. Unlike the example of normal automaticity described in Figure 1.3, there was no noticeable suppression of the abnormal automatic rhythm following this period of stimulation. The amount of suppression of spontaneous diastolic depolarization causing abnormal automaticity by overdrive is directly related to the level of membrane potential at which the automatic rhythm occurs (Hoffman and Dangman 1982; Dangman and Hoffman 1983). For example, Purkinje fibers showing automaticity at moderately depolarized membrane potentials of -60 to -70 mV still manifest some overdrive suppression, although less than those fibers with automaticity at -90 mV. Automaticity in Purkinje fibers with membrane potentials less than -60 mV as shown in Figure 1.11, is only slightly suppressed by short periods of overdrive, if at all. These differences in the effects of overdrive may be related to the reduction in the amount of sodium entering the cell as membrane potential decreases as we described for overdrive of the sinus node. At low levels of membrane potential, Na^+ channels are inactivated, decreasing the fast inward Na^+ current, and therefore there is a reduction in the amount of Na^+ entering the cells during overdrive and the degree of stimulation of the sodium-potassium pump (Falk and Cohen 1984). For markedly depolarized tissue showing no suppression after brief periods of overdrive, long periods of rapid overdrive can suppress automaticity either because enough Na^+ eventually enters the cell through calcium channels to stimulate the pump (Falk and Cohen 1984) or because Ca^{2+} entering during the upstroke of slow response action potentials occurring at the low level of membrane potential is exchanged for Na^+, thereby elevating the intracellular Na^+ concentration (Mullins 1981) which stimulates the pump. As described before, an increase in intracellular calcium can also suppress spontaneous diastolic depolarization by increasing K^+ conductance.

Unlike the effects of overdrive stimulation, the effects of prematurely stimulated impulses on abnormally automatic rhythms do not appear to be significantly different than the effects on normally automatic ones. In experiments on Purkinje fibers with abnormal automaticity, the cycle length following prematurely stimulated impulses was nearly the same as the cycle length prior to stimulation and remained nearly constant (and less than compensatory) over a wide range of premature coupling intervals (Dangman and Hoffman 1985).

Arrhythmias Caused by Abnormal Automaticity   At normal sinus rates there may be little overdrive suppression of pacemakers with abnormal automaticity. As a result of the lack of overdrive suppression, even transient sinus pauses or occasional long sinus cycle lengths may permit an ectopic focus with a slower rate than the sinus node to capture the heart for one or more beats. On the other hand, ectopic pacemakers with normal automaticity would probably be quiescent during relatively short, transient sinus pauses because they are overdrive-suppressed. It is also possible that the depolarized level of membrane potential at which abnormal automaticity occurs might cause entrance block into the focus and prevent it from being overdriven by the sinus node, even when impulses initiated in the focus could leave it (unidirectional block) (Ferrier and Rosenthal 1980). This would lead to parasystole, an example of an arrhythmia caused by a combination of an abnormality of impulse conduction and initiation. All these features of abnormal automaticity are evident in the Purkinje fibers that survive in regions of transmural myocardial infarction and that cause ventricular arrhythmias during the subacute phase (see Chapter III).

The firing rate of an abnormally automatic focus might also be enhanced above that of the sinus node leading to arrhythmias in the absence of sinus node suppression or conduction block between the focus and surrounding myocardium. The automatic rate is a direct function of the level of membrane potential—the greater the depolarization, the faster the rate as illustrated in Figures 1.9 and 1.10 (Brown and Noble 1969; Imanishi 1971; Cranefield 1975; Imanishi and Surawicz 1976; Katzung and Morgenstern 1977). Experimental studies have shown firing rates in muscle and Purkinje fibers of 150–200/min at membrane potentials less than -50 mV and these rates should be sufficiently rapid to enable these pacemakers to sometimes control the heart. Catecholamines also increase the rate of firing caused by abnormal automaticity (Hume and Katzung 1980) and therefore, may contribute to a shift in the pacemaker site from the sinus node to a region with abnormal automaticity.

We cannot identify with any certainty which clinical arrhythmias are caused by abnormal automaticity. Occasional reports in the literature have described atrial or ventricular arrhythmias that have electrocardiographic characteristics consistent with an automatic mechanism, are not overdrive-suppressed but may be reduced or abolished by a slow channel blocking drug. These features are consistent with characteristics expected of an arrhythmia caused by abnormal automaticity. Among those arrhythmias is accelerated idioventricular rhythm after myocardial infarction (see Chapter III).

Triggered Activity

Triggered activity is a term used to describe impulse initiation in cardiac fibers that is dependent on afterdepolarizations (Cranefield and Aronson 1974; Cranefield 1977; Cranefield and Aronson 1988). Afterdepolarizations are oscillations in membrane potential that follow the upstroke of an action potential. There are two kinds of afterdepolarizations that may cause triggered activity. One occurs early; that is, during repolarization of the action potential (early afterdepolarization). The other is delayed until repolarization is complete or nearly complete (delayed afterdepolarization). When either kind of afterdepolarization is large enough to reach the threshold potential for activation of a regenerative inward current, action potentials result that are referred to as "triggered". Therefore, a key characteristic of triggered activity discriminating it from automaticity is that for triggered activity to occur, at least one action potential must precede it (the trigger). Automatic rhythms can arise *de novo* in the absence of any prior electrical activity such as following long periods of quiescence, whereas triggered activity cannot (Cranefield 1975; Cranefield and Aronson 1988).

Triggered activity will cause arrhythmias when the site of impulse initiation shifts from the sinus node to the triggered focus. In order for this to occur, the rate of triggered impulses should be faster than the sinus rate either transiently or persistently. This might result when firing of the sinus node is slowed or inhibited, there is block of sinus impulses, or the rate of triggered activity is faster than normal sinus node impulse initiation. The factors causing the shift in the site of impulse initiation should be very similar to those we described in our discussion of automaticity.

It has yet to be definitely established that triggered activity causes arrhythmias in the *in situ* human heart. Triggered activity can be readily induced in both normal and diseased isolated cardiac tissue preparations when exposed to an environment not unlike that expected to exist *in situ*, for example an environment containing catecholamines, ischemia, or excess digitalis (see discussion in the following paragraphs). Therefore, because there is reasonable evidence that isolation and superfusion of cardiac tissue *in vitro* does not drastically change its basic electrophysiological properties, we see every reason to believe that triggered activity should occur *in situ*. Identification of afterdepolarizations in cardiac fibers of the arrhythmic heart should provide irrefutable proof that they are an arrhythmogenic mechanism. However, Bozler, after concluding in 1943 that extrasystoles and tachycardias might be caused by oscillatory afterpotentials, went on to say that "unfortunately, the study of these weak and localized potentials in the heart *in situ* presents great technical difficulties". This statement still holds true today. Much of the evidence for triggered activity as an arrhythmogenic mechanism in the heart *in situ* is indirect and is derived from studies on the effects of drugs and electrical stimulation on arrhythmias, but afterdepolarizations have also been recorded using extracellular recording techniques.

Delayed Afterdepolarizations and Triggered Activity

Figure 1.12A shows an example of a delayed afterdepolarization recorded with a microelectrode in a superfused preparation of atrial muscle exposed to catecholamines. The delayed afterdepolarization is an oscillation in membrane potential that occurs after repolarization of the action potential (indicated in the figure by the unfilled arrow). The delayed afterdepolarization is caused by events occurring during the action potential that will be described later. Also shown in Figure 1.12A is that a delayed afterdepolarization may be preceded by an afterhyperpolarization (black arrow), in which case the membrane potential transiently becomes more negative after the action potential than it was just before it. However, afterhyperpolarizations do not always precede delayed afterdepolarizations. The transient nature of the delayed afterdepolarization

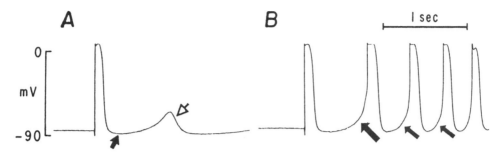

Figure 1.12: An example of a delayed afterdepolarization recorded with a microelectrode from an atrial fiber in the canine coronary sinus is indicated by the unfilled arrow in panel A, while the solid arrow indicates an afterhyperpolarization. The onset of triggered activity is indicated by the large solid arrow in panel B, while the smaller arrows indicate subsequent triggered impulses. (Reproduced from Wit and Rosen (1989) with permission.)

clearly distinguishes it from normal spontaneous diastolic (pacemaker) depolarization during which the membrane potential declines almost monotonically until the next action potential occurs (compare Figure 1.12A with Figure 1.1). All oscillations in membrane potential that occur during diastole are not delayed afterdepolarizations because some oscillations may not be coupled to the action potential, but may occur at random. In addition to microelectrode recordings such as the one shown in Figure 1.12A, delayed afterdepolarizations can also be identified using techniques for recording extracellular potentials (Cramer et al. 1977; Wit et al. 1979). Because the extracellular current that flows during the afterdepolarization is relatively weak and the frequency components of the signal relatively slow, high amplification of the extracellular signal with a low value for the low frequency cutoff in the amplifier is required. When these conditions are fulfilled, afterdepolarizations can be clearly seen in extracellular recordings from isolated cardiac tissue. Figure 1.13 shows delayed afterdepolarizations in simultaneous extracellular (top trace) and microelectrode (bottom trace) recordings from an isolated, superfused preparation of atrial muscle. However, a major problem that exists when this technique is used to locate delayed afterdepolarizations in the *in situ* heart is discriminating the extracellular voltage deflections caused by afterdepolarizations from deflections that are a result of the motion of the heart since movement alone can mimic delayed afterdepolarizations in extracellular recordings (Olsson et al. 1990). A second important problem is the difficulty in locating focal sites at which afterdepolarizations and triggered activity may be originating. Nevertheless, extracellular electrodes have been used to demonstrate what appear to be delayed afterdepolarizations occurring in the *in situ* heart (Priori et al. 1988).

A triggered impulse is initiated when a delayed afterdepolarization depolarizes the membrane potential to the threshold potential for activation of the inward current responsible for the upstroke of the action potential. Triggered

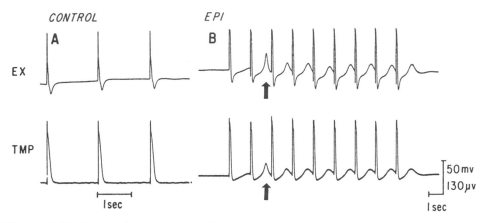

Figure 1.13: Comparison of extracellular recording of electrical activity from atrial muscle in the canine coronary sinus (top trace, labeled "EX") with intracellular recording (bottom trace, labeled "TMP"). Panel A shows control records obtained during superfusion with normal Tyrode's solution. Membrane potential during diastole is steady. Panel B shows records obtained after epinephrine was added to the superfusate to cause delayed afterdepolarizations. The afterdepolarizations are indicated by the arrows on both the extracellular and intracellular records. (Reproduced from Wit et al. (1979) with permission.)

impulses are shown by the arrows in Figure 1.12B. Afterdepolarizations do not always reach threshold so that triggerable fibers may sometimes be stimulated at a regular rate without becoming rhythmically active, e.g., the stimulated action potential in Figure 1.12A. The conditions under which delayed afterdepolarizations may reach threshold will be discussed in detail later. However, as a prelude to that discussion we mention here that probably the most important influence that causes subthreshold delayed afterdepolarizations to reach threshold is a decrease in the cycle length (an increase in the rate) at which action potentials occur. Therefore, arrhythmias triggered by delayed afterdepolarizations can be expected to be initiated by either a spontaneous or pacing-induced increase in the heart rate.

A triggered action potential is also followed by an afterdepolarization that may or may not reach threshold. When it does not reach threshold, only one triggered impulse occurs. Quite often the first triggered action potential is followed by a short or long "train" of additional triggered action potentials each arising from the afterdepolarization caused by the previous action potential (Figure 1.12B). The merging of the rising phase of the afterdepolarization with the upstroke of the action potential during triggered activity may be smooth and, as a result, the fiber may show phase 4 depolarization that is indistinguishable from the phase 4 depolarization seen during automatic activity.

Causes of Delayed Afterdepolarizations and Triggered Activity   Delayed afterdepolarizations usually occur under a variety of conditions in which there is an increase in Ca^{2+} in the myoplasm and the sarcoplasmic reticulum (SR) above normal levels (sometimes referred to as "Ca overload"). Abnormalities in the sequestration and release of Ca^{2+} by the SR also may contribute to their occurrence. The proposed mechanisms by which an increase in intracellular Ca^{2+} may cause delayed afterdepolarizations will be discussed in detail later. There is evidence that the fluctuations in Ca^{2+} cause an oscillatory inward current (called the transient inward current) that is responsible for the afterdepolarization. Because there is an increase in intracellular Ca^{2+} during ischemia, delayed afterdepolarization-dependent triggered activity may play a role in the generation of some ischemic arrhythmias. To provide an overview of their properties, we shall mainly discuss some conditions other than ischemia in which delayed afterdepolarizations have been observed. The role of delayed afterdepolarizations in causing ischemic arrhythmias is discussed in subsequent chapters.

The most widely recognized cause of delayed afterdepolarization-dependent triggered activity is digitalis toxicity (Davis 1973; Ferrier et al. 1973; Ferrier and Moe 1973; Hashimoto and Moe 1973; Hogan et al. 1973; Rosen et al. 1973a; 1973b; Aronson and Cranefield 1974). Toxic concentrations of cardiac glycosides induce one or more oscillations in membrane potential following stimulated action potentials in Purkinje fibers, ventricular muscle and atrial muscle studied *in vitro*. Figure 1.14 shows a microelectrode recording from a

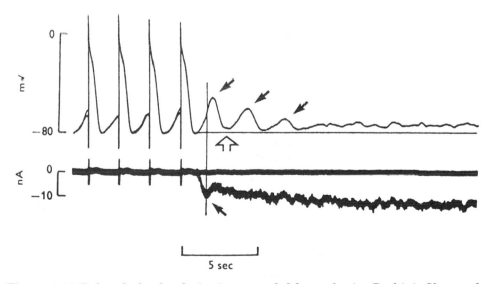

Figure 1.14: Delayed afterdepolarizations recorded from a bovine Purkinje fiber made toxic with strophanthidin. The top trace shows four stimulated action potentials followed by delayed afterdepolarizations (solid arrows). The trace below the action potential recording shows the membrane current measured when a voltage clamp was applied to clamp membrane potential at the maximum diastolic level (unfilled arrow) following another series of four stimulated action potentials. The solid arrow on the bottom (current) trace shows the transient inward current. (Reproduced from Lederer and Tsien (1976) with permission.)

bovine Purkinje fiber (top trace) intoxicated with 1 mmol/L of the digitalis compound strophanthidin. Four stimulated impulses are shown, after which stimulation was stopped. The last stimulated impulse is followed by three oscillations in the membrane potential (black arrows), the digitalis-induced delayed afterdepolarizations. One of these afterdepolarizations may sometimes reach threshold to cause triggered action potentials, particularly if the rate of stimulation is sufficiently rapid. Ventricular arrhythmias (repetitive responses) caused by digitalis in the heart *in situ* can also be initiated by pacing at rapid rates (Zipes et al. 1974). As toxicity progresses, the duration of the trains of repetitive responses induced by pacing increases. Rapid pacing can also induce arrhythmias in the digitalis-toxic human heart (Castellanos et al. 1967; Lown et al. 1967b; Lown 1968), which we assume are caused by delayed afterdepolarizations. It has also been found that endogenous digitalis-like substances produced by the human body and secreted in the bile can induce delayed afterdepolarizations and triggered activity (Kieval et al. 1988). It was proposed that such endogenous substances might under certain circumstances, contribute to paroxysmal tachycardias previously thought to be idiopathic.

Cardiac glycosides cause delayed afterdepolarizations by inhibiting the Na/K pump. In toxic amounts, this effect results in a measurable increase in intracellular Na^+ (Deitmer and Ellis 1978; Lee and Dagostino 1982). An increase in intracellular Na^+, in turn, causes an increase in intracellular Ca^{2+} (Lee and Dagostino 1982); when intracellular Na^+ is increased the concentration-dependent driving force for Na^+ across the sarcolemma is decreased, that in turn diminishes Ca^{2+} extrusion from the cell by Na/Ca exchange. Hence, there is a net inward Ca^{2+} movement (Reuter and Seitz 1968; Mullins 1979; 1981). Other pharmacological agents that increase intracellular Na^+ by either inhibiting Na^+ extrusion or by increasing Na^+ entry into cells may also lead to an increase in cell Ca^{2+} and delayed afterdepolarizations for a similar reason. For example, delayed afterdepolarizations and triggered activity occur in ventricular muscle superfused with a K^+-free solution containing normal or elevated Ca^{2+} (Eisner and Lederer 1979; Hiraoka et al. 1979; 1981; Hiraoka and Kawano 1984). Superfusates lacking K^+ cause delayed afterdepolarizations by inhibiting the Na/K pump much the same as digitalis (Eisner and Lederer 1979). Na^+ entry into cardiac cells can also be enhanced by other agents such as aconitine (Sawanobori et al. 1987) or grayanotoxin that can cause delayed afterdepolarizations and triggered activity (Kimura et al. 1984; Brown et al. 1981).

In addition to digitalis and Na pump inhibition, catecholamines are probably the next most widely recognized cause of delayed afterdepolarizations. Delayed afterdepolarizations and triggered activity caused by catecholamines have been recorded with microelectrodes in atrial fibers of the mitral valve (Wit and Cranefield 1976), atrial fibers lining the coronary sinus (Wit and Cranefield 1977), atrial fibers in the inferior right atrium (Rozanski and Lipsius 1985) and atrial fibers from hearts with cardiomyopathy (Boyden et al. 1984). The delayed afterdepolarizations in Figures 1.12 and 1.13 were caused by catecholamines in atrial fibers of the canine coronary sinus. Infusion of catecholamines through a catheter into the coronary sinus in the dog causes atrial tachycardia that has all the characteristics of triggered activity (Malfatto et al. 1988) and therefore, some naturally occurring atrial tachycardias caused by triggered activity are probably induced by the sympathetic nervous system. Ventricular muscle and Purkinje fibers can also develop delayed afterdepolarizations in the presence of catecholamines (Belardinelli and Isenberg 1983; Lazzara and Marchi 1989). Sympathetic stimulation may, therefore, also cause triggered ventricular arrhythmias, possibly some of the ventricular arrhythmias that accompany exercise (Lerman et al. 1986) and some ventricular arrhythmias during ischemia and infarction (El-Sherif et al. 1980; 1983b).

Catecholamines may cause delayed afterdepolarizations by increasing the slow inward, L-type calcium current (Reuter 1974). Studies in canine coronary sinus have attributed the catecholamine-induced delayed afterdepolarizations in part to the traditional receptor-effector pathway involving the β-adrenergic receptor, signal transduction via the GTP-regulatory protein, Gs, and stimulation of adenylate cyclase activity (Horn et al. 1989). The net effect of β-adrenergic stimulation is an increase in transsarcolemmal calcium entry into cardiac cells (Vassalle and Mugelli 1981; Tseng and Wit 1987a). In addition to increasing the inward calcium current, catecholamines enhance uptake of Ca^{2+} by the SR leading to increased Ca^{2+} stored in the SR and the subsequent release of an increased amount of Ca^{2+} from the SR during the twitch (Morad and Rolett 1972; Fabiato and Fabiato 1975; Fabiato 1983). The increased Ca^{2+} in the SR induced by catecholamines also may lead to the occurrence of delayed afterdepolarizations.

Other pharmacological agents or natural humors that increase intracellular calcium may also cause delayed afterdepolarizations or increase the amplitude of delayed afterdepolarizations that already exist. Examples are the experimental calcium current agonist drug, Bay K 8644 (January and Fozzard 1988), α-adrenergic agonists (Kimura et al. 1984; Tajima and Dohi, 1985) and histamine (Levi et al. 1981; Tajima and Dohi 1985; Cameron and Antonik 1988).

The phenomenon of overdrive excitation in Purkinje fibers is most likely the result of delayed afterdepolarization-dependent triggered activity. The usual effect of overdrive stimulation is to suppress spontaneous diastolic depolarization and automaticity by increasing the electrogenic Na/K pump current (overdrive suppression, see section on automaticity and Figure 1.3) (Vassalle 1970). Increasing extracellular Ca^{2+} over the range of 2–10 mmol/L also decreases the rate of automatic activity by shifting the threshold potential towards more positive levels (Weidmann 1955). However, when superfused with Tyrode's solution containing elevated Ca^{2+} (8.1 mmol/L), Purkinje fibers develop what appears to be enhanced spontaneous diastolic depolarization during a period of stimulation (Temte and Davis 1967) followed by persistent rhythmic activity after stimulation is stopped (overdrive excitation) (Vassalle and Carpentier 1972; Wald and Waxman 1981; Valenzuela and Vassalle 1983; 1985). A similar phenomenon occurs in the presence of norepinephrine that normally inhibits overdrive suppression (Vassalle and Carpentier 1972). Overdrive excitation is demonstrated in Figure 1.15. Panel A shows action potentials recorded

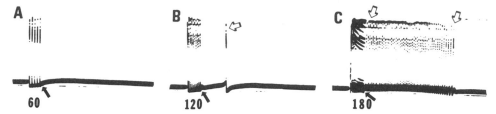

Figure 1.15: Overdrive excitation in a Purkinje fiber in the presence of low Na, norepinephrine, and theophylline in the superfusate. The preparation was stimulated for 5 seconds at rates of 60 (A), 120 (B), and 180 (C) per minute. (Reproduced from Valenzuela and Vassalle (1985) with permission).

from a Purkinje fiber during a short period of stimulation at 60/min. After stimulation was stopped, the fiber was quiescent. In panel B following stimulation at 120/min for the same period of time a single nondriven action potential followed the last stimulated one. Finally, in panel C, after a similar period of stimulation at a rate of 180/min a long period of overdrive excitation occurred. The rate of the rhythmic activity in panel C was fastest immediately after drive and then progressively slowed, accompanied by a decrease in the slope of the diastolic depolarization (which cannot be seen because of the slow oscilloscopic sweep speed). As illustrated in Figure 1.15, the period of overdrive excitation was longer after faster drive rates (Valenzuela and Vassalle 1983). Although during rhythmic activity delayed afterdepolarizations are not apparent, an oscillatory potential (delayed afterdepolarization) can be recognized after the last action potential (panel C). The combination of high Ca^{2+} (8.1 mmol/L) and norepinephrine is even more effective in causing overdrive excitation and increases the amplitude of the oscillatory potentials (Valenzuela and Vassalle 1983).

Overdrive excitation is probably a result of delayed afterdepolarizations that cause the steepening of the diastolic depolarization during and after a period of drive. The combination of a period of drive (Lado et al. 1982), norepinephrine (Reuter and Scholz 1977) and elevated extracellular Ca^{2+} (Reuter and Scholz 1968; Valenzuela and Vassalle 1985) all bring about an increase in Ca^{2+} influx in the Purkinje fibers and the increase in intracellular Ca^{2+} necessary to cause the appearance of delayed afterdepolarizations.

Overdrive excitation also can be demonstrated in the heart *in situ*. After acute AV block caused by surgical ligation of the His bundle in the canine heart, a period of rapid stimulation of the ventricles is followed by rhythmic activity that is faster than the idioventricular rhythm (Vassalle et al. 1976; Vassalle 1977; Ilvento et al. 1982). Figure 1.16 shows electrocardiograms recorded from the canine heart with AV block. The first two complexes at the left of the top trace indicate the spontaneous idioventricular rate. These complexes are followed by two stimulated impulses at a more rapid rate (underlined). The stimulated impulses are followed by the faster rhythm of overdrive excitation (beginning at the arrow). In general, decreasing the duration of

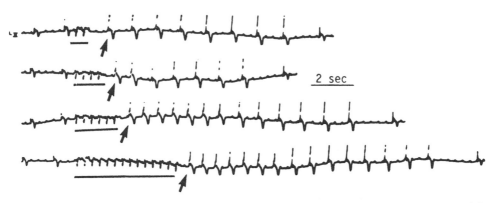

Figure 1.16: Ventricular rhythm induced by overdrive pacing in canine heart with surgically-induced heart block. Each trace is a lead II ECG. At the left of each trace is one cycle (two QRS complexes) of the idioventricular rhythm prior to overdrive. The period of overdrive is underlined and the first QRS of the rhythm that ensued after overdrive is shown by the arrow beneath each trace. Note that the rhythm that occurred after overdrive was faster than the idioventricular rhythm (overdrive excitation). (Reproduced from Vassalle et al. (1976) with permission.)

diastole during overdrive and increasing the number of driven beats (both to a maximum point beyond which suppression occurs) increase the rate and duration of the induced rhythmic activity. This is shown in each of the subsequent traces in Figure 1.16 where the duration of the period of stimulation is increased (underlined). The rhythm induced by the periods of stimulation then slows before stopping (Vassalle et al. 1976). The overdrive excitation in this experimental model may result from the increased catecholamine levels found acutely after surgery causing AV block. Sympathetic stimulation or norepinephrine administration and Ca^{2+} infusion enhance overdrive excitation *in situ*, as they do *in vitro*, making the induced rhythms faster and longer lasting (Vassalle et al. 1976). A relationship of this experimental phenomenon to the occurrence of ventricular arrhythmias caused either by the sympathetic nervous system or pathological influences is not established, but it may be of some importance in causing ventricular tachycardia that arises in Purkinje fibers during the subacute phase of infarction (see Chapter III).

Delayed afterdepolarizations and triggered activity occur in rat ventricular muscle that is hypertrophic secondary to renovascular hypertension, particularly if extracellular Ca^{2+} is elevated (7.2–12.0 mmol/L) (Aronson 1981). The occurrence of delayed afterdepolarizations may be related to abnormalities of membrane Ca^{2+} currents or to abnormalities of SR uptake and release of Ca^{2+} that occurs concomitantly with hypertrophy (Aronson 1981). Ventricular myocardium from diabetic rats is also more prone to develop delayed afterdepolarizations under conditions believed to cause myoplasmic Ca^{2+} overload such as ouabain and increased extracellular Ca^{2+} (Nordin et al. 1985).

Delayed afterdepolarizations and triggered activity may also occur in the absence of pharmacological agents or an increase in extracellular Ca^{2+}. Triggerable fibers have been found in the upper pectinate muscles bordering the crista terminalis in the rabbit heart, in branches of the sinoatrial ring bundle, or in transitional fibers between the ring bundle and ordinary pectinate muscle (Saito et al. 1978). Apparently normal fibers in human atrial myocardium (resting potentials of -70 mV to -75 mV) have been shown to have delayed afterdepolarizations and to be triggered (Mary-Rabine et al. 1980). These atrial fibers can become automatic at relatively slow rates because of spontaneous diastolic depolarization. Delayed afterdepolarizations in these spontaneously active fibers are superimposed on the spontaneous diastolic depolarization that causes the automatic activity. When a delayed afterdepolarization reaches threshold it triggers a more rapid rhythm. Spontaneous diastolic depolarization, delayed afterdepolarizations and triggered activity also are evident in human atrial fibers with very low membrane potentials (< -60 mV) and slow response action potentials (Hordof et al. 1976; Ten Eick and Singer 1979; Mary-Rabine et al. 1980). Such abnormal preparations have been obtained from atria that are dilated as a result of cardiac disease. Catecholamines are sometimes necessary for the afterdepolarizations to occur.

Parenthetically, a corollary to delayed afterdepolarizations being caused by an increase in intracellular calcium is that substances and drugs that reduce intracellular calcium diminish or abolish delayed afterdepolarizations. Examples are acetylcholine in atrial fibers (Ten Eick et al. 1976; Wit and Cranefield 1977), drugs that block fast Na^+ channels such as Class I antiarrhythmic drugs (Elharrar et al. 1978; Rosen and Danilo 1980; Karagueuzian and Katzung 1981; Wasserstrom and Ferrier 1981; Hewett et al. 1983; Sheu and Lederer 1985), drugs that block slow (L-type) calcium channels such as verapamil (Ferrier et al. 1973; Wit and Cranefield 1977; Mary-Rabine et al. 1980; Gough et al. 1984), drugs that block Na/Ca exchange such as adriamycin (Binah et al. 1983), and drugs that alter the release of calcium from the SR such as caffeine and ryanodine (Paspa and Vassalle 1984; Aronson et al. 1985).

In the next section, we discuss the specific membrane current that results from calcium overload and causes delayed afterdepolarizations, the transient inward current. However, oscillations in membrane potential occurring after an action potential and resembling delayed afterdepolarizations caused by this current, might also result from passive interactions among cells in a syncytial sheet having different kinds of action potentials and might not be dependent on an elevation of intracellular calcium. These interactions have been simulated by Van Capelle and Durrer (1980) in a computer model using a sheet of excitable elements coupled together by passive resistances. When cells with spontaneous diastolic depolarization and pacemaker activity were coupled to nonpacemaker cells by a critically low resistance in this model, the repetitive activity of the pacemaker cells was completely inhibited. A single stimulus then evoked an action potential and started sustained rhythmic activity. The rhythmic activity was stopped by a single stimulus. When the coupling resistance was lowered a bit more, the action potential evoked by the stimulus was followed by oscillatory activity resembling afterdepolarizations. These apparent afterdepolarizations resulted from the electrotonic effect of the nonpacemaker cell on the pacemaker cell. The diastolic membrane potential of the pacemaker cells began to depolarize, but then returned to the maximum diastolic level before reaching threshold because of current flow from the nonpacemaker cell. When threshold potential was reached, repolarization of the triggered action potential was followed by spontaneous diastolic depolarization to threshold if coupling resistance between the two kinds of cells was not low enough to prevent it (Van Capelle and Durrer 1980). Such interactions may occur at the border zone of an acutely ischemic region as is discussed in Chapter II.

Properties of Delayed Afterdepolarizations and Ionic Mechanisms   Delayed afterdepolarizations and triggered activity are usually caused by an oscillatory membrane current called the transient inward current, which is distinct from the pacemaker currents (Aronson et al. 1973; Lederer and Tsien 1976; Aronson and Gelles 1977; Hiraoka 1977; Kass et al. 1978a; 1978b; Eisner and Lederer 1979; Vassalle and Mugelli 1981; Karagueuzian and Katzung 1982; Lipsius and Gibbons 1982; Lipp and Pott 1988; Tseng and Wit 1987a). Under any of the conditions that cause delayed afterdepolarizations the transient inward current is elicited by the action potential that precedes the delayed afterdepolarization. This is evident from studies showing that the transient inward current can be recorded after a depolarizing voltage-clamp pulse. In the area enclosed by the dashed rectangle, Figure 1.17 shows a square wave pulse used to depolarize the cell membrane in an experiment on a calf Purkinje fiber (top trace v) and the membrane currents during and after the pulse (bottom trace). The time course of the membrane depolarization follows the square pulse and to some extent mimics an action potential. Following the end of the pulse, the membrane potential was clamped and the current that flowed at this time was measured. The time course of this current is shown by the arrow in the current trace. The current that flows into the cell (inward current is downward) rises quickly to a peak and then declines. This transient inward current causes delayed afterdepolarizations because when the membrane is not clamped, a transient depolarization results after the action potential. The transient inward current is also shown in Figure 1.14 during a different kind of experimental protocol. We described the oscillatory changes in membrane potential after a period of stimulation in the Purkinje fiber bundle that was exposed to a toxic amount of strophanthidin (arrows in the top trace). Following a subsequent period of stimulation, membrane potential was clamped at the diastolic level preventing the oscillations (unfilled arrow) and the membrane current was measured. The oscillatory transient inward current that occurred during this time is indicated by the arrow in the bottom trace.

The level to which depolarization must occur from the resting potential during the voltage-clamp square wave pulse in order to elicit the following transient inward current (the threshold potential) has varied widely in different tissues, ranging from -60 mV in atrial muscle from the coronary sinus (Tseng and Wit 1987a) to -13 mV in ferret papillary muscle exposed to toxic

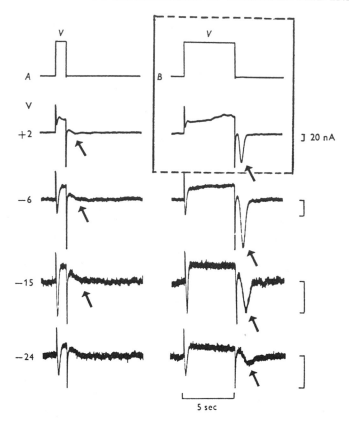

Figure 1.17: Effects of depolarizing voltage-clamp pulse duration and magnitude on the amplitude of the transient inward (TI) current in a calf Purkinje fiber exposed to 1 μmol/L strophanthidin. The holding potential was −41 mV. The top trace in each column is the clamp pulse. Below this trace are the current records. Effects of pulses 1 second in duration to membrane potential levels of +2, −6, −15, and −24 mV are shown in column A (left) and effects of pulses 4 seconds in duration to the same potential levels are shown in column B (right). The arrows indicate the TI current in each of the current traces. (Reproduced from Lederer and Tsien (1976) with permission.)

amounts of digitalis (Karagueuzian and Katzung 1982). The threshold level of depolarization probably depends to some extent on the intracellular Ca^{2+} levels. Raising extracellular Ca^{2+}, (and thereby intracellular Ca^{2+}) shifts the level of depolarization necessary to elicit the transient inward current in a negative direction (Vassalle and Mugelli 1981). The transient inward current has been elicited after voltage-clamp pulses applied from membrane potentials (holding potentials) of around −80 to −20 mV (Lederer and Tsien 1976; Vassalle and Mugelli 1981). At holding potentials less negative than −60 mV, the pacemaker current does not occur, yet a large transient inward current may occur after an appropriate clamp pulse applied from this level (Lederer and Tsien 1976), indicating that the transient inward current is distinct from the pacemaker current. Similarly, the transient inward current has been elicited after the fast inward current was first inactivated by voltage-clamp steps to potentials less negative than -60 to -50 mV (Lederer and Tsien 1976; Vassalle and Mugelli 1981), indicating that afterdepolarizations can occur in fibers with slow as well as fast response action potentials. Even though the transient inward current occurs over this wide range of membrane potentials, its amplitude and kinetics are affected by the level of membrane potential at which it is elicited. This has been shown in experimental voltage-clamp studies with a clamp protocol in which a fixed depolarization step was used to elicit the current and the level of repolarization (membrane potential at which the current is measured) was varied over a wide range. The data from these studies show that the transient inward current is maximal at around -60 mV and diminishes at more positive and more negative membrane potentials (Kass et al. 1978b; Karagueuzian and Katzung 1981; Vassalle and Mugelli 1981; Arlock and Katzung 1985).

As a result of the dependence of the transient inward current on the level of membrane potential, the amplitude of delayed afterdepolarizations and therefore, the possibility of triggered activity are influenced by the level of membrane potential at which the action potentials occur. In the digitalis-toxic Purkinje system there is a "window" of membrane voltage for maximum diastolic potential, which is between approximately -75 to -80 mV, at which the amplitude of delayed afterdepolarizations tends to be greatest (Ferrier 1980, Wasserstrom and Ferrier 1981). (This is not the exact same membrane potential at which the transient inward current was maximum in the voltage-clamp studies described above because other factors such as membrane resistance at different levels of potential also influence the afterdepolarizations occurring in the absence of voltage clamp.) When delayed afterdepolarizations occur at the membrane potentials that favor a maximum amplitude, any intervention that hyperpolarizes or depolarizes the membrane (such as rapid pacing, a spontaneous change in rate, or intracellular application of hyperpolarizing or depolarizing current) tends to reduce their magnitude and to suppress any rhythms the afterdepolarizations might induce. Similarly, when there are no delayed afterdepolarizations in the presence of digitalis and the membrane potential is at a voltage less than or greater than the "window", interventions that bring membrane potential into this voltage range often induce delayed afterdepolarizations. A similar dependence on membrane potential has been shown for delayed afterdepolarizations in atrial fibers of the coronary sinus (Henning and Wit 1981) and in Purkinje fibers from infarcts (Le Marec et al. 1985; Gough and El-Sherif 1989).

In addition to the effects of the resting or maximum diastolic potential, the results of voltage-clamp studies also explain other ways in which the time course of voltage change of action potentials control the characteristics of delayed afterdepolarizations. In these studies, increasing the magnitude of a depolarizing voltage-clamp pulse enhanced the amplitude of the transient inward current that followed the pulse and caused the current to develop more rapidly (Lederer and Tsien 1976; Vassalle and Mugelli 1981; Karagueuzian and Katzung 1982; Tseng and Wit 1985). This is shown by the records in Figure 1.18

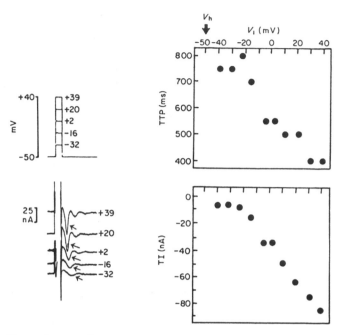

Figure 1.18: Dependence of the time-to-peak (TTP) and amplitude of the transient inward (TI) current on the depolarization level of voltage-clamp pulses (V_1 level). Left top shows superimposed voltage traces obtained during a voltage-clamp protocol. Depolarizing pulses of 0.5-second duration were applied from a holding potential of -50 mV to levels ranging from -32 to $+39$ mV every 15 seconds. Left bottom shows the current traces following the depolarization steps (depolarization levels of voltage steps are also marked at the right of the voltage and current traces). The current traces during the depolarization steps are largely omitted and only that part of the current trace following return of membrane potential to the holding potential is shown. The arrows indicate the TI current. Right top shows the relation between TI current time-to-peak (TTP, ordinate) and V_1 levels (abscissa). Right bottom shows the relation between the TI current amplitude (TI, ordinate) and V_1 levels (abscissa). (Reproduced from Tseng and Wit (1987a) with permission.)

from an experiment on an atrial fiber from the canine coronary sinus. At the top left, the voltage-clamp pulses are shown, ranging from -32 mV to $+39$ mV. Below are the superimposed current traces recorded during each clamp pulse, with the transient inward current indicated by the arrows. The largest amplitude transient inward current occurred after the largest clamp pulse to $+39$ mV and the smallest amplitude transient inward current occurred after the smallest clamp pulse to -32 mV. The graphs at the right show plots of the time-to-peak (TTP) of the transient inward current and the transient inward current amplitude (TI) versus depolarization voltage amplitude (V_1). Time-to-peak decreased while transient inward current amplitude increased with increasing amplitude of depolarization. On the basis of these data, action potentials with larger amplitudes are expected to have larger delayed afterdepolarizations, while a decrease in the amplitude of the action potential should decrease the delayed afterdepolarization. The effects of the amplitude of depolarization on the transient inward current may depend on the effects of the depolarizing pulses (or action potentials) on intracellular Ca^{2+}. Ca^{2+} influx via the inward current through L-type calcium channels plays some role. The steep part of the curve relating the increase in transient inward current amplitude to the increased level of depolarization occurs over a range of membrane potentials at which the Ca^{2+} inward current is activated and also increases in amplitude with an increase in the level of depolarization (Coraboeuf 1980). However, depolarizing clamp steps that do not activate the L-type calcium current may also activate the transient inward current (see Vassalle and Mugelli 1981 for details) and the slope factor for the transient inward current may be more positive and steeper than the activation curve for the Ca^{2+} current (Karagueuzian and Katzung 1982). Therefore, other mechanisms such as Na/Ca exchange (Eisner and Lederer 1985) or release of Ca^{2+} from internal stores, both of which occur during the action potential, may also play a role in causing the increasing transient inward current that follows depolarizations of increasing amplitude.

At fixed levels of depolarization, increasing the duration of a voltage-clamp pulse, which increases the time that the membrane is in the depolarized state, increases the amplitude of the transient inward current and accelerates the time course at which it achieves maximum amplitude (Lederer and Tsien 1976; Vassalle and Mugelli 1981; Karagueuzian and Katzung 1982; Tseng and Wit 1987a). This property is shown in Figure 1.17 in records from an experiment on a Purkinje fiber bundle exposed to a toxic concentration of digitalis, where the effects of clamp pulses 1 second in duration in the left column are compared with the effects of clamp pulses of 4 seconds duration shown in the right column. The membrane potential was depolarized to levels of $+2$, -6, -15, and -24 mV with clamp pulses of each duration. After the short (1 second) duration clamp pulses, the transient inward current is barely noticeable at the different levels of membrane depolarization (left column, arrows), while it is much larger after the long (4 seconds) duration clamp pulses (right column, arrows). This figure also shows the effects of different levels of membrane depolarization on the amplitude of the transient inward current that we discussed before; maximum transient inward current occurred after clamp pulses to -6 mV in the Purkinje fiber bundle. The prolongation of the clamp pulse and duration of membrane depolarization increases intracellular Ca^{2+} by increasing the flow of inward calcium current leading to an increase in the transient inward current (Coraboeuf 1980; Kass and Scheuer 1982). Other mechanisms may also be involved. Therefore, delayed afterdepolarizations are influenced by the action potential duration with longer action potential durations favoring the occurrence of delayed afterdepolarizations (Henning and Wit 1984). One example of the influence of action potential duration on delayed afterdepolarization amplitude is the observation that during digitalis toxicity, the amplitude of delayed afterdepolarizations at the area of maximum action potential duration in the Purkinje system (the gate of Myerburg et al. 1970) tends to be greater than at sites more proximal or distal where action potential duration is shorter

(Rosen MR, personal communication). Another example is that drugs like quinidine that prolong action potential duration may increase delayed afterpolarization amplitude (Wit et al. 1990b) while drugs such as lidocaine that shorten action potential duration may decrease delayed afterpolarization amplitude (Sheu and Lederer 1985).

The relationship between the duration of depolarizing clamp pulses and the amplitude of the transient inward current described above shows that increasing the amount of time the membrane is maintained in the depolarized state enhances the amplitude of the transient inward current and causes it to occur more quickly. For the same reason, the amplitude of the transient inward current has been shown to increase after repeated voltage-clamp pulses. The amplitude is inversely related to the interval between pulses and directly related to the number of pulses (Lederer and Tsien 1976; Vassalle and Mugelli 1981; Tseng and Wit 1987a). This explains several important properties of delayed afterpolarizations. First, the amplitude of delayed afterpolarizations is dependent on the number of action potentials that precede them. That is, after a period of quiescence, the initiation of a single action potential may be followed by either no afterpolarization or only a small one. With continued stimulation, the afterpolarizations increase in amplitude and triggered activity may eventually occur (Ferrier et al. 1973; Rosen et al. 1973b; Wit and Cranefield 1976; 1977; Aronson 1980; Henning and Wit 1984). Second, the amplitude of delayed afterpolarizations and their coupling interval to the previous action potentials are dependent upon the cycle length at which action potentials are occurring and triggered activity can be induced by a critical decrease in the drive cycle length (Ferrier et al. 1973; Rosen et al. 1973b; Wit and Cranefield 1976; 1977; Saito et al. 1978; Aronson 1981; El-Sherif et al. 1983b; Nordin et al. 1985). This is illustrated by the effects of the stimulus cycle length on the amplitude of delayed afterpolarizations recorded from an atrial fiber in the canine coronary sinus, shown in Figure 1.19. The transmembrane potentials, at the left, were recorded when the stimulus cycle length was 2000 msec; the afterpolarization amplitude following the last stimulated impulse is 5 mV. In the center, the stimulus cycle length was 1500 msec and afterpolarization amplitude after the last stimulated impulse is 15 mV. At the right, at a stimulus cycle length of 1200 msec, afterpolarization amplitude reached 20 mV after the third stimulated action potential before triggered activity was initiated. In cardiac fibers that have automaticity in addition to delayed afterpolarizations such as human atrial fibers, a spontaneous increase in the rate of automatic activity can cause an increase in afterpolarization amplitude and triggering in the same way as increasing the extrinsic drive rate (Mary-Rabine et al. 1980). Digitalis-induced delayed afterpolarizations occur either singly or as two or more "damped" oscillations following the action potential (see Figure 1.14) (Ferrier et al. 1973; Rosen et al. 1973b). When two or more afterpolarizations are present their relationship to the drive cycle length is complex. As drive cycle length decreases, the amplitude of the first afterpolarization increases, reaching a peak at a cycle length of about 500 msec and triggered activity may occur. If it does not, at shorter drive cycle

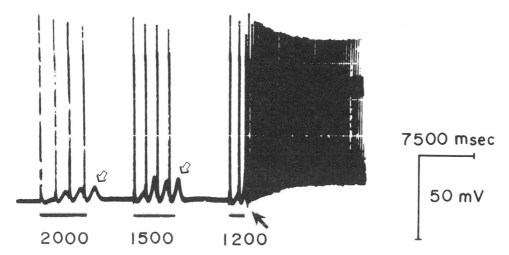

7500 msec

50 mV

2000   1500   1200

Figure 1.19: Effects of stimulation rate on delayed afterdepolarizations and triggered activity. Transmembrane action potentials were recorded from an atrial fiber in the canine coronary sinus superfused with Tyrode's solution containing norepinephrine. The stimulus cycle lengths and the periods of stimulation are indicated by the horizontal black bars. Triggered activity occurred at the black arrow during stimulation at a cycle length of 1200 msec. The rate of triggered activity is so rapid that the individual action potentials cannot be seen at the slow oscilloscopic sweep speed. (Reproduced from Wit and Cranefield (1977) with permission.)

lengths the magnitude of this first afterdepolarization decreases. However, the second delayed afterdepolarization continues to increase in magnitude as drive cycle length shortens further and may eventually reach threshold and induce triggered activity.

A decrease in the length of even a single drive cycle (i.e., a premature impulse) also results in an increase in the amplitude of the delayed afterdepolarization that follows the premature cycle. This is demonstrated in Figure 1.20 in recordings from an atrial fiber in the canine coronary sinus. In panel A, the last two action potentials in a series of ten driven at a cycle length of 4000 msec is followed by a prematurely stimulated action potential with a coupling interval of 2500 msec. The afterdepolarization following the premature action potential (black arrow) is larger than the afterdepolarization following the previous stimulated action potentials. As the premature action potential occurred earlier after the previous impulse (panel B), the amplitude of the afterdepolarization that followed it increased (arrow). In panel C, at a premature coupling interval of 1000 msec, the afterdepolarization reached threshold initiating triggered activity at the arrow. The premature coupling interval at which triggered activity occurs is also dependent on the basic drive cycle length. As the basic drive cycle length decreases, the premature coupling interval needed to induce triggered activity increases (Moak and Rosen 1984).

Decreasing the drive cycle length, in addition to increasing amplitude, also tends to decrease the coupling interval of delayed afterdepolarizations to the

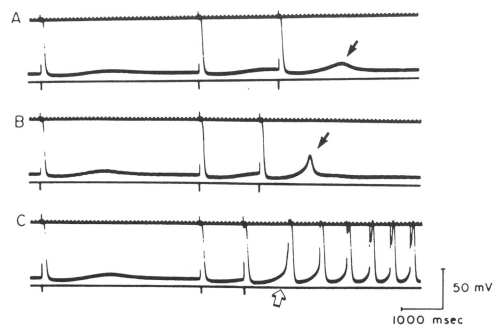

Figure 1.20: Effects of premature stimulation on afterdepolarization amplitude and triggering. Each panel shows transmembrane potentials recorded from a Tyrode's super-fused preparation of atrial muscle from the canine coronary sinus. The bottom trace shows the stimulus pulse. The first two action potentials, from left to right, are the last action potentials in a train of ten stimulated at a basic cycle length of 4000 msec. The third action potential results from a premature stimulus. The afterdepolarizations following the prematurely stimulated action potentials are indicated by the arrows. (Reproduced from Wit and Cranefield (1977) with permission.)

action potential upstroke or terminal phase of repolarization by increasing the rate of depolarization of the afterdepolarization, (Ferrier et al. 1973; Rosen et al. 1973b; Wit and Cranefield 1977; Saito et al. 1978). As a result there is a direct relationship between the drive cycle length at which triggered impulses are initiated, and the coupling interval between the first triggered impulse and the last stimulated impulse that induced them, e.g., as the drive cycle length is reduced the first triggered impulse occurs earlier with respect to the last driven action potential. This characteristic property forms the basis for one of the indirect ways that triggered activity induced by a decrease in the drive cycle length in the whole heart is sometimes distinguished from reentrant activity induced by a decrease in the drive cycle length since the relationship for reentrant impulses initiated by rapid stimulation is often the opposite, e.g., as drive cycle length is reduced, the first reentrant impulse occurs later with respect to the last driven action potential (see section later in this chapter on Identifying Mechanisms of Arrhythmias in the Heart). A decrease in the coupling interval of premature impulses that initiate triggered activity is also sometimes associated with a decrease in the coupling interval of the triggered impulse, but this effect is not consistent so that it cannot be stated that there is a direct relationship between premature coupling interval and coupling interval of the triggered impulse. In general, the coupling interval between the stimulated premature impulse and the triggered impulse remains constant as the premature coupling interval is decreased (Johnson and Rosen 1987).

The increased time during which the membrane is in the depolarized state at shorter stimulation cycle lengths or after premature impulses increases Ca^{2+} in the myoplasm and the SR, thereby increasing the transient inward current that is responsible for the increased afterdepolarization amplitude and causing the current to reach its maximum amplitude more rapidly, decreasing the coupling interval of triggered impulses. The repetitive depolarizations can increase intracellular Ca^{2+} because of repeated activation of the inward Ca^{2+} current that flows through L-type calcium channels. Repetitive voltage-clamp pulses to low potentials that do not activate the inward Ca^{2+} current can also lead to an increase in the transient inward current, and therefore, there is an additional mechanism for increasing intracellular Ca^{2+} that is not yet elucidated (Vassalle and Mugelli 1981). In addition, Na^+ enters the cell during the upstroke of each action potential and intracellular Na^+ may rise at rapid rates of stimulation. Intracellular Ca^{2+} then might also rise through Na/Ca exchange secondary to the increase in intracellular Na^+ (January and Fozzard 1984). Other factors may also contribute to the increase in afterdepolarization amplitude following a period of stimulation. Rapid stimulation may cause a decline in the maximum diastolic potential (Saito et al. 1978; Aronson 1981; Valenzuela and Vassalle 1983; Kline 1990) because of accumulation of K^+ in the extracellular space (Kline and Kupersmith 1982; Kline 1990). Depolarization may enhance the amplitude of the transient inward current and afterdepolarization if the membrane potential is shifted into a range more optimum for the occurrence of delayed afterdepolarizations (described above) (Henning and Wit 1981; Wasserstrom and Ferrier 1981). In addition, the decrease in maximum diastolic potential may bring the afterdepolarization closer to threshold, favoring the occurrence of triggered activity at more rapid rates of stimulation.

Subcellular Mechanism of Delayed Afterdepolarizations   As we mentioned earlier, the occurrence of delayed afterdepolarizations is usually associated with a situation in which intracellular Ca^{2+} levels are elevated. On depolarization of the membrane during an action potential the intracellular free Ca^{2+} normally increases primarily by Ca^{2+} influx through the L-type calcium channels. Initially, this rapid rate of change of intracellular Ca^{2+} triggers Ca^{2+} release from the sarcoplasmic reticulum (SR), which causes a further rise in intracellular free Ca^{2+} and contraction (Fabiato and Fabiato 1975). Repolarization then induces a synchronous Ca^{2+} uptake by the SR in the cell and relaxation. If intracellular Ca^{2+} is very high or if catecholamines or cyclic AMP are present, both of which enhance calcium uptake by the SR, the Ca^{2+} in the SR may rise during repolarization to a critical level at which a secondary spontaneous and synchronous release of Ca^{2+} from the SR occurs after the action potential and relaxation of contraction (Fabiato and Fabiato 1975). This secondary release of Ca^{2+} generates an aftercontraction as well as the transient inward current and the afterdepolarization. After one or several afterdepolarizations myoplasmic Ca^{2+} may decrease because Na/Ca exchange extrudes Ca^{2+} from the cell, and membrane potential stops oscillating.

The exact mechanism by which the secondary rise in myoplasmic Ca^{2+} after repolarization causes the transient inward current is unclear and is still a source of controversy. Two possibilities are being actively considered. The first is that the calcium released from the SR after repolarization acts on the sarcolemma to increase its conductance to ions (mainly Na^+) that flow into the cell down a concentration gradient through membrane channels. The channels are not specific for Na^+ however, because in experiments on digitalis, toxic Purkinje fibers in which the reversal potential of the transient inward current was measured, it was found to be around -5 mV (Kass et al. 1978b). The reversal potential for Na^+, (E_{Na}) is normally about $+79$ mV. The reversal potential of the transient inward current in these experiments did not correspond specifically to the equilibrium potential of any major ion, being more negative than E_{Na} and more positive than E_K or E_{Cl}. Therefore, ions other than Na^+, with more negative equilibrium potentials, such as K^+ or Cl^-, were also proposed to act as charge carriers and it was suggested that the transient inward channel was a nonselective channel (Kass et al. 1978b; Colquhoun et al. 1981; Cannell and Lederer 1986; Ehara et al. 1988). The second mechanism proposed for the origin of the transient inward current is that the rise in calcium causes the transient inward current through an electrogenic (rheogenic) exchange of Ca^{2+} for Na^+. According to this hypothesis, the transient rise in myoplasmic Ca^{2+} that is released from the SR after the action potential is expected to result in "transport" of Ca^{2+} out of the cell across the sarcolemma by the Na/Ca exchanger. Such an efflux is coupled to a Na^+ influx. If more than two Na^+ ions are exchanged for each Ca^{2+} ion, a net inward current occurs (Baker et al. 1969; Mullins 1979; Eisner and Lederer 1985). If the transient inward current is caused by electrogenic Na/Ca exchange, theory predicts that the current will not have a reversal potential and that an increase in the free internal Ca^{2+} will only lead to a net inward current (Mullins 1979; 1981; Noble 1984; Arlock and Katzung 1985; DiFrancesco and Noble 1985). A reversal potential has not been found in a number of studies on the transient inward current (other than the one by Kass et al. 1978b mentioned above) supporting the view that it is caused by a Na/Ca exchange mechanism. Also, substitution of extracellular Na^+ with Li^+ decreased afterdepolarization amplitude or abolished the transient inward current, effects that should not have occurred if this current is dependent on a nonselective cation channel (Fedida et al. 1987; Lipp and Pott 1988; Tseng and Wit 1987b) because Li^+ should freely pass through the channel. However, Li^+ is not transported by the Na/Ca exchanger.

The charge carrier for the transient inward current that causes delayed afterdepolarizations in a normal extracellular environment appears to be mainly Na^+. This has been elucidated by changing the concentration of ions in the extracellular fluid. Removal of Na^+ leads to a decrease in the afterdepolarizations and transient inward current (Karagueuzian and Katzung 1982; Arlock and Katzung 1985; Tseng and Wit 1987b). If the transient inward current flows through a nonselective cation channel, the fact that the current is carried by Na^+ can be explained by the preponderance of this ion in the extracellular environment. That the current is carried by Na^+ is also consistent with a Na/Ca exchange mechanism.

The Rate of Triggered Activity   The rate and rhythm of triggered activity has a pattern that is characteristic for the specific cause. The patterns of triggered activity have been mostly elucidated in experimental studies on isolated tissues. The recognition of these patterns might sometimes be useful for identifying triggered activity in the heart *in situ* and for distinguishing it from other mechanisms of arrhythmogenesis, as we will discuss later on.

Once the drive cycle length is decreased to the critical value that causes an afterdepolarization to reach threshold and trigger an action potential, a train of triggered action potentials, rather than only one, often occurs. In Purkinje fibers made toxic with digitalis, the rate of triggered activity is dependent on the preceding drive cycle length; as the drive cycle length used to trigger decreases, the rate tends to increase (Moak and Rosen 1984). This increase in rate is most prominent during the first few beats. The rate may remain constant thereafter, increase still further or decrease. The stimulus rate that is used to trigger may also influence the rate of triggered activity of Purkinje fibers surviving in infarcts (Le Marec et al. 1985) (see Chapter III) and Purkinje fibers exposed to elevated Ca^{2+} and catecholamines (Valenzuela and Vassalle 1983; 1985) in the same way that it influences digitalis-induced triggered activity. In atrial fibers exposed to catecholamines only the first triggered beat shows this cycle length dependence (shorter cycle length at faster drive rates), but the fastest rate attained during triggered activity is not related to the cycle length of the basic drive (Johnson et al. 1986). Comparable data are not available for catecholamine-induced triggered activity in ventricular fibers, although they might be predicted to behave the same as atrial fibers.

The increase in amplitude of the transient inward current with increasing activity is largely responsible for the perpetuation of triggered activity, once the first nondriven (triggered) action potential has occurred. If the first triggered action potential arises from the peak of the delayed afterdepolarization, then the coupling interval (cycle length) between the upstroke of this action potential and the last driven one often is shorter than the drive cycle length. Hence, the afterdepolarization following the first triggered action potential will be even larger than the afterdepolarization from which it arose (recall that the rate of rise of the transient inward current and the afterdepolarization increases at shorter cycle lengths) and a second nondriven (triggered) action potential will occur at a short coupling interval. The continuation of triggered activity is then dependent on the delayed afterdepolarization after each triggered action potential reaching threshold.

Once established, triggered activity occurring under different conditions may have different characteristics. For example, triggered activity caused by digitalis toxicity has different characteristics than triggered activity caused by catecholamines. The differences in the characteristics of triggered activity after digitalis and after catecholamines may be related to the function of the Na/K pump, partly or mostly inhibited during the former but still active during the latter. Catecholamine-induced triggered activity in atrial fibers can be subdivided into several well defined phases that are shown in Figure 1.21 (Wit et al. 1981b; 1987). There is an initial phase of 5–10 seconds during which a marked increase in rate occurs that is sometimes associated with membrane depolarization (labeled "a" in the figure). Then, there is a second phase during which rate accelerates more gradually and that is associated with membrane depolarization (labeled "b"). This is followed by a third phase during which maximum diastolic potential hyperpolarizes, rate slows, and triggered activity eventually terminates (labeled "c"). During a final phase following termination, maximum diastolic potential hyperpolarizes relative to the maximum diastolic potential prior to triggering and then returns to the control value (labeled "d"). Triggered arrhythmias in the *in situ* heart caused by this mechanism would be expected to go through these same phases.

The initial rapid increase in rate occurring with the first few triggered beats results from the influence of the short cycle length of the first triggered beats on afterdepolarization amplitude and rate of depolarization, e.g., there is an increase in amplitude and rate of depolarization of afterdepolarizations at the short cycle lengths. After triggered activity is initiated there is an increase in extracellular K^+ that begins during the first few beats (Kline 1990; Henning et al. 1987). This increase in extracellular K^+ is shown in the bottom trace in Figure 1.21, which is the measured level of K^+ obtained with a K^+-sensitive

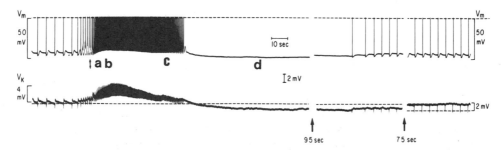

Figure 1.21: Changes in membrane potential and extracellular K^+ during triggered activity in an atrial fiber of the canine coronary sinus. The top trace is the transmembrane potential recording, cut off at the dashed line so that 0 potential is not shown. The fiber was first stimulated at a long cycle length (at the left), and then stimulus cycle length was abruptly decreased to cause triggered activity at the arrow. After triggered activity terminated, stimulation was resumed at the right. The bottom trace is a record of extracellular K^+ activity recorded with a K^+-selective microelectrode inserted into the extracellular space of the triggered fiber. The 4-mV voltage scale is equivalent to 2 mmol/L K^+. (Reproduced from Wit and Rosen (1986) with permission.)

microelectrode inserted into the interstitial space of the tissue. The increase in K^+ most likely results from K^+ efflux during the action potential and the inability of diffusion out of the extracellular space and the Na/K pump to balance this efflux (Kline and Kupersmith 1982). After the first 5–10 beats, as extracellular K^+ continues to increase, maximum diastolic potential declines simultaneously. Subsequent to the first few triggered impulses, the rest of the increase in rate during triggered activity parallels the progressive rise in extracellular K^+ and depolarization of the maximum diastolic potential (Henning et al. 1987). As we have described, a decrease in the membrane potential from levels of around -80 mV to around -60 mV increases the afterdepolarization amplitude and its rate of depolarization that is responsible for the acceleration of the rate of triggered activity. The decrease in membrane potential also accelerates the rate by shifting maximum diastolic potential closer to threshold potential. In addition, it is predicted that with each beat, Na^+ and Ca^{2+} enter during depolarization of the action potential resulting in an increase in intracellular Na^+ and Ca^{2+} (Cohen et al. 1982; Lado et al. 1982; January and Fozzard 1984). This increase in the intracellular Ca^{2+} should also increase the rate by increasing the transient inward current.

Soon after depolarization brings the maximum diastolic potential to a minimum level, membrane potential slowly starts to hyperpolarize (Figure 1.21). Extracellular K^+ begins to decrease after hyperpolarization begins. Activation of an outward current from the electrogenic Na/K pump (activated as intracellular Na^+ continues to accumulate during triggered activity) is expected to contribute to the hyperpolarization and the decrease in extracellular K^+ (Gadsby and Cranefield 1979a; 1979b) in much the same way as hyperpolarization occurs during prolonged rapid overdrive stimulation of cardiac fibers (Vassalle 1970; Browning et al. 1979). The increase in maximum diastolic potential and the outward electrogenic current both play a role in slowing and eventually stopping triggered activity (Wit et al. 1981b).

After an episode of triggered activity there is further hyperpolarization of the maximum diastolic potential to levels usually negative to those prior to triggering (Figure 1.21). Both hyperpolarization and further depletion of extracellular K^+ are associated with enhanced Na pumping driven by intracellular Na^+ accumulated during rapid activity (Vassalle 1970; Kunze 1977; Browning et al. 1979; Kline and Kupersmith 1982). The electrogenic Na/K pump hyperpolarizes the membrane that may be further hyperpolarized by the direct action of reduced extracellular K^+ on the membrane. The return of membrane potential and extracellular K^+ to control levels is due then to return of the pump rate to its original baseline value as extrusion of intracellular Na^+ is completed.

After the termination of triggered activity in atrial fibers, the stimulated action potentials at the hyperpolarized membrane potential are followed by afterdepolarizations of reduced amplitude, and triggering is more difficult to induce (Saito et al. 1978; Henning et al. 1987). The decrease in the amplitude of delayed afterdepolarizations following a period of triggered activity is shown in the right panels in Figure 1.21. Several possible reasons for the decrease in amplitude include (1) a decrease in transient inward current at hyperpolarized membrane potentials (Lederer and Tsien 1976), (2) a decrease in intracellular Na^+ and Ca^{2+} following a period of rapid activity (Cohen et al. 1982; Lado et al. 1982), (3) the direct opposing effect of increased outward electrogenic Na^+ pump current on the afterdepolarization, (4) a decrease in action potential duration caused by enhanced electrogenic pump current (Gadsby and Cranefield 1979b; 1982) that in turn decreases afterdepolarization amplitude (Henning and Wit 1984). From this characteristic it is predicted that immediately after a paroxysm of triggered tachycardia terminates in the heart it should be very difficult to initiate another paroxysm until the effects of the period of triggered activity have worn off.

The changes in maximum diastolic potential and rate during triggered activity caused by digitalis in Purkinje fibers are different than in the atrial fibers described above. During the course of triggered activity, maximum diastolic potential may decrease and there may be further depolarization as the rhythm stops (Rosen and Danilo 1980). During this time there may be an increase in the rate of triggered activity associated with the depolarization and no gradual slowing as described above. However, there also may be gradual slowing of the rate of digitalis-toxic Purkinje fibers before triggered activity stops (Johnson and Rosen 1987). Purkinje fibers in an environment of elevated Ca^{2+} and catecholamines also have a different pattern of triggered activity (Valenzuela and Vassalle 1983; 1985). Triggered activity, induced by rapid stimulation, progressively slows without the initial acceleration. After a fast rate of drive the first triggered impulse occurs at a cycle length longer than the drive cycle length because of the long time needed for the afterdepolarization to reach threshold. The afterdepolarization following the triggered action potential is somewhat smaller because of the long cycle length and takes even longer to reach threshold. Slowing of the triggered rate occurs gradually because of the decreasing oscillatory potential. In addition, the activation of an outward current due to electrogenic sodium extrusion may contribute to cessation of activity (Valenzuela and Vassalle 1983).

Effects of Electrical Stimulation on Established Triggered Activity   We have discussed how triggered activity caused by delayed afterdepolarizations is initiated by stimulation. These characteristics may be of use in identifying triggered activity in the *in situ* heart (described later). Also of importance in identifying triggered arrhythmias *in situ* are the effects of electrical stimulation on established triggered activity.

In general, triggered activity is markedly influenced by overdrive stimulation (stimulation at a rate faster than the triggered rate). The effects of overdrive have been studied in only several experimental situations: on triggered activity caused by catecholamines in atrial fibers and by digitalis or myocardial infarction in Purkinje fibers. These effects are dependent both on the rate and duration of overdrive (Wit et al. 1981b; Johnson et al. 1986). Figure 1.22 shows the effects of overdrive on triggered activity caused by catecholamines in atrial fibers. In this experiment, during a short period of overdrive at a rate only

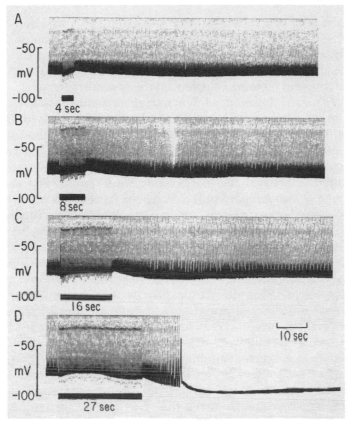

Figure 1.22: Effects of overdrive on maximum diastolic potential and triggered activity of an atrial fiber in the canine coronary sinus superfused with Tyrode's solution containing norepinephrine. The records are displayed at high amplification to emphasize the changes in maximum diastolic potential so the tops of the action potentials are not shown. The cycle length of triggered activity prior to overdrive was 400 msec. The horizontal bars below each panel indicate the periods of overdrive at a cycle length of 300 msec. (Reproduced from Wit et al. (1981b) with permission.)

moderately faster than the triggered rate (underbar in panel A), there was a decrease in the maximum diastolic potential; following the period of overdrive triggered activity continued, and the rate was faster than it was before overdrive (overdrive acceleration), because of the decrease in the maximum diastolic potential. The decrease in maximum diastolic potential may result, at least partly, from additional K^+ accumulation in the extracellular space during overdrive (Kline and Wit, unpublished observations). The postoverdrive acceleration lasted for several seconds and then the rate of triggered activity gradually slowed and maximum diastolic potential increased until preoverdrive values were attained. Panels B, C and D of Figure 1.22 show the effects of longer periods of overdrive. Eight and 16 seconds of overdrive were accompanied by a decrease in maximum diastolic potential, and overdrive acceleration followed. Maximum diastolic potential and triggered rate then returned to the preoverdrive values. However, when overdrive stimulation was done for a critical duration of time (27 seconds in panel D), the maximum diastolic potential following the overdrive increased to levels more negative than before, and during the increase in membrane potential the rate of triggered activity slowed until the triggered rhythm stopped. When triggered activity stops after a period of overdrive at a moderate rate, as shown in Figure 1.22, some 10–50 impulses may occur after termination of the overdrive before termination of the triggered activity. The increase in maximum diastolic potential and the slowing and termination of triggered activity following a period of overdrive are caused by an enhanced activity of the electrogenic Na/K pump (Wit et al. 1981b). During a period of overdrive there is a transient increase in intracellular Na^+ because of the increased number of action potentials that stimulates the pump (Vassalle 1970; Browning et al. 1979; Gadsby and Cranefield 1979b; Cohen et al. 1982). This same series of events shown in Figure 1.22 also occurs if the duration of overdrive is kept constant and the rate of overdrive is increased. As the overdrive rate increases, the postoverdrive hyperpolarization of maximum diastolic potential and slowing of rate increase until triggered activity stops. We assume that overdrive stimulation will have similar effects on catecholamine-dependent triggered activity in ventricular or Purkinje fibers and on triggered activity resulting from other causes not related to digitalis toxicity. Experimental data are not available at the present time. When the rate at which coronary sinus fibers are overdriven is very fast, triggered activity may stop immediately upon termination without the prior increase in maximum diastolic potential or gradual slowing that is shown in Figure 1.22 (Wit et al. 1979).

In digitalis-toxic Purkinje fibers, overdrive stimulation can also terminate triggered activity and this effect is dependent on the overdrive cycle length, but not the overdrive duration (Moak and Rosen 1984; Johnson and Rosen 1987); termination occurs more frequently at more rapid overdrive rates and may not be immediate, e.g., several triggered impulses may continue to occur after stimulation is stopped before triggered activity stops (Moak and Rosen 1984). When overdrive is not rapid enough to terminate the triggered rhythm, it can cause overdrive acceleration. Termination by overdrive is not accompanied by hyperpolarization of the maximum diastolic potential and is probably not caused by increased Na/K pump activity because the pump is partially inhibited by digitalis. The exact mechanism for termination has not been elucidated.

Premature stimuli may also terminate triggered rhythms as shown in digitalis-toxic Purkinje fibers (Moak and Rosen 1984), Purkinje fibers in myocardial infarcts (Dangman and Hoffman 1985), or atrial fibers exposed to catecholamines (Wit and Cranefield 1976; Johnson et al. 1986), although termination is much less frequent than by overdrive (Johnson and Rosen 1987). It has not been demonstrated that the premature impulse must occur at a critical point in the cycle length of triggered activity caused by digitalis. In the investigation on digitalis-toxic Purkinje fibers, premature stimuli terminating triggered activity appeared to occur at random locations in diastole (Moak and Rosen 1984). In triggered activity caused by catecholamines in atrial fibers, a critical premature coupling interval that terminates triggered activity can sometimes be found (Johnson et al. 1987). In a study on triggering in the mitral valve, it was shown that a premature impulse that terminated triggered activity was followed by an increased afterhyperpolarization which, in turn, was followed by an afterdepolarization that did not reach threshold, perhaps because it arose from the more negative membrane potential of the preceding afterhyperpolarization (Wit and Cranefield 1976). The premature impulses that had this effect occurred late in diastole. Whether this mechanism applies to other kinds of triggered activity is not known. Triggered activity could not be terminated by single premature stimuli in rabbit pectinate muscle (Saito et al. 1978).

There is only a limited amount of data from studies on isolated tissues, of the effects of premature stimuli that fail to terminate triggered activity on the return (post-premature) cycle length of the triggered rhythm. For the most part, they resemble the effects of premature impulses on abnormal automaticity; the return cycle length is often similar to the basic triggered cycle length and less than compensatory (Moak and Rosen 1984; Dangman and Hoffman 1985; Johnson et al. 1986). In catecholamine-induced triggered activity in atrial fibers, longer coupled premature impulses may be followed by a shorter return cycle, while short coupled prematurely stimulated impulses may result in a significant prolongation of the return cycle (Johnson et al. 1986).

Early Afterdepolarizations and Triggered Activity

Early afterdepolarizations are manifested as a sudden change in the time course of repolarization of an action potential; membrane potential does not follow the trajectory characteristic of normal repolarization but suddenly shifts in a depolarizing direction. This is illustrated in the example of an early afterdepolarization recorded with an intracellular microelectrode in a superfused Purkinje fiber shown in Figure 1.23. The normal time course of repolarization of the action potential is shown in panel A. The arrow in panel B shows the deviation in membrane potential that constitutes the early afterdepolarization. Early afterdepolarizations may appear at the plateau level of membrane potential that is usually more positive than -60 mV as in Figure 1.23B or they may appear later during phase 3 of repolarization. In Figure 1.24B, trace 1 shows the normal time course of repolarization of a Purkinje fiber action potential while trace 2 shows a deviation from this normal time course late during phase 3, which is the early afterdepolarization. Early afterdepolarizations occurring late in repolarization occur at membrane potentials more negative than -60 mV in atrial, ventricular, or Purkinje cells that have normal resting potentials. Both Figures 1.23B and 1.24B also show that membrane potential is moving toward the resting potential during the early afterdepolarization, meaning that

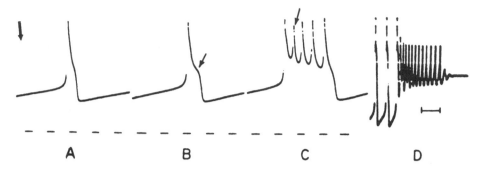

Figure 1.23: Early afterdepolarizations (EADs) and triggered activity during repolarization in a Purkinje fiber. **A** shows the transmembrane potential with normal repolarization of a spontaneously active Purkinje fiber. **B** shows an early afterdepolarization at the arrow occurring during the plateau phase of the action potential. **C** shows triggered action potentials (arrow) during the plateau. **D** shows arrest of repolarization at a low level of membrane potential after a period of triggered activity. (Reproduced from Cranefield (1977) with permission.)

net membrane current is still outward. Occasionally, the repolarizing change in membrane potential may be transiently arrested at the second level of resting potential and net membrane current during the early afterdepolarization is zero (Cranefield and Aronson 1988) or there is a small depolarization indicating net inward membrane current (Damiano and Rosen 1984; Davidenko et al. 1989). Under certain conditions early afterdepolarizations can lead to "second upstrokes" (Cranefield 1975; 1977) or action potentials; when an early afterdepolarization is large enough, the decrease in membrane potential leads to an increase in net inward (depolarizing) current and a second action potential occurs prior to complete repolarization of the first as shown in panel C (arrow) of Figure 1.23 and by trace 3 in panel B of Figure 1.24. The second action potential occurring during repolarization is triggered in the sense that it is evoked by an early afterdepolarization that in turn, is induced by the preceding action potential. The second action potential may also be followed by other action potentials, all occurring at the low level of membrane potential characteristic of the plateau (Figure 1.23C) or at the higher level of membrane potential of late phase 3 (Figure 1.24 panel Ac). Without the initiating action potential there could be no triggered action potentials. The sustained rhythmic activity may continue for a variable number of impulses and terminates when repolarization of the initiating action potential returns membrane potential to a high level (Figure 1.23C). As repolarization occurs the rate of the triggered rhythm slows because the rate is dependent on the level of membrane potential in the same way as is abnormal automaticity. Sometimes repolarization to the high level of membrane potential may not occur and membrane potential may remain at the plateau level or at a level intermediate between the plateau level and the resting potential (the second level of membrane potential) (Gadsby and Cranefield 1977) (Figure 1.23D). The sustained rhythmic activity may then

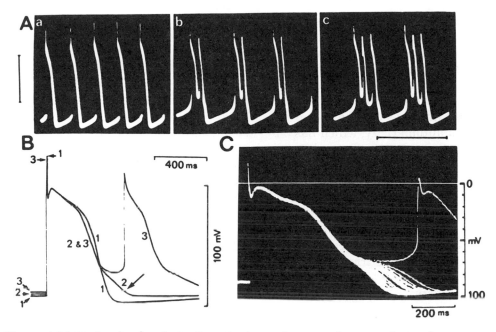

Figure 1.24: Early afterdepolarizations (EADs) and triggered activity during late repolarization in a Purkinje fiber. In **A**, three panels are shown: (a) shows a spontaneously firing Purkinje fiber with prominent phase 4 depolarization; (b) shows the occurrence of a single triggered action potential caused by an EAD occurring during repolarization of each spontaneous action potential; (c) shows the occurrence of two triggered action potentials caused by an EAD occurring during repolarization of each spontaneous action potential. In **B** the development of an EAD and a triggered action potential in three superimposed traces is shown. Trace 1 is the normal Purkinje fiber action potential; trace 2 shows alteration in the time course of late repolarization leading to the occurrence of an EAD (arrow); trace 3 shows further alteration in late repolarization, leading to a triggered action potential. **C** shows superimposed traces recorded from a Purkinje fiber in the course of developing EADs and a triggered action potential. (Reproduced from Coulombe et al. (1985) with permission.)

continue at the reduced level of membrane potential (Cranefield 1977; Cranefield and Aronson 1988).

The level of membrane potential at which the triggered action potentials occur determines the rate of triggered activity and whether the triggered action potentials can propagate and excite adjacent normal regions. At the more positive membrane potentials of the plateau, the rate of triggered activity is more rapid than later during phase 3. Triggered action potentials occurring at the plateau level have slow upstrokes and, therefore, conduction of these action potentials may sometimes block (Kupersmith and Hoff 1985; Mendez and Delmar 1985), while the faster upstrokes of triggered action potentials occurring later during phase 3 enable them to propagate more easily.

The major differentiation between triggered activity caused by early afterdepolarizations and abnormally automatic rhythms may be that the former results from interruption of repolarization and the latter from steady depolarization of the membrane to a similar range of potentials. Otherwise, some of the mechanisms and characteristics of triggered rhythms caused by early afterdepolarizations may be identical to those of abnormal automaticity (see below). The rhythmic activity that is triggered by an early afterdepolarization may well be triggered in its mechanism of onset but automatic during the subsequent impulses (Damiano and Rosen 1984). With this in mind, the term triggered automaticity, which has often been misused as a synonym for triggered activity, probably is a good description of that sustained rhythm that is triggered by an early afterdepolarization (Wit and Rosen 1986). There is also a possibility that once triggered, the sustained rhythmic activity is perpetuated by delayed afterdepolarizations (Cranefield and Aronson 1988).

Causes of Early Afterdepolarizations and Triggered Activity   Early afterdepolarizations and triggered activity have been produced in experimental studies under a variety of conditions, some of which would never be expected to be associated with naturally occurring arrhythmias in the heart *in situ*. Most of these conditions somehow delay repolarization of the action potential by increasing inward current or by decreasing outward current during the repolarization phases. Most often, early afterdepolarizations occur more readily in Purkinje fibers than in ventricular or atrial muscle.

Experimental drugs such as aconitine (Matsuda et al. 1959; Schmidt 1960) and veratrin (Goldenberg and Rothberger 1937; Matsuda et al. 1953) cause early afterdepolarizations in isolated superfused preparations of Purkinje fibers by increasing Na^+ conductance and inward current during the plateau phase of the action potential (Peper and Trautwein 1966). Administration of aconitine to the canine by Scherf (1929) induced extrasystoles (usually bigeminy) occurring during the T wave and coupled to a sinus beat, a characteristic that is expected of early afterdepolarization-dependent triggered impulses since they occur during repolarization. Direct application of aconitine to the atrial or ventricular epicardium resulted in rapid tachycardias that, in the ventricles, had the characteristics of ventricular flutter (Scherf and Schott 1973). Slowing of the sinus rhythm with vagal stimulation facilitated the occurrence of the arrhythmias while total inhibition of sinus rhythm prevented their occurrence. This is another expected characteristic of early afterdepolarization-dependent triggered activity because the initiation of the triggered rhythm is dependent on the occurrence of an action potential with prolonged repolarization (facilitated by a slow rate), the trigger, and total inhibition of the sinus rhythm prevents the occurrence of this trigger.

Early afterdepolarizations may occur when the rate of stimulation is markedly slowed, reducing the outward current generated by the Na/K pump, especially when K^+ in the extracellular fluid is lower than normal, also reducing outward current (Cranefield and Aronson 1988). In contrast to agents like aconitine that appear to act by increasing inward current, cesium (Brachmann et al. 1983b; Damiano and Rosen 1984) causes early afterdepolarizations and triggered activity by blocking outward K^+ current, which also delays repolarization (Isenberg 1976). Here, the superimposition of normally occurring inward current during the period of prolonged repolarization can account for the early afterdepolarizations (see below for an additional description of possible ionic mechanisms causing early afterdepolarizations). Pleomorphic ventricular tachycardias that sometimes resemble torsades de pointes have been induced by infusing dogs with cesium (Brachmann et al. 1983b). Occurrence of tachycardia is preceded by Q-T interval prolongation, a consequence of delayed repolarization, as is commonly seen in patients with torsades (Coumel et al. 1984). The initial beat of the tachycardia caused by cesium often occurs during repolarization, e.g., during the T wave. Early afterdepolarizations and triggered activity have been seen in monophasic action potentials recorded from the ventricles in dogs with cesium-induced ventricular tachycardia (Levine et al. 1985; Ben David and Zipes 1988; Hanich et al. 1988b). An example of these recordings is shown in Figure 1.25. Monophasic action potentials showing early afterdepolarizations and triggered activity have also been recorded during ventricular extrasystoles in the canine ventricle subjected to ventricular outflow obstruction at end diastole (Franz et al. 1989), and during acute occlusion of the right ventricular outflow tract in patients undergoing valvuloplasty for pulmonic stenosis (Levine et al. 1988). Because the experimental arrhythmias caused by agents known to induce early afterdepolarizations such as cesium do resemble

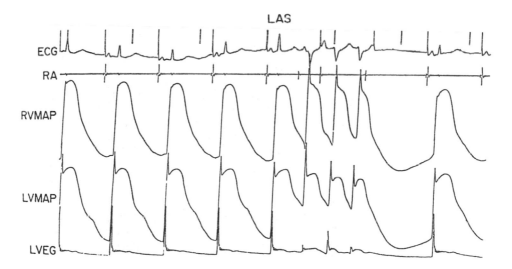

Figure 1.25: Triggered activity caused by early afterdepolarizations (EADs) in the canine heart. The top two traces are the ECG and a right atrial electrogram (RA). The traces labeled RVMAP and LVMAP are monophasic action potentials recorded from the right and left ventricle. The bottom trace is an electrogram recorded from the left ventricle (LVEG). LAS indicates stimulation of the left ansae subclaviae activating the sympathetic nervous system. When this was done, repetitive activity occurred during the plateau of the action potential, which was interpreted to result from triggered activity. (Reproduced from Ben-David and Zipes (1988) with permission.)

torsades de pointes, it has been proposed, which clinically occurring torsades is caused by early afterdepolarizations (discussed in more detail later) although probably not caused by too much cesium.

Other chemicals that can cause early afterdepolarizations and triggered activity are used as therapeutic agents and therefore, triggered activity is likely to be a cause of arrhythmias associated with drug toxicity. Antiarrhythmic drugs that prolong the duration of the action potential of Purkinje fibers (e.g., sotalol (Strauss et al. 1970; Carmeliet 1985; Hiromosa et al. 1988), N-acetyl procainamide, (Dangman and Hoffman 1981), clofilium (Gough et al. 1988), and quinidine (Roden and Hoffman 1985; Davidenko et al. 1989) can cause early afterdepolarizations and triggered activity when administered to isolated preparations of Purkinje fibers, particularly when the rate of stimulation is low and the K^+ concentration in the superfusate is less than normal, e.g., < 4 mM. Figure 1.26 shows an example of early afterdepolarizations caused by quinidine in a canine Purkinje fiber. The preparation was first stimulated at a cycle length of 1000 msec and the action potential with the shortest duration was recorded (filled arrow). The stimulus cycle length was then increased to 8000 msec, causing the action potential to lengthen progressively as can be seen by the superimposed traces recorded after the increase in cycle length. The deviation of the latter phase of repolarization from the normal trajectory

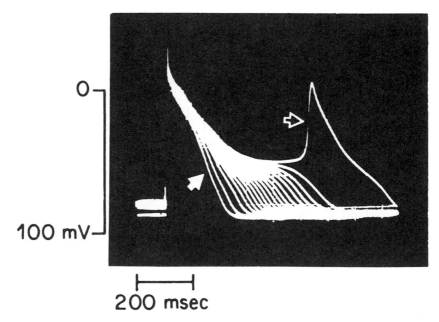

Figure 1.26: Quinidine-induced early afterdepolarizations (EADs) recorded from an isolated superfused bundle of canine Purkinje fibers. A number of superimposed traces are shown. The solid white arrow indicates the normal time course of repolarization before quinidine exerted its effect. The black arrow indicates the triggered action potential. (Reproduced from Roden and Hoffman (1985) with permission.)

constitutes the early afterdepolarizations that led to a triggered impulse (unfilled arrow). The mechanisms by which these effects are exerted have been studied in detail for only some of these drugs. Both the d (no β-receptor blockade) and the l (β blocking) forms of sotalol prolong the action potential duration by inhibiting the repolarizing K current, I_K, (Carmeliet 1985). The prolongation of the action potential by quinidine leading to early afterdepolarizations is also related to quinidine's blocking effect on the outward membrane repolarizing K^+ current, and not to quinidine's well known effect to block the Na^+ channel (Colatsky 1982). In fact, $\dot{V}_{max}$ of the action potential upstroke is unchanged at low concentrations (1 μmol/L) of quinidine that can cause early afterdepolarizations in Purkinje fibers (Roden and Hoffman 1985). The blocking effect of quinidine on K^+ channels is also potentiated at slower heart rates while the blocking effect on I_{Na} is reduced at slower heart rates. The lack of blockade of Na^+ channels at low concentrations of quinidine may favor the development of early afterdepolarizations because the inward Na^+ window current may be important for their occurrence (see section on ionic mechanisms). Quinidine is known to cause ventricular tachyarrhythmias in patients undergoing antiarrhythmic therapy with the drug. Interestingly, the arrhythmias may occur at low plasma quinidine concentrations that do not cause QRS widening (Selzer and Wray 1964), consistent with the observations in the isolated Purkinje fibers of afterdepolarizations occurring without depression of the action potential upstroke. Hypokalemia and bradycardia both predispose to the occurrence of quinidine-induced torsades de pointes (Smith and Gallagher 1980) and both have been shown to potentiate induction of early afterdepolarizations in vitro by quinidine (Roden and Hoffman 1985; Davidenko et al. 1989). Torsades has also been associated with N-acetylprocainamide (Olshansky et al. 1982; Chow et al. 1984; Stratmann et al. 1985) and sotalol administration (Kuck et al. 1984). Magnesium can abolish EAD-dependent triggered activity in experimental studies (Bailie et al. 1988; Davidenko et al. 1989) and has been shown to be antiarrhythmic when used to treat some clinical cases of drug-induced torsades de pointes (Tzivoni et al. 1984; Perticone et al. 1986), further evidence that the clinical arrhythmia is really a manifestation of triggered activity.

Early afterdepolarizations leading to triggered activity in isolated cardiac preparations may also be caused by factors that are present in the heart in situ during acute ischemia and myocardial infarction. Hypoxia or the combination of hypoxia and acidosis, with or without catecholamines, can induce early afterdepolarizations in Purkinje fibers (Trautwein et al. 1954; Adamantidis et al. 1986; Kupersmith et al. 1986). Increasing CO_2 in Tyrode's solution to 20% causes early afterdepolarizations in Purkinje fibers (Coraboeuf and Boistel 1953; Coraboeuf et al. 1976; 1980; Coraboeuf 1980). High concentrations of catecholamines have been shown to cause early afterdepolarizations and triggered activity in Purkinje fibers (Brooks et al. 1955; Hoffman and Cranefield 1960). Under certain conditions stretch might also cause early afterdepolarizations and triggered activity (see Lab 1978; 1982; 1987 for details). Stretch of the ventricles might occur during acute heart failure or in a ventricular aneurysm. We will discuss the roles of hypoxia, acidosis, CO_2, catecholamines and stretch, all of which might be present in the ischemic environment, in causing acute ischemic arrhythmias in Chapter II.

We have discussed only a few of the causes of early afterdepolarizations. For a complete review of the experimental conditions that may cause early afterdepolarizations and triggered activity we refer our readers to two excellent monographs, one by Cranefield (1975) and the other by Cranefield and Aronson (1988).

Ionic and Membrane Mechanisms for Early Afterdepolarizations   During the plateau phase of the action potential, net membrane current is outward throughout the range of membrane potentials between approximately 0 mV and the resting potential. The net repolarizing current results from an imbalance between inward and outward membrane currents. Inward current components include a background Na^+ current (Gadsby and Cranefield 1977), Na^+ current flowing through incompletely inactivated Na^+ channels (the Na^+ window current) (Dudel et al. 1967a; Attwell et al. 1979; Coraboeuf et al. 1979) and the L-type calcium current (Carmeliet 1980; Coraboeuf 1980). An inward current may also be generated by the Na/Ca exchanger. One of the outwardly directed membrane currents is a K^+ current flowing in a gated channel whose permeability is both time and voltage-dependent (the delayed rectifier, i_K) (McAllister and Noble 1966; DiFrancesco and Noble 1985; Gintant et al. 1991). Other contributions to outward membrane current in the plateau range are a time-independent K^+ current that is small because of inward rectification (Dudel et al. 1967b) and the current generated by the electrogenic Na/K pump (Isenberg and Trautwein 1974; Gadsby and Cranefield 1979b; 1982). Normally the net outward membrane current shifts membrane potential progressively in a negative direction and the final rapid phase of action potential repolarization takes place. An early afterdepolarization occurs when, for some reason, the current voltage relationship is altered to cause outward current during repolarization to approach or attain 0, at least transiently. Cranefield and Aronson (1988) pointed out that if membrane potential remains unchanging for a short period of time during repolarization to cause an early afterdepolarization, it is analogous to a fiber at the low level of resting potential at which net membrane current is 0. Such a shift can be caused by any of the factors discussed previously, which either decrease outward current or increase inward current to cause early afterdepolarizations. If the change in the current-voltage relationship results in a region of net inward current during the plateau range of membrane potentials (Trautwein 1970), it could lead to a secondary depolarization (a triggered action potential) during the plateau or phase 3 by activating a regenerative inward current.

The early afterdepolarizations that occur during late repolarization, at membrane potentials negative to about −60 mV (phase 3), probably have different ionic mechanisms than those that occur earlier during the plateau phase. They result when I_{K1} is modified (blocked, for example, by cesium) to prolong repolarization (Coulombe et al. 1980). In addition, these early afterdepolarizations appear to result at least partly from a Na^+ current flowing through TTX sensitive channels (Coulombe et al. 1980). This current is the Na^+ window current that occurs in a potential range more negative than approximately -50 mV (Attwell et al. 1979). When early afterdepolarizations reach a noticeable size as the result of simultaneous reduction in i_{K1} and an increase in the Na^+ window current, they become very sensitive to further changes in i_{K1}; a small additional decrease triggers premature action potentials. A reduction of the delayed repolarizing K current i_K, which occurs mainly during the late plateau phase, also increases early afterdepolarization amplitude and causes repetitive activity during phase 3 of repolarization (Coulombe et al. 1980). A similar effect is expected from a reduction in the Na/K pump current. Inhibition of the pacemaker current, i_f, either by experiments using low concentrations of cesium, or in a computer model did not depress early afterdepolarization amplitude, probably because i_f increases slowly during diastole after the occurrence of the early afterdepolarization (Coulombe et al. 1980). Thus the mechanism causing early afterdepolarization-dependent triggered activity during late repolarization is distinct from the mechanism causing normal automaticity.

Early afterdepolarizations occurring in the plateau range of membrane potentials (-50 mV to 0 mV) can result from increased activation of the L-type calcium current. Evidence for this includes the experimental results showing that early afterdepolarizations and the current transient associated with them are enhanced by Bay K 8644 (a chemical that increases L-type calcium current) and blocked by the L-type calcium channel blocker, nitrendipine (Marban et al. 1986; January and Riddle 1989), and that the early afterdepolarizations at positive membrane potentials are not abolished by TTX or low-sodium solutions. Early afterdepolarizations induced by elevated extracellular calcium concentrations are also unaltered by ryanodine or by chelating intracellular calcium (Marban et al. 1986). This is evidence for the hypothesis that early afterdepolarizations occurring at the plateau level of membrane potentials depend on the transsarcolemmal calcium current. Other outward and inward currents may also be involved in the control of early afterdepolarizations occurring during the plateau, for example, the inward current responsible for delayed afterdepolarizations (the transient inward current) that is also activated during the plateau phase (Coulombe et al. 1980). Electrogenic Na-Ca exchange might also induce oscillations at the plateau level (Fischmeister and Vassort 1981). Reduction of outward current generated by the Na/K pump is also expected to enhance early afterdepolarization at the plateau level of membrane potential.

Triggered activity initiated by an early afterdepolarization may consist of only a second upstroke or it may be more sustained. When it persists for a number of action potentials, the mechanism for the perpetuation of the rhythmic activity is uncertain. It may involve the same membrane currents that cause abnormal automaticity or the membrane currents that cause delayed afterdepolarizations (Cranefield and Aronson 1988).

The ionic current responsible for the upstrokes of the action potentials during triggered activity caused by early afterdepolarizations is determined by the level of membrane potential at which the action potentials occur. Triggered action potentials occurring during the plateau phase and early during phase 3, at a time when most fast Na^+ channels are still inactivated, most likely have upstrokes caused by the inward L-type calcium current (Cranefield 1975; Wit et al. 1976). At higher membrane potentials during late phase 3 of repolarization, where there is partial reactivation of the fast Na^+ channels, fast Na^+ responses predominate. Current flowing through both L-type calcium channels and partially reactivated fast Na^+ channels may be involved over intermediate ranges of membrane potential.

Characteristic Properties of Early Afterdepolarizations and Triggered Activity   From the experiments on early afterdepolarizations and triggered activity in isolated preparations of cardiac tissue, we can summarize the characteristics that are useful in identifying this arrhythmogenic mechanism in the heart *in situ*. Later we will compare these characteristics with those of arrhythmias caused by other mechanisms to provide an overview for how arrhythmias generated by different arrhythmogenic mechanisms might be identified.

Early afterdepolarizations, like delayed afterdepolarizations, show a cycle length dependence; they are markedly influenced by the rate at which the triggering action potentials occur (Damiano and Rosen 1984). However, the relationship between cycle length and the occurrence of triggered activity caused by early afterdepolarizations is opposite to the relationship between cycle length and triggered activity caused by delayed afterdepolarizations. At a "physiological range" of cycle lengths (a range that encompasses the normal sinus rhythm of the adult human heart—1000 to 700 msec), early afterdepolarizations have rarely occurred in the studies on isolated preparations of cardiac fibers, even in the presence of such powerful inducing agents as cesium. As cycle length is increased and repolarization prolongs, early afterdepolarizations are more likely to occur. In Figure 1.27 action potentials that were recorded from a Purkinje fiber bundle exposed to cesium chloride, are shown. At a stimulus cycle length of 2 seconds (panel A) repolarization appears normal and there are no apparent early afterdepolarizations. When stimulus cycle length was prolonged to 4 seconds (panel B) early afterdepolarizations appeared (arrows), finally leading to a triggered action potential. Further prolongation of the stimulus cycle length to 6 seconds (panel C) resulted in a triggered action potential (arrows) following every stimulated action potential while a prolongation of stimulus cycle length to 10 seconds (panel D) caused a train of triggered action potentials to follow each stimulated action potential. This effect of cycle length on triggered arrhythmias also was seen in the studies in which cesium was administered systemically to dogs that we discussed earlier. In studies of cesium-induced early afterdepolarizations in Purkinje fibers such as the one shown in Figure 1.27 the early afterdepolarizations increased to achieve peak triggered activity as drive cycle length increased and then, as cycle length was prolonged still further, they decreased in magnitude (Damiano

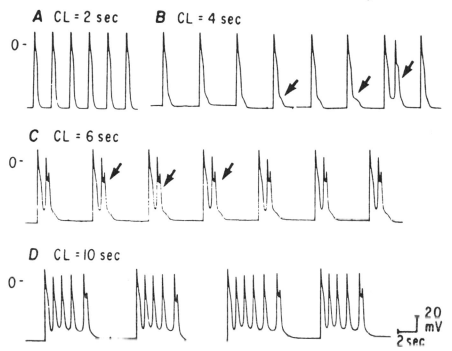

Figure 1.27: Effects of drive cycle length (CL) on early afterdepolarizations (EADs) and triggered activity caused by cesium in a bundle of canine Purkinje fibers. Arrows indicate EADs and triggered action potentials. (Reproduced from Damiano and Rosen (1984) with permission.)

and Rosen 1984) (not shown in the Figure). Therefore, there appears to be a range of cycle lengths at which early afterdepolarizations are likely to occur and the balance of inward and outward currents is less favorable for their occurrence above or below this range.

Once early afterdepolarizations have achieved a steady state magnitude at a constant drive cycle length, any event that even transiently shortens drive cycle length tends to reduce their amplitude (Damiano and Rosen 1984). Hence, initiation of a single premature depolarization, which is associated with an acceleration of repolarization, will reduce the magnitude of the early afterdepolarizations that accompany the premature action potential and as a result triggered activity is not expected to follow premature stimulation.

As drive cycle length is prolonged, the level of membrane potential at which early afterdepolarizations occur becomes more positive and the interval between the primary (triggering) action potential upstroke and the early afterdepolarization or triggered action potential decreases. Thus, there is a tendency with increasing bradycardia, for the coupling interval between the afterdepolarization-induced ectopic impulse and the stimulated impulse to decrease. The triggered impulse also conducts more slowly and aberrantly (a reflection of the more positive membrane potential). The result is a bradycardia-induced tachycardia during which there may be very slow conduction (Damiano and Rosen 1984). The ectopic impulses generated by early afterdepolarizations tend to have consistent (fixed) coupling to the impulses that induce them, if the cycle length of these impulses is constant.

Another important characteristic is that the longer the basic drive cycle length, the greater the number of impulses that are triggered by early afterdepolarizations. This characteristic is also shown in Figure 1.27. Once a triggered rhythm is induced it may be sustained or it may slow gradually and then terminate with a subthreshold early afterdepolarization.

The effects of overdrive pacing and premature stimulation on established and sustained early afterdepolarization-dependent triggered rhythms can be differentiated from their effects on the initiation of triggered rhythms. These effects have been investigated on Purkinje fibers superfused with Tyrode's containing cesium (Damiano and Rosen 1984) in an attempt to provide information that might be helpful for identifying triggered rhythms in the *in situ* heart by stimulation techniques. The likelihood of termination of prolonged periods of triggered activity by stimulation depends largely on the membrane potential at which the rhythm is occurring. A single premature depolarization can sometimes terminate triggered rhythms occurring at membrane potentials more negative than about -65 mV because, following a stimulated premature impulse, there may be acceleration of repolarization and hyperpolarization of the membrane to the maximum diastolic potential at which triggered activity does not occur. Premature stimuli usually are unable to terminate rhythms caused by early afterdepolarization-induced triggered activity at membrane potentials more positive than -50 to -55 mV because repolarization to the maximum diastolic potential is not induced; although there may be some hyperpolarization following the premature impulse, membrane potential remains at the low level at which there is triggered activity. Therefore, in this situation, the effects of premature stimulation on triggered activity are similar to its effects on abnormal automaticity.

The level of membrane potential at which triggered activity occurs also influences the effects of overdrive stimulation. At a low level characteristic of triggered activity during the plateau, relatively short periods of overdrive have no effect on the membrane potential or the triggered rate following stimulation (unlike the effects of overdrive on normal automaticity and similar to its effects on abnormal automaticity). Longer periods of overdrive hyperpolarize the membrane and cause some transient overdrive suppression, similar to that which occurs after long periods of overdrive of a focus with abnormal automaticity (Dangman and Hoffman 1983). Long periods of overdrive may even stop the triggered rhythm if membrane potential hyperpolarizes to the maximum diastolic potential, but this is not the usual effect. The more positive the maximum diastolic potential of the triggered rhythm, the more difficult it is to overdrive-suppress it. At the more negative levels of membrane potential associated with triggered activity arising during phase 3 of repolarization, overdrive suppression and termination occurs more easily (Damiano and Rosen 1984).

A mechanism for the effects of overdrive on triggered activity caused by early afterdepolarizations can be proposed based on what is known about over-drive suppression of automatic rhythms (Vassalle 1970; Dangman and Hoffman 1983). At the low levels of membrane potential of the plateau at which triggered rhythms sometimes occur, the fast inward Na^+ current is largely inactivated. Overdrive for a short period of time probably causes little additional Na^+ accumulation in the cells, no appreciable increase in activity of the electrogenic Na/K pump and no overdrive suppression (Falk and Cohen 1984). With an increased duration of overdrive the amount of Na^+ that enters the cells through L-type Ca channels increases, stimulating activity of the electrogenic Na/K pump, causing hyperpolarization. The triggered rhythm slows both because of the increased outward pump-generated current that opposes the net inward current causing diastolic depolarization, and the increase in membrane potential. Ca^{2+} influx through L-type Ca^{2+} channels could also lead to an inrease in intracellular Na^+ through Na/Ca exchange and contribute to the increase in Na/K pump activity. Triggered activity may terminate if membrane potential increases to a stable high level after the overdrive, caused by the electrogenic pump current. At the more negative levels of membrane potential during phase 3 of repolarization, at which triggered activity sometimes occurs, Na^+ does enter the cell during the action potential upstroke and pump activity is expected to increase during overdrive. The increased current generated by the pump should slow the rate of diastolic depolarization following overdrive and the hyperpolarization caused by the pump can terminate the triggered activity. However, after a period of time, pump current should return to normal and triggered activity should reoccur.

Arrhythmias Caused By Reentry

The second major heading of arrhythmia mechanisms in Table 1 is abnormal impulse conduction. One means whereby conduction abnormalities can cause arrhythmias has already been discussed, namely, the escape of subsidiary pacemakers that occurs when there is sinoatrial or atrioventricular block. Abnormal impulse conduction also causes reentrant excitation, a mechanism causing arrhythmias that does not depend on the generation of impulses by cells.

In the heart driven by the sinus rhythm, the conducting impulse normally stops propagating after sequential activation of atria and ventricles. It dies out because it is surrounded by refractory tissue that it has just excited and because it runs into the inexcitable fibrous annulus. A new impulse must arise in the sinus node for subsequent activation. Under special conditions, the propagating impulse may persist after complete activation of the heart to reexcite atria or ventricles after the end of their refractory periods. This is called reentrant excitation. The studies of Mayer (1906), Mines (1913; 1914) and Garrey (1914) early in this century clearly defined the mechanisms by which an electrical impulse can continue to propagate and reexcite tissue it has previously excited.

Their conclusions were for the most part based on studies of simple experimental models, i.e., using rings of excitable tissue in which the circulating impulse could easily be followed. Here is a description of such an experiment as written by Mines in the *Transactions of the Canadian Royal Academy* (1914). The style is his and is common for papers written at that time. The paper was presented by T.G. Brodie at the meeting of the Academy after Mines' death in 1914. "Large dog-fish (Acanthias). Killed by decapitation. Spinal cord pithed. Heart excised and placed in a dish with blood . . . After half-an-hour the heart is beating well. Cut away sinus: the auricle and ventricle stop. Cut off auricle, slit it up to form a ring, spread it out on a glass plate, pour on serum and cover up with a vaseline watch-glass. Pricking with a needle point provokes a strong contraction. Wave runs round ring in each direction; the waves meet on the opposite sides of the ring and die out. Repeated the stimulus at diminishing intervals and after several attempts started a wave in one direction and not in the other. The wave ran all the way round the ring and then continued to circulate going round about twice a second. After this had continued for two minutes, extra stimuli were thrown in. After several attempts the wave stopped." Our schematic diagram of this experiment is shown in Figure 1.28. As shown in panel A, if a ring of excitable tissue is stimulated at one point, indicated by the black dot, two waves of excitation progress in opposite directions around the ring (shown by the arrows), but only one excitation of the ring occurs since the waves collide and die out. By temporarily causing conduction block near the site of stimulation (at the shaded area in panel B), however, an excitation can be induced to progress in only one direction around the ring, the area of block preventing the conduction of a wave in the other direction. (In Mines' experiment, block occurred because of the rapid stimulation). Once an impulse is conducting in one direction around the ring (long arrow in panel B), if the conduction is restored in the region of the block, the impulse can than return to its site of origin and reenter tissue it previously has excited (panel C). The impulse can also continue to circulate. Circular conduction of this kind has been called circus movement. In a more modern version of this (Mines') experiment, Frame et al. (1987) induced reentry around an isolated ring composed of the circumferential muscle bundles around the tricuspid valve. Basic pacing initiated two impulses that conducted around the ring in opposite directions and collided (as in Figure 1.28A) while rapid pacing caused block of one of the impulses, allowing the other to conduct around the entire ring (as in Figure 1.28B). Circus movement then continued for 30 minutes to 1 hour in some experiments. Similar circus movement could also be induced *in situ* to cause atrial flutter (Frame et al. 1987).

It is apparent from the results of the early studies such as the one performed by Mines, that for reentry to occur, a region of block must be present, at least transiently. The block is necessary to launch propagation of the impulse in one direction and to prevent excitation of the return pathway that the impulse eventually uses to reenter the region it is to reexcite. Transient block, causing reentry, can occur in the heart after rapid stimulation (Mines' experiment) or after premature excitation. It exists only during the initiating impul-

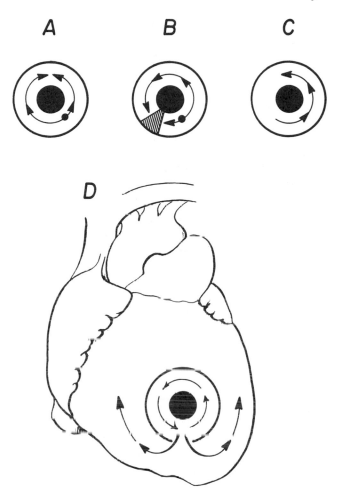

Figure 1.28: Schematic representation of reentry in a ring of cardiac tissue. In panels A, B, and C, the pattern of impulse propagation is indicated by the arrows, and the small dot indicates the area in which a stimulus was applied to the ring. Panel D places the ring of tissue into the ventricles where the circulating impulse can cause rapid arrhythmias.

ses and then disappears. Reentry also may occur when there is permanent block, but the block must then be unidirectional. In the ring experiment shown in Figure 1.28, identical circus movement would occur if, instead of transient block caused by rapid stimulation, permanent unidirectional conduction block were present in the shaded area of panel B. This means that conduction is blocked in one direction (from right to left in the diagram), but can proceed in the other (from left to right). It is obvious that if permanent block occurred in both directions reentry could not occur. Unidirectional block often occurs in cardiac fibers in which excitability and conduction are depressed. The electrophysiological mechanisms are discussed later in this chapter.

In addition, for reentry to occur, the impulse that is conducting around the circuit must always find excitable tissue in the direction in which it is propagating. The conduction time around the ring must be longer than the effective refractory period of the cardiac fibers that comprise the ring. In other words, the wavelength of the reentrant impulse that is the product of the conduction velocity and the effective refractory period must be shorter than the length of the pathway of the reentrant circuit (Mines 1914; Smeets et al. 1986). If it is not, conduction of the reentering impulse would be blocked because the impulse returns to regions it has previously excited before they recover excitability. In reality, conduction velocity and refractory period may vary from site to site in a reentrant circuit, causing changes in the wavelength in different locations. However, the average wavelength must still be less than the path length. Normal heart muscle (excluding nodal fibers) has a refractory period that ranges from about 150–500 msec and a conduction velocity that can range from about 0.5–2.0 m/s. Therefore, the impulse conducting at a normal velocity of at least 0.5 m/s in a reentrant pathway must conduct for at least 150 msec before it can return and reexcite a region it previously has excited. This means the conduction pathway must be at least 7.5 cm long for reentry to occur. Such long reentrant pathways, functionally isolated from the rest of the heart, rarely exist. Clearly, the length of the pathway necessary for reentry can be shortened if the conduction velocity is slowed and/or the refractory period is reduced. For example, if conduction velocity is slowed to 0.05 m/s (as can occur in diseased cardiac fibers, in the normal sinus or AV node, or because of anisotropy in normal atrial or ventricular muscle) the reentrant circuit need be no more than 7.5 mm in length. Circuits of this size can readily exist in the heart. Therefore, slowed conduction permits reentry to occur more easily (Cranefield and Hoffman 1971).

The "ring" of tissue in which reentry occurs as diagrammed in Figure 1.28 is called the reentrant circuit. It can be located almost anywhere in the heart and can assume a variety of sizes and shapes. The circuit may be an anatomical structure, such as a loop of fiber bundles in the peripheral Purkinje system. The anatomical circuit has a central obstacle that prevents the impulse from taking a "short-cut" that would stop reentry. The circuit may also be functional and its existence, size, and shape be determined by electrophysiological properties of cardiac cells rather than an anatomically defined pathway. The central inexcitable region of a functional circuit is often the result of refractoriness of cells in the center of the circuit rather than a real obstacle. The size and location of an anatomically defined reentrant circuit obviously remains fixed and results in what may be called "ordered reentry." The size and location of reentrant circuits dependent on functional properties rather than anatomy may also be fixed (ordered), but they also may change with time leading to random reentry. Random reentry is probably most often associated with atrial or ventricular fibrillation, whereas ordered reentry can cause most other types of arrhythmias (Hoffman and Rosen 1981). We discuss examples of each kind of reentry later in this chapter.

It is difficult to demonstrate with certainty that reentry is the cause of an arrhythmia in the heart *in situ*, or even in a piece of isolated cardiac tissue. In general, the criteria for proving that an arrhythmia is caused by reentry as established by Mines in 1913 and 1914 should be followed as closely as possible. These criteria are: (1) an area of unidirectional block should be demonstrated so that the impulse conducts in one direction only. As described, unidirectional block may be transient or permanent. Unidirectional block is a prerequisite for the initiation of most reentrant rhythms (except a form of reflection described later). (2) The impulse should be shown to propagate along alternate pathways around the area of unidirectional block, to activate the tissue beyond the block with delay, and then to reexcite the tissue proximal to the block. During a sustained reentrant rhythm, the movement of the excitatory wave should be observed to progress through the pathway, to return to the point of origin, and then to follow the same pathway again. In the early experiments on rings of jellyfish subumbrella tissue (Mayer 1906) or on cooled turtle or dogfish heart muscle (Mines 1914), this could be accomplished by observing the slow movement of the wave of contraction with the eye. In more complex isolated preparations or the *in situ* heart, electrical recordings are needed to "map" the activation sequence. Mines warned against a potential pitfall, even when the complete sequence of activation is mapped and the impulse is shown to return to the point of origin in a reentrant pathway: "The chief error to be guarded against is that of mistaking a series of automatic beats originating at one point in the ring and traveling around it in one direction only owing to complete block close to the point of origin of the rhythm on one side of this point" (Mines 1914). Therefore, he stressed a third criterion for proving that reentry is occurring; (3) "The best test for circulating excitation (circus movement) is to cut through the ring at one point. If the impulse continues to arise in the cut ring, circus movement as a cause can be ruled out" (Mines 1914). It is very difficult, and often impossible, to fulfill all these criteria in studies in complex isolated preparations of cardiac muscle or in intact hearts. Many of the experimental works in which the goal was to show that reentry was the cause of an arrhythmia concentrated on satisfying the first two of Mines' criteria. The first studies in which an attempt was made to demonstrate reentry in the intact heart were described by Lewis and coworkers (1920), and we will show an example of their work in our discussion on "mapping" in Chapter II (see Figure 2.29 in that chapter). Many of the experimental results discussed in subsequent chapters on ischemic arrhythmias rely on indirect evidence to suggest that reentry occurred. Sometimes this conclusion is reached without fulfilling any of Mines' criteria (for example, see the discussion on the use of electrical stimuli to identify mechanisms of arrhythmias later in this chapter).

Role of Slow Conduction

A condition necessary for reentry is that the impulse be sufficiently delayed in the alternate pathway(s) to allow elements proximal to the site of unidirectional block to recover from refractoriness. In Figure 1.28B, the impulse traveling around the ring in one direction because of the transient block, must not return to this site of block before it and the regions around it recover excitability if reentry is to succeed. In the case of rapidly conducting impulses, sufficient delay might occur if the pathway is long enough so that while the impulse is traveling at a normal velocity, enough time can pass to allow recovery of excitability. Reentry is facilitated when conduction is slow because such long pathways are not then necessary. A low conduction velocity can be a consequence of active membrane properties determining the characteristics of inward currents depolarizing the membrane during the action potential, or it can be a consequence of passive properties governing the flow of current between cardiac cells.

An important feature of the transmembrane action potentials of atrial, ventricular, and Purkinje fibers that governs the speed of propagation, is the magnitude of the inward Na^+ current flowing through the fast Na^+ channels in the sarcolemma during the upstroke. The magnitude of this current flow is reflected in the rate at which the cell depolarizes (V_{max} of phase 0) (Fozzard 1979). The depolarization phase or upstroke of the action potential results from the opening of specific membrane channels (fast Na^+ channels) through which Na^+ ions rapidly pass from the extracellular fluid into the cell. The detailed process of channel opening and closing was described by a model formulated by Hodgkin and Huxley (1952) for the nerve action potential, which has recently been revised to describe cardiac Na^+ channels (Fozzard 1990).

During conduction of the impulse, the inward transmembrane Na^+ current flowing during the depolarization phase (0) of the action potential, results in the flow of axial current along the cardiac fiber through the cytoplasm and the intercalated disks connecting the cardiac cells. The current flows out of the cells through the membrane ahead as resistive and capacitive current. The conduction velocity depends both on how much capacitive current flows out of the cell at unexcited sites ahead of the propagating wavefront and the distance at which the capacitive current can bring membrane potential to threshold. One important factor that influences the amount of current flowing through the sarcoplasm of a muscle fiber (axial current) and, therefore, capacitive current, is the amount of fast inward Na^+ current causing the propagating action potential. A reduction in this inward current, leading to a reduction in the rate and amplitude of depolarization during phase 0, may decrease axial current flow, slow conduction, and lead to conduction block. Such a reduction may result from inactivation of Na^+ channels. The intensity of the inward Na^+ current depends on the fraction of Na^+ channels that open when the cell is excited and the size of the Na^+ electrochemical potential gradient (relative concentration of Na^+ outside the cell in the extracellular space, compared to Na^+ concentration inside the cell (Weidmann 1955)). The fraction of Na^+ channels available for opening is determined largely by the level of membrane potential at which an action potential is initiated (Weidmann 1955; Grant and Starmer 1987). Na^+ channels are inactivated either after the upstroke of an action potential or if the steady state resting membrane potential is reduced.

Immediately after the upstroke, cardiac fibers are inexcitable because of Na$^+$ channel inactivation at the positive level of membrane potential. During repolarization, progressive removal of inactivation allows increasingly large Na$^+$ currents to flow through the still partially inactivated Na$^+$ channels when the cells are excited. The inward Na$^+$ current, amplitude, and rate of rise of premature action potentials initiated during this relative refractory period is reduced because the Na$^+$ channels are only partly reactivated (Weidmann 1955). In Figure 1.29A premature action potentials 2 and 3 have low amplitudes and slow rates of depolarization because they were initiated prior to repolarization of action potential 1. Hence the conduction velocity of these premature action potentials is low. Premature activation of the heart can, therefore, induce reentry because premature impulses conduct slowly in regions of the heart where the cardiac fibers are not completely repolarized (where Na$^+$ channels are to some extent inactivated) and their conduction may also block in regions where cells have not yet repolarized to about -60 mV. Hence the prerequisites for reentry, slow conduction, and block, can be brought about by premature activation.

Conduction that is slow enough to facilitate reentry might also occur in cardiac cells with persistently low levels of resting potential (that may be between -60 and -70 mV) caused by disease. At these resting potentials, about 50% of the Na$^+$ channels are inactivated (Weidmann 1955) and therefore unavailable for activation by a depolarizing stimulus. Also, at these resting membrane potentials, recovery from inactivation is markedly prolonged and ex-

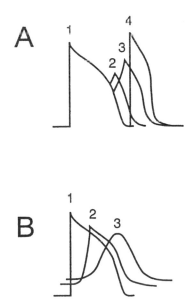

Figure 1.29: Diagram of the appearance of prematurely stimulated action potentials in panel A, and action potentials arising at different levels of resting membrane potential in panel B.

tends beyond complete repolarization (Gettes and Reuter 1974). The magnitude of the inward Na^+ current during phase 0 of the action potential is reduced and consequently both the speed and amplitude of the upstroke are diminished (Figure 1.29B, action potentials 2 and 3), decreasing axial current flow and slowing conduction significantly. Such action potentials with upstrokes dependent on inward current flowing via partially inactivated Na^+ channels are sometimes referred to as "depressed fast responses". Further depolarization and inactivation of the Na^+ channels may decrease the excitability of cardiac fibers to such an extent that they may become a site of unidirectional conduction block (Dodge and Cranefield 1982) (see discussion of geometrical factors causing unidirectional block later in this chapter). Thus, in a diseased region with partially depolarized fibers, there may be some areas of slow conduction and some areas of conduction block, depending on the level of resting potential. This combination may cause reentry. The chance for reentry in such fibers is even greater during premature activation, or during regular rhythms at a rapid rate because slow conduction velocity or the possibility of block is increased even further, owing to the prolonged time needed for the channels to recover from inactivation.

After the upstroke of the normal action potential, membrane potential begins to return to the resting level because the Na^+ channels are inactivated and the fast (depolarizing) Na^+ current ceases to flow. However, this return is slowed by a second inward current that is smaller and slower than the fast Na^+ current and probably is carried by both Na^+ and Ca^{2+} ions (Tsien 1983). This secondary inward current flows through L-type Ca^{2+} channels that are distinct from the fast Na^+ channels (Bean 1985). The threshold for activation of the L-type Ca^{2+} current is in the range of -30 mV to -40 mV compared with about -70 mV for the fast Na^+ current. This current inactivates much more slowly than the fast Na^+ current and gradually diminishes as the cell repolarizes. Under special conditions, this Ca^{2+} current may also underlie the occurrence of the slow conduction that causes reentrant arrhythmias (Cranefield 1975). Although the fast Na^+ channel may be largely inactivated at membrane potentials near -50 mV, the L-type Ca^{2+} channel is not inactivated and is still available for activation (Cranefield 1975; Tsien 1983). Under certain conditions, in cells with resting potentials less than -60 mV (such as when membrane conductance is very low or when catecholamines are present), this normally weak inward Ca^{2+} current may give rise to regenerative action potentials that propagate very slowly and are prone to block. The propagated action potential, dependent on inward Ca^{2+} current, is referred to as the "slow response" (Cranefield 1975). Slow response action potentials can occur in diseased cardiac fibers with low resting potentials, but they also occur in some normal tissue of the heart, such as cells of the sinus and AV nodes where the maximum diastolic potential is normally less than about -70 mV (Zipes and Mendez 1973; Cranefield 1975). Elsewhere (Chapter II), we discuss whether slow response action potentials play a role in the genesis of reentrant arrhythmias caused by acute ischemia.

The slow conduction that facilitates the occurrence of reentry can also be caused by factors other than a decrease in inward current during the upstroke of the transmembrane action potential. An increased resistance to axial current flow, which can be expressed as "effective axial resistance" (defined by Spach et al. (1981; 1982) as resistance to current flow in the direction of propagation) decreases the magnitude and spread of axial current along the myocardial fiber and may decrease conduction velocity. Although the effective axial resistance is dependent on both the intracellular and extracellular resistance to current flow, experimental studies have been mostly concerned with how changes in intracellular resistance can lead to slow conduction and reentry. During conduction of the impulse, axial current flows from one myocardial cell to the adjacent cell through the gap junctions of the intercalated disks that form a major source of intracellular resistance to current flow along a fiber bundle (Fozzard 1979). Therefore, the structure of the myocardium that governs the extent and distribution of these gap junctions has a profound influence on axial resistance and conduction. This influence can be seen in normal atrial or ventricular myocardium. The atria and ventricles are composed of bundles of myocardial cells that have been called unit bundles by Sommer and Dolber (1982). Such bundles are comprised of 2–30 cells surrounded by a connective tissue sheath. Within a unit bundle, cells are tightly connected or coupled to each other through intercalated disks that contain the gap junctions. All the cells of a unit bundle are connected to each other within the space of 30 to 50 μm down the length of a strand (Sommer and Dolber 1982). An individual cardiac myocyte may be connected to as many as nine other myocytes through one or more intercalated disks (Hoyt et al. 1989). These connections are mainly at the ends of the myocytes rather than along the sides, but the overlapping nature of the junctions effectively connects myocytes within a bundle in the transverse as well as the longitudinal direction. This overlap is shown in the diagrams in Figure 1.30A, which are camera lucida drawings from 2-μm thick sections of epicardial muscle. The shaded areas are prominent interstitial vessels and connective tissue septae, and the disks are represented by the wavy lines, only at the ends of the cells (Hoyt et al. 1989). Despite the absence of lateral connections at the sides of the cells, activation can still occur in the lateral direction, for example from cell F to cell C in the middle drawing, through the connections at the ends of the cells (arrows). Therefore, as a consequence of the many intercellular connections, the myocytes in a unit bundle are activated uniformly and synchronously as an impulse propagates along the bundle. The unit bundles are also connected to each other. Unit bundles lying parallel to each other in normal atrial and ventricular muscle are connected in a lateral direction at intervals in the range of 100–150 μm (Sommer and Dolber 1982). A diagram of two unit bundles is shown in Figure 1.30B. Extracellular spaces between the cells within a unit bundle are denoted by the thick black lines while extracellular spaces between unit bundles are denoted by areas shaded with oblique lines. The gap junctions between the cells are indicated by the perforations in the wavy lines representing intercalated disks. It can be seen in the diagram that as a consequence of this structure, the myocardium is better coupled in the direction of the long axis of its cells and bundles

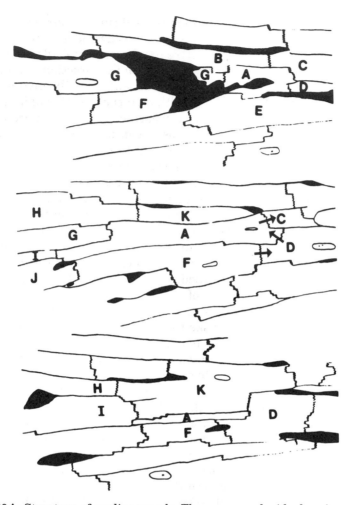

Figure 1.30A: Structure of cardiac muscle. Three camera lucida drawings of epicardial ventricular muscle demonstrating numerous interconnections of the myocytes at intercalated disks are shown. Individual cells are labeled A-K (Reproduced from Hoyt et al. (1989) with permission).

(because of the high frequency of the gap junctions within a unit bundle) than the direction transverse to the long axis (because of the low frequency of interconnections between the unit bundles, the arrow shows one of these interconnections). According to the diagram in panel B, "current flow going laterally from one unit bundle into the next must proceed in a labyrinthine path, whereas current flow in a longitudinal direction can proceed in a straight line" (Sommer and Dolber 1982). This is reflected in a lower axial resistivity in the longitudinal direction than in the transverse direction in cardiac tissues that are composed of many bundles (Clerc 1976; Roberts et al. 1979). For example, gross tissue longitudinal resistivity measured *in situ* by Roberts et al. (1979)

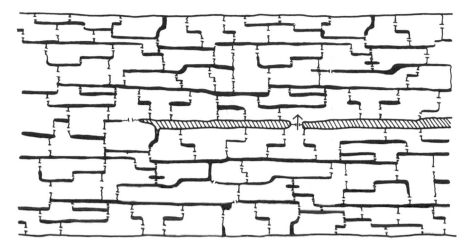

Figure 1.30B: Structure of cardiac muscle showing a schematic drawing of two adjacent "unit bundles" of cardiac muscle cells and their interconnections. (Reproduced from Sommer and Dolber (1982) with permission.)

in epicardial muscle of the canine heart was 199 Ω/cm in the longitudinal direction and 625 Ω/cm in the transverse direction, a ratio of 3.1:1. As stated above, the effective axial resistivity is an important determinant of the conduction velocity, and therefore, conduction through atrial and ventricular myocardium is much more rapid in the longitudinal direction because of the lower resistivity than in the transverse direction. Thus, cardiac muscle is anisotropic; its conduction properties vary depending on the direction in which they are measured.

It is largely through a series of studies published by Spach and colleagues throughout the 1980s that we have been informed about the detailed anisotropic conduction properties of cardiac muscle. We review the major concepts here because slow conduction resulting from anisotropic properties is an important cause of some ischemic arrhythmias that we discuss in subsequent chapters. Spach et al. (1981; 1982; 1985) have classified anisotropy into two major subdivisions: uniform and nonuniform. Uniform anisotropy is characterized by an advancing wavefront that is smooth in all directions (longitudinal and transverse to fiber orientation) indicating relatively tight coupling between groups of fibers in all directions (although coupling is "tighter" in the longitudinal than in the transverse direction because of the myocardial structure discussed in the previous paragraph) (Spach et al. 1988). Uniform anisotropy is exemplified by the conduction properties of normal septal ventricular muscle shown in Figure 1.31A. The muscle was stimulated in the center (pulse symbol) and activation spread away from this site in all directions as indicated by the arrows. In the direction of the longitudinal axis of the fibers (along the length of the unit bundle) (from top to bottom) the isochrones are widely spaced indicating rapid conduction, in this case 0.51 m/s. There is a relatively broad area

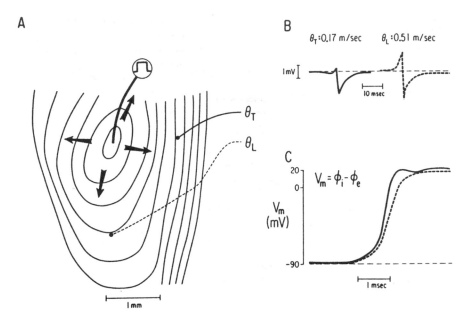

Figure 1.31: Relationship between the spread of excitation in uniform anisotropic ventricular muscle (A) and the extracellular and transmembrane potential waveforms (B and C). The excitation sequence in panel A was constructed from the extracellular waveforms measured at 100 positions on the endocardial surface of the right ventricular septum. The extracellular waveforms in panel B were measured at the sites indicated by the solid dots superimposed on the isochrones of panel A. The direction of propagation at a single transmembrane potential recording site was altered by initiating propagation at different locations, one to produce propagation along the longitudinal axis of the impaled fiber and the other to produce propagation along the transverse axis. Panel C shows the effects of the different directions of propagation on the upstroke of the action potential. (Reproduced from Spach and Dolber (1985) with permission.)

of fast conduction with an elliptic shape of the isochrones that is characteristic of uniform anisotropy (Spach and Dolber 1986). In the direction transverse to the long axis (between unit bundles) (to the right and to the left) the isochrones are spaced close together indicating slower conduction, 0.17 m/s in this example. As the direction of propagation changes between these two axes, the apparent conduction velocity changes monotonically from fast to slow, another characteristic of uniform anisotropy (Spach et al. 1981). The slow conduction in the direction transverse to the longitudinal fiber axis occurs despite action potentials with normal resting potentials and upstroke velocities. Associated with the differences in conduction velocity based on direction of propagation are, however, unexpected changes in the action potentials. That is, when going from fast longitudinal conduction to slow transverse conduction, the rate of depolarization during the upstroke of the action potential ($\dot{V}_{max}$) increases and the time constant of the foot of the upstroke decreases without any change in the resting potential as shown in Figure 1.31C; the upstroke that is dashed was recorded from a cell during longitudinal propagation while the upstroke indicated by the solid line was recorded from the same cell during transverse propagation (Spach et al. 1981). These characteristics are opposite to the changes in the action potentials associated with slowing of conduction when the membrane currents are altered (such as by membrane depolarization) (Dominguez and Fozzard 1970; Hunter et al. 1975) as discussed previously. Despite the increase in $\dot{V}_{max}$ when conduction is slowed in the transverse direction, the slowing of conduction is associated with a decrease in the amplitude of the extracellular electrogram showing that there is a decrease in the extracellular current flow as a result of the increased axial resistivity. In uniform anisotropic tissue the extracellular unipolar wave form has a large amplitude, smooth biphasic, positive-negative morphology during propagation in the fast longitudinal direction that is shown in Figure 1.31B (dashed line) and a low-amplitude smooth triphasic (negative-positive-negative) morphology in the transverse direction shown in Figure 1.31B by the solid line (Spach et al. 1979). The initial negativity of the electrogram in the transverse direction is a reflection of distant activity rapidly propagating along the longitudinal axis (Spach et al. 1979).

Nonuniform anisotropy has been defined by Spach et al. (1982) as tight electrical coupling between cells in the longitudinal direction, but recurrent areas in the transverse direction in which side-to-side electrical coupling of adjacent groups (unit bundles) of parallel fibers is absent. Therefore, propagation of normal action potentials transverse to the long axis is interrupted such that adjacent bundles are excited in a markedly irregular sequence or "zigzag conduction" (Spach et al. 1982; Spach and Dolber 1986). In nonuniformly anisotropic muscle there is also an abrupt transition in conduction velocity from the fast longitudinal direction to the slow transverse direction, unlike uniform anisotropic muscle in which intermediate velocities occur between the two directions. For example, in the nonuniform anisotropic atrial pectinate bundles from older patients, Spach and Dolber (1986) described a narrow zone of fast longitudinal conduction with the rest of the bundles excited by slow transverse spread and no zone of intermediate conduction velocities at different angles to the long fiber axis. This pattern of excitation is diagrammed in Figure 1.32A. The white arrow on the outline of the preparation indicates the narrow region of fast conduction down the long axis of the fibers when the bundle was excited at the asterisk. The zigzag arrow indicates the irregular course of excitation across the fibers, that occurred all along the length of the zone of fast conduction. The zone of fast conduction was shifted to another longitudinal pathway when the stimulus site was shifted (not shown). Conduction in the transverse direction in these nonuniformly anisotropic bundles was nearly as slow as the slowest conduction associated with membrane depolarization and slow response action potentials (Cranefield 1975). In pectinate muscles from older patients, mean fast velocity was 0.69 m/s and slow velocity was 0.07 m/s, a ratio of almost 10:1 (Spach and Dolber 1986) despite the normal resting potential and the fast action potential upstroke of the atrial cells. As in uniform anisotropy, the upstroke velocity of the action potential is more rapid in the slow direction

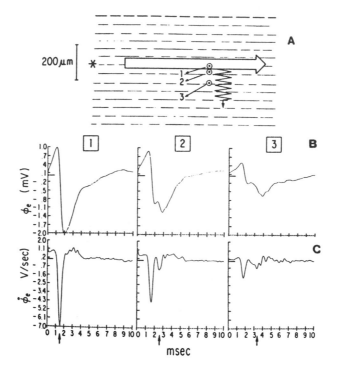

Figure 1.32: In panel A, a nonuniform anisotropic atrial muscle bundle with the long axis of the myocardial fibers indicated by the dashed lines is diagrammed. The bundle was stimulated at the asterisk at the left. Propagation of the longitudinal wave front is shown by the large open arrow. Transverse propagation occurred as diagrammed by the "zigzag" arrow. Electrograms shown in B were recorded from sites 1, 2, and 3 on the diagram. The first derivative of these electrograms is shown in panel C. (Reproduced from Spach and Dolber (1986) with permission.)

transverse to the long axis of the fibers than in the fast direction parallel to the long axis. The morphologic basis for the nonuniform anisotropic properties in human atrial muscle is that the fascicles of muscle bundles are separated in the transverse direction by fibrous tissue which proliferates with aging to form longitudinally oriented insulating boundaries. Intercellular connections cannot occur where the cardiac fibers are separated by connective tissue septae and there is uncoupling between parallel oriented groups of fibers (Spach et al. 1982; Spach and Dolber 1986). Part of the reduction of the conduction velocity in this transverse direction may be a result of the tortuous path length necessary for the wavefront to propagate transversely from one bundle to another because of these septae, accounting for the zigzag activation pattern. Similar connective tissue septae cause nonuniform anisotropy in other normal cardiac tissues such as crista terminalis, the interatrial band in adult atria and ventricular papillary muscle, as well as in pathological situations in which fibrosis in the myocardium occurs (chronic ischemia). The irregular activation is evident transversely in the extracellular electrogram that is characterized by a sequence of multiple deflections, each representing activation of a separate bundle of fibers. The largest most rapid intrinsic deflection is produced by local excitation and less rapid and lower amplitude deflections are produced by excitation of adjacent fascicles (Spach et al. 1982). In Figure 1.32B, the multiple deflections can be seen in electrograms recorded from sites 2 and 3 in the atrial pectinate muscle and are even more prominent in the derivatives of these electrograms (Figure 1.32C). During longitudinal propagation large biphasic electrograms are still evident (electrogram at site 1).

The increase in the upstroke velocity ($\dot{V}_{max}$) of the action potential associated with a change in the direction of propagation from longitudinal to transverse in uniform and nonuniform anisotropic myocardium is not predicted by theory developed to explain propagation in a continuous cable (Hodgkin 1954) as cardiac muscle has often been treated. In a continuous cable model, $\dot{V}_{max}$ remains constant as axial resistance increases to slow conduction. Rather, the increase in $\dot{V}_{max}$ can be explained if there are discontinuities along the propagation pathway (Spach et al. 1981; Rudy and Quan 1987). The discontinuous conduction in the transverse direction of uniformly anisotropic muscle is postulated to be a result of the necessity for intracellular current to pass through localized regions of high resistance relative to the cytoplasm (the gap junctions). As a result of the regions of high resistance, the active membrane is separated into patches and propagation of the impulse halts momentarily while the current from one patch discharges the capacitor of the next patch with depolarizing current. This is actually an exaggeration of the characteristics of conduction that is normally discontinuous but is made more discontinuous in the transverse direction in uniform anisotropy because of the sparse gap junctions. In nonuniform anisotropy, the structural changes can cause the discontinuities. Computer models (Roberge et al. 1986; Rudy and Quan 1987) have shown that $\dot{V}_{max}$ increases as the resistance to intracellular current flow increases at the disks. Computer models of propagation do not, however, show the decrease in the time constant of the foot of the action potential associated with higher axial resistivity and slower conduction. Rather they show the expected increase (Roberge 1986; Rudy and Quan 1987) unless a directional difference in the effective membrane capacitance is incorporated such that there is less capacitance in the transverse than the longitudinal direction (Spach et al. 1987). The proposed effect of the increased longitudinal capacitance is that the Na^+ current has to discharge more downstream capacitance through local circuit currents slowing down the foot of the action potential. The structural basis of the directional difference of capacitance is a mystery. Other explanations other than discontinuous propagation have also been offered to explain the increase in $\dot{V}_{max}$ and the decrease in the time constant of the foot of the upstroke during transverse conduction. One possibility that has been suggested is that during transverse propagation, particularly in nonuniformly anisotropic tissue, there is an increased number of collisions among dissociated wavefronts (Rudy and Quan 1987). It has been shown that at the sites of collisions of propagating wavefronts, the upstroke velocity of the action potential is increased (Spach et al. 1973). The shape of the leading edge of the wavefront is also predicted to influence the rate of depolarization during the action potential upstroke (Suenson 1985). Propagation in the longitudinal direction that is initiated by stimulation at a single point is characterized by very curved isochrones with the leading edge in the shape of a narrow cone (Figure 1.31). Therefore, cells in the leading edge of the wavefront are not only electrically loaded by the cells ahead of them that they must excite, but also by cells to the side that are lagging behind and have not yet been excited. The larger the load on these leading cells, the larger the time constant of the foot and the smaller the $\dot{V}_{max}$. On the other hand, during transverse propagation, the wavefront plane is more normal to the direction of propagation (it is not cone shaped) and the neighboring cells at the head of the wavefront are not lagging behind (Figure 1.31). The lower electrical load should be associated with a faster foot and a faster action potential upstroke (Suenson 1985).

Anisotropy on a macroscopic scale can also influence conduction at sites where a bundle of cardiac fibers branches or where separate bundles coalesce. Marked slowing can occur when there is a sudden change in the fiber direction causing an abrupt increase in the effective axial resistivity (Spach et al. 1982). Figure 1.33 illustrates this point. The drawings show a small branch of an atrial pectinate muscle from the crista terminalis. The general direction of the fiber orientation is indicated by the thin broken lines and the pattern of propagation is illustrated by the thick solid lines and arrows. In A (1) at the left, wavefronts imitated by stimulation at the top propagate down the crista and into the branch along the longitudinal axis of the fibers throughout and so there is no delay entering the branch. At the right in A (2), wavefronts initiated by stimulation at the bottom propagate up the crista and into the branch, but they encounter a marked change in direction of the fibers from longitudinal to transverse while entering the branch, slowing conduction because of the sudden increase in axial resistance. Conduction block, which sometimes may be unidirectional, may occur at such junction sites particularly when the inward current is decreased. (We discuss this in the next section in relation to the rest of this figure.)

The structural features of the cellular interconnections influence axial current flow and conduction as exemplified by the anisotropic properties of cardiac muscle. The intracellular resistance may also increase because of an increase in gap junctional resistance that results from a decrease in the conductance of the junctions, e.g., a decrease of the ease with which the ions that carry axial current move through the junctions. If cardiac muscle is modeled as a continuous linear cable, the conduction velocity is inversely proportional to the square root of the axial resistance. However, in the model of Rudy and Quan (1987), at very high disk resistances, there was a greater decrease in velocity than predicted by this relationship because the cable is no longer continuous. It is periodically interrupted by the high-resistance disks. In the model, conduction velocity could be reduced by a factor of 20 by increasing disk resistance and decremental conduction and block occurred, whereas velocity was only reduced by one third when Na^+ channel conductance alone was decreased (Rudy and Quan 1987; Quan and Rudy 1990). The effects of increasing gap junctional resistance on conduction velocity is also apparent from experiments

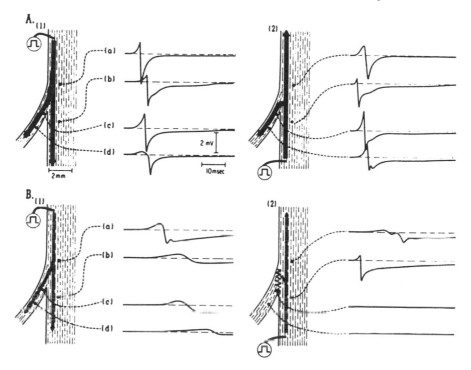

Figure 1.33: Conduction characteristics and unidirectional block at branch sites. The drawings represent a small branch formed by the origin of a pectinate muscle from the larger crista terminalis. The general direction of the fiber orientation is indicated by the broken lines. The patterns of propagation are shown by the solid arrows. Extracellular waveforms recorded at sites indicated by the dashed lines are also shown. (Reproduced from Spach et al. (1982) with permission.)

in which octanol and heptanol have been studied. These alcohols supposedly have a somewhat selective effect on the gap junction and can markedly slow conduction velocity. In experiments on anisotropic muscle, conduction slowing caused by heptanol was more prominent in the transverse than longitudinal direction and block occurred transversely before longitudinally (Delmar et al. 1987; Balke et al. 1988), because of the initial high resistance in this direction. Perhaps the most important influence on gap junctional resistance in pathological situations is the level of intracellular calcium; a significant rise increases resistance to current flow through the junctions and eventually leads to physiological uncoupling of the cells (DeMello 1975; Hess and Weingart 1980). Intracellular calcium increases during ischemia and may be a factor causing slow conduction and reentry (see Chapter II).

Mechanisms of Unidirectional Block of Impulse Conduction

Unidirectional block—block of conduction in one direction along a bundle of cardiac fibers, but maintained conduction in the other direction—is necessary for the occurrence of most forms of reentry. Unidirectional block in part of the circuit leaves a return pathway through which the impulse conducts to reenter previously excited areas. There are a number of mechanisms that might cause unidirectional block. They involve both active and passive electrical properties of cardiac cells.

Regional Differences in Recovery of Excitability

One cause of the unidirectional block that enables the initiation of reentry is regional differences in recovery of excitability. When differences in effective refractory period duration exist in adjacent areas, conduction of an appropriately timed premature impulse may be blocked in the region with the longest refractory period, which becomes a site of unidirectional block, while continuing through regions with shorter refractory periods. Figure 1.34 is a schematic

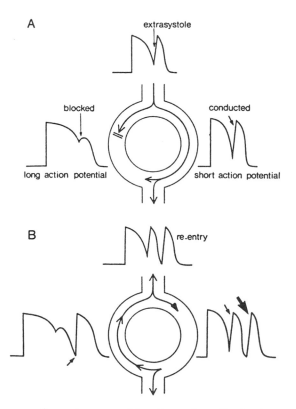

Figure 1.34: Diagram of reentry caused by dispersion of refractory periods. A ring of cardiac muscle is shown and the pattern of conduction is indicated by the arrows. Action potentials with different durations, located in different regions of the ring are diagrammed.

representation of the initiation and continuation of circus movement reentry in an anatomically defined circuit, with differences in effective refractory period duration resulting from differences in the time course of action potential repolarization being the cause for unidirectional block in one of the pathways. The action potentials in various parts of the circuit are shown. In the upper panel (A), a premature extrasystole (that can be either induced by electrical stimulation or that may occur "spontaneously") is blocked in the pathway with the long action potentials and refractory periods (to the left) referred to as the blocked pathway, and conducts in the other pathway with shorter action potentials and refractory periods (to the right). This pattern of activation is indicated by the arrows. In order for block to occur, the premature impulse must also arise in a region with a short refractory period, so that it occurs before the action potentials in the left pathway repolarize. In the lower panel, which shows a continuation of these events, the blocked pathway is retrogradely invaded by the impulse conducting from the right, to cause the second action potential (arrow at the left), the proximal region where the premature impulse originated is then reexcited (reentry), the impulse once again enters the right pathway and continues to circulate in the reentrant circuit causing another action potential in the right pathway (large arrow). As mentioned in our description of Figure 1.28, for successful reexcitation of the region where the extrasystole was initiated, elements in the circuit at the region of block and proximal to it (toward the site of origin) must have regained their excitability by the time the impulse that is conducting through the pathway arrives there. If the longest refractory period in this example is 0.3 seconds at the site of block in the region of long action potential duration, and conduction velocity of the premature impulse is 40 cm/s, the minimal length of the circuit (the "wavelength") to the site of block must be $40 \times 0.3 = 12$ cm in order to allow sufficient time for it to recover excitability. The region where block occurs is available for reexcitation when these appropriate conditions are present. Also, because electrotonic current flows from unexcited cells distal to the region of block to regions proximal to the block during antegrade conduction of the extrasystole, repolarization in the last cells to be activated by the premature impulse before block occurs is accelerated, making it more likely that the returning (retrograde) reentrant impulse will successfully propagate through this region (Janse et al. 1969; Mendez et al. 1969; Sasyniuk and Mendez 1971).

Continuation of reentry induced by a premature impulse is also facilitated because refractory period duration of the premature action potential is shortened. Therefore, on the next excursion of the reentrant impulse around the circuit, the impulse conducts in a circuit with a shorter refractory period. Finally, conduction velocity of premature impulses is decreased, shortening the wave length (Van Dam 1960; Rensma et al. 1988) and facilitating successful excitation of the region proximal to the unidirectional block.

Therefore, the unidirectional block caused by regional differences in excitability is actually a result of transient block—block that occurs in the antegrade direction in the left pathway while conduction is successful in the retrograde direction. This kind of unidirectional block not only can cause initiation of reentry in anatomical circuits as shown in Figure 1.34, but also in functional circuits as described below. For reentrant arrhythmias to arise because of regional differences in refractory periods, a premature depolarization that initiates reentry is as necessary a requirement as the conditions allowing perpetuation of reentrant activation; both a "trigger" (the premature impulse) and a "substrate" (the reentrant circuit) are needed. The mechanism causing the premature depolarization may be quite different from the arrhythmia it initiates; it might arise spontaneously by automaticity or it might be a result of triggered activity. The premature impulse might also be induced by an electrical stimulus during programmed stimulation protocols (see discussion later in this chapter).

The degree of nonuniformity in effective refractory period duration necessary for a properly timed premature stimulus to cause reentry may be quite small. This degree of nonuniformity is often referred to as the dispersion in refractory periods or dispersion in recovery of excitability, meaning the difference between the shortest and longest refractory period. In isolated left atrial preparations from the rabbit heart, the difference between longest and shortest refractory period is normally in the order of 30 msec (Allessie et al. 1976) meaning that a premature impulse can arise in one region 30 msec before recovery of excitability of another region. When stimuli were delivered at the border of two areas with different refractory periods in atrial tissue in the experiments of Allessie et al. (1976), the minimal difference in refractory period needed to cause block of an appropriately timed stimulated premature impulse was between 11 msec and 16 msec, well within the normal physiological range of variation of refractory period durations. A properly timed single premature stimulus can initiate reentry in the atria because the differences in refractory period may cause unidirectional block (Allessie et al. 1976). In the ventricles, where refractory periods are much longer than in the atria, the physiological differences between longest and shortest refractory period duration is in the order of 40 msec (Han and Moe 1964; Janse 1971). This is true both for a regularly driven rhythm (basic cycle length 600 msec, average refractory period duration in the order of 200 msec) and also after a premature impulse that shortens the refractory period. An example of the effects of premature stimulation on the dispersion of refractoriness in the ventricle is shown in Figure 1.35. In this experiment, the refractory periods at 12 different intramural sites of the left ventricle of a canine heart were measured during steady state conditions by stimulating through intramural needle electrodes. These needles are shown at the left of the upper panel; the electrode numbers increase from endocardium to epicardium. The stimulus protocol is shown below. Refractory periods were measured during a basic driven rhythm of 600 msec by a single test stimulus (A); after a single premature impulse with a coupling interval of 240 msec by applying a second premature test stimulus (B); and by similarly applying test stimuli after 2 premature impulses (C); after 3 premature impulses (D); and after 4 premature impulses (E). These refractory periods are plotted above for the different recording sites. There is a dispersion of refractory periods among sites in the order of 20 msec during regular drive of

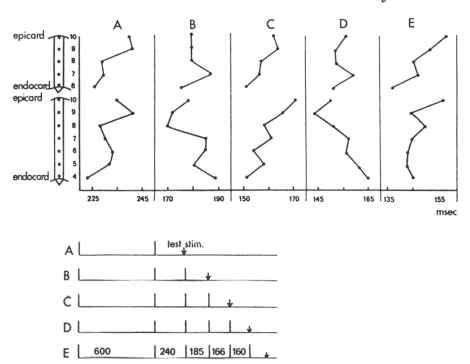

Figure 1.35: Distribution of refractory periods at multiple sites in the canine left ventricle during a regularly driven rhythm and after the application of premature stimuli. The stimulation protocol is shown below; the basic drive cycle was 600 msec. A test stimulus (arrow) was applied after the basic drive (A) or after 1 (B), 2 (C), 3 (D), or 4 (E) premature stimuli to determine the refractory period at 12 sites. These refractory periods are plotted above with the site on the ordinate, and the refractory period on the abscissa. (Reproduced from Janse (1971) with permission.)

the ventricles (A) and after one or more premature impulses (B-E). Despite this dispersion in refractory period duration, no area of unidirectional block was observed during application of up to five successive premature stimuli to the left ventricle of normal canine hearts, and no reentrant arrhythmias could be induced (Janse 1971). Therefore, unlike the atria, dispersion of refractory periods in normal ventricles is not sufficiently large to allow initiation of reentry by premature impulses. When dispersion of refractory periods is increased by local cooling of the ventricles and a critical difference between shortest and longest refractory period ranging from 95 to 145 msec is reached, premature stimuli delivered at the site with the shortest refractory period can induce repetitive activity in the canine left ventricle, presumably because of block of the premature impulses in the regions of long refractory period and reentry (Wallace and Mignone 1966; Kuo et al. 1983). Similarly, critical increases in the dispersion of refractory periods that are caused by acute or prolonged ischemia result in reentrant arrhythmias as discussed in later chapters. When normal ventricles are stimulated at increasingly faster rates, ventricular fibrillation may eventually occur (MacWilliam 1923; Brooks et al. 1964), possibly because reentry is initiated on the basis of conduction block caused by local differences in refractory period duration and on shortening the wavelength because of the shortening of the refractory period.

As emphasized by Allessie et al. (1976), the difference between longest and shortest refractory period is not the only factor determining whether premature stimuli will induce reentry. If the regions of long and short refractory periods are separated by a large distance, an early premature impulse arising in a region of short refractoriness may not be able to arrive in the region of long refractoriness sufficiently early to cause block because conduction between the regions may be slow. Regions of long and short refractory periods must, therefore, be relatively close to one another for block to occur. In addition, if block does occur, the size of the area of unidirectional block is of crucial importance. Even in the presence of large differences in refractory period duration, reentry may not occur when the area with long refractory periods is small, because the impulse traveling around the area of unidirectional block along alternate pathways will not be delayed sufficiently and may arrive at the site distal to the area of block before it has had a chance to recover. Thus, "dispersion in recovery of excitability" is in itself not a complete index for describing the propensity for induction of reentrant arrhythmias.

The regional differences in recovery of excitability that lead to unidirectional conduction block might also occur in the absence of regional differences in action potential duration. Computer models have shown that the activation sequence of a propagating impulse can lead to asynchronous repolarization and refractoriness even when membrane properties are homogeneous (Van Capelle and Durrer 1980; Quan and Rudy 1990). A stimulated premature impulse can block in a region that has been depolarized most recently by a prior wave of excitation, and that is still refractory, but may conduct into another region that was excited much earlier by the prior wave of excitation and that has had time to recover excitability. The conducting premature excitation wave then can later return to excite the area of block after it recovers resulting in reentry.

Asymmetrical Depression of Excitability

Unidirectional conduction block in a reentrant circuit can also be persistent and independent of premature activation. Persistent unidirectional block is often associated with depression of the transmembrane potentials and excitability of cardiac fibers. An example of persistent unidirectional block caused by depression of the action potentials in an isolated, superfused bundle of Purkinje fibers is shown in Figure 1.36. The center segment of the bundle was depressed by superfusing only this region with a solution high in K^+. The action potentials recorded from this region are shown in the middle traces of A and B. They had a low resting potential, slow upstroke velocity, and small amplitude because of the elevated K^+. The ends of the bundle had normal action poten-

A   **B**

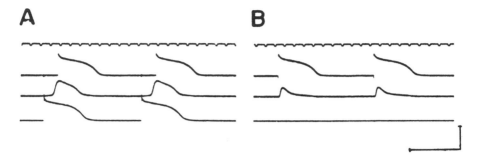

Figure 1.36: Unidirectional conduction block in the segment of a bundle of canine Purkinje fibers depressed with high K^+ (middle trace). (A) Stimulation at one end of the bundle results in conduction. The recording sites shown in the lower, middle, and top traces were activated in that order. (B) Stimulation at the other end of the bundle results in activation of recording site in top trace (nearest stimulating electrode), but conduction block in the depressed area (middle trace) so that the opposite end of the bundle was not activated (bottom trace). Calibrations: vertical: 100 mV; horizontal: 500 msec. (Reproduced from Cranefield et al. (1973) with permission.)

tials because they were superfused with a normal solution; the transmembrane potentials from these regions are in the top and bottom traces. The records in panel A were obtained while stimulating the bundle through the electrodes on the left end. The impulse successfully propagated to the right end of the bundle as indicated by depolarization in the bottom, middle, and top traces in that order. The records in panel B were obtained while stimulating the bundle on the right end. The impulse could not conduct to the other end, but blocked in the center depressed region, as indicated by the very small depolarization in the center trace (Schmitt and Erlanger 1928; Cranefield et al. 1971).

There are several possible mechanisms for the persistent unidirectional block in a region where action potentials are depressed. In 1895, in studies in which unidirectional block was produced by applying cold or poisons locally to frog sartorius muscle, Engelmann was the first to postulate that unidirectional block may occur because of asymmetrical depression of excitability. Experimental unidirectional block resulting from asymmetrical depression of excitability caused by a crushing probe was produced by Downar and Waxman (1976) in studies on isolated bundles of Purkinje fibers. Such asymmetrical depression of the action potential might also occur because of asymmetrical distribution of a pathological event. As a simple example, the action potential upstrokes in a bundle of fibers may be diminished as a result of a reduction of perfusion after coronary occlusion, but the depression of the upstroke may be more severe towards one end of the bundle than the other. This situation is diagrammed in Figure 1.37. A propagating impulse consisting of an action potential with a normal upstroke velocity (1) enters the poorly perfused region (stippled in the diagram) and propagates through this region with decrement (from left to right or from site 2 to 4). That is, as it conducts from the less depressed end (1) to the more severely depressed end (4), the action potential upstroke velocity and

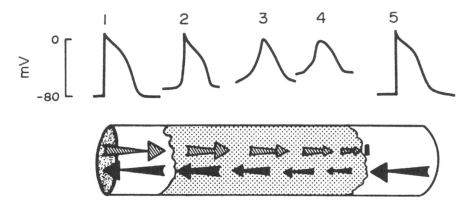

Figure 1.37: Asymmetrical depression of excitability as a mechanism for unidirectional conduction block in a bundle of cardiac muscle fibers. Above are shown diagrams of action potentials that were recorded along the fiber bundle. Stippled part of the bundle is depressed. Conduction from left to right along the bundle is indicated by the striped arrows, conduction from right to left by the black arrows. (Reproduced from Wit and Rosen (1989) with permission.)

amplitude progressively decrease, as does the axial current flowing towards cells to be excited by the upstroke (as indicated by the decreasing size of the striped arrows). When the impulse arrives at the opposite end of the depressed segment of the bundle where there is suddenly a normal perfused bundle with normal action potentials (between action potential 4 and 5), the action potential amplitude is markedly reduced and the weak axial current from site 4 is not sufficient to depolarize the normal membrane at site 5 to threshold. Therefore, conduction blocks even though the normally perfused region is excitable. Conduction in the opposite direction (from right to left) however, might still succeed. The large axial current generated by the normal action potential at site 5 can flow for a considerable distance through the depressed region and may depolarize to threshold fibers at some distance from the most severely depressed region (perhaps as far as site 3). These cells, in turn, may be able to excite adjacent fibers in the direction of propagation (from right to left) and as a result the impulse successfully propagates from site 3 to site 1 as indicated by the black arrows. Propagation continues because there are no large differences in the action potentials at adjacent sites that cause block (Wennemark et al. 1968; Downar and Waxman 1976; Van Capelle and Janse 1976). In the experimental example of unidirectional block described in Figure 1.36, the increase in K^+ in the superfusate might have caused asymmetrical depression of excitability as diagrammed in Figure 1.37.

Geometrical Factors Causing Unidirectional Block

Geometrical factors related to tissue architecture may also influence impulse conduction and under certain conditions lead to unidirectional block. An impulse can conduct rapidly in either direction along the length of a bundle of atrial, ventricular, or Purkinje fibers with normal electrophysiological properties. However, there is usually some asymmetry in the conduction velocity, meaning that conduction in one direction may take slightly longer than in the other direction (Cranefield 1975; Fozzard 1979; Dodge and Cranefield 1982). This is of no physiological significance. The asymmetry of conduction can be the result of several factors. Bundles of cardiac muscle are composed of interconnecting myocardial fibers with different diameters, packed in a connective tissue matrix. These bundles branch frequently (although the individual myocardial fibers do not branch). An impulse conducting in one direction encounters a different sequence of changes in fiber diameter, branching, and frequency and distribution of gap junctions than it does when traveling in the opposite direction. The "configuration of pathways" in each direction is not the same (Cranefield 1975). These structural features influence conduction by affecting the axial currents that flow ahead of the propagating wave front. Some of these influences are diagrammed in Figure 1.38. Results of theoretical analyses indicate that the conduction velocity of an impulse passing abruptly from a fiber of small diameter to one of large diameter (from left to right in panel A as indicated by the black arrow) transiently slows at the junction because the larger cable results in a larger sink for the longitudinal axial current (there is more membrane for this current to depolarize to threshold if conduction of the impulse is to continue) (Goldstein and Rall 1974; Fozzard 1979; Dodge and Cranefield 1982; Joyner et al. 1984b; Quan and Rudy 1990). Depolarizing current flow from the region with the small membrane area to the one with the large membrane area is indicated by the striped arrows in the diagram. A similar slowing occurs when an impulse conducts into a region where there is an abrupt increase in branching of the myocardial syncytium; conduction transiently slows because of the larger current sink provided by the increased membrane area that must be depolarized. In the opposite direction, it can be predicted that conduction will speed transiently as the impulse moves from a larger to a smaller cable because the small sink for axial current results in more rapid depolarization of the membrane to threshold (Goldstein and Rall 1974; Fozzard 1979; Joyner et al. 1984b). Theoretically, if there is a large enough difference in the diameter of the two cables, an impulse conducting from the small cable to the large cable should block at the junction as shown by membrane potentials 1 and 2 above the diagram in Figure 1.38A; there is a propagating action potential at site 1 but only a subthreshold depolarization at site 2, indicating block. In the opposite direction, excitation will proceed from the large diameter fiber to the small one. For this model to explain unidirectional block, once the abrupt change in cell diameter or membrane area has occurred it cannot abruptly return to its original diameter. If the abnormalities of that region are symmetrical around its midpoint (an abrupt increase in fiber diameter followed later by an abrupt decrease) block would occur irrespective of direction. For example, the diagram in Figure 1.38 (panel A) shows an abrupt increase in fiber diameter and then an abrupt decrease. An impulse conducting from left to right might block as we have explained, but an impulse conducting

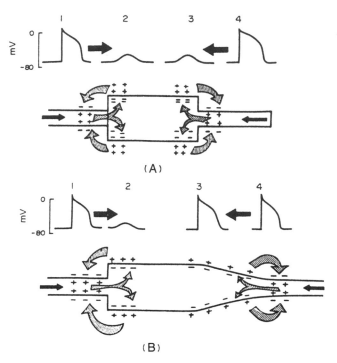

Figure 1.38: Conduction of an impulse at the junction of a bundle of cardiac fibers with different diameters. In panel A, a small fiber bundle, connected to a large fiber bundle, connected to a small fiber bundle is diagrammed. When the impulse conducts from left to right (black arrow), it encounters a sudden increase in fiber diameter and membrane area that the current flow (striped arrows) must depolarize to threshold for conduction to succeed. If the membrane is not depolarized to threshold, conduction blocks as indicated by membrane potentials 1 and 2 above. The change in membrane area in A is symmetrical; that is, the large diameter cable is connected at the other end to another small diameter cable. Therefore, an impulse conducting from right to left would also block for the same reason (membrane potentials 4 to 3). Panel B shows an asymmetrical nonuniformity that might cause unidirectional block. Conduction from left to right blocks at the region where there is an abrupt increase in fiber diameter as in A (membrane potentials 1 and 2 above). However, the transition from small to large cable at the opposite end is gradual. An impulse conducting from right to left can still depolarize the membrane to threshold despite a gradual increase in membrane area (action potentials 3 and 4 above). (Reproduced from Wit and Rosen (1989) with permission.)

from right to left would also block (membrane potential 4 to 3) for the same reason. An asymmetrical nonuniformity, however, such as the one shown in Figure 1.38B, would result in unidirectional block and one-way conduction (Dodge and Cranefield 1982). In the diagram, there is an abrupt increase in fiber diameter followed by a gradual return to the original diameter. In this model, block would occur in the direction in which there is an abrupt increase in the sink (from left to right, between action potentials 1 and 2) for the reasons described above. However, in the opposite direction (from right to left), the gradual increase in diameter would not cause block (action potentials 4 to 3) because the axial current would actually increase; there is a gradual decrease in the internal resistance of the cable as its diameter increases as well as an increase in transmembrane current because of the larger membrane area (Goldstein and Rall 1974).

A probable example of unidirectional block based on similar geometrical factors in the normal heart is at the junctions between Purkinje and muscle cells. At certain sites, propagation from muscle to Purkinje fibers is possible while propagation from Purkinje fibers to muscle is not (Overholt et al. 1984). This asymmetry of conduction might result from the difference in mass of the Purkinje and muscle layers. The smaller mass Purkinje fiber bundles is represented by the small diameter cable at the left in Figure 1.38B, while the larger mass muscle is represented by the larger diameter cable. It is unlikely that in normal circumstances these localized sites of unidirectional block predispose to reentry because the myocardium is quickly excited via the many other Purkinje to muscle junctions where the geometrical differences are not sufficient to cause block. It is possible, however, when conduction in ischemic myocardium is slow and coupling resistance at the junctions increases, that such sites of unidirectional block may become important in initiating reentry (Gilmour et al. 1984, 1985, Janse et al. 1985d).

It is doubtful that abrupt changes in geometrical properties, such as fiber diameter, of the magnitude required to cause block of the normal action potential often exist (except at some Purkinje muscle junctions as described above) because the safety factor for conduction is large; there is a large excess of activating current over the amount required for propagation (Fozzard 1979). Dodge and Cranefield (1982) have pointed out that "only if an action potential is a relatively weak stimulus and the unexcited area is not easily excited will plausible changes in membrane resistance, cell diameter, or intercellular coupling produce block". There is a necessity for interaction of abnormal action potentials and decreased excitability with the preexisting anatomical impediments. As will be discussed later, in acute ischemia such conditions will occur. When the resting potential of fibers in a muscle or Purkinje bundle is decreased, the reduced action potential upstroke results in a decreased axial current and therefore, the action potential is a weak stimulus. The normal directional differences in conduction are then exaggerated. At a critical degree of depression of the action potential upstroke, conduction may fail in one direction while being maintained in the other (although it may be markedly slowed). At this critical degree of depression the reduced axial current might not be sufficient to depolarize the membrane to threshold where the current sink is increased because of the structural changes described above (increased fiber diameter), but the axial current is still more than adequate during conduction in the opposite direction.

The anisotropic properties of cardiac muscle also represent a geometrical factor that may sometimes contribute to the occurrence of unidirectional block. As we have described, Spach et al. (1981) have indicated that in anisotropic muscle the safety factor for conduction is lower in the longitudinal direction of rapid conduction than in the transverse direction of slow conduction (opposite to that predicted on the basis of continuous cable theory). The low safety factor longitudinally is a result of the proposed large current load on the membrane associated with the low axial resistivity and large membrane capacitance in the longitudinal direction. The low safety factor may result in preferential conduction block of premature impulses in the longitudinal direction under certain conditions. In uniform anisotropic muscle, a decrease in inward current during the depolarization phase of an action potential, such as might result from premature activation, results in slowing of conduction in the longitudinal direction more than in the transverse direction but propagation still continues as a spatially smooth process as shown in Figure 1.39. At the left side of panel A, is a drawing of a bundle of atrial fibers with uniform anisotropic properties, which was stimulated at the site indicated by the pulse symbol at a basic cycle length of 800 msec. The isochrones show the more rapid impulse spread in the longitudinal direction (wide spacing) than in the transverse direction (narrow spacing). Representative electrograms recorded from site 1 in the transverse direction and sites 2 and 3 in the longitudinal direction are shown to the right of the diagram. An activation map of the spread of an early premature impulse with a coupling interval of 345 msec is shown at the far right in panel A. Conduction velocity slowed in both longitudinal and transverse directions (isochrones are closer together) but velocity in the longitudinal direction remained higher than in the transverse direction even at the earliest coupled premature impulse that still propagated. The electrograms shown to the immediate left of the diagram have a reduced amplitude reflecting the decreased extracellular current associated with the premature activation, but they essentially maintained their original morphology. Conduction block of early premature impulses (not shown in the figure) occurs in both longitudinal and transverse directions nearly simultaneously in uniform anisotropic muscle (Spach et al. 1988). In nonuniform anisotropic atrial muscle, however, premature activation in the experiments of Spach et al. (1988), resulted in conduction block in the longitudinal direction even though the impulse was conducting from a region with a long refractory period into a region of shorter refractory period, while conduction in the transverse direction continued. The results of an experiment demonstrating this property are shown in Figure 1.39, panel B (1). The diagram of the bundle of nonuniform anisotropic atrial muscle is at the left with the site of stimulation indicated by the pulse symbol; the electrograms recorded from the labeled sites are to the immediate right of the diagram. Activation during basic pacing at an 800-msec cycle length occurred rapidly in the longitudinal direction along a narrow band indicated by the broad, unfilled, arrow and large biphasic electrograms (3 and 4), and activation occurred slowly in the transverse direction as indicated by the zigzag arrows and polyphasic electrograms (1 and 2). The activation pattern of an early premature impulse initiated at a coupling interval of 327 msec is shown in the diagram at the far right of panel B(1). Block occurred in the longitudinal direction as indicated by the depolarization at site 3 but not at site 4, while conduction continued in the transverse direction to sites 1 and 2. Action potentials, and thus refractory periods, are also shorter when the impulse propagates in the transverse direc-

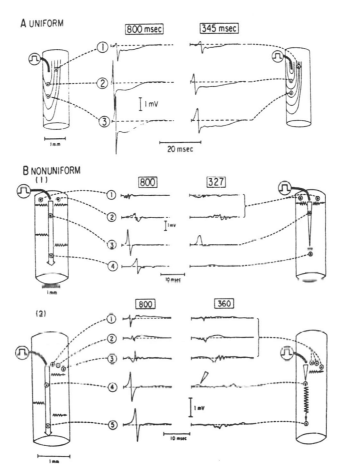

Figure 1.39: Propagation of premature impulses in human atrial muscle bundles with uniform (A) and nonuniform (B) anisotropic properties. In each panel, the excitation sequence during regularly stimulated impulses at a cycle length of 800 msec and several extracellular wave forms are shown on the left while excitation sequences and extracellular wave forms of premature beats with the premature coupling interval above are shown on the right. In panel A isochrones represent time differences of 1 msec. The bundle was from a 12-year-old patient. In panel B, the excitation sequence was so complex that it was not possible to draw isochrones. The long unfilled arrows at the left in B_1 and B_2 represent narrow regions of fast conduction along the longitudinal axis of the fibers. On the right, the unfilled elongated triangles represent decremental conduction. Zigzag arrows represent irregular spread of excitation. Bundles in panel B were obtained from older (> 50 years) patients. (Reproduced from Spach et al. (1988) with permission.)

tion, compared to longitudinal propagation because of an electrotonic effect on repolarization (Osaka et al. 1987). The shorter action potential duration in the transverse direction may contribute to continued conduction of premature impulses. The site of block between 3 and 4 can become a site of unidirectional block that leads to reentry, much like the block of premature impulses caused by a sudden increase in action potential duration and effective refractory period. It can be excited by an impulse propagating in the opposite direction as we describe later in Figure 1.43. Sometimes, prior to the conduction block of the premature impulse in the longitudinal direction, there is a sudden transition of the large extracellular biphasic waveform to a small polyphasic waveform as shown in Figure 1.39 panel B(2). At the left, the activation pattern of the nonuniform anisotropic atrial bundle and the electrograms during basic pacing at the cycle length of 800 msec is shown; at the right is the activation pattern and electrograms during conduction of a premature impulse initiated at a coupling interval of 360 msec, a coupling interval just longer than that needed to cause block. Electrograms 4 and 5, recorded from the longitudinal pathway, changed from high-amplitude, biphasic deflections during the basic drive to low-amplitude polyphasic deflections during the premature excitation (see traces 4 and 5 at the right). Spach et al. (1988) proposed that this change was caused by asynchronous firing "as a depolarization progressed longitudinally in a zigzag manner" caused by longitudinal dissociation (dissociated microscopic longitudinal conduction), as indicated by the zigzag arrow from site 4 to 5 in Figure 1.39B(2). It was also proposed that propagation along the longitudinal axis was actually occurring more in the transverse direction as the impulse weaved back and forth, resulting in slower conduction with a high safety factor (Spach et al. 1988). Such dissociation was associated with a marked decrease in the longitudinal conduction velocity. Block has also been shown to occur preferentially in the longitudinal direction in experiments in which the ability of the membrane to supply depolarizing current was reduced after exposure to high extracellular K^+ concentration (Tsuboi et al. 1985).

In contrast to the findings of Spach et al. (1981; 1982) are results of a simulation study in a computer model in which excitable elements with identical electrophysiological properties were connected to each other and coupling resistance was made higher in the transverse than in the longitudinal direction to simulate the anisotropic properties of cardiac muscle. Conduction of premature impulses failed first in the transverse direction and succeeded in the longitudinal direction (Van Capelle 1983), opposite to the results of the experiments in atrial bundles described above. This computer model did not incorporate the nonuniform anisotropy nor the directional differences in membrane capacitance that was proposed to be an integral cause of preferential longitudinal block by Spach et al. (1987). In experiments on epicardial ventricular muscle in which fibers were partially uncoupled with heptanol, block occurred more promptly for transverse than for longitudinal propagation (Delmar et al. 1987; Delgado et al. 1990). Thus, it appears that a decrease in the strength of the depolarizing currents such as during premature stimulation favors longitudinal block in nonuniform anisotropic muscle but an increase in axial resistance is more likely to cause slowing of conduction and block first in the transverse direction (Balke et al. 1988; Delgado et al. 1990).

Anisotropy can also result in unidirectional block at sites of muscle bundle branching or at the junction of muscle bundles (Spach et al. 1982). It was shown in Figure 1.33A(2) that when a wavefront propagating in a bundle of parallel fibers enters a branch that is formed at an acute angle, the direction of propagation is quickly altered from longitudinal to transverse causing an abrupt increase in the effective axial resistance in the direction of propagation and a slowing of conduction velocity. If the inward current is also reduced by partial depolarization such as after premature stimulation or elevation of extracellular K^+, conduction block may occur (Spach et al. 1982). This is shown in Figure 1.33B(2) where extracellular K^+ concentration was increased from 4.6 to 9.0 mEq/L. Failure of the stimulated impulse to enter the branch is shown by the absence of electrical activity at sites c and d. On the other hand, as shown in Figure 1.33B(1), propagation from the other direction into the branch does not involve a change in the direction of the wavefront relative to the fiber orientation since it continues in a parallel direction, and therefore, there is no block in this direction when inward current is reduced by the elevation of extracellular K^+ (Spach et al. 1982). These sites can become areas of unidirectional block that are instrumental in the occurrence of reentry as described later in this chapter.

Alterations in Refractory Period

In addition to the slow conduction and unidirectional block, alterations of the effective refractory period may contribute to the occurrence of reentry. As indicated previously, a decrease in the effective refractory period decreases the wavelength of the reentrant impulse and therefore, the necessary size of the reentrant circuit. If the refractory period is decreased, the degree of slow conduction needed for successful reentry is diminished. The effective refractory period of cardiac fibers in a reentrant circuit may be decreased during rapid tachycardias because of rate-dependent shortening of the action potential duration (Frame et al. 1987; Quan and Rudy 1990). The computer model of Quan and Rudy (1990) predicts that in circuits with a small or no excitable gap, electrotonic interaction between the head and the tail of the reentrant wave front can also shorten action potential duration. If the effective refractory period is decreased sufficiently, more than one reentrant circuit can exist at a time in some regions (Moe 1962; Moe et al. 1964). The effective refractory period of atrial muscle, for example, is decreased by the acetylcholine released during vagal stimulation. As a result, reentry in atrial muscle causing atrial fibrillation is more easily induced during vagal stimulation (Coumel et al. 1978). Several reentrant circuits exist simultaneously during this arrhythmia (Moe et al. 1964; Allessie et al. 1985). Action potential duration and effective refractory period are decreased in the ventricle during reperfusion after brief periods of ischemia as described in Chapter II or in some of the ventricular muscle cells in chronically ischemic areas (Chapter IV), probably contributing to the occurrence of reentry.

Ordered Reentry

A distinction has been made between ordered and random reentry by Hoffman and Rosen (1981). Ordered reentry implies a circuit that has a fixed size and location. The circuit is usually comprised of a well defined anatomical pathway—an anatomical circuit. Functional circuits (dependent on cellular electrophysiological properties rather than anatomy) might also cause ordered reentry if the electrophysiological properties crucial for reentry are confined to a specific location, and reentry only occurs in that location. During random reentry, propagation occurs in reentrant pathways that can change their size and location. For this to occur, the circuits must be functional rather than anatomical.

There are several examples of anatomical circuits that cause ordered reentry. The essential requirements for anatomical reentry have been illustrated in Figures 1.28 and 1.34. They are the presence of two discrete conducting pathways, which communicate at their proximal and distal ends and the occurrence of transient or unidirectional block in one of the pathways while conduction is maintained in the other pathway. As we have discussed, for reentry to occur, all cells in the reentrant circuit must have recovered their excitability before being invaded again by the circulating wave. This can only occur if the path length in the reentrant circuit is greater than the average wavelength of the propagating impulse in the circuit, which is given by the product of the average conduction velocity and effective refractory period. If conduction velocity and/or refractory period change in different parts of the circuit, wavelength in different parts of the circuit may also change. However, average wavelength for the entire circuit must still be less than path length. In the example shown in Figure 1.34, if a uniform conduction velocity of 40 cm/s is assumed, the wavelength is 40 cm/s × 0.3 sec (the effective refractory period) = 12 cm, meaning that the path length must be greater than 12 cm for reentry to succeed. Therefore, if conduction velocity is not severely depressed, the path length must be long. Long anatomical reentrant circuits involving normal cardiac muscle may be formed in the Wolff-Parkinson-White (WPW) syndrome. Reentrant circuits in the WPW syndrome are comprised of the atria, AV conducting system (AV node and His bundle), ventricles and an accessory pathway connecting atria and ventricles; the normal AV conducting system and the accessory pathway being the two discrete conducting pathways that communicate at their proximal end through the atria, and distal end through the ventricles (Durrer et al. 1967; Gallagher et al. 1978). Reentry can be initiated by an atrial premature impulse that blocks in the accessory pathway but succeeds in conducting to the ventricles through the normal AV conducting pathway (similar to the block diagrammed in Figure 1.34). Once the premature impulse reaches the ventricles, it returns to the atria by retrograde conduction through the accessory pathway which has recovered excitability. The wave front, now circulating in one direction, can continue propagating through atria, AV junction, ventricle, accessory pathway, and back to the atria. However, although the reentrant excitation wave is propagating in normal myocardium, conduction is not rapid through the entire circuit, but rather, slows in the part of the circuit through the AV node, facilitating the occurrence of ordered reentry.

The long reentrant circuit comprised of the bundle branches that communicate proximally through the His bundle, and distally through ventricular myocardium is another example of an anatomical circuit causing ordered reentry (Janse 1971; Akhtar et al. 1974; Lyons and Burgess 1979). Reentry may occur in the specialized conducting system of the ventricles because of the normal differences in refractory periods between the two major bundle branches. In a study of functional bundle branch block by Moe et al. (1965), early coupled premature impulses were stimulated in the His bundle of the canine heart. Such impulses propagated into the right and left bundle branches. At appropriately short coupling intervals, block of a stimulated premature impulse occurred in the right bundle branch but not in the left bundle branch because the effective refractory period of the right bundle is longer than the left. Since the right ventricle was not activated through the right bundle branch, the impulse that activated the left ventricle through the left bundle branch spread into the right ventricle and caused retrograde activation of the right bundle. The His bundle could also be retrogradely excited by the reentrant impulse from the right bundle. Conduction of a premature impulse around the long reentrant pathway comprised of the bundle branches may be slow enough to permit recovery of excitability in the proximal bundle branch and His bundle because the prematurely stimulated impulse conducts in relatively refractory tissue. Reentry caused by this mechanism might also occur after spontaneously occurring atrial or junctional premature impulses and cause atrial echoes or ventricular tachycardia. Premature stimulation of the ventricles also may be followed by repetitive ventricular depolarizations resulting from reentrant excitation through the bundle branches (Akhtar et al. 1978). When a premature stimulus is applied to the right side of the interventricular septum, the stimulated impulse may block in the right bundle branch that has a longer refractory period than the ventricular muscle. It still may conduct through the septal myocardium into the left bundle branch and activate the left bundle retrogradely to the His bundle. Conduction can then occur antegradely through the right bundle to reactivate the ventricles as a reentrant impulse (Lyons and Burgess 1979). Usually only one or two successive reentrant responses caused by bundle branch reentry follow the stimulated premature impulse and this mechanism does not cause sustained ventricular arrhythmias in normal ventricles. However, sustained ventricular tachycardia involving bundle branch reentry can occur when cardiac disease slows intraventricular conduction (Caceres et al. 1989). Tachycardia has been prevented by surgical resection of part of the left bundle branch (Spurrell et al. 1973), or by electrical ablation of the right bundle branch (Tchou et al. 1988), an application of Mines' experimental studies on the tortoise heart (cutting the reentrant circuit) to clinical arrhythmias.

A third example of a long anatomical circuit in which the reentrant wavefront propagates in normal myocardium is the band of circumferential muscle bundles around the natural obstacle provided by the orifice of the tricuspid valve (Frame et al. 1986; 1987; Boyden et al. 1989b). Reentry causing atrial flutter can be initiated in this region in a canine model by premature or rapid atrial stimulation after a lesion is made in the atria between the venae cava and a second lesion is made from the intercaval region to the base of the right atrial appendage. The reentrant impulse conducts in partially refractory tissue around the orifice at velocities of around 50 cm/s. Tightening a ligature around the muscle bundles just above the tricuspid ring terminated the reentry by interrupting the circuit, another example of fulfillment of Mines' criteria. The function of the lesions is to protect the circus movement from being interrupted; the lesions prevent waves of excitation spreading out of the circuit path from one point into the atria, from returning to preexcite part of the circuit at another point (Frame et al. 1987). This experimental model shows that a second barrier, in addition to the one providing a central inexcitable region around which the reentrant wave front circulates, may also be needed to provide protection so that reentry is not interrupted by an impulse that short circuits the pathway. Such protective barriers are probably important for maintaining sustained reentry in other regions of the heart but they have not been studied in any detail.

If conduction is markedly slowed, and/or refractory period duration considerably shortened as discussed previously, the length of reentrant circuits causing anatomical reentry may be very much shorter than the examples described in the previous paragraphs. Slowing of conduction and alterations of refractory periods may occur under pathological conditions including ischemia. In experiments *in vitro*, reentry was demonstrated in small anatomical circuits (circumference of 10–20 mm) composed of Purkinje bundles from the ventricular conduction system, when conduction was depressed by exposure of the bundles to an environment containing elevated K^+ concentration (Wit et al. 1972b). Ordered reentry in a small anatomical loop comprised of Purkinje fiber bundles and ventricular muscle depressed by elevated K^+, is shown in Figure 1.40. The experimental preparation is drawn at the top of the figure and the location of three microelectrodes and two stimulating electrodes (S_1 and S_2) are shown. In panel A, while being perfused with a normal Tyrode's solution, basic drive stimuli were applied through electrode S_1, leading to action potential generation at all recording sites. Conduction was rapid as indicated by the nearly simultaneous occurrence of the action potential upstrokes at all recording sites, precluding the occurrence of reentry. The records in panels B-E were obtained after the action potentials were depressed (resting potential reduced and upstroke velocity decreased) by superfusing the entire preparation with a solution containing elevated K^+ (15 mmol/L) and epinephrine, a combination that causes slow response action potentials (Carmeliet and Vereecke 1969;

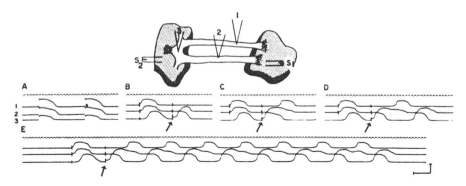

Figure 1.40: Circus movement reentry in a "loop" comprised of Purkinje fiber bundles connected by ventricular muscle (diagram above). The locations of three microelectrodes are indicated on the diagram along with two stimulating electrodes (S_1 and S_2). Transmembrane potentials recorded with the three microelectrodes are shown in the panels below. (Reproduced from Wit et al. (1972b) with permission.)

Cranefield 1975). In the three traces in each panel, the first two action potentials were stimulated (stimulus artifacts are evident); the first action potential was elicited by the last of a train of basic stimuli at S_1, and the second was a result of premature stimulation at S_2 (arrows). The delay in activation between sites 1 and 2, and site 3 during the last basic stimulus, was considerable as shown in panel B. Also shown in B is that a premature impulse (arrow) initiated at S_2 activated site 3 and 2 but blocked before reaching site 1. In panel C the premature impulse (arrow) activated sites 3, 2, and 1 in that order. Conduction of the premature impulse, originating at S_2, blocked in the antegrade direction before it reached site 1 as in panel B, but activated site 1 in the retrograde direction after traveling through the branch in which site 2 was located. In panel D the premature impulse (arrow) activated 3, 2, 1, returned to 3 as a reentrant impulse and then activated 2 again. In panel E, the premature impulse (arrow) initiated a sustained reentrant rhythm in which the sequence of activation was sites 3, 2, 1, 3, 2, 1, etc., showing that the activation wave was continuously circulating around the loop of tissue. Therefore, it is possible that small reentrant circuits in the distal ventricular conducting system might sometimes cause arrhythmias if their action potentials are depressed. This might occur under conditions of acute ischemia where extracellular K^+ is also elevated (see Chapter II).

Other mechanisms for slow conduction that we discussed (anisotropy and cellular uncoupling) may also operate in anatomical circuits, thereby allowing reentry to occur in a small circuit. If an impulse must conduct transversely to the long axis of the muscle fiber bundles that comprise the circuit, conduction velocity will be slow, as is characteristic of transverse conduction (Brugada et al. 1990). A combined mechanism of dispersion of refractoriness responsible for unidirectional block of premature impulses and slow anisotropic conduction was shown to cause reentry through small anatomical circuits in isolated preparations of canine atrium by Spach et al. (1989). An increase in gap junctional resistance and the resultant decrease in axial current flow, can also cause conduction slow enough to allow reentry in small anatomical circuits (Quan and Rudy 1990). Conduction is also slowed in regions of a circuit with abrupt increases in effective axial resistance as may be caused by a sudden change in fiber orientation.

An important feature of an anatomically defined, ordered reentrant circuit is that there often exists a gap of either partially or completely excitable tissue between the crest of the circulating reentrant impulse and the relatively refractory "tail". This means that there is a segment of the reentrant circuit that is excitable while the reentrant impulse is traveling around the circuit. As a result, impulses originating outside the reentrant circuit can invade the circuit through this gap and influence the reentrant rhythm. Such invading impulses may arise spontaneously outside the circuit or may be initiated artificially, either by electrical stimulation or mechanically ("chest thump"). Figure 1.41 illustrates the concept of an excitable gap in a model circuit with a uniform conduction velocity and uniform refractory periods and the effect of an impulse arising outside the circuit on the reentrant wave front. An anatomical circuit with fixed dimensions and a single entrance pathway is diagrammed. In this diagram the entrance pathway also serves as an exit pathway for the reentrant wavefront to enter surrounding myocardium, but other models may have separate entrance and exit pathways. The black arrow in the reentrant circuit represents the reentrant impulse with the arrow point being the crest of the depolarizing wave and the end of the arrow being the tail. The length of the arrow is the absolutely refractory part of the circuit, the dotted area that trails it is the relatively refractory part and the clear region is the completely excitable gap. (In some instances there may be no completely excitable region in an anatomical circuit (Frame et al. 1986).) The transit time of the reentrant impulse around the circuit determines one cycle length of tachycardia (the $R_1 \rightarrow R_1$ interval). In panel A(1) a (stimulated) premature impulse (R_2) (unfilled arrow from above) is shown to reach the circuit and enter it in the region of the completely excitable gap. The stimulated premature wave front may then propagate both in the antegrade (to the right) and retrograde (to the left) direction in the reentrant pathway. In the retrograde direction it collides with the oncoming reentrant wave front, extinguishing both stimulated and reentrant impulses at the point of collision. In the antegrade direction, the stimulated impulse becomes the reentrant impulse and propagates through the circuit in completely excitable tissue of the gap (which also moves around the circuit), shown in A(2). This stimulated, e.g., reentrant wave front would leave the circuit through the normal exit route and become the next tachycardia impulse (R_3). Since the stimulated impulse traveled through the circuit in completely excitable tissue at normal velocity, the interval between the stimulated impulse (R_2) and the next impulse of tachycardia that it causes (R_3) is equal to the normal transit time around the circuit or the normal tachycardia cycle length ($R_1 \rightarrow R_1$). However the rhythm is reset, e.g., the sum of the curtailed (premature) cycle length and the return cycle length (first post-stimulus cycle)

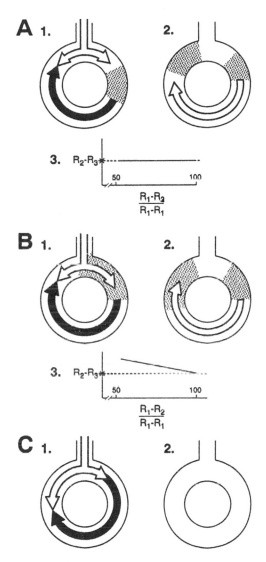

Figure 1.41: Effects of premature impulses on a reentrant circuit with an excitable gap. In each panel diagrams are shown of an anatomical circuit with a single entrance route from above. The black arrows in A1, B1, and C1 represent the reentrant impulse causing tachycardia; the length of the black arrows are the wavelength of the impulse and shows the part of the circuit that is absolutely refractory. The part of the circuit that is stippled is relatively refractory, and the part of the circuit that is not stippled is completely excitable and is the fully excitable gap. The unfilled arrows in all panels represent a prematurely stimulated impulse initiated outside the circuit. The graphs in A3 and B3 show the expected relationship between the return cycle length (following the premature impulse) (R_2-R_3) and premature coupling interval (R_1-R_2/R_1-R_1) for premature impulses conducting in the fully excitable gap (A3) and in relatively refractory tissue of a partially excitable gap (B3).

($R_1 \rightarrow R_2 + R_2 \rightarrow R_3$) is less than two cycle lengths of the tachycardia ($2(R_1 \rightarrow R_1)$). This holds throughout the range of premature coupling intervals at which the stimulated premature impulse is able to conduct around the circuit at a normal velocity in completely excitable tissue. Thus, a plot showing the relationship between the premature coupling intervals and the return, post-stimulus cycles over this range appears as a flat line. This plot is shown in Figure A(3). The post-stimulus cycle length is the R_2-R_3 interval on the y axis. The normalized premature coupling interval is represented by R_1-R_2/R_1-R_1 on the x axis where R_1-R_1 is the basic cycle length of the tachycardia. In this graph, R_2-R_3 remains constant (and equal to R_1-R_1) over the entire range of premature coupling intervals, indicating conduction of the premature impulse in completely excitable tissue. Premature impulses entering the circuit in the relatively refractory part of the excitable gap (stippled region in the circuit) shown by the unfilled arrow in B(1) also collide with the reentrant impulse in the retrograde direction, extinguishing it while conducting in the antegrade direction, but conduction around the circuit is slower than normal because it is in relatively refractory tissue, indicated by the stippled area in B(2). Therefore, the return (post-stimulus) cycle that is dependent on the conduction time of the stimulated impulse in the circuit, is longer than the tachycardia cycle. As the coupling interval of the stimulated, premature, impulse is decreased and this impulse enters the circuit earlier and earlier in the relatively refractory gap, conduction time around the circuit and the return cycle progressively increase. Thus a plot showing the relationship between the premature coupling interval and the return cycle length appears as shown in Figure 1.41, B(3). The line representing the R_2-R_3 interval increases as the normalized premature coupling interval (R_1-R_2/R_1-R_1) decreases. It is also apparent on the graph that conduction time of the premature impulse around the circuit as measured by the R_2-R_3 interval, is greater than conduction time of the normal tachycardia impulse around the circuit that is indicated by the dashed line. The sum of the premature and return cycle may either be less than compensatory or greater than compensatory depending on how slow conduction of the premature impulse is around the circuit. Extremely slow conduction may prolong the return cycle to such an extent that the sum of the premature and return cycles is greater than the sum of two spontaneous cycles. However, more often, despite slowing of conduction of the premature impulse in the circuit, the prolonged return cycle does not compensate for the shortened premature cycle (Almendral et al. 1986a; 1986b; Stamato et al. 1987; Bernstein and Frame 1990). Panel C shows what happens when an earlier premature impulse, indicated by the unfilled arrow, reaches the circuit when it is even less excitable. It conducts retrogradely into the circuit and collides with the wavefront of the reentrant impulse but cannot excite the antegrade path because it expires in refractory tissue (black tail of the reentrant impulse). Thus, reentry is terminated (C2). The range of coupling intervals over which there is evidence that the premature impulse entered the reentrant circuit to reset the tachycardia prior to termination of reentry, is a rough measurement of the duration of the excitable gap if the premature stimuli are applied close to the circuit (Bernstein and Frame 1990). Therefore, fixed reentrant circuits with excitable gaps have patterns of responses to premature stimulation that are characteristic for this mechanism. These patterns can be compared to the responses of other arrhythmogenic mechanisms to premature stimulation that we have already described and are often useful to identify the mechanism of an arrhythmia in the heart *in situ.* These patterns, however, would not be expected if the circuit had no excitable gap preventing entrance of the stimulated impulse, or if the circuit was functional and able to change its size or shape and hence the length of the conducting pathway, after a premature impulse. Later we discuss how arrhythmia mechanisms are sometimes distinguished based on the response of the arrhythmias to applied stimuli.

Rarely, during premature stimulation, the stimulated impulse may enter and activate the circuit without extinguishing the reentrant wavefront that is already in the circuit, resulting in two separate wavefronts traveling around the circuit simultaneously (Brugada et al. 1990). This can effectively double the rate of the reentrant tachycardia. This phenomenon may occur if the stimulated impulse only conducts in one direction after entering the circuit as described above, but failure to conduct in the other direction is not a result of collision with the wavefront already in the circuit. Rather, it results from block of the premature impulse before it encounters the reentrant wavefront, allowing the reentrant wavefront to persist.

In addition to ordered reentry in circuits with anatomically defined conducting pathways, ordered reentry may also occur in functional circuits, e.g., circuits that are formed because of electrophysiological properties of the cardiac cells and not by a predetermined anatomical pathway. Allessie and coworkers (1973; 1976; 1977) were able to induce stable reentrant tachycardia in small pieces of isolated rabbit left atrium by precisely timed premature impulses in regions that were activated normally at regular rates of stimulation. Initiation of reentry was made possible by the different refractory periods of atrial fibers in close proximity to one another. The premature impulse that initiated reentry, blocked in fibers with long refractory periods and conducted in fibers with shorter refractory periods, eventually returned to the initial region of block after excitability recovered there. The impulse then continued to circulate around a central area which was kept refractory because it was constantly bombarded by impulses propagating toward it from all sides of the circuit. Activation of a preparation of atrial myocardium during this leading circle reentry is shown in Figure 1.42. The upper right drawing shows the isochrones from 0 to 100 during one complete revolution of the reentrant impulse. The drawing below is a simplified diagram using an arrow to depict the reentrant excitation wave, and also shows the bombardment of the central area by impulses from the circuit. This central area provides a functional obstacle that prevents excitation from propagating across the fulcrum of the circuit. At the left are representative transmembrane potentials recorded from sites A, 1–5, and D on the drawing of the tissue. Recordings from sites 3 and 4 at the center of the circuit show low-amplitude deflections characteristic of collision and block. No anatomical obstacles or anatomically defined conducting pathways are present in the leading circle and the reentrant circuit is completely defined by the electrophysiological properties of the tissue involved. The circumferences

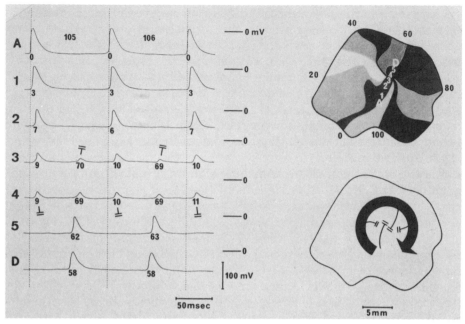

Figure 1.42: Leading circle reentry in atrial myocardium. At the top right is a diagram of activation of a piece of left atrial muscle during tachycardia that was induced by premature stimulation. The activation pattern is indicated by the isochrones (0 to 100 msec) for one complete revolution of the wave front. The diagram at the bottom right is the same piece of atrial myocardium with the reentrant pattern of activation indicated by the thick black arrow. The small curved lines towards the center indicate wave fronts colliding in the center of the circuit. The transmembrane potentials recorded at the seven sites indicated on the upper right diagram (A,1–5,D) are displayed at the left. (Reproduced from Allessie et al. (1977) with permission.)

of the smallest (leading) circle around the functional obstacle may be as little as 6–8 mm and represents a pathway in which the efficacy of stimulation of the circulating wavefront is just sufficient to excite the tissue ahead which is still in its relative refractory phase. Conduction through the functional reentrant circuit is slowed, therefore, because impulses are propagating in partially refractory tissue. In the leading circle model no gap of fully excitable tissue exists between crest and tail of the circulating wave and resetting by prematurely stimulated impulses might not be possible. Reentrant excitation that has been mapped in the atria of canine models of atrial flutter may be caused by the leading circle mechanism (Allessie et al. 1984; Boyden 1988). Functional reentrant circuits of the leading circle type may also change their size and location and if they do, would fall under the general category of random reentry (discussed later).

We have already mentioned that anisotropy can cause conduction slow enough to result in reentry in small anatomical circuits. Reentrant circuits caused by anisotropy can also occur without well defined anatomical pathways and might be classified as functional. However, unlike the functional characteristic that leads to the leading circle type of reentry, that is a difference in refractory periods in adjacent areas, in functional reentry caused by anisotropy, the functional characteristic is the difference in effective axial resistance to impulse propagation dependent on fiber direction. We have classified this mechanism as anisotropic reentry in contrast to the leading circle mechanism. In its pure form both the unidirectional conduction block and the slow conduction through the reentrant circuit is a result of anisotropic, discontinuous propagation and there is no need for variations in membrane properties such as regional differences in refractory periods or depression of the resting and action potential (Spach et al. 1988). An example of anisotropic reentry initiated by premature stimulation in a bundle of nonuniform anisotropic atrial fibers is shown in Figure 1.43. A diagram of the isolated, superfused preparation is

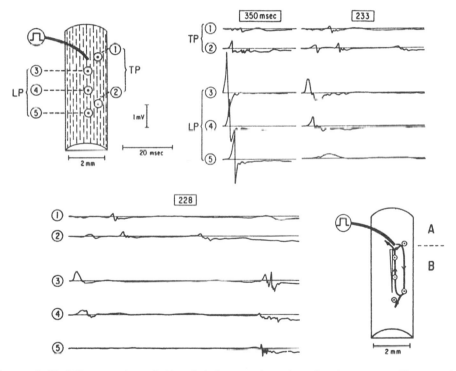

Figure 1.43: Microreentry of stimulated premature impulse in a nonuniform anisotropic bundle of atrial muscle. A diagram of the isolated preparation is at the upper left, showing the location of the stimulating electrode (pulse symbol) and the recording electrodes (1, 2, 3, 4, 5). LP: longitudinal propagation; TP: transverse propagation. The electrograms at the right were recorded from those sites during basic pacing at a 350-msec coupling interval, and premature stimulation at a 233-msec coupling interval. Electrograms recorded at the lower left during premature stimulation at a coupling interval of 228 msec show reentry. The pattern of reentry is diagrammed at the lower right. On the diagram, the unfilled elongated triangle indicates decremental longitudinal conduction of the premature impulse that blocked. Black arrow shows the reentrant pattern of excitation. (Reproduced from Spach et al. (1988) with permission.)

shown at the top left with the location of recording electrodes in the longitudinal direction (LP) at sites 3, 4, and 5 and the electrodes in the transverse direction (TP) at sites 1 and 2. At a basic stimulus cycle length of 350 msec (to the right of the drawing), propagation succeeded in the longitudinal direction as indicated by the large biphasic waveforms in traces 3, 4, and 5, and in the transverse direction as indicated by the small, fractionated waveforms in traces 1 and 2. At a premature coupling interval of 233 msec (at the top right), conduction in the longitudinal direction failed as indicated by the low-amplitude depolarization at site 5, but continued in the transverse direction (traces 1 and 2) for reasons that we have discussed earlier—the higher safety factor for transverse conduction. Fractionation of the electrogram is, however, increased. At a coupling interval of 228 msec (bottom left panel) conduction block also occurred in the longitudinal direction as indicated by a failure to excite site 5 and continued in the transverse direction but site 5, and then sites 4 and 3 were reexcited retrogradely. The reentrant circuit is diagrammed at the lower right. The open elongated triangle indicates the decremental longitudinal conduction of the premature impulse to block. The black arrow shows the successful transverse propagation near the stimulus site with subsequent longitudinal, antegrade, and then retrograde conduction to form a reentrant circuit. The circuit was limited to the region marked by the solid lines with the arrows. On the basis of the longitudinal and transverse conduction velocities of premature impulses in nonuniform anisotropic muscle and measurements of refractory periods in these experiments, Spach et al. (1988) calculated that circuits in nonuniform anisotropic bundles can be as small as 2–4 mm² (transverse velocity of 0.5 m/s, dissociated longitudinal velocity of 0.2 m/s) in the absence of nonuniformities in repolarization. Furthermore, anisotropic circuits are elliptical or rectangular because of the directional differences in conduction velocities with the long axis of the ellipse in the fast, longitudinal direction. Circuits with this shape can have a smaller dimension than circular circuits such as the leading circle (Spach et al. 1988). Anisotropic reentry, like other types of functional reentry must still occur around a central barrier formed by refractoriness of cells at the center of the circuit. Although in the experiments on atrial muscle only single reentrant beats were shown, sustained reentry based on anisotropy has been documented in a thin sheet of epicardial ventricular myocardium produced by freezing the inner two thirds of the left ventricle in the rabbit heart (Allessie et al. 1988; Schalij 1988). The muscle fiber bundles in the epicardial sheet are arranged parallel to one another and are separated by connective tissue septa, but anisotropy is relatively uniform except in some regions where there may be fibrosis. Sustained reentry causing ventricular tachycardia was induced by rapid pacing. Figure 1.44A shows an activation map of an anisotropic reentrant circuit in this model. The activation times are plotted on a representation of the multiple electrode array on the anterior and lateral left ventricle. Activation begins in the region within the 10-msec isochrone indicated by the asterisk (activation times of 3–6 msec) and progresses, as shown by the arrows, to the 140-msec isochrone (activation times of 132 msec), closing the reentrant loop. The shape of the circuit is oval as is

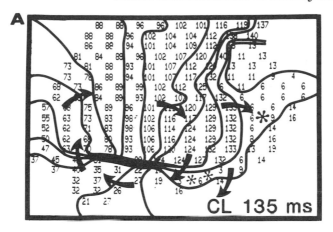

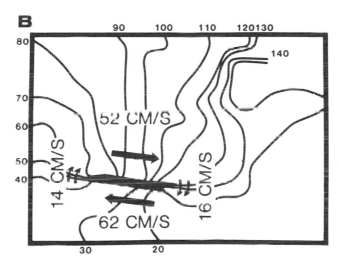

Figure 1.44: Anisotropic reentry in ventricular myocardium. The activation map in panel A is of the epicardial surface of the left ventricle of the Langendorf-perfused rabbit heart after the inner two thirds of the ventricular wall was frozen with a cryoprobe. The direction of the long axis of the myocardial fibers is from left to right in the figure. Isochrones are drawn at 10-msec intervals, the direction of activation is shown by the arrows. The cycle length (CL) of the tachycardia was 135 msec. Panel B shows the estimated conduction velocities in centimeters per second in different parts of the reentrant circuit. Arrows show the direction of propagation corresponding to the adjacent conduction velocity. Numbers around the perimeter are the values of the isochrones. (Reproduced from Schalij (1988) with permission.)

characteristic of anisotropic reentry. The oval shape results from the rapid conduction in the direction of longitudinal fiber orientation (52 cm/s from left to right; Fig. 1.44B) where the isochrones are widely spaced, and the slow conduction in the transverse direction (16 cm/s from top to bottom; Fig. 1.44B) where the isochrones are bunched closely together. Activation in the direction transverse to the fiber long axis provides the slow conduction that enables reentry to occur. At the center of the circuit there are also collisions of wavefronts similar to the leading circle mechanism (not shown in the figure) (Schalij 1988).

Anisotropic reentrant circuits usually remain in a fixed position to cause ordered reentry (Dillon et al. 1988). The degree of anisotropy (ratio of longitudinal to transverse conduction velocity) varies in different regions of the ventricle and the circuit can only reside in a region where the conduction transverse to the longitudinal axis is sufficiently slow to allow reentry. Stability of anisotropic reentrant circuits is also assisted by the presence of an excitable gap that does not occur in the leading circle functional circuit. The excitable gap is caused by the sudden slowing of conduction velocity and decrease in the wavelength of excitation as the reentrant impulse turns the corner from the fast longitudinal direction to the slow transverse direction or from the slow transverse direction to the fast longitudinal direction (Lammers et al. 1987; Schalij 1988).

Random Reentry

In random reentry the location of the reentrant circuit is not fixed, but rather, the circuit may change size, shape, and location for each reentrant revolution. Therefore, the reentrant circuit must be a functional one. Either the leading circle mechanism or anisotropic reentry might sometimes be random. Changes in size and location of leading circle reentry can result from changes in refractory period. In the atria, activation of parasympathetic nerves shortens the refractory period that decreases the size of the leading circle reentrant circuit and therefore, might allow several circuits to exist simultaneously.

Experiments have shown that functional reentry caused by the leading circle mechanism can be initiated in the atrium because of inhomogeneities in refractory periods that result from different time courses of repolarization of adjacent cells. The excitation wave circulates around a region of intact tissue that is inexcitable because it is continuously bombarded by centripetal wave fronts from the reentrant impulse, and the time required for one complete revolution of the reentrant wave is determined by the refractory period of the tissue. There is no fully excitable gap because the head of the reentrant wave front is propagating in the relative refractory tissue of the tail (Allessie et al. 1973; 1976; 1977). In anisotropic reentry, functional reentry is a result of inhomogeneities in conduction properties resulting from structural features of the myocardium. The excitation wave may circulate around a functional obstacle similar to the one in leading circle reentry or around a small anatomical obstacle (Spach et al. 1982; Dillon et al. 1988; Schalij 1988). Another model of functional reentrant excitation that can cause random reentry does not require any inhomogeneities of the transmembrane action potentials or conduction properties or a central obstacle, functional or anatomical. Vortex reentry or spiral waves have been initiated in computer models of homogeneous elements or in various kinds of homogeneous excitable media (properties do not vary throughout the media), an example of which is molecular diffusion in a chemical system. Under appropriate circumstances a pulse in two-dimensional, homogeneous, excitable media can be made to circulate as a rotor with a wavelength that is proportional to the square root of the diffusion coefficient of the media (Winfree 1989; 1990a; 1990b; 1990c; Courtemanche and Winfree 1991). Preexisting functional heterogeneities in conduction (or diffusion) properties or refractoriness (time course of recovery of excitability) are not prerequisites for the initiation of spiral waves in excitable media. The heterogeneity that allows initiation can be the result of a previous excitation wave and the pattern of recovery from that wave. When heterogeneities in recovery exist, the application of a second stimulus over a large geometrical area to initiate a second excitation wave only excites a region where there has been sufficient time for recovery from the previous excitation and not regions that are not yet recovered. An excitation wave is elicited at the excitable site that is in the form of a rotor because the wave cannot move in the direction of the wake of the previous wave but only in the opposite direction, moving into adjacent regions as they in turn recover. The inner tip of the rotor wavefront circulates around a disk of quiescent medium; the size of this disk expands as the medium is made less excitable (Winfree 1989; 1990a; 1990b; 1990c; Courtemanche and Winfree 1991). By definition the rotor has a marked curvature, and this curvature slows down its propagation. In the case of a curved depolarization wave front (rotor) in excitable tissue such as cardiac muscle, slowing may be the result of an increased electrical load, e.g., a curved wavefront must depolarize not only cells in front of it in the direction of propagation, but current also flows to cells on its sides. The slow activation by a rotor is not dependent on conduction in relatively refractory myocardium and therefore, there is an excitable gap despite the functional nature of the reentry (Winfree 1989). The location of the rotor can occur anywhere the second stimulated excitation encounters the wake of the first excitation with the appropriate characteristics (Winfree 1990a; 1990b; 1990c). The reader is referred to the many excellent publications of Arthur T. Winfree for a clearer, more detailed, and quantitative description of this interesting and important phenomenon. Although the occurrence of rotors in excitable media of various kinds is proven, whether rotors and spiral waves are a cause of arrhythmias in the heart is still uncertain and a subject of active investigation. It has been argued that reentrant excitation initiated by premature stimuli in small pieces of epicardial muscle (Davidenko et al. 1990; Jalife et al. 1991) and in the *in situ* ventricles during the initiation of ventricular fibrillation by strong electrical shocks (Chen et al. 1988; Shibata et al. 1988) is a result of rotors and not preexisting heterogeneities in anisotropy, or refractoriness. The appearance of reentrant patterns resembles the spiral waves in the computer simulations. Although stable in terms of location and cycle length in small pieces of tissue where they are bounded by the edges of the preparation, in the *in situ* normal ventricles, the small circulating rotors are not stable, meet the criteria of random reentry, and lead to ventricular fibrillation. Even though nonuniform dispersions of refractoriness or anisotropy are not necessary for the initiation of reentrant excitation caused by rotors in excitable media, the myocardium, even when normal, is never homogeneous and the heterogeneities are influential in the initiation and perpetuation of reentry as discussed in the previous sections of this chapter.

Random reentry is associated mostly with atrial or ventricular fibrillation. Experimental studies in which excitation patterns have been mapped during these arrhythmias have shown that it is exceptional if an impulse follows the same route more than once. Rather, areas are continuously reexcited by different wavefronts (Janse et al. 1980c; Allessie et al. 1985). This was originally recognized by McWilliam in 1887 who described ventricular fibrillation as a peristaltic contraction wave along the complexly arranged and intercommunicating bundles: "For apart from the possibility of rapid spontaneous discharges of energy by the muscular fibers, there seems to be another probable cause of continued and rapid movement (observed during fibrillation). The peristaltic contraction traveling along such a structure as that of the ventricular wall must reach adjacent muscle bundles at different points of time, and since these bundles are connected by anastomosing branches, the contraction would naturally be propagated from one contracting fiber to another over which the contraction wave had already passed. Hence, if the fibres are sufficiently excitable and ready to respond to contraction waves reaching them, there would evidently be a more or less rapid series of contractions in each muscular bundle . . . the movement would tend to go on until the excitability of the muscular tissue had been lowered so that it failed to respond with a rapid series of contractions." Later, MacWilliam wrote: "Any influence cutting down the refractory period or lengthening the conduction time disproportionately must naturally favour the process of reexcitation; a combination of such changes is, of course, still more effective. Hence the development of fibrillation is witnessed at one time as an apparently "spontaneous" event in a vigorous heart manifesting signs of extreme irritability (for example from chloroform, digitalis etc.) or in a normal heart subjected to stimulation—excessive rapidity of excitation playing an essential part by shortening the refractory period and slowing the conduction time" (MacWilliam 1923). It is of interest that MacWilliam's descriptions were for the most part based on visual observation of the fibrillating heart. In addition to clearly indicating that ventricular fibrillation can occur in a normal heart when it is subjected to what we now would call an "aggressive stimulation protocol", as mentioned in our introduction, he was one of the first to suggest that death from sudden coronary artery obstruction in man is due to ventricular fibrillation.

Important early contributions to our understanding of fibrillation were made by Garrey in 1914, who stated that the nature of fibrillation lies in the existence of "blocks of transitory character and shifting location" resulting in "propagation of the contraction wave in a series of ring-like circuits of multiple complexity." The importance of an adequate tissue mass for the occurrence and maintenance of fibrillation was demonstrated by Garrey (1914) who showed that small pieces of tissue ceased to fibrillate when isolated from fibrillating atria or ventricles. He wrote: "The larger the mass, the greater the probability

that each impulse will circulate until it reaches tissue which has once contracted but has passed out of the refractory state". This accounts for the fact
that large hearts fibrillate more easily than small ones, and that ventricular
fibrillation in small hearts, such as those of cats, rabbits, mice, etc., may stop
spontaneously, whereas it usually does not terminate spontaneously in larger
hearts such as the dog heart, as noted by McWilliam in 1887.

In this century, insight into the mechanism of fibrillation had been obtained largely through theoretical analysis and the study of computer models,
before it became possible to simultaneously record from multiple sites in fibrillating atria or ventricles. Moe (1962), utilizing a computer model, formulated
the multiple wavelet hypothesis, according to which fibrillation may be initiated by a rapid series of impulses arising by any mechanism, be it reentrant
or automatic. The persistence of fibrillation then results from fractionation of
the wavefronts in partially and irregularly excitable tissues, so that independent wavelets occur that course around multiple islets of refractory tissue, that
continuously shift their location, causing the pattern of conduction to shift as
well (Moe 1962). According to this hypothesis a small mass of tissue cannot
support a number of wavelets sufficient to maintain fibrillation, although individual circus movements may still be supported. Moe (1962) added that "direct
test of this hypothesis is difficult if not impossible in living tissue,"

Allessie and coworkers (1985) tested the multiple wavelet hypothesis by
simultaneously recording from 192 electrodes spaced at regular distances of 3
mm on the endocardial surface of right and left atria of isolated canine hearts,
perfused through the coronary arteries according to the Langendorff technique.
Atrial fibrillation was induced by premature stimuli while acetylcholine
(which shortens the atrial refractory period) was continuously administered in
the perfusion fluid. Fibrillation was maintained as long as acetylcholine was
infused, and terminated spontaneously as soon as the infusion was stopped.
During maintained fibrillation, the presence of multiple independent wavelets
was demonstrated, each of which represented part of a reentrant circuit. The
width of the wavelets could be as small as a few millimeters, but broad wavefronts propagating uniformly over large segments of the atria were observed
as well. Each individual wavelet existed only for a short time, no longer than
a few hundred milliseconds. Extinction of a wavelet could be caused by fusion
or collision with another wavelet, by reaching the border of the atria, or by
meeting refractory tissue. New wavelets could be formed by division of a wave
at a local area of conduction block, or by an offspring of a wave traveling
towards the other atrium. The major difference between the excitation patterns
observed in these experiments and those in Moe's computer model (Moe 1962;
Moe et al. 1964) was that the number of wavelets (reentrant circuits) was much
smaller in the canine atria. It was estimated by Allessie et al. (1985) that the
critical number of wavelets in both atria to maintain fibrillation was between
3 and 6. Figure 1.45, taken from this work of Allessie et al. (1985), shows 30
consecutive "snapshots" of electrical activity in the right atrium (schematically
outlined) during stable atrial fibrillation. Each panel represents a time frame
of 10 msec. The black contours indicate the areas of the atrium that were

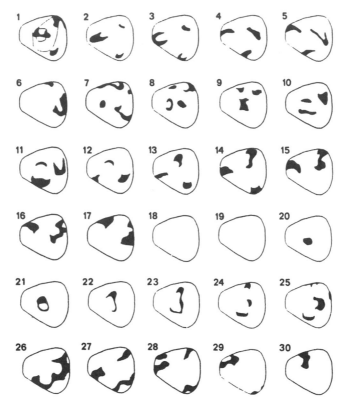

Figure 1.45: Thirty consecutive "snapshots" of electrical activity of the right atrium during stable atrial fibrillation induced by acetylcholine in the canine heart. Each panel represents a time frame of 10 msec and the black contours indicate the areas of the atrium that were excited during the corresponding 10-msec time window. Black areas may represent parts of reentrant circuits that move around the atria during fibrillation. (Reproduced from Allessie et al. (1985) with permission.)

excited during the corresponding 10-msec time window. On the average, 3 wavelets were often present in the right atrium as shown in snapshots 1–5, but both size and number of the wavelets varied considerably with time. At time frames 18 and 19, electrical activity in the right atrium had completely stopped, showing that when there is such a small number of wavelets, the statistical chance of cancellation of all wavelets is rather high. Fibrillation in the right atrium alone would not have been sustained; the critical number of wandering wavelets required for self-perpetuating fibrillation must therefore be higher than 3. However in this example, fibrillation did not terminate at time frames 18 and 19; new wavelets subsequently appeared that probably originated from the left atrium.

Three-dimensional activation maps have also shown random, functional reentrant circuits at the site of stimulation during initiation of ventricular fibrillation with a premature electrical stimulus (Chen et al. 1988). Complete activation maps of the ventricles during later stages of fibrillation have not been obtained.

As we have discussed, the reentrant mechanisms causing the multiple wavelets associated with atrial or ventricular fibrillation are uncertain. They may result from leading circle reentry, anisotropic reentry, or spiral waves caused by rotors.

Reflection

The term reflection has been used to describe a form of reentry in a linear bundle in which two excitable regions are separated by an area of depressed conduction (Cranefield 1975). During reflection, excitation occurs slowly in one direction along the bundle and is followed by continued propagation and excitation occurring in the opposite direction. One form of reflection may in fact be microreentry based on a functional longitudinal dissociation within the depressed segment (Schmitt and Erlanger 1928; Wit et al. 1972a; Cranefield et al. 1973). How this might occur is diagrammed in Figure 1.46. The diagram at the top of the figure depicts two adjacent fibers in a bundle. The entire shaded area is depressed (reduced membrane potential and slow action poten-

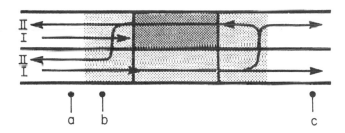

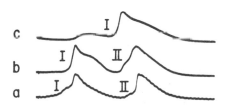

Figure 1.46: Diagram of reflection based on microreentry. At the top is a schematic representation of two adjacent myocardial fibers. Shaded region indicates area of depressed conduction. Arrows show pattern of activation, arrows labeled I are an antegradely conducting wave front and arrows labeled II are a retrogradely conducting reflected wave front. Action potentials shown below were recorded at sites a, b, and c on the diagram. (Modified from Wit and Bigger (1975) with permission.)

tial upstrokes), the darker area in the upper fiber indicating more severe depression than the lighter area in the lower fiber. Unidirectional conduction block occurs in the more severely depressed region. The mechanisms for unidirectional block in depressed regions have been discussed. Arrows labeled "I" show the impulse entering the two fibers from the left end. Conduction of the impulse (I) blocks in the fiber at the top, in the severely depressed region, but continues in the fiber at the bottom that is not as depressed. Once past the region of severe depression, the impulse conducts transversely from the bottom fiber to the top fiber. It then conducts retrogradely through this severely depressed region in the top bundle. Arrows labeled "II" show the reflected impulse returning to reexcite the left end of the bundle. Action potentials that were recorded from sites a, b, and c in the bottom fiber are shown below: action potentials labeled I were recorded as the impulse conducted from left to right; action potentials labeled II were recorded as the impulse conducted from right to left, returning to its origin.

A fundamentally different mechanism for reflection has been proposed, where antegrade and retrograde transmission along the bundle occurs through the same fibers, as compared to functional longitudinal dissociation where antegrade and retrograde transmission are in different fibers (Cranefield et al. 1971; Cranefield 1975). This kind of reflection has been produced experimentally in linear bundles of Purkinje fibers in which there was a central segment of inexcitability resulting in conduction block. Inexcitability was caused by superfusing the center segment of the bundle with sucrose or an "ischemic" solution containing high levels of K^+ (Antzelevitch et al. 1980; Jalife and Moe 1981; Rozanski et al. 1984a). Such a bundle with an inexcitable segment is diagrammed in Figure 1.47C. An impulse initiated proximal (P) to the inexcitable region (at the left), propagates to the border of the inexcitable region and blocks there (membrane potentials 1, 2, and 3 in A and B). Axial current flows through the inexcitable cable to depolarize electrotonically the membrane of fibers distal to the inexcitable segment (action potentials 4, 5, 6, 7 in A). This electrotonic manifestation of the blocked impulse decays along the cable in the inexcitable segment according to the length constant, which is dependent to a large extent on the intracellular and extracellular resistances to current flow. If the inexcitable segment is sufficiently short relative to the length constant (less than 2 mm in the experiments of Antzelvitch et al. (1980) and of Jalife and Moe (1981)), the current flow across the inexcitable region can depolarize the excitable fibers distal to this region and can excite an action potential (potentials 6, 7, in B). The time delay before the occurrence of the distal action potential is dependent to a large extent on the time course and amplitude of the electrotonic current flow. The action potential initiated distal to the point of block not only will conduct distally along the fiber as shown in B (action potentials 6, 7, and 8) but can itself cause retrograde axial current flow through the inexcitable gap to depolarize the part of the fiber proximal to the gap at the site of the original block. This depolarization progressing retrogradely through the inexcitable region is indicated by the vertical lines drawn on action potentials 5, 4, and 3 in panel B. If the sum of excitation times in both antegrade

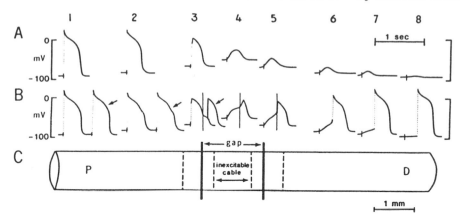

Figure 1.47: Schematic representation of a bundle of Purkinje fibers is shown in panel C with a central inexcitable segment (inexcitable cable). The proximal end of the bundle near the stimulating electrodes is indicated by "P", the distal end of the bundle is indicated by "D". Above are shown simulated transmembrane potentials when propagation across the inexcitable segment fails (A) and when electrotonic transmission across the inexcitable segment succeeds (B), resulting in reflection. (Modified from Antzelevitch and Moe (1981) with permission.)

and retrograde directions across the inexcitable gap exceeds the refractory period of the proximal segment, an action potential will be elicited in the proximal segment, which propagates retrogradely along the fiber (arrows at sites 3, 2, and 1 in B). This reflected action potential reenters the part of the bundle that already was excited. Thus impulse transmission in both directions occurs over the same pathway unlike the types of reentry discussed previously.

It has been questioned whether the delay in excitation of the distal region caused by purely electrotonic transmission across an inexcitable segment, would be sufficient to allow time for the proximal region to repolarize sufficiently to recover excitability so that reexcitation by retrograde electrotonic current flow would be possible (Janse and Van Capelle 1982a). Additional delays provided by slow conduction may be necessary. At the boundary of the inexcitable gap (made inexcitable by exposure to 35 mmol/L K^+ for example) diffusion of K^+ ions will occur into adjacent tissue so that a transition zone between normal tissue and the area of inexcitability will be created where both slow responses and depressed fast responses may occur. These responses should conduct very slowly, and account for an extra delay over and above that caused by electrotonic transmission alone. From the *in vitro* experiments it appears that because of the existence of such a transition zone of reduced excitability, delays of 100 msec to 200 msec may result across a small (1 to 2 mm) segment of inexcitable tissue before the segment distal to the inexcitable gap is excited (Antzelevitch and Moe 1981; Rozanski et al. 1984a). This delay is long enough to allow proximal cells to recover their excitability and be available for reexcitation. Such a situation may exist in hearts with regional ischemia where local inhomogeneities due to local variations in extracellular K^+ may give rise to similar conditions present in the *in vitro* studies. The presence of phase 4 depolarization in the tissue distal to the inexcitable segment facilitates reflection by making possible even longer delays in activation of the distal tissue (Janse and Van Capelle 1982a). Subthreshold depolarizations transmitted electrotonically across the inexcitable segment may, depending on their timing with respect to the intrinsic cycle length of the tissue exhibiting phase 4 depolarization, accelerate or delay the firing of the automatic cells. When delayed, such automatic impulses may reexcite the tissue proximal to the inexcitable segment after it has completely recovered excitability (Jalife and Moe 1976; Moe et al. 1977; Jalife and Moe 1979).

Identifying Mechanisms of Arrhythmias in the Heart

In the study of arrhythmias in the *in situ* heart, it is not routinely possible to obtain the direct electrical recordings from the arrhythmogenic source that enable one to determine the electrophysiological mechanism causing the arrhythmias, such as microelectrode recordings of spontaneous diastolic depolarization or afterdepolarizations, or activation maps showing the presence of reentrant circuits. Therefore, indirect approaches have evolved that can be used to provide information that suggests, although not beyond a shadow of a doubt, what is the mechanism causing the arrhythmia. Among these approaches is (1) the characterization of the appearance of the arrhythmia on the electrocardiogram, (2) the effects of electrical stimulation of the heart on the arrhythmia, and (3) the effects of certain pharmacological agents on the arrhythmia. Because electrical stimulation of the heart has been an important tool in the study of mechanisms causing both clinical and experimental ischemic arrhythmias, we will take time here to describe the technique and its logic in some detail.

Electrical Stimulation of the Heart to Determine Arrhythmogenic Mechanisms

The mechanism causing an arrhythmia in the *in situ* heart can sometimes be deduced from a determination of the response of the arrhythmia to various patterns of electrical stimulation. The translation of the effects of electrical stimuli on the cardiac rhythm into conclusions concerning the electrophysiological mechanisms causing an arrhythmia is based largely on studies in which the effects of electrical stimulation were determined on transmembrane action potentials recorded with microelectrodes in isolated and superfused cardiac tissues, many of which we have described in previous sections of this chapter. It must be kept in mind that when using electrical stimulation to study arrhythmia mechanisms, the stimulated impulses must reach the site of arrhythmia origin in order for this approach to be valid. This might not always be the case, particularly when the site of stimulation is at a distance from the site of origin as might occur, for example, when the site of stimulation is in the right ventricle during study of ventricular tachycardia caused by infarction, originating in the left ventricle. The stimulated impulse(s) then might not reach the site at which the arrhythmia arises because of the electrophysiological properties of the intervening tissue in the conduction pathway between the stimulus site and the site of arrhythmia origin (Wellens 1971). An intervening region of prolonged refractoriness or depressed conduction might cause stimulated impulses to block before they reach the site of origin. If conduction time from the stimulation site to the site of arrhythmia origin is prolonged, impulses generated in the arrhythmogenic focus also may be able to leave that focus and depolarize large regions of myocardium around it, preventing the stimulated impulse from reaching the site of origin. Even when the stimulation site is close to the site of arrhythmia origin, areas of depressed conduction may prevent the stimulated impulses from reaching the arrhythmogenic cells.

Techniques

Two basic patterns of stimulation are generally used to study the mechanisms of arrhythmias, overdrive stimulation and programmed premature stimulation. Overdrive stimulation protocols entail stimulating the heart at a rate more rapid than the rate of the spontaneous rhythm for a period of time and then observing the effects of the period of stimulation on the spontaneous rhythm immediately after the overdrive is stopped. Overdrive stimulation can be implemented during sinus rhythm to determine whether the period of stimulation can induce the occurrence of an arrhythmia that has sometimes appeared spontaneously. Overdrive stimulation can also be implemented during the arrhythmia to determine if the overdrive can terminate it, or if it does not, to determine the effect of the overdrive on characteristics of the arrhythmia, most important of which is the rate. The overdrive stimuli can be applied to either the atria or the ventricles. In general, there are two variables in the overdrive protocol: the number of stimuli in the overdrive train and the cycle length at which the stimuli are delivered to the heart. A typical study might begin using overdrive with the longest cycle length at which the heart can be stimulated without escape of the spontaneous rhythm from control of the stimuli. The initial period of overdrive stimulation might be short, no longer than 10 to 15 impulses as is illustrated in Figure 1.48, panel A. Here the electrocardiogram recorded from a normal canine heart during a short period of overdrive applied to the left ventricle during sinus rhythm is shown. Sinus rhythm continued after the overdrive without any discernible alteration. After this period of stimulation, and observance of the effects of the stimulation on the rhythm, the rate of subsequent periods of stimulation was progressively increased. In the example in Figure 1.48, the rate of overdrive in panels B and C is increased, but the number of overdrive impulses remains constant. The protocol might

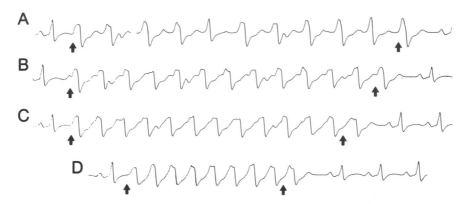

Figure 1.48: Electrocardiogram recorded from a canine heart during overdrive stimulation of the ventricles. The first complex in each panel is a sinus beat. Overdrive stimulation starts at the first arrow and ends at the second arrow. The last overdrive impulse is followed by sinus rhythm. In panels A-C overdrive was for 13 impulses at an increasing rate (there is a break in the trace in A where two paced impulses are omitted). In panel D overdrive was for 9 impulses.

then be repeated, using different durations of overdrive, also at different rates (panel D). The only effect of the overdrive in the example shown in Figure 1.48 was a transient suppression of the rate of the spontaneous rhythm after overdrive stops and no new rhythm was induced. This is, in general, the expected behavior of a normal heart. Arrhythmias may occur after the overdrive in hearts that have spontaneously occurring arrhythmias or in diseased hearts, even when no arrhythmias occur spontaneously. Examples are shown in later chapters.

Programmed stimulation of the heart refers to the application of single or multiple premature stimuli during the cycle length of the dominant rhythm; premature stimuli meaning that a stimulus is applied and a response is elicited earlier than the next expected beat. In the absence of an ongoing arrhythmia, programmed stimulation is used to determine if an arrhythmia can be induced. Most frequently during programmed stimulation protocols, the heart is stimulated at a regular cycle length (the basic stimuli) that can capture the rhythm and control the rate rather than allowing sinus rhythm to control the rate. One or more premature stimuli are introduced during this basic rhythm at different coupling intervals to a basic stimulus. In attempting to initiate an atrial arrhythmia, the atria are usually stimulated and in attempting to initiate a ventricular arrhythmia the ventricles are usually stimulated although this is not always the case. The premature stimuli are not applied after every basic stimulus but only after a number of basic stimuli that may vary from about 7 to 15 in different studies. The number of basic stimuli between premature stimuli should be sufficient to allow the heart to recover from the effects of the premature stimulus and to be in a steady state condition. An example of this protocol is shown in Figure 1.49. Panel A shows the ECG that was recorded while the basic drive stimuli were applied to the right ventricle of a canine heart at a regular cycle length of 300 msec. The basic stimuli are labeled "S_1".

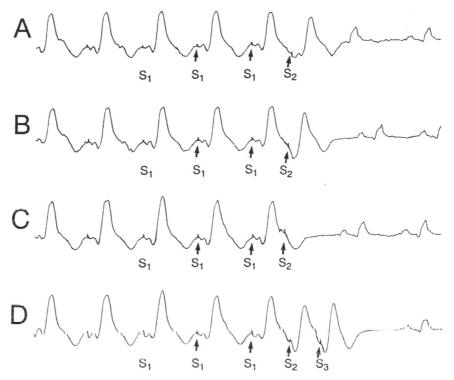

Figure 1.49: Electrocardiogram recorded from a canine heart during programmed premature stimulation protocol. The first five impulses from left to right were initiated during the basic drive (S_1). In panels A-C, the coupling interval of the premature impulse (S_2) was progressively decreased. In panel D, two successive premature impulses (S_2 and S_3) follow the last basic drive impulse.

A premature stimulus was applied at a long coupling interval of 250 msec to the tenth basic drive impulse in the train (S_2). There was a pause in the stimulation after the premature stimulus that allowed for observance of the effects of the premature impulse on the spontaneous rhythm before stimulation was continued. In this case, sinus rhythm continued after the pause. The premature stimulus was then gradually moved towards the previous basic drive stimulus, that is, the coupling interval between the premature stimulus and the basic drive stimulus was decreased during subsequent periods of stimulation. The decrease in coupling interval continues until the refractory period of the ventricle is reached or the stimulus initiates an arrhythmic event. After ten more basic drive stimuli, the premature stimulus (S_2) occurred with a coupling interval of 200 msec in panel B and 160 msec in panel C. In panel C, the premature stimulus was not followed by a response, indicating that the effective refractory period had been reached. No arrhythmias were initiated by the premature stimuli in this heart. More than one premature stimulus may also be applied after a basic stimulus with different coupling intervals to each other as shown in panel D. S_2 and S_3 are the two successive premature stimuli coupled to the basic drive stimulus S_1. There are several reasons for using more than one premature stimulus for the induction of an arrhythmia. One reason may be that a single stimulated impulse is not able to reach the site of the arrhythmia origin because there is an intervening region of prolonged refractoriness caused by a prolonged action potential duration. When this occurs, the first premature impulse is sometimes able to decrease the duration of the refractory period because of the decreased action potential duration of a premature response, enabling the second premature impulse to propagate to the site of arrhythmia origin (Almendral et al. 1986a; Stamato et al. 1987). In clinical studies, electrogram recordings from a catheter have shown the failure of single premature impulses stimulated in the right ventricle from reaching reentrant circuits in the left ventricle, while the second of two premature stimulated impulses succeeded (Josephson et al. 1978b). This phenomenon is called "peeling back" of the refractory period. Another reason that a second premature impulse can sometimes improve the efficacy for the induction of an arrhythmia is that it intensifies the effects of the first premature impulse; that is, two premature impulses in a row make delayed afterdepolarizations larger than one premature impulse, or enlarge regions of conduction block or slow conduction necessary for the initiation of reentry. More complex programmed stimulation protocols are illustrated in Chapter IV where we discuss arrhythmias in healing and healed infarcts. Single or multiple premature stimuli can also be applied to the atria or ventricles during a spontaneously occurring rhythm, without using a basic drive. This can be done during sinus rhythm in attempting to initiate an arrhythmia, or during a sustained arrhythmia in an attempt to stop the arrhythmia or measure the effects of the stimuli on the rate or characteristics of the arrhythmia. Multiple premature stimuli rather than single premature stimuli are used during an arrhythmia for the same reasons as described above for initiation: to either improve the chance of the stimulated impulse to reach the site of origin or to intensify the effects of the first premature impulse.

Effects of Electrical Stimulation on Arrhythmias Caused by Automaticity

In our discussion of automaticity as an arrhythmogenic mechanism, we considered how the sinus node pacemaker and electrical stimulation (pacing) influence subsidiary pacemakers with different automatic mechanisms. We showed that overdrive either by the sinus node or by electrical stimuli exerts an inhibitory effect on the normal automatic mechanism of subsidiary pacemakers (overdrive suppression), which is primarily the result of enhanced Na/K pump activity but has less inhibitory effects on the abnormal automatic mechanism of subsidiary pacemakers. These known effects of overdrive on pacemaker mechanisms, determined from careful and detailed studies on isolated, superfused preparations of cardiac tissue, are sometimes useful in distinguishing automatic arrhythmias from arrhythmias caused by reentry or triggered activity in the *in situ* heart. The effects of overdrive stimulation can also be of use in distinguishing arrhythmias caused by normal automaticity from those caused by abnormal automaticity (Hoffman and Dangman 1982).

Based on the results of the experimental studies, it can be assumed that arrhythmias caused by normal or abnormal automaticity in the *in situ* heart cannot be initiated by overdrive stimulation. In the experimental microelectrode studies on isolated superfused pacemaker tissues, application of overdrive stimuli has not shown that stimuli can induce rhythmic firing caused by automaticity when these tissues are quiescent. When overdrive is applied during an ongoing arrhythmia caused by normal automaticity, the rate of the arrhythmia is expected to be transiently suppressed immediately after overdrive is stopped. The transient pause after overdrive should be followed by a gradual speeding up of the rhythm until the original rate is resumed. The duration of the transient pause and the time required for resumption of the original rate is expected to be directly related to the rate and duration of the overdrive, based on the previously described studies on isolated, superfused Purkinje fiber bundles. It is important to stress that the arrhythmia caused by normal automaticity cannot be terminated, but only suppressed transiently as was also shown in the microelectrode studies. This behavior is mainly a result of the increased activity of the Na/K pump that is dependent both on the rate and duration of stimulation as discussed previously. This characteristic behavior of normally automatic pacemakers has been demonstrated in some clinical and experimental electrophysiological studies on both atrial and ventricular tachycardias (Goldreyer et al. 1973; Scheinman et al. 1974; Le Marec et al. 1985). An example is shown in Figure 1.50 of a clinical ventricular tachycardia that responded in this predicted way to overdrive and, therefore, might be caused by a normal automatic mechanism. Each panel shows three leads of the electrocardiogram; panel A shows records obtained while pacing (St) for 4 beats. The last stimulated impulse, shown by the arrows, was followed by a pause before tachycardia resumed. Panel B shows records obtained while pacing for a slightly longer period of time. The ventricular pacemaker was transiently suppressed, allowing a short period of sinus rhythm before tachycardia resumed (large arrow).

On the other hand, arrhythmias caused by abnormal automaticity should not be suppressed by overdrive unless the overdrive period is long and the rate of overdrive is fast (Hoffman and Dangman 1982). The difficulty in suppressing such arrhythmias stems from the lesser amount of Na^+ entering the cells during the upstroke of the action potential and therefore, less intense Na pump stimulation by overdrive as previously mentioned. Short periods of overdrive can even result in a transient speeding of the rate of impulse generation (overdrive acceleration) (Hoffman and Dangman 1982). Accelerated idioventricular rhythms or tachycardia occurring within the first 24 hours of myocardial infarction are not easily overdrive-suppressed and therefore may be caused by abnormal automaticity (see Chapter III). Like normal automaticity, arrhythmias caused by abnormal automaticity cannot be started or stopped by overdrive stimulation.

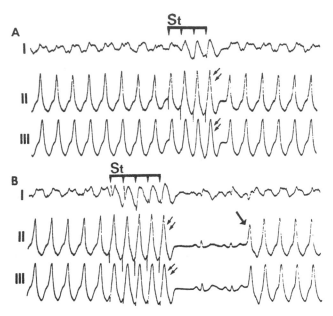

Figure 1.50: Overdrive stimulation of ventricular tachycardia that may be caused by automaticity. Each panel shows three electrocardiographic leads. In panel A there is a short period of stimulation (St), the last stimulated impulse (arrows) is followed by a short pause and then recurrence of tachycardia. In panel B, a longer period of stimulation (St) is followed (after the small arrows) by greater suppression of tachycardia, allowing the occurrence of two sinus beats before tachycardia reappears (large arrow). (Reproduced from Fontaine et al. (1984) with permission.)

The characteristics of the response of arrhythmias caused by automaticity to premature stimulation is also sometimes useful in distinguishing automaticity from other arrhythmogenic mechanisms. Of major importance is the fact that automatic rhythms caused by either normal or abnormal automaticity cannot be started or terminated by stimulated, premature impulses (based on data obtained from the microelectrode studies on pacemaker tissue), in contrast to reentry and triggered activity discussed in the following sections. Other than that, premature impulses induced at different times during diastole may transiently perturb an automatic rhythm for a few cycles, and the characteristics of the perturbation may sometimes distinguish automaticity from other arrhythmogenic mechanisms. The response of normal and abnormal automaticity to premature stimulation may be somewhat similar. The characteristic response of an automatic pacemaker to premature stimulation is best exemplified by the response of the sinus node to atrial premature stimulation (Strauss et al. 1973). In Figure 1.51 is plotted the normalized return cycle (cycle following the premature impulse) on the y axis versus the normalized premature cycle (test cycle) on the x axis for a study in which premature stimuli were applied to the atria of the human heart during sinus rhythm. The solid line (A) represents the line of identity; points falling on this line are compensatory (the

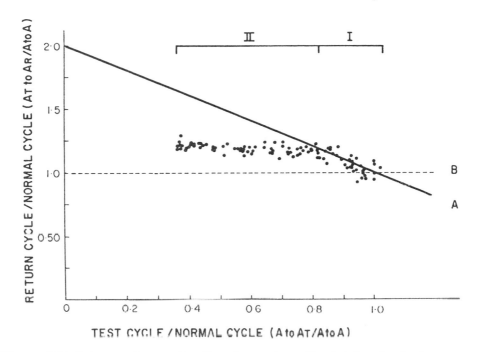

Figure 1.51: Return cycles as a function of premature stimulated cycles during premature atrial stimulation in a patient in sinus rhythm. The graph depicts the relationship of the normalized return cycle to the degree of prematurity of the test cycle, which is also normalized. Points falling on line A represent non-reset of the sinus pacemaker (fully compensatory pause). Line B projecting from the y axis is a reference line indicating the spontaneous sinus cycle length. The distance the points that are reset (points that fall below line A) are above line B is interpreted to indicate conduction time into and out of the sinus node assuming the sinus node pacemaker cycle immediately following the premature depolarization is identical to the preceding sinus node pacemaker cycle (see text for discussion). (Reproduced from Strauss et al. (1973) with permission.)

sum of the premature cycle and the return cycle is equal to the sum of two spontaneous cycles). Premature impulses delivered late in the cycle length were followed by a compensatory pause and fall on this line (as the test cycle shortens, the return cycle lengthens in a reciprocal manner) because the premature impulses collided with the impulse emanating from the sinus node pacemaker without reaching and resetting the pacemaker. Therefore, the pacemaker discharge following the premature impulse occurs exactly on time. As the premature coupling interval is decreased, a point is reached in the basic cycle where the premature impulse reaches the pacemaker before it has spontaneously depolarized to threshold and depolarizes it early. The pacemaker is reset. When this occurs the postextrasystolic cycle (which is a result of the stimulated or reset pacemaker cells spontaneously depolarizing to threshold) is less than compensatory and the points fall below the line of identity. For the most part, the postextrasystolic cycle length is expected to be equal to the unperturbed spontaneous cycle length, as explained in our discussion on the effects of premature stimulation on spontaneous diastolic depolarization, earlier in this chapter. The dashed line (B) on the graph in Figure 1.51 indicates the cycle length of the basic rhythm so that the return cycle length relative to the basic cycle length can be seen to be somewhat longer in this study. The prolonged return cycle has been proposed to result from slowed conduction of the premature impulse into the pacemaker site, and the pacemaker impulse out of this site (Strauss et al. 1973). It also might result, at least partly, from depression of the rate of spontaneous diastolic depolarization. Further shortening of the premature coupling interval to midcycle results in points parallel to the dashed line and possibly slightly above it, which indicates no change in the postextrasystolic cycle length over a wide range of coupling intervals. If the rate of the rhythm is slow enough so that shortening of the postextrasystolic cycle length can occur (as seen in some of the microelectrode studies described earlier), the points at very short premature coupling intervals would dip below the dashed line on the graph. Finally, conduction of very early premature impulses might block prior to reaching the pacemaker and the next pacemaker discharge would, again, occur on time. Of course, this relationship might be upset by changes in conduction of impulses into and out of the pacemaker site.

This same relationship between premature and return cycle length, found in studies on sinus rhythm, has also been shown in studies on some ectopic tachycardias and when found, indicates that the tachycardias are likely to be caused by automaticity (Goldreyer et al. 1973; Scheinman et al. 1974; Gillette and Garson 1977). Figure 1.52 shows the effects of atrial premature depolarizations induced by stimulation on a sustained atrial tachycardia in the human heart (Goldreyer et al. 1973). The return atrial cycle length following the atrial premature depolarization (A_2A_3) is plotted as a function of the coupling interval of the stimulated premature impulse (A_1A_2). The diagonal line is the line of identity and indicates where points fall when there is a fully compensatory pause following the premature impulse. The cycle length of the tachycardia was approximately 400 msec. As with the sinus node, the plot shows that late coupled premature impulses are followed by compensatory return cycles while earlier premature impulses are followed by return cycles that are equal to or slightly longer than the cycle length of the arrhythmia and less than compensatory. The return cycles also remain relatively constant over a wide range of premature coupling intervals. In this study the return cycle following some very early premature impulses was shorter than the basic cycle as predicted by some of the experimental studies described earlier. Ectopic pacemakers might also exist in an extensive region of slow conduction, much as the pacemaker in the sinus node, and conduction delays into and out of the pacemaker site may influence to some extent the relationship between return cycle and premature cycle. Conduction delays might cause some of the prolongation of the return cycle. However, when the above relationship is seen, it is probably indicative of automaticity (either normal or abnormal) since triggered activity and reentry are expected to show a different behavior (see next section).

In addition to the atrial arrhythmias that we have discussed, some ventric-

APD during AET

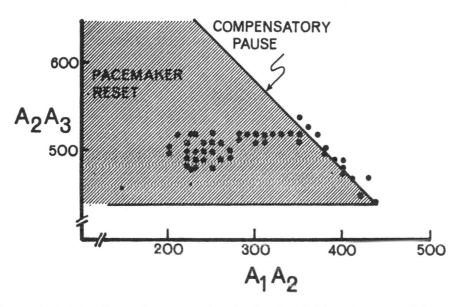

Figure 1.52: The effects of prematurely stimulated atrial impulses on atrial ectopic tachycardia (AET). The atrial interval (return cycle) following the atrial premature depolarization (APD) is plotted on the y axis in milliseconds (A_2A_3), as a function of the coupling interval of the stimulated APD (A_1A_2) in milliseconds on the x axis. The diagonal line indicates a fully compensatory atrial pause following the APD. The cycle length of tachycardia was approximately 400 msec. (Reproduced from Goldreyer et al. (1973) with permission.)

ular arrhythmias are likely to be caused by automaticity. Idioventricular rhythms in patients with complete heart block respond to premature stimulation in the manner shown in the microelectrode studies on slowly beating Purkinje fibers described earlier; the postextrasystolic cycle following late premature impulses is longer than the cycle length of the basic rhythm but less than compensatory, while it is shorter than the basis cycle length following early premature impulses (and obviously less than compensatory) (Klein et al. 1972). Some exercise provoked ventricular tachycardia might also be caused by normal automaticity (Palileo et al. 1982; Sung et al. 1983). On the other hand, there is some evidence that accelerated idioventricular rhythms in the clinical setting of myocardial infarction might be caused by abnormal automaticity. We discuss the mechanism for this arrhythmia in Chapter III.

Effects of Electrical Stimulation on Reentrant Excitation

We will discuss the effects of electrical stimulation on reentry before discussing its effects on triggered activity because historically, electrical stimulation was originally used as a tool to identify reentrant excitation and to distinguish reentry from arrhythmias caused by automatic impulse initiation. There is a stark contrast between the effects of stimulation on the two mechanisms that made identification of the cause of an arrhythmia relatively simple. This simplicity was not upset until the 1970s when the arrhythmogenic mechanism of triggered activity was rediscovered. The hallmark feature of reentry was that it could be induced and stopped by electrical stimuli (overdrive or premature stimuli) unlike automaticity. Discovery of this feature of reentry can be traced to the experiments of the physiologist George Ralph Mines (1913; 1914) on isolated rings of cardiac tissue, cut from a variety of animal hearts that we described earlier, in which he showed that stimulation at rapid rates at one point on a ring of heart muscle could initiate reentry. It is interesting to keep his experiments in mind when reading the recent results of clinical studies on programmed stimulation of the heart in patients with ischemic heart disease. One cannot help but be amazed at how such simple experiments found their way into the clinic and were eventually responsible for over 400 papers with the words "programmed electrical stimulation" in the title alone in the last 10 years. Both Mines (1913; 1914) and Garrey (1914), who were performing similar experiments independently at the same time, recognized that reentry can be induced by stimulation because the inciting stimuli produce unidirectional block in one limb of the reentrant circuit as well as cause a critical amount of slow conduction. Within the past 20 years this mechanism has been directly demonstrated as a mechanism for the initiation of reentry in a variety of isolated tissue preparations, using microelectrode recording techniques as we described in a previous section of this chapter, as well as in the *in situ* heart using multiple electrode mapping techniques. Mines (1913) also showed that stimulation during a reentrant rhythm could terminate the rhythm (" . . . extra stimuli were thrown in. After several attempts the reentrant wave was stopped"). A record from one of his experiments on a ring of auricle and ventricle, in which he stopped reentry with a stimulus is shown in Figure 1.53. Mines

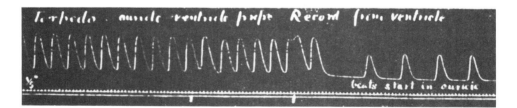

Figure 1.53: Records of contraction obtained from a ring of auricle and ventricle from the heart of an electric ray by G.R. Mines. " . . . the preparations were, before stimulation, either quiescent or giving infrequent spontaneous beats. After the application of rhythmic stimuli . . . the cessation of the stimuli was followed by a quick reciprocating movement of auricle and ventricle . . ." shown by the rapid series of contractions in the record. This rapid series was caused by circus movement around the ring. Single shocks were then applied to the ring during the rapid activity at the times indicated by the markers on the bottom trace. The properly timed second shock terminated the rapid rhythm. (Reproduced from Mines (1913) with permission.)

recognized that termination of the reentrant rhythm resulted from making the conducting pathway refractory to the circulating impulse. During subsequent years Mines' observation that reentry could be initiated and terminated by applying stimuli to cardiac tissue was utilized by experimental electrophysiologists to initiate reentrant arrhythmias in animal hearts *in situ*. For example, Thomas Lewis initiated atrial flutter in the canine heart by rapidly stimulating the atria, which he then mapped in an attempt to show that it resulted from reentry around the venae cavae (Lewis 1920; Lewis et al. 1920). However, as far as we can determine, the use of programmed premature stimuli coupled to a basic drive to initiate and terminate reentrant arrhythmias should be attributed to Gordon K. Moe in papers published in 1956 and 1963. Moe and colleagues (1956; 1963) were studying the conduction properties of the AV junction in dog hearts by applying premature stimuli to the atria to determine how they were conducted to the ventricles. This had been a standard procedure for a long time to investigate refractoriness and the excitability properties of excitable tissue (for example see Forbes et al. 1923; Krayer et al. 1951; Brooks et al. 1955; Van Dam et al. 1956). In the course of these studies Moe produced atrial echo beats after appropriately timed premature atrial beats that he attributed to reentry in the AV junction. Undoubtedly he had the experiments of Mines in mind when he interpreted the results of this study. In fact, Moe showed that single properly timed premature stimuli could initiate and terminate a tachycardia (supraventricular) in one dog that he presented as a case report in the American Heart Journal in 1963 (Moe et al. 1963). This marked the beginning of the use of programmed stimulation techniques to study the mechanisms of arrhythmias and, in particular, to identify reentrant arrhythmias.

The study of arrhythmia mechanisms in man with programmed electrical stimulation began in 1967 when the groups of Durrer in Amsterdam and Coumel in Paris independently, and simultaneously published their initial results obtained by intracardiac stimulation and recording with multiple catheters (Coumel et al. 1967; Durrer et al. 1967). To appreciate the impact this technique had on the study of arrhythmias in the 20 years that followed, the reader is referred to a volume on cardiac arrhythmias edited by Brugada and Wellens (1987), appropriately titled *Cardiac Arrhythmias: Where To Go From Here?*

Initially it was sufficient to show that an arrhythmia could be started or stopped by overdrive or programmed stimulation in order for a strong case to be made for a reentrant mechanism (Wellens 1971). That is because until the 1970s, the only other mechanism that was widely considered to be a cause of arrhythmias was automaticity, and automaticity cannot be started or stopped by stimulation. After the early 1970s when the concept of afterdepolarization-induced arrhythmias was revived and expanded, these criteria alone were not sufficient and had to be strengthened with additional ones, because triggered activity caused by delayed afterdepolarizations can also be started and stopped by stimulation.

The initiation of arrhythmias by overdrive or programmed stimulation can be used as an indicator of a reentrant mechanism if other characteristics (described below) are also present that eliminate the probability of triggered activity dependent on delayed afterdepolarizations. An example of the initiation of an arrhythmia by atrial premature stimulation in the human heart is shown in Figure 1.54. We are using the initiation of supraventricular tachycar-

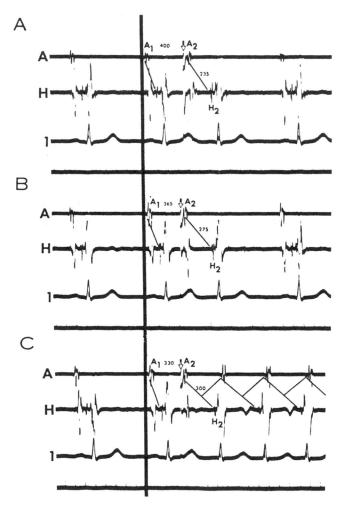

Figure 1.54: Initiation of reentry in the atrioventricular (AV) node by atrial premature stimulation causing supraventricular tachycardia. In each panel an atrial electrogram (A), a His bundle electrogram (H), and a lead I electrocardiogram are shown along with 100-msec time marks (bottom trace). The heavy vertical bar aligns the tenth atrial beat of sinus origin (A₁) prior to the introduction of the stimulated atrial premature beat at the arrow (A₂). The A₁A₂ interval is given above each atrial electrogram in milliseconds. The His bundle depolarizations resulting from conduction of A₂ are labeled H₂ and the A₂-H₂ intervals are given in milliseconds on the diagonal lines. (Reproduced from Goldreyer and Damato (1971) with permission.)

dia for this example even though later on, in discussing ischemic arrhythmias, we concentrate on ventricular tachycardia. However, some of the characteristics that identify an arrhythmia as reentrant (in addition simply to its initiation by stimuli) are more clearly manifested during initiation of some supraventricular tachycardias than ventricular tachycardia. In each panel in Figure 1.54, an atrial electrogram (A), a His bundle electrogram (H), and a lead I electrocardiogram are shown. The heavy vertical bar aligns the tenth atrial beat of sinus origin (A_1) prior to the induction of the stimulated atrial premature beat (A_2, shown by the arrow). In panel A, the premature coupling interval (A_1-A_2) is 400 msec and was followed by resumption of sinus rhythm. In panel B, the premature coupling interval is 365 msec and was also followed by resumption of sinus rhythm. However, in panel C after a premature impulse at a coupling interval of 330 msec, atrial tachycardia was initiated. It is proposed that the arrhythmia results because, at this critical premature coupling interval; unidirectional block occurs in a potential reentrant circuit and slow conduction is induced to occur around that circuit in accordance with the results of Mines' experiments. Likewise, unidirectional block and slow conduction is expected when there is overdrive stimulation at a critical rate and for a critical duration, accounting for the initiation of a tachycardia after a period of overdrive. However, it might also be argued that the arrhythmia is triggered, caused by delayed afterdepolarizations reaching threshold at the critical rate and duration of overdrive or prematurity of stimulation. In the study of supraventricular tachycardia shown in Figure 1.54, there is additional evidence that reentry, rather than triggering occurred. It is known from the results of a large body of research that the supraventricular tachycardia shown in Figure 1.54 originates in the AV node. We will not discuss this evidence here but refer the reader to several publications (Bigger and Goldreyer 1970; Goldreyer and Bigger 1971; Goldreyer and Damato 1971; Wit et al. 1971; Janse et al. 1971; 1976). It can be seen in Figure 1.54, that as the premature stimulus cycle length was decreased, conduction through the AV node became slower as indicated by an increase in the A-H interval of the His bundle electrogram. In panel A, 235 msec were required for the premature atrial impulse to conduct through the AV node before the His bundle was depolarized; in panel B, 275 msec were required; and in panel C 300 msec were required. The initiation of tachycardia was associated with a critical prolongation of the A-H interval to 300 msec. The ability to directly demonstrate that induction of the arrhythmia is related to a critical amount of slow conduction in the region where the arrhythmia originates adds credence to the interpretation that the arrhythmia is caused by reentry. Similarly, at the pacing rate that induces supraventricular tachycardia, AV nodal conduction is slowed also to a critical degree (Goldreyer and Damato 1971). The induction of triggered activity caused by delayed afterdepolarizations is not dependent on slowed conduction and should not show this relationship.

In some studies, not only is supraventricular tachycardia (nonsustained or sustained) induced by the appropriately timed premature atrial impulse with the critical degree of AV nodal conduction slowing, but also further decreases in the premature coupling interval continue to induce tachycardias. Similarly, when tachycardia is initiated spontaneously by spontaneous premature depolarizations, it may be initiated over a wide range of coupling intervals (Bigger and Goldreyer 1970). When this occurs there is an inverse relationship between the premature impulse coupling interval and the interval from the premature impulse to the first impulse of tachycardia, which is shown in Figure 1.55A (Bigger and Goldreyer 1970; Goldreyer and Bigger 1971). In the figure, the A_2A_3 interval that represents the time from the premature impulse to the first impulse of tachycardia, increases as the premature coupling interval (A_1A_2) decreases. This inverse relationship has been proposed to be a specific characteristic for the initiation of reentrant arrhythmias. The proposed mechanism is explained in Figure 1.55B, which shows schematic diagrams of a reentrant circuit that might cause supraventricular tachycardia (for simplicity the circuit is depicted as an anatomical ring although the anatomy of reentrant circuits in the AV node is not known in any detail). Panel A shows the activation pattern that might occur during propagation of the basic impulse; both limbs of the circuit are activated in the antegrade direction as the impulse enters this region (black arrows in A1), and the activation wave is followed by a wake of effectively (dark black) and relatively (stippled) refractory tissue (panel A2) as it leaves the region. In the diagram, the effective refractory period is inhomo-

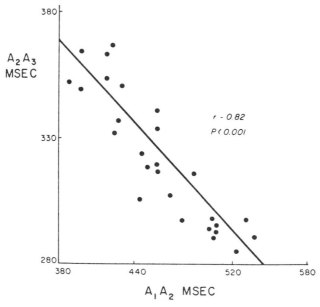

Figure 1.55A: In the top panel, the reciprocal relationship between the coupling intervals of premature impulses (A_1A_2) that induced supraventricular tachycardia in a patient, and the first cycle length following the premature impulse (A_2A_3) is shown. In this case, the premature atrial impulses occurred spontaneously. (Reproduced from Bigger and Goldreyer (1970) with permission.)

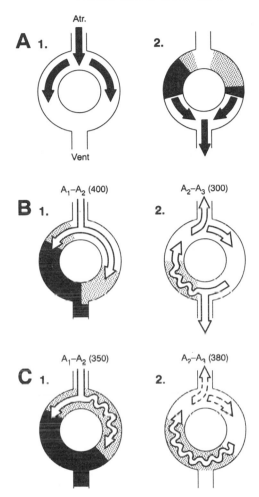

Figure 1.55B: Diagrams of a hypothetical reentrant circuit in the atrioventricular (AV) junction that explain why the A_2A_3 interval prolongs as A_1A_2 decreases. In A, the black arrows indicate activation by the last basic impulse. The activation wave is followed by an effectively refractory (black) and a relatively refractory (stippled) period (A_2). The effective refractory period is longer in the left pathway than in the right. Panels B and C show activation by premature impulses (unfilled arrows) initiating reentry. Conduction of the earlier premature impulse in C around the circuit is slower than in B accounting for a longer A_2-A_3 interval.

geneous, being longer in the left pathway than in the right. A premature impulse at a coupling interval of 400 msec that initiates tachycardia (panel B1) blocks in one limb of the circuit because of refractoriness (indicated by the arrow to the left) and conducts around the circuit through the other limb in relatively refractory tissue (arrow to the right), to reexcite the atria (panel B2). The transit time around the circuit, which is 300 msec determines the cycle length to the first tachycardia impulse following the stimulus (A_2-A_3) (panel

B2). An even earlier premature impulse (shorter A_1-A_2 coupling interval of 350 msec), still blocks in the left pathway and conducts more slowly around the circuit through the right pathway (panel C1) because it is propagating in tissue that is more refractory. Transit time around the circuit is longer (380 msec), the time for reemergence into the atrium is longer, and the A_2-A_3 interval is longer. Therefore, at shorter premature coupling intervals, slower conduction around the circuit results in the inverse relationship.

In the example of AV nodal reentry, the hypothesis is that, at a critical overdrive rate or premature coupling interval, unidirectional block occurs, as well as the necessary degree of slow conduction that is needed to cause reentry. The block and slow conduction are not present during normal rhythm. The occurrence of block is not evident from the electrical recordings but is equated with a critical degree of conduction slowing in the AV node. In patients with the Wolff-Parkinson-White (WPW) syndrome, the occurrence of block as well as slow conduction in the reentrant circuit can be seen in electrocardiographic and local electrogram recordings when supraventricular tachycardia is initiated by programmed stimulation (Durrer et al. 1967). However, the application of these rules to the ventricle, which is our concern when discussing ischemic arrhythmias, is sometimes problematical because not only can occurrence of unidirectional block not usually be seen, but often recordings are not obtained from the area of slow conduction in the reentrant circuit, comparable to the AV node in the examples described above. An inverse relationship between the coupling interval of the initiating stimuli and the first impulse of tachycardia is, however, sometimes evident on the electrocardiogram, indicating a reentrant mechanism. When this relationship is not seen on the ECG, it is still possible that such a relationship might be seen in the region of slow conduction (reentrant circuit) when recordings are obtained there.

Another feature of reentrant arrhythmias is that they can be terminated by overdrive or premature stimulation as predicted by Mines' experiments on rings of cardiac tissue. This is not specific for reentry because triggered activity caused by delayed afterdepolarizations can also be terminated (described in the next section). The termination of reentry by stimulation can only be demonstrated in stable, sustained tachyarrhythmias, the initiation of which is dependent on the transient block and slow conduction caused by an initiating event such as a premature impulse. If the unidirectional block and slow conduction is a permanent property of the circuit, reentry may immediately reoccur after stimulation. As with initiation, termination by overdrive requires a critical rate and duration of the stimulation train while termination with stimulated premature impulses requires a critical coupling interval between the premature impulse and the previous impulse of the tachyarrhythmia. An example of termination by a stimulated premature impulse of supraventricular tachycardia caused by AV nodal reentry is shown in Figure 1.56. An atrial electrogram (AE), His bundle electrogram (HBE), and electrocardiogram (ECG) are shown in each panel. The first cycle length at the left (420 msec) in each panel is during the supraventricular tachycardia. The last spontaneous impulse of tachycardia prior to the prematurely stimulated impulse is indicated by the black bar. A

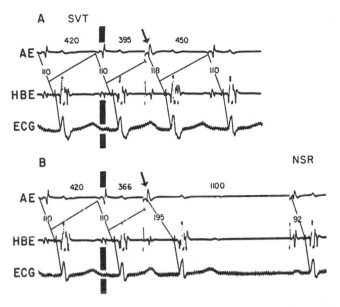

Figure 1.56: Termination of reentrant supraventricular tachycardia with programmed stimulation. An atrial electrogram (AE), His bundle electrogram (HBE), and electrocardiogram (ECG) are shown in each panel. Numbers above AE trace indicate atrial cycle lengths, numbers between AE and HBE traces indicate AV nodal conduction time. Black bar is positioned at last tachycardia impulse prior to a single prematurely stimulated impulse (arrow) that did not terminate tachycardia in A but did terminate it in B. (Reproduced from Goldreyer and Bigger (1971) with permission.)

single premature impulse was stimulated at a coupling interval of 395 msec in panel A and did not terminate the tachycardia; it was followed by a tachycardia impulse at a cycle length of 450 msec. A single premature impulse was stimulated at a coupling interval of 366 msec in panel B and terminated the tachycardia. Conduction of the premature impulse that terminated tachycardia through the AV node was slower (195 msec) than the premature impulse that did not terminate the arrhythmia (118 msec). This observation is taken as indirect evidence that the premature impulse that terminated tachycardia conducted slowly and eventually blocked in the AV nodal reentrant circuit. We described the mechanism by which a stimulated impulse can enter a reentrant circuit and stop the circulating wavefront earlier. Demonstration of slow conduction and block of premature impulses in reentrant circuits causing ventricular tachycardia is much more difficult in the *in situ* heart because the circuit cannot always be precisely located, particularly in clinical studies (see Chapter IV).

Failure to terminate an arrhythmia by stimulated impulses does not alone eliminate reentry as a mechanism for the arrhythmia. Termination of reentry requires that the stimulated impulse is able to enter the reentrant circuit to cause the block of the reentrant wavefront. This requires the circuit to have an excitable gap. As we discussed in a previous section of this chapter, functional circuits caused by the leading circle mechanism and some anatomical circuits may not have a gap of excitability that allows a premature impulse to penetrate into the circuit. If a tachycardia is very rapid, the excitable gap may also be very small, preventing easy penetration by stimulated impulses. Reentrant tachycardias that are dependent on circuits without a fully excitable gap are still predicted to be terminated by application of countershock, but this may entail a different mechanism than described above. Shock may prolong the duration of action potentials in the circuit (Dillon 1991) and cause the reentrant wavefront to block in refractory tissue (Sweeney et al. 1990; Dillon 1991). This may also be the basis for the termination of fibrillation by shock since fibrillation is probably the result of multiple, functional, reentrant circuits.

In general, overdrive or programmed stimulation is not used to explore the mechanisms of extrasystoles. A limited amount of experimental data suggests a complex relationship between the rate of overdrive and the frequency of extrasystoles (Wit et al. 1972b). Extrasystoles may be increased in number when increasing the rate of overdrive slows conduction in the reentrant circuit and then abolished if a further increase in rate causes conduction block in the circuit. However, when stimulation is stopped, the arrhythmias should return if there is a persistent region of slow conduction and block that is the cause of reentry.

Resetting and Entrainment The response of an arrhythmia to a prematurely stimulated impulse or to a period of overdrive that does not terminate it may still provide information useful for determining the mechanism of the arrhythmia. Reentrant rhythms can be reset by both kinds of stimulation patterns in a characteristic way that is sometimes different (at least theoretically) from the response of other arrhythmogenic mechanisms.

Some information on the effects of stimulated premature impulses on reentry comes from studies on experimental preparations of isolated tissues or hearts in which reentrant excitation has been mapped. Other predictions concerning the effects of premature impulses on reentry are based mainly on theoretical considerations, using a model of a reentrant circuit with a fixed pathway in which the circuit cannot change its dimensions, and in which there is an excitable gap as we previously described in Figure 1.41. Such circuits may have a single entrance and exit pathway leading into and out of the circuit as in Figure 1.41 or the entrance and exit pathways may be separate. These characteristics will influence the characteristics of the resetting response as seen on the electrocardiogram. The theoretically possible responses of a tachycardia caused by reentrant excitation to premature stimulation are diagrammed in Figure 1.41. The stable tachycardia cycle length (R_1-R_1) is determined by the time it takes the reentrant wavefront to travel one complete revolution around the circuit and reach an exit pathway to the ventricles. When such a circuit is the cause of a tachycardia, premature depolarizations (R_2) delivered late in the cycle length are often followed by a postextrasystolic pause that is compensatory for the same reason as described for automatic tachycardias; the stimulated impulse may not be able to reach the reentrant circuit, possibly due to collision between the stimulated impulse and the impulse coming from the circuit. The next tachycardia impulse then comes precisely on time. In this case the tachycardia is not reset because the sum of the premature cycle length (R_1-R_2) and the return cycle length (R_2-R_3) is equal to two successive tachycardia cycle lengths. Over the range of premature coupling intervals that does not reset the tachycardia, the relationship between premature coupling interval and the following (return) cycle falls along the line of identity (see Figures 1.51 and 1.52.) Premature impulses delivered earlier in the tachycardia cycle might have several different effects that are dependent on some of the characteristics of the reentrant circuit. If there is no excitable gap, as might be expected of some functional circuits, no resetting of the tachycardia will occur because the stimulated impulse cannot enter the circuit and the return cycle will remain compensatory. If the excitable gap is partially excitable, e.g., composed of relatively refractory tissue, premature impulses that succeed in entering the circuit and traveling around it will do so at reduced conduction velocities as diagrammed in Figure 1.41B (Frame et al. 1986; 1987). When they emerge from the circuit they cause the first postextrasystolic (tachycardia) impulse. As a result of the slowing of conduction of the premature impulse around the circuit the postextrasystolic cycle (R_2-R_3) is longer than the basic cycle (R_1-R_1) represented by the dashed line in Figure 1.41B3. Conduction time of the premature impulse around the circuit should continue to increase as the premature impulse is delivered earlier and earlier in the cycle, because the premature impulse conducts in more refractory tissue, causing an inverse relationship between the premature coupling interval (R_1-R_2) and the postextrasystolic cycle (R_2-R_3) (Figure 1.41B3). In the study by Bigger and Goldreyer (1970) on AV nodal reentrant tachycardia, the prolongation of the postextrasystolic cycle over the entire range of premature coupling intervals was sufficient to result in a greater than compensatory pause following the premature impulse. However, the postextrasystolic cycle length can be less than compensatory. An inverse relationship between the premature interval and the return cycle interval caused by slowing of conduction of the premature impulse in the reentrant circuit, as shown in Figure 1.41B3, is indicative of reentry because this type of response does not occur with automaticity (or triggered activity, which is described later). Recall that for automatic impulse initiation, the return cycle length is fairly constant over a wide range of premature coupling intervals and may even decrease at short coupling intervals (Figures 1.51 and 1.52).

If there is a large fully excitable gap (a gap comprised of completely excitable tissue), premature impulses reaching the circuit are expected to conduct around the circuit with the same velocity as the reentrant wave front that is causing the tachycardia and the postextrasystolic cycle would be equal to the tachycardia cycle and less than compensatory (Figure 1.41A). This could occur over a relatively wide range of coupling intervals resulting in a relationship similar to that expected from a pacemaker over the intermediate range of coupling intervals; the line describing the relationship of the return cycle (R_2-

R_3) to the premature cycle (R_1-R_2) would be flat (Figure 1.41A3). However, it is expected that stimulated extrasystoles that are sufficiently premature would eventually invade the circuit when it is relatively refractory, resulting in prolonged return cycles, inversely related to the premature coupling intervals. The prolongation of the postextrasystolic cycle after early premature impulses is opposite to that which occurs during automaticity. Thus, a curve might be plotted that consists of a segment that is compensatory at long premature coupling intervals (because the stimulated impulse does not reach the circuit), a segment that is less than compensatory and flat at intermediate premature coupling intervals (when the stimulated impulse is conducting in completely excitable tissue in the circuit) (Figure 1.41A3), and a segment that is ascending at short premature coupling intervals (when the stimulated impulse is conducting in relatively refractory tissue in the circuit) (Figure 1.41B3). Still earlier premature impulses might block prior to reaching a circuit resulting in interpolation as described for an automatic focus. A sufficiently early premature impulse could also terminate the tachycardia by blocking in the circuit and causing block of the reentrant wavefront as we described previously, and this is not expected of automatic impulse initiation.

As mentioned previously, the entrance route that a stimulated impulse takes into a circuit and the exit route from the circuit may be separate. When this occurs, the return cycle following a premature impulse may be less than the tachycardia cycle because the premature impulse, after entering the circuit, need not conduct around the entire circuit before exiting. The return cycle may still show any of the relationships to the premature cycle that is described in Figure 1.41. That is it may be flat or show an inverse relationship to the premature coupling interval depending on whether it is conducting in partially or fully excitable tissue. This expected effect of premature impulses on the cycle length of reentry might also be altered in a functional circuit if the premature impulse can somehow cause a change in the size or shape of the circuit. It is not possible to easily predict what the effects would be.

In summary, the relationship between the postextrasystolic cycle and the curtailed cycle when premature impulses are stimulated during a tachycardia caused by reentry may be different than during automaticity. Therefore, premature stimulation during the study of a tachycardia may provide useful information that helps determine whether reentry is the mechanism. However, there are a number of confounding influences to upset the theoretically predicted relationships. These influences include the absence of an excitable gap, and the properties of intervening tissue between the stimulus site and the site of the circuit that can slow or block conduction of premature impulses into and out of the circuit. Therefore, failure to find the relationships expected for a reentrant mechanism does not necessarily mean that the arrhythmia is not caused by reentry.

The concept of entrainment describes the effects of overdrive stimulation on tachycardias caused by reentrant excitation. Waldo et al. (1987) defined entrainment as an increase in the rate of all tissue responsible for sustaining tachycardia to the faster pacing rate (during overdrive) with the resumption of the same tachycardia at its original rate upon abrupt cessation of pacing or slowing of the pacing rate below that of the tachycardia. A description of the basic characteristics of entrainment of a reentrant tachycardia follows. It does not take into account all of the subtleties that have been described during years of continued study. We will point out how these characteristics of entrainment differ from overdrive of other arrhythmogenic mechanisms and how they can be used to indicate a reentrant mechanism. Later, in Chapter IV, we will discuss how entrainment has provided evidence that some of the clinical arrhythmias caused by ischemic heart disease are caused by reentry.

Overdrive pacing resulting in entrainment of a reentrant tachyarrhythmia accelerates the heart rate to the pacing rate. This is not a surprising statement because acceleration of the heart rate should be expected to occur during overdrive of a tachyarrhythmia caused by any arrhythmogenic mechanism. However, there is a fundamental difference between the response of reentry and the other mechanisms. During overdrive of an automatic or triggered focus for example, the excitation wave spreads from the site of pacing over the cardiac chamber to activate it in a pattern that is dependent on the site of stimulation and the way that the impulse spreads from that site. The electrocardiographic wave form of the stimulated chamber (atrial P wave or ventricular QRS) is characteristic of the site of stimulation and the pattern of impulse spread from that site and is not significantly influenced by the arrhythmogenic focus. The focus is activated by the spreading excitation wave and the tissue in the region of the focus simply acts as a part of the conducting pathway. It no longer acts as the site of impulse initiation. After stimulation is discontinued, impulse initiation shifts back to the original site of impulse generation if the mechanism for impulse initiation has not been extinguished (in the case of triggered activity). During overdrive stimulation of a reentrant tachycardia (entrainment), the chamber of the heart that is stimulated is not activated with a pattern only characteristic of the site of stimulation and pattern of impulse spread from that site. The activation pattern occurring during the tachycardia, which is dependent on the location of the reentrant circuit and how the reentrant impulse exits from the circuit is, at least partly retained. Impulses are still emanating from the site of tachycardia origin (the reentrant circuit) during overdrive, but at a faster rate caused by the pacing. As a result, during entrainment the ECG wave form of the chamber in which the circuit is located should be a fusion complex, because it is partly activated by the pacing excitation wave and partly by the reentrant impulse. We will describe how this occurs in the next pages.

The occurrence of fusion between the paced wave front and the reentrant wave front is the first criterion of entrainment; overdrive accelerating the rate of the arrhythmia is demonstrated by the occurrence of consistent fusion complexes. The occurrence of acceleration of the rate of a reentrant arrhythmia during overdrive with the resultant fusion ECG complexes has been shown to occur for a number of different kinds of clinical arrhythmias. However, its occurrence during paroxysmal atrial tachycardia associated with the preexcitation syndrome provides the strongest evidence that it is an important hallmark of reentry (Waldo et al. 1983), since the evidence that this arrhythmia is caused by reentry (involving the AV conducting system and a bypass tract) is the strongest for any clinical arrhythmia (Gallagher et al. 1978). Figure 1.57 explains what the overdrive pacing is doing to the reentrant circuit, why the rate of tachycardia increases and how the fusion occurs. Our description is based on the classical paper of Waldo et al. (1983) and the other publications by this group (MacLean et al. 1981; Waldo et al. 1984; 1987). Diagrams of the reentrant circuit in the preexcitation syndrome are shown as a simple loop with that part of the circuit above the AV node being the atria (A) and that part below, the ventricles (V). The AV node which is a region of slow conduction connects the two at the left and an AV bypass pathway connects them at the right. During tachycardia excitation occurs around the loop as shown by the arrows labeled x in the left panel (spontaneous PAT) traveling from the atria to the ventricles through the AV conducting system and back from the ventricles to the atria via the bypass tract (Wellens and Durrer 1975; Gallagher et al. 1978). The middle panel shows the first stimulated impulse of an overdrive train (PACE Atria), represented by the large unfilled arrow, that reaches and enters the circuit. In order to enter into the circuit as shown, there must be an excitable gap and therefore, entrainment will only occur when an excitable gap is present. The stimulated impulse that enters the circuit (shown by arrows x + 1) propagates both in the antegrade (orthodromic) direction (with respect to the

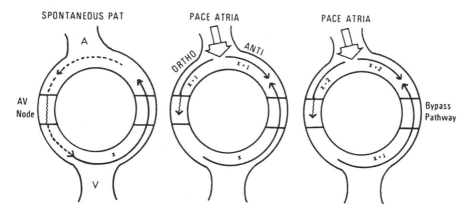

Figure 1.57: Diagram of events occurring during entrainment of a reentrant circuit causing supraventricular tachycardia. A diagram of the reentrant circuit comprised of atrium (A), atrioventricular (AV) node, ventricle (V), and bypass pathway is shown during the arrhythmia (spontaneous PAT) and during overdrive pacing (PACE Atria). The arrows show activation sequences in the reentrant circuit. In the left panel, arrow (x) shows the pattern of activation during the tachycardia. In the center panel, the large unfilled arrowhead above represents the paced atrial impulse entering the circuit to divide into two wave fronts, one represented by arrow x + 1 in the orthodromic direction and the other by arrow x + 1 in the antidromic direction. The antidromic paced wave front (x + 1) continues in the reentrant circuit (as shown in the right panel) only to collide with the next paced wave front (x + 2). (Reproduced from Waldo et al. (1983) with permission.)

direction of propagation of the reentrant excitation wave) and in the retrograde (antidromic) direction. In the antidromic direction, it collides with the reentering impulse already in the circuit (arrow x), extinguishing this reentrant excitation wave. However, the stimulated impulse also continues to propagate through the circuit in the orthodromic direction (x + 1, ortho) starting a new reentrant wave. This is similar to the pattern of activation of reentrant circuits by premature impulses that reset the tachycardia as we described in Figure 1.41. The next stimulated impulse is shown in the right panel (large unfilled arrow and arrows x + 2) to arrive at the circuit and enter in the same way as the first one. In the antidromic direction it collides with the excitation wave from the previous stimulus (arrow x + 1) that is moving around the circuit. This second stimulated impulse also propagates around the circuit in the orthodromic direction (arrow x + 2). This process continues with each stimulated excitation that reaches the circuit during overdrive; collision extinguishes the reentrant wave from the previous stimulus with initiation of a new reentrant excitation wave. Therefore, the rate of the arrhythmia is increased; that is, reentry is occurring more frequently, dictated by the rate of overdrive. The fusion in this model occurs in the atrial part of the circuit where the stimuli are applied and is dependent on the site of collision between the stimulated impulse and the reentrant impulse (initiated by the previous stimulus). As shown in the diagrams in the middle and right panels in Figure 1.57, because of the site of collision (opposing arrowheads at the right), the atria are activated both by the stimulated impulse and the reentrant impulse causing the fusion. The P wave during entrainment of a supraventricular tachycardia of this kind has a positive initial component caused by the stimulated excitation and a following negative component from the retrograde impulse from the reentrant circuit. (During stimulation from this site during sinus rhythm, the P wave is entirely positive, while during the tachycardia it is entirely negative.) We must emphasize that the diagrams represent an interpretation of the results that were initially based on the recording of the electrocardiogram and local electrograms that show a general sequence of activation but not on detailed excitation maps. Subsequently, studies on several experimental arrhythmias in which detailed mapping of reentrant circuits has been accomplished, have confirmed many of the proposals that were originally based on electrogram recordings and electrocardiographic characteristics alone (El-Sherif et al. 1987; Boyden et al. 1989b; Waldecker et al. 1993). Important evidence for the events diagrammed in Figure 1.57 in the studies on WPW was that the site at which an electrogram was recorded in the left atrium in the region of the bypass tract was activated in a retrograde direction during tachycardia by the impulse coming through the bypass tract from the ventricles and that the direction of activation did not change during entrainment with fusion as indicated by an unchanging electrogram morphology. On the other hand, electrograms recorded from the high right atrium were changed during pacing because they were directly activated by the pacing excitation wave and no longer by the reentrant excitation wave (Waldo et al. 1983).

Another characteristic of entrainment is that the original tachycardia resumes when overdrive pacing is stopped. The first QRS after pacing, which has the same ECG morphology as prior to overdrive is actually the last paced impulse without fusion. It was also originally proposed that this first unfused QRS should occur at a cycle length, measured to the last fusion beat, which is equal to the pacing cycle length (Waldo et al. 1983). The explanation for these characteristics is shown in Figure 1.58. The left panel shows the activation sequence during entrainment that is the same as diagrammed in Figure 1.57; there is collision of the stimulated impulse in the antidromic direction (arrow x + 1) with the reentrant impulse (arrow x) emerging from the bypass pathway and conduction of the stimulated impulse in the orthodromic direction through the AV node (arrow x + 1). The last paced impulse initiated in the orthodromic direction continues around the circuit (arrow Xn in the right panel), but is not met by another stimulated impulse since overdrive is stopped; there is no fusion. The last stimulated impulse can continue to propagate around the circuit (dashed arrow in the right panel) and cause the tachycardia to continue. The cycle length to the first unfused QRS after overdrive is the same as the pacing cycle length since this impulse was initiated by the last stimulus in the overdrive train (Waldo et al. 1983).

A third characteristic of transient entrainment is that it may sometimes be demonstrated over a range of overdrive stimulus cycle lengths, and when it is, the degree of fusion increases in favor of the paced activation sequence at the faster pacing rates. This feature can be explained using the diagrams of Figure 1.57. The center and right panels, which show the activation pattern during entrainment, demonstrate the site of collision (and thus the degree of

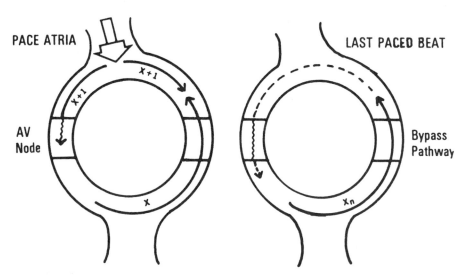

Figure 1.58: Diagram of events occurring at the end of a period of entrainment. The diagram at the left shows the activation patterns during the last paced beat and the diagram at the right shows how reentry continues. The format is similar to Figure 1.57. (Reproduced from Waldo et al. (1983) with permission.)

fusion) in the atrial end of the circuit of the antidromic paced wave front, and the wave front already in the circuit at this stimulus rate. The site of collision is where arrowhead x + 1 in the center panel collides with arrowhead x, and where arrowhead x + 2 in the right panel collides with arrowhead x + 1. When the stimulus rate is increased, this general pattern of activation remains the same. The stimulated excitation wave enters the circuit and collides with the reentrant impulse in the antidromic direction while propagating in the ortho-dromic direction, but the site of collision in the antidromic direction is moved further towards the bypass pathway because, at the faster rate, the paced impulse is initiated earlier with respect to the reentrant impulse and thus has more time to activate the atrium. In order for this to occur, the assumption must be made that conduction time around the circuit is the same or slower for the reentrant impulses initiated at the faster rate of stimulation and that the stimulated impulse arrives in the circuit earlier because of the decreased stimulus cycle length. Because more of the atria is activated directly by the paced impulse, the degree of fusion has increased. In the experiments on atrial tachycardia that led to this explanation, it was shown that the electrogram recorded from the left atrium near the bypass tract (coronary sinus region), which was activated in the retrograde direction by the reentrant impulse dur-ing entrainment at the slower pacing cycle length, was activated in the ante-grade direction during entrainment at the faster pacing rate because the region of collision moved distal to this recording site. In addition, slower conduction in the AV node, which forms part of the reentrant circuit delayed the returning reentrant excitation wave (Waldo et al. 1983).

The final important characteristic of entrainment of a reentrant tachycar-dia is that when the overdrive pacing rate is increased to a critical value, fusion no longer occurs, the ECG morphology becomes characteristic of the pacing site, and tachycardia does not continue when pacing is stopped. All these char-acteristics result from termination of reentry by the overdrive stimulation. In Figure 1.58, the left panel shows the usual pattern of collision in the antidromic direction and propagation in the orthodromic direction during entrainment. If this were the last paced atrial impulse, continuation of tachycardia would be dependent on the orthodromic paced impulse, represented by arrow x + 1, continuing to propagate through the AV node and around the reentrant circuit as indicated by arrow Xn in the right panel. An increase in the rate of overdrive to some critical value can also cause conduction block of the orthodromically conducting impulse (x + 1 in the left panel) in the same way that an early premature impulse blocked in the circuit diagrammed in Figure 1.41C. In the studies on the tachycardia associated with preexcitation, orthodromic block often occurred in the AV node because of its rate sensitivity. Since, when block occurs, there is no conducting reentrant excitation wave, tachycardia does not continue. The region of the reentrant circuit is then activated normally by the next stimulated wavefront causing a change in the ECG morphology to that characteristic of the pacing site. It is necessary to achieve block of both ortho-dromic and antidromic paced wavefronts to terminate the tachycardia. The electrogram recordings in the clinical studies documented the occurrence of block in the AV node as a failure of occurrence of the His bundle electrogram after the stimulated impulse. The region of block was then activated from another direction during the next paced impulse, by the stimulated impulse that spread rapidly into the ventricles over the bypass tract. As part of this third criterion for entrainment, therefore, there is the demonstration of the occurrence of block to a local recording site concomitant with the change in the ECG, followed by activation of that local site from a different direction during the next impulse.

The failure to demonstrate all the criteria for entrainment that we discussed does not necessarily mean that the arrhythmia under study is not caused by reentrant excitation. We have already mentioned that an excitable gap must be present in the circuit for entrainment and termination of an arrhythmia to occur. Reentrant tachycardias caused by the leading circle mechanism, therefore, would not be expected to be entrained and might not be terminated by overdrive although detailed studies of effects of overdrive on this reentrant mechanism are not available. Fusion on the electrocardiogram during overdrive of a reentrant tachycardia might also not be seen, depending on the site of stimulation (Okumura et al. 1985) or the rate of the tachycardia. Pacing from sites distal to the area of slow conduction may prevent the delay of the stimulated impulse in the circuit which is necessary for fusion with the next stimulated activation wave. Also, when pacing proximal to the area of slow conduction, excessive delay of the stimulated impulse in the circuit may allow activation of most of the chamber by the next stimulated excitation wave and fusion would not be seen on the ECG. Fusion might still be seen in the morphology of the electrogram recorded at the site of collision of the reentrant and the stimulated impulse. If the tachycardia rate is very rapid, tachycardia may immediately be terminated at overdrive rates that are fast enough to capture the circuit and thus, the other features of entrainment would not be demonstrated under these circumstances.

Effects of Electrical Stimulation on Arrhythmias Caused by Triggered Activity

Triggered arrhythmias are caused by both early and delayed afterdepolarizations. From our previous discussion of these mechanisms in this chapter it is predicted that the response of arrhythmias caused by each mechanism to stimulation, should be different.

Arrhythmias Caused by Delayed Afterdepolarizations   We described how the amplitude of delayed afterdepolarizations increases with a decrease in the cycle length at which the action potentials occur until the afterdepolarizations reach threshold to cause triggered activity. Therefore, triggered arrhythmias caused by delayed afterdepolarizations in the *in situ* heart should be initiated by either overdrive stimulation or programmed premature stimulation. We have already indicated that automatic arrhythmias are not initiated by stimulation and on this basis, triggered arrhythmias should be readily distinguishable from automatic ones. However, reentrant arrhythmias can also be induced by the same stimulation protocols, so it is important to consider the question of whether there are any other characteristics during initiation that might enable a distinction between triggered activity and reentry. An attempt to distinguish between the two mechanisms is further complicated by experiments showing that triggered activity resulting from different causes, e.g., digitalis, catecholamines, etc., also has different characteristics. The following guidelines have been proposed to assist in distinguishing delayed afterdepolarization-induced triggered activity from other causes of arrhythmias (Rosen et al. 1980; Rosen and Reder 1981). The guidelines are based on the characteristics of triggered activity determined from the *in vitro* studies with microelectrodes.

Triggered activity caused by delayed afterdepolarizations has been more easily induced by rapid pacing or by several successive premature stimuli than by a single premature stimulus in studies on isolated tissue preparations, and therefore, this characteristic is also expected to occur in the heart. Rapid pacing or a number of premature stimuli are more effective in increasing intracellular Ca^{2+} levels, which control the afterdepolarization amplitude, than a single premature stimulus. Also, arrhythmias caused by triggered activity should be more easily induced by premature stimuli superimposed on a rapid drive rate than on a slow one because during rapid pacing, the afterdepolarization amplitude is larger and membrane potential at the peak of the afterdepolarization is closer to threshold. In contrast, reentrant rhythms in humans seem to be more easily and reproducibly induced by premature impulses than by rapid pacing, although several premature impulses in succession are sometimes necessary (Wellens 1978; Akhtar 1984; Brugada and Wellens 1984a; Wellens and Brugada 1984). One reason may be that premature impulses block more effectively in areas with long refractory periods than impulses during rapid pacing, a prerequisite for initiation of reentry, because rapid pacing can shorten refractory period duration.

Extrasystoles or the first beat of tachycardias caused by delayed afterdepolarization-dependent triggered activity initiated by stimulation are predicted to occur late in the cardiac cycle or with long coupling intervals (Rosen et al. 1980). This proposal is based on the experimental data from studies on isolated tissue that show that delayed afterdepolarizations rarely reach their peak amplitude at less than 50% of the cardiac cycle when the drive cycle length is less than 1000 msec. In contrast, reentrant beats often occur early in the cycle (Wit et al. 1982a).

One would expect a direct relationship between the cycle length of a period of stimulation that induces triggered activity dependent on delayed afterdepolarizations and the coupling interval of the first beat of tachycardia caused by triggered activity to the last stimulated impulse. As the pacing cycle length decreases, the coupling interval from the last stimulated impulse to the first impulse of tachycardia should decrease, because at short cycle lengths the coupling interval of the afterdepolarizations to the preceding action potential decreases. A direct relationship between pacing cycle length and coupling of the first impulse of tachycardia has been shown to occur in hearts with arrhythmias caused by digitalis toxicity (Gorgels et al. 1987). This relationship might sometimes be complicated by the presence of two afterdepolarizations and the possibility of a triggered impulse arising from either one (Wit and Rosen 1986). The direct relationship has also been shown in some cases of idiopathic ventricular tachycardia believed to be caused by triggered activity (Lerman et al. 1986). Such a direct relationship is not expected during initiation of reentrant arrhythmias. Failure to show the direct relationship, however, cannot be taken as proof that the arrhythmia is not caused by triggered activity because slow conduction into or out of the triggerable focus can distort it. During initiation of triggered activity with premature stimuli in the microelectrode studies described earlier, there were no significant effects of the premature stimulus coupling interval on the coupling interval of the first triggered impulse to the premature impulse (Johnson and Rosen 1987). On the basis of these data it is expected that, during initiation of arrhythmias caused by triggered activity *in situ* with programmed premature stimulation, the coupling interval of the first beat of tachycardia should remain relatively constant over a range of coupling intervals of premature impulses. The response to premature stimulation is also contrary to that predicted during initiation of reentrant arrhythmias where an inverse relationship is expected between premature stimulus coupling interval and the coupling interval between the premature impulse and first impulse of tachycardia.

Although other characteristics of the initiation of triggered arrhythmias caused by delayed afterdepolarizations have been proposed, we do not think that they are useful for identifying those triggered arrhythmias caused by ischemia or infarction. For example, the cycle length of a tachycardia caused by digitalis-induced delayed afterdepolarizations diminishes when the cycle length of the basic rhythm that induces it is decreased (Wittenberg et al. 1970; Zipes et al. 1974; Gorgels et al. 1983; 1987). However, the cycle length of triggered rhythms resulting from causes other than digitalis has not been shown to have this relationship to the cycle length of the inducing rhythm (Johnson et al. 1986).

Triggered arrhythmias caused by delayed afterdepolarizations, unlike automatic arrhythmias and like reentrant arrhythmias, are predicted to be terminated by electrical stimulation. Single premature impulses may terminate triggered arrhythmias but, based on the results of microelectrode studies, termination should be infrequent and not usually reproducible at the same critical premature cycle length. In contrast, single premature impulses often terminate reentrant arrhythmias in a reproducible manner and over a consistent range of premature cycle lengths in any one individual as long as the reentrant circuit has an excitable gap (Wellens 1978; Akhtar 1984; Josephson et al. 1984; Wellens and Brugada 1984). Therefore, an arrhythmia that is readily terminated by a single prematurely stimulated impulse is more likely to be caused by reentry than by triggered activity. The effects of premature impulses that do not terminate sustained triggered activity have also been determined. The response is almost identical to that of automaticity (Dangman and Hoffman 1985). The return cycle length remains fairly constant over a wide range of premature coupling intervals and nearly the same as the cycle length of the basic triggered rhythm (less than compensatory).

On the other hand, overdrive stimulation should reproducibly terminate triggered arrhythmias. Termination requires a critical rate and duration of overdrive as it does with reentry (Wit et al. 1981b; Moak and Rosen 1984; Johnson et al. 1986). Overdrive stimulation may cause acceleration of triggered arrhythmias followed by gradual slowing and termination or rapid overdrive may cause abrupt termination. A gradual slowing of the rate prior to termination is not expected of reentrant arrhythmias, although reentrant rhythms might be accelerated. Overdrive stimulation that does not terminate triggered activity, such as when the cycle length of overdrive is too long or when the trains of stimuli are too short, does not entrain the arrhythmia (Vos et al. 1989; Furukawa et al. 1990). Although the heart rate is accelerated to the rate of the overdrive, progressive fusion is not realistically expected as during entrainment of a reentrant arrhythmia because the entire chamber of the heart should be activated by the overdrive wave front. One could devise models where some fusion between the overdrive wave front and an activation wave front emanating from the triggered focus could occur, but this would require entrance block into the focus and perhaps other extensive regions of block. While this might occasionally happen, there is no reason to believe that it would occur in the majority of cases. Other characteristics of entrainment as discussed before, are not expected of triggered activity caused by delayed afterdepolarizations. If triggered activity is not terminated by a period of overdrive, the first cycle length following the overdrive may be decreased. There also may be a direct relationship between this first cycle length and the cycle length of overdrive. This is demonstrated in Figure 1.59 that shows experimental data obtained from the digitalis-toxic canine heart (Gorgels et al. 1983). The panels show five simultaneously recorded electrocardiographic leads (I, II, III, V_1, V_6). In the top left panel, the experimental protocol is demonstrated; during ventricular tachycardia (Va), a period of overdrive stimulation (indicated by S) is followed by resumption of tachycardia (V). At the bottom left, it can be seen that after overdrive at a cycle length of 290 msec, the last stimulated impulses (Vs) are followed by a tachycardia impulse with a coupling interval of 395 msec. The bottom middle panel shows that the coupling interval to the first tachycardia impulse decreased to 365 msec after pacing at a cycle length of 250 msec, and the bottom right panel shows that the coupling interval to the first tachycardia impulse decreased even further to 295 msec after a shorter pacing cycle length of 200 msec. This direct relationship between pacing cycle length (Vs-Vs) and cycle length of the first tachycardia impulse (Vs-V) is also shown in the graph at the top right.

It is therefore apparent that although the response of triggered arrhythmias caused by delayed afterdepolarizations to stimulation can be predicted from the experimental studies, there is no single feature that would positively

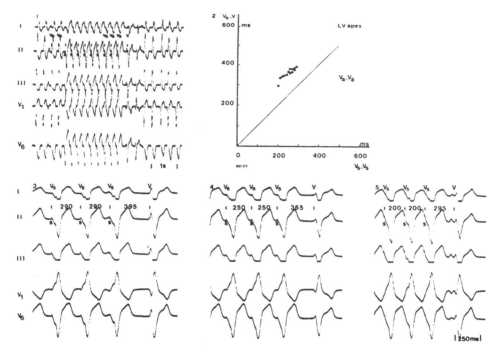

Figure 1.59: Effects of overdrive stimulation on tachycardia caused by delayed afterdepolarization-dependent triggered activity in the digitalis-toxic canine heart. The panel at the upper left shows the experimental protocol. Five electrocardiographic leads are shown (I, II, III, V_1, V_6). "S" beneath complexes of lead II indicates period of overdrive pacing during tachycardia. V_a are ventricular complexes prior to onset of overdrive. V_s indicates the last three stimulated ventricular complexes; V is first postpacing ventricular complex. The three bottom panels show, at an expanded time scale, the last three stimulated complexes during the overdrive train (S) and the first postpacing ventricular complex (V). Overdrive cycle lengths are 290 msec (bottom left panel); 250 msec (bottom middle panel); and 200 msec (bottom right panel). A graph showing the direct relationship between pacing cycle length (V_s-V_s) and first postpacing cycle length (V_s-V) is shown at the upper right. (Reproduced from Gorgels et al. (1983) with permission.)

enable a triggered rhythm to be distinguished from reentry. Since the characteristics of initiation and termination of triggered rhythms by stimulation are very different from the characteristics of automatic rhythms, it should be easier to distinguish between these mechanisms by pacing techniques. However, this differentiation may be made more difficult when an arrhythmia is persistent and the initiation cannot be studied. Also, entrance block of stimulated impulses into arrhythmogenic foci, whether automatic or triggered, may negate the use of pacing techniques to distinguish between these mechanisms.

The characteristics of some clinical arrhythmias occasionally conform to those expected of delayed afterdepolarization-dependent triggered activity (Brugada and Wellens 1984b; Cranefield and Aronson 1988). In addition to digitalis toxicity, an example is some cases of exercise-induced ventricular tachycardia in patients with no structural heart disease (Sung et al. 1983;

Lerman et al. 1986). This tachycardia, which occurs spontaneously during exertion, can sometimes be initiated by overdrive pacing or programmed premature stimulation. An isoproterenol infusion during stimulation may be required for successful initiation. Lerman et al. (1986) have proposed that the tachycardias are caused by a catecholamine-induced increase in cyclic AMP, which is known to cause delayed afterdepolarizations. The termination of tachycardias by intravenous injection of adenosine, which antagonizes the electrophysiological effects of catecholamines mediated through the adenylate cyclase-cyclic AMP system supports this hypothesis. Adenosine does not significantly effect other arrhythmogenic mechanisms (Rosen et al. 1983). Jackman et al. (1984) have also proposed that some forms of ventricular tachycardia associated with the congenital long QT syndrome, and that are dependent on adrenergic stimulation, are a result of triggered activity caused by delayed afterdepolarizations. Cranefield and Aronson (1988) have provided a detailed review of the clinical arrhythmias that may be caused by triggered activity.

Arrhythmias Caused by Early Afterdepolarizations   Arrhythmias caused by early afterdepolarizations should not be inducible by overdrive pacing, similar to automatic arrhythmias and unlike arrhythmias caused by delayed afterdepolarizations or reentry. Similarly, triggered activity that is dependent on early afterdepolarizations is not expected to immediately follow the short cycle length of one or several prematurely stimulated impulses. As shown in the experimental studies, the appearance of early afterdepolarization-induced triggered activity is facilitated by long cycle lengths and therefore, this kind of triggered activity should be initiated by slowing the basic heart rate. Of course, if an increase in heart rate caused by pacing, for example, caused entrance block into a focus where early afterdepolarizations occur, the block could cause a prolongation of the cycle length in that focus that might result in triggered activity (Cranefield and Aronson 1988). Prematurely stimulated impulses might also initiate triggered activity caused by early afterdepolarizations if there is a long compensatory pause following the stimulated impulse. The long cycle might trigger an arrhythmia that would follow it (Cranefield and Aronson 1988). In the absence of such entrance block, bursts of tachycardia caused by early afterdepolarizations should occur more frequently when the heart rate is slowed, and pacing the heart at faster rates than the basic underlying rhythm is predicted to cause disappearance of the periods of tachycardia. Increasing the basic heart rate shortens action potential duration and thereby suppresses early afterdepolarizations. When the pacing is stopped arrhythmias should reappear as the action potential returns to its original duration. However, the reappearance of the arrhythmias may not be immediate because it requires some time for the action potential duration to lengthen, owing to the enhanced pump current that follows a period of rapid stimulation.

Many of these characteristics have been shown to apply to the experimental triggered arrhythmias caused be cesium in the *in situ* canine heart (Brachmann et al. 1983b; Levine et al. 1985; Hanich et al. 1988b) and have been demonstrated in some cases of torsade de pointes in patients. As previously discussed, torsade de pointes is ventricular tachycardia characterized by QRS complexes with peaks that twist around the isoelectric line in patients with a prolonged QT interval (Coumel et al. 1984). Acquired forms of the syndrome (prolonged QT and torsade caused by quinidine for example) exhibit all the features expected of triggered activity caused by early afterdepolarizations whereas other forms (congenital) may not be due to this mechanism (Schechter et al. 1984). Torsade de pointes invariably occurs after a preceding long R-R interval (Kay et al. 1983; Roden et al. 1986), is unlikely to be initiated by programmed stimulation (Bhandari et al. 1985; Coumel et al. 1984) and can be prevented from occurring by pacing the heart at a rapid rate (Kay et al. 1983; Coumel et al. 1984). Cranefield and Aronson (1988) have also proposed that repetitive monomorphic ventricular tachycardia, described by Coumel et al. (1985) and Zimmermann et al. (1986), is caused by early afterdepolarizations. These tachycardias also occur after a long R-R interval and their occurrence is prevented during and after a period of overdrive pacing. Other kinds of arrhythmias with these characteristics might also be caused by early afterdepolarizations. In contrast, as we have described, triggered arrhythmias caused by delayed afterdepolarizations may become more frequent as heart rate increases (Rosen et al. 1980) and the effects of increasing the heart rate on reentry may be variable; reentry might be exacerbated or it might stop (Wit et al. 1972b). However, there may be some difficulty in distinguishing early afterdepolarization-dependent triggered arrhythmias from automatic ones only on the basis of their response to electrical stimulation since the occurrence of automatic arrhythmias is facilitated by slow heart rates and increasing the basic heart rate by overdrive pacing may cause disappearance of automatic arrhythmias during the periods of pacing. The electrocardiographic characteristics of arrhythmias caused by the triggered activity and by automaticity might be of additional help. The triggered rhythms are more likely to occur in bursts or salvos of different lengths with the first few cycle lengths of a burst decreasing progressively and the last few cycle lengths increasing progressively.

Triggered arrhythmias caused by early afterdepolarizations might not only occur in bursts, but might also be sustained. When sustained, their response to a single premature stimulus or overdrive pacing can be predicted on the basis of the results of the *in vitro* studies described before. Some arrhythmias might be terminated by premature stimuli, but this should be a relatively rare occurrence. The effects of premature stimulated impulses that do not terminate the arrhythmia are expected to be the same as their effects on automatic impulse initiation. Some arrhythmias also might be terminated by overdrive pacing but termination should not be the usual effect. When termination occurs it is expected to immediately follow the overdrive, whereas termination of triggered activity caused by delayed afterdepolarizations may sometimes be preceded by up to ten triggered "afterbeats" (Moak and Rosen 1984; Wit et al. 1981b). When termination does not occur, overdrive is not expected to cause any significant effect on the rhythm; the response should be more similar to an arrhythmia caused by abnormal automaticity (Dangman and Hoffman

1983) than normal automaticity, which is readily overdrive-suppressed (Vassalle 1970). Because of this variability of response, stimulation during a sustained tachycardia caused by early afterdepolarizations is not much help in determining the mechanism.

Therefore, like the triggered arrhythmias caused by delayed afterdepolarizations, there is no single feature in the response to electrical stimulation that would positively enable an early afterdepolarization-induced triggered rhythm to be distinguished from other arrhythmogenic mechanisms. Early afterdepolarization-induced nonsustained arrhythmias can usually be differentiated by pacing from rhythms induced by delayed afterdepolarizations or automaticity at high membrane potentials and sometimes from reentry, but the response of sustained triggered activity to pacing is often indistinguishable from abnormal automaticity occurring at low membrane potentials.

Summary of Effects of Electrical Stimulation

Despite the fact that there are exceptions and inconsistencies to all the rules that can be proposed to distinguish among the different arrhythmogenic mechanisms using stimulation techniques, determining the effects of electrical stimulation is really quite useful. We will summarize the most important points.

1. Initiation of a tachycardia by stimulation most often indicates that the arrhythmia is caused either by reentry or delayed afterdepolarization-induced triggered activity. Other characteristics of initiation that we described are then useful in distinguishing between the two. Other mechanisms for arrhythmias such as automaticity and triggered activity caused by early afterdepolarizations are usually eliminated.

2. Termination of a tachycardia by overdrive or premature stimulation is expected of reentry or triggered activity caused by delayed afterdepolarizations, but not of automaticity and rarely of early afterdepolarization-dependent triggered activity. Overdrive suppression is expected of arrhythmias caused by normal automaticity and overdrive acceleration may occur with arrhythmias caused by abnormal automaticity.

3. Entrainment of a tachycardia during overdrive is indicative of a reentrant mechanism and is not expected of other mechanisms.

4. The pattern of the response to premature stimulation is expected to be different during arrhythmias caused by automaticity and those caused by reentry (when it is not terminated). During automatic arrhythmias the return cycle length should not increase and might even decrease as the premature coupling interval decreases. The return cycle should be less than compensatory. During reentrant arrhythmias the return cycle length should increase as the premature impulse occurs earlier in the dominant cycle. The increase may sometimes begin to occur with late coupled premature impulses or it may not occur until premature impul-

ses are early coupled. The return cycle length is often less than compensatory.

Electrical Stimulation of the Normal Ventricles

Now that we have defined the effects of electrical stimulation on different arrhythmogenic mechanisms, we briefly consider how the normal (nonischemic) heart responds to stimulation. Since ischemic and infarcted hearts are prone to arrhythmia induction by stimulation techniques, it is necessary to be sure that these arrhythmias are not induced in normal hearts in order to attribute their occurrence to the effects of ischemia and infarction.

Induction of Ventricular Fibrillation

It has been known for a long time that a single electrical stimulus, if strong enough and properly timed in the cardiac cycle, can induce ventricular fibrillation in the normal heart (King 1934). Mines (1914) also applied his concepts on the initiation of reentry to the initiation of fibrillation by the application of stimuli to the heart. He described that, "It was found in a number of experiments that a single tap of the Morse key if properly timed would start fibrillation . . . In the production of fibrillation just described, the stimulus apparently arrives at some part of the ventricular muscle just at the end of the refractory phase and probably before the refractory phase has ended in some other regions of the muscle". The initiation of fibrillation, by analogy, was attributed to the same mechanism as the initiation of rhythmic beating in the rings of cardiac muscle: unidirectional block and slow conduction around the circuit.

This phenomenon of induction of fibrillation by single stimuli was studied subsequently in several laboratories (Williams et al. 1934; Wiggers and Wégria 1940), the most influential publication being that of Wiggers and Wégria (1940) in which the term "vulnerable period" was introduced. The vulnerable period corresponds to the end of the T wave and is related to the so-called "dip" phenomenon, a period of hyperexcitability during the relative refractory period (Brooks et al. 1955) that is due to anodal excitation (Van Dam 1960). During this phase, stimuli of increasingly greater intensity first produce single responses, then multiple responses, ventricular fibrillation, and finally no response at all (the "no-response" phenomenon (Brooks et al. 1955)). Fibrillation can only be induced by bipolar stimulation and is due to excitation at the anode (Harris and Moe 1942; Cranefield et al. 1957; Hoffman and Cranefield 1960; Hoffman and Cranefield 1964). However, Van Dam (1960) was unable to induce fibrillation by applying strong anodal pulses alone during the vulnerable period via small electrodes, and he concluded that a large area had to be stimulated for fibrillation to occur. Opinions about the necessary intensity of the stimuli differ, possibly because electrodes of different sizes have been used. Sometimes fibrillation thresholds are about 20 times as great as those for diastolic stimulation (Hoffman and Cranefield 1964; Matta et al. 1976; Gang et al. 1982) while other reports give a figure of several hundred times diastolic threshold (Moe et al. 1941). In any case, the induction of ventricular fibrillation in a normal heart by a single stimulus requires that it has a strong intensity and that it is delivered during the vulnerable period.

There are several possible mechanisms for the initiation of ventricular fibrillation by shocks delivered during the vulnerable period. One is that during the vulnerable period, there exists a heterogeneous state of excitability or nonuniform dispersion of refractoriness. Some myocardial fibers are in their absolute refractory period, others are partially refractory, and still others have regained full excitability due in large part to different time courses of repolarization. Anodal current has been proposed to increase this heterogeneity in excitability by inducing repolarization in fibers in their plateau phase, and by hyperpolarizing fibers already repolarized, even to such an extent that impulses will not be propagated (Brooks et al. 1955). Anodal break-excitation can occur at the end of the pulse, cathodal make-excitation at the beginning (Dekker 1970). Since the currents are strong, and the bipolar arrangements of the fairly large electrode ensures that a large amount of tissue is involved, the inhomogeneities induced by the procedure could well set the stage for local reentry that begins the fibrillatory process. Another mechanism has been proposed by Chen et al. (1988), based on the results of three-dimensional activation maps in a limited region of ventricular myocardium. This mechanism is described by the schematic diagram shown in Figure 1.60. Activation during the regular rhythm begins at S_1 and moves away from this site in a pattern indicated by the solid line isochrones in the left panel. The sequence of isochrones from e-a is also the sequence of repolarization with the earliest activated area (e) repolarizing first and the latest activated area, (a), repolarizing last. When a shock is given at S_2, the shock field is distributed in a pattern illustrated by the dashed lines with the strength of the potential gradient strongest closest to the electrodes and weakest furthest from the electrodes (decreasing from 1 to 5). In the vicinity of the S_2 electrode, the shock cannot excite the myocardium because it has not yet repolarized, and instead prolongs refractoriness by either eliciting graded responses (Kao and Hoffman 1958) or by prolonging the action potential duration (Dillon 1991). The region of prolonged refractoriness is shown by the black area in the middle panel. At a distance from the S_2 electrode, where excitability is recovered sufficiently (diagonal lines in the middle panel), S_2 can initiate excitation waves, which as shown by the arrow in the right panel, may then propagate away from the border of the directly depolarized region, around the area of block, and enter the blocked region from the opposite side after it is no longer refractory to cause reentry. This mechanism is analogous to the formation of rotors in excitable media because it does not rely on preexisting heterogeneities in the properties of the myocardial cells, but on the heterogeneities introduced by the prior excitation wave.

The feeling that the technique of applying strong shocks to the heart may

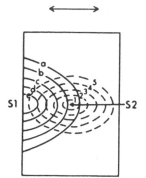 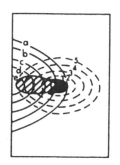 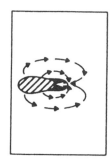

Figure 1.60: Schematic diagram of proposed mechanism for reentry induced by a shock that causes ventricular fibrillation. The left panel shows the sequence of repolarization (indicated by solid isochrones a, b, c, d, e) after a wave front initiated at S_1. Solid lines e-a indicate increasing degrees of recovery. Also superimposed on this sequence is the location and strength of the field (dashed ellipses) generated by a premature stimulus S_2. Dashed lines 1–5 indicate decreasing strength of the S_2 field. In the center panel, the region indicated by hatching is directly depolarized by the S_2 stimulus. The region indicated in black undergoes a graded response that causes prolongation of refractory periods. Arrows in the right panel show pathway of activation following premature stimulation at S_2. Activation conducts away from border of directly depolarized region in all directions except towards the region undergoing a graded response in which refractory periods were prolonged. This region is activated later (white arrow). Activation then reenters the directly depolarized region. (Reproduced from Chen et al. (1988) with permission).

be too far removed from the events occurring in either normal hearts that are put under some form of stress or in diseased hearts led to other techniques by which it was hoped to measure "electrical instability". Thus, the finding that the threshold for fibrillation was only slightly higher than that for multiple responses to a single stimulus (Hoffman et al. 1951) led to the use of the "multiple response threshold" (Han and Moe 1964). Nevertheless, it is still necessary to apply strong stimuli during the vulnerable period to obtain multiple responses. Later, it was found that by introducing two premature stimuli at only twice diastolic threshold, the intensity of a third premature stimulus necessary to induce multiple ventricular responses, or even fibrillation, could be much reduced (Thompson and Lown 1972; Matta et al. 1976). Thus, the use of the term "vulnerability" may mean different things, such as the intensity of a single shock applied during the vulnerable period, or the intensity of the third of a series of three premature stimuli, which results in either ventricular fibrillation or multiple ventricular responses. The common denominator of these different techniques is that bipolar stimulation is used. Since in most studies, both cathodal and anodal electrodes have had the same dimensions, both cathodal and anodal currents have their effects, those of the anode being more important because the vulnerable period coincides with the phase in the cardiac cycle when excitability for anodal currents is lowest. It is also important to note that ventricular tachycardias lasting for more than just several beats are not induced in normal hearts by these stimulation procedures.

Induction of Ventricular Arrhythmias

Although the classical investigations described above carefully defined the conditions needed for induction of ventricular fibrillation in normal hearts by strong stimuli, they do not address the important question of whether "physiological stimuli" (defined as being low-intensity electrical stimuli of 2–10 times diastolic threshold that elicit a response in the vicinity of small diameter cathodal or bipolar stimulating electrodes) can induce arrhythmias in the normal ventricle. These physiological stimuli produce propagating impulses rather than the complex excitation patterns resulting from anodal and cathodal currents flowing through large amounts of tissue.

The effects of single premature stimuli applied to the ventricles of a normal human heart or the heart of an experimental animal either during sinus rhythm or while driving the ventricle at a constant rate are clear and consistent. When the duration of the premature stimuli is kept less than 5 msec, the strength less than 10 times diastolic threshold, and the stimuli are applied to regions other than the interventricular septum, arrhythmias of any kind including ventricular fibrillation are rarely induced no matter where the stimuli are applied in the cardiac cycle, even during the vulnerable period (Janse 1971; Karagueuzian et al. 1979; Moore et al. 1980; Echt et al. 1983; Hamer et al. 1984; Garan et al. 1985). Similarly, overdrive stimulation at cycle lengths greater than about 200 msec does not initiate arrhythmias. It can be concluded, therefore, that either triggered activity caused by delayed afterdepolarizations or reentry are not easily initiated in the normal ventricles. The exception is that a single premature stimulus delivered to the right ventricular septum of the canine or human heart may induce a nonstimulated response following the stimulated response, that is, caused by bundle branch reentry, that is, reentry involving a circuit that includes the His bundle and the bundle branches (Moe et al. 1956) by the mechanism that was described earlier in this chapter. Occasionally, two or three successive bundle branch reentrant beats occur. In about 6% of patients in whom a sustained ventricular tachycardia can be induced by programmed stimulation, the underlying mechanism is bundle branch reentry (Caceres et al. 1989). However, in order for sustained tachycardia to occur, there must be some disease of the conducting system that slows conduction. Sustained tachycardia does not occur in circuits comprised of the bundle branches when the conducting system is normal.

In general it appears that more aggressive stimulation protocols, meaning when more than one premature stimulus is applied in succession or more rapid rates of overdrive stimulation, can sometimes induce arrhythmias in the normal ventricles even when the stimuli are only slightly greater than threshold intensity. In dogs, 2–5 successive ventricular premature stimuli rarely (1.5%

to 12% incidence) induce repetitive ventricular responses or ventricular fibrillation if the stimulus durations are short (< 5 msec) and the stimulus strengths are low (less than 1.5–4 times diastolic threshold) (Janse 1971; Michelson et al. 1981d; Hamer et al. 1984; Garan et al. 1985; Scherlag et al. 1985). Repetitive ventricular responses are classified as 1–5 nonstimulated responses following the stimulated premature impulses, which are caused by intramyocardial rather than bundle branch reentry. The mechanism may depend on the normal dispersion of refractoriness that occurs in ventricular muscle resulting in unidirectional block, slow conduction, and reentry of the premature impulses. Although originally described as being a specific arrhythmia in hearts with ischemic disease that are susceptible to severe tachyarrhythmias and sudden death (Greene et al. 1978), numerous subsequent studies have shown that these arrhythmias can be initiated in normal as well as ischemic hearts (Brugada et al. 1984; Buxton et al. 1984a; 1984b). Ventricular fibrillation has also been induced in experimental animal hearts (Wetstein et al. 1982; Hamer et al. 1984) and in patients without ischemic heart disease by programmed ventricular stimulation with low-intensity stimuli (Brugada et al. 1984; Morady et al. 1984b). It is rare that it is induced by one or two premature stimuli and more likely to be induced by three or four premature stimuli. However, induction of ventricular fibrillation by even four low-intensity premature stimuli is relatively rare in normal hearts. Very rapid overdrive stimulation might also induce repetitive responses or fibrillation in the normal heart, particularly if coronary perfusion is decreased during stimulation, causing a period of ischemia.

Nonsustained ventricular tachycardia, usually defined as six beats to about 30 seconds of polymorphic or monomorphic tachycardia (rate more than 100/min) can be induced by programmed stimulation in up to about 45% of human hearts without ischemic disease (Brugada et al. 1984; Morady et al. 1984b). It is rarely induced by a single premature stimulated impulse, more frequently induced by two successive premature stimulated impulses, and more frequently still by three premature stimulated impulses; in the majority of cases, three premature stimuli are needed (Brugada et al. 1984; Morady et al. 1984a; Kudenchuk et al. 1986). Like repetitive responses, the mechanism for this arrhythmia is probably dependent on dispersion of ventricular muscle refractoriness leading to reentry. In our experience, such nonsustained tachycardias can rarely be induced in normal canine hearts by 1–3 premature stimuli of low intensity.

Sustained monomorphic or polymorphic ventricular tachycardia cannot be induced by programmed stimulation in normal experimental animal hearts. Sustained monomorphic ventricular tachycardia also cannot be induced in human hearts without ischemic or structural heart disease when there is no evidence of spontaneously occurring tachyarrhythmias (Brugada et al. 1984; Buxton et al. 1984a; Morady et al. 1984b). Unlike nonsustained tachycardia, it is not seen as a nonclinical arrhythmia caused by reentry in normal myocardial tissue. Sustained monomorphic ventricular tachycardia can be induced in human hearts without clinical evidence of ischemic or structural heart disease when there is documented spontaneous occurrence of the arrhythmia (Lerman 1988). We suspect that these hearts have pathological changes or a biochemical abnormality that cannot be detected with standard clinical techniques. Sustained polymorphic ventricular tachycardia may be induced in human hearts without evidence of ischemic heart disease by aggressive stimulation protocols (Brugada et al. 1983; 1984).

In summary, some general conclusions can be made concerning the effects of stimuli on the rhythm of the normal ventricles, to provide a basis for comparison with the effects of stimuli on ischemic or infarcted ventricles. Single strong stimuli with appropriate characteristics (long duration greater than 10 msec and up to several hundred times diastolic threshold) applied during the vulnerable period induce ventricular fibrillation. Fibrillation may also be induced by a series of 3–4 premature stimuli of only several times diastolic threshold or by overdrive stimulation at very rapid rates. Reentry is the most likely mechanism that causes fibrillation. Single premature stimuli even during the vulnerable period do not induce arrhythmias when the strength of the stimuli is limited to several times that which is necessary to excite a propagated response during diastole. Multiple premature stimuli with a short pulse duration and several times diastolic threshold, or overdrive stimulation at cycle lengths at which reasonable coronary perfusion is maintained, rarely induce arrhythmias. When they do, the arrhythmias are often short runs of very rapid and irregular nonsustained ventricular tachycardia or ventricular fibrillation. Therefore, the distinguishing feature between those premature stimuli that induce ventricular fibrillation in normal hearts and those that do not is the magnitude of the current applied to the heart. Long periods of nonsustained tachycardia (greater than a few seconds), or sustained uniform ventricular tachycardias cannot usually be induced in normal hearts no matter what the stimulation protocol or the strength of the stimuli (including strong stimuli applied during the vulnerable period).

Chapter II

Ventricular Arrhythmias in the Acute Phase of Myocardial Ischemia and Infarction

Arrhythmias in Man: Relationship to Sudden Death

The term acute phase of myocardial ischemia refers to events occurring within the first 2–4 hours after the sudden onset of a reduction of blood flow through a coronary artery. There is compelling clinical evidence that acute myocardial ischemia is one of the most important causes of ventricular arrhythmias in humans. Sudden cardiac death, which in the great majority of cases is due to ventricular fibrillation, occurs almost exclusively in people with coronary artery disease (Davies 1981; Goldstein et al. 1981). Only a minority of those individuals who have been successfully resuscitated from sudden ventricular fibrillation subsequently developed a myocardial infarction (Cobb et al. 1980; Goldstein et al. 1981) suggesting that if indeed myocardial ischemia was involved, it was transient. In two thirds of the population that developed ventricular fibrillation outside the hospital, collapse occurred almost instantly (within 1 minute) after the onset of symptoms (chest pain or dyspnea) (Liberthson et al. 1974; 1982), indicating that if the onset of symptoms can be equated with the onset of ischemia, ischemia need only exist for a short time in order to induce arrhythmias. This proposed relationship between transient ischemia and arrhythmias has been corroborated by studies in patients with transient coronary artery spasm in whom ventricular arrhythmias, including ventricular fibrillation, occur within minutes after the beginning of electrocardiographic signs of myocardial ischemia caused by the spasm (Maseri et al. 1982). Most often, arrhythmias develop when ST segment elevation is either still growing or when it has reached maximal levels, but there are reports in which arrhythmias were found to occur after ST segment changes had returned to normal (Maseri et al. 1982; Araki et al. 1983; Previtali et al. 1983; Tzivoni et al. 1983). Thus, arrhythmias can result both from transient ischemia during the ST segment changes and from reperfusion (after return of the ST segment to normal). In a study in which more than 7,000 transient ischemic periods were monitored using ST segment changes as an indicator of ischemia, single ventricular premature depolarizations and bigeminy were quite frequent. Severe arrhythmias

161

(ventricular tachycardia and fibrillation) occurred in 18% of the patients, but in only 3.6% of the ischemic episodes (Maseri et al. 1982).

Evidence from ambulatory ECG recordings in patients dying suddenly does, surprisingly, not always unequivocally indicate that transient ischemia is the main culprit. It is true that the majority of these patients have coronary artery disease. It is also true that in these patients ventricular fibrillation is the cause of death in more than 90% of cases. Most frequently, a ventricular tachycardia, which may be initiated by either an early or a late ventricular premature beat, eventually degenerated into ventricular fibrillation. However, ST segment changes preceding the fatal event were observed in a minority of cases in some studies (10% to 20%) (Bayés de Luna et al. 1985; 1989; Leclercq et al. 1986; 1988). It may be argued that these were selected patients (otherwise they would not have been on ambulatory monitoring) and that the presence of ischemia was not detected by a single monitor ECG lead. There are also other reports indicating that 50% to 64% of patients on ambulatory monitoring developed signs or symptoms of ischemia (ST segment elevation or depression, T wave inversion, anginal complaints) shortly before the fatal arrhythmia (Liberthson et al. 1982; Roelandt et al. 1984). The relationship between ischemia and sudden death is further supported by the finding of Goldstein et al. (1986) that of 227 patients with coronary artery disease who were successfully resuscitated after out-of-hospital arrest, 40% had an acute myocardial infarction, 37% an ischemic event, whereas 18% were classified as a "primary arrhythmic event". Another study in survivors of out-of-hospital cardiac arrest revealed a high incidence of painless ST depression following exercise that might have been associated with the "fatal" arrhythmia (Sharma et al. 1987). Finally, the frequency of ischemic episodes increases in the early morning and wanes in the early afternoon and evening. The onset of myocardial infarction and of sudden death have a similar circadian variation, implying that sudden death occurs when ischemia is most common (Muller et al. 1985; 1987). Still, factors other than ischemia must be considered. While it is admitted that these may largely be unknown, an increase in sympathetic tone seems to be an important factor in initiating fatal arrhythmias (Lown 1979b; Leclercq et al. 1988).

When coronary artery occlusion is not transient but persists (because of for example occlusive thrombi or long-lasting spasm), ischemic cells become irreversibly damaged and myocardial infarction results. The relationship between total occlusion of a coronary artery and infarction has been documented in both clinical and postmortem pathological studies (DeWood et al. 1980; Davies and Thomas 1984). The incidence of ventricular arrhythmias during the acute phase of myocardial infarction (first 24 hours after onset of symptoms) is higher than for transient ischemic episodes although it varies widely in different reports: ventricular premature depolarization 10% to 93%; ventricular tachycardia 3% to 39%; ventricular fibrillation 4% to 36% (for a review see Bigger et al. 1977). These differences might be explained if different time intervals elapsed between onset of symptoms (which may indicate the onset of the occlusion) and the moment the patient was examined. Arrhythmias are severe only during certain time periods and not continuously. The true incidence of ventricular fibrillation must, of course, be higher than reported since many patients succumb before medical examination is possible (Pisa 1980). Therefore, there is no doubt that myocardial ischemia, whether transient and causing reversible changes, or permanent and resulting in myocardial infarction, causes arrhythmias in humans.

It is generally accepted that the occurrence of lethal arrhythmias in humans is the result of the interplay between several factors, which are called substrate, trigger, and modulating factors (Coumel 1987). As a substrate one may consider the functional changes brought about by acute ischemia creating the setting for functional reentrant circuits within the ischemic myocardium, or the anatomical arrangement of surviving myocardial fibers within a healed infarct that provide an anatomically defined reentrant circuit. Arrhythmias in the setting of acute ischemia or infarction will only become manifest in the presence of appropriate triggers, such as ventricular premature depolarizations (Lown and Wolf 1971), especially when they occur after a long pause (Leclercq et al. 1988), or increases in heart rate. Modulating factors, such as the activity of the sympathetic nervous system, electrolyte disturbances (for example low serum K^+ levels (Nordrehaug and von der Lippe 1983)), or impaired left ventricular function may modify both the substrate and the trigger. The different experimental models that have been used to study the arrhythmias resulting from ischemia and infarction vary in respect to substrate, triggers and modulating factors.

Animal Models of Acute Ischemic Arrhythmias

The study of electrophysiological changes in cardiac muscle and mechanisms of arrhythmias caused by acute ischemia cannot easily be done in patients and, therefore, experimental models are used. The majority of studies in these models involve obstructing flow through a coronary artery to cause ischemia. The experimental animal that is most often used for investigations on electrophysiological mechanisms of arrhythmias caused by ischemia is the dog, but pigs, cats, rabbits, ferrets, guinea pigs, and rats have been studied as well. It is sometimes difficult to compare the results of studies on the different species because of differences in electrophysiological properties of the heart, and differences in cardiac and coronary artery anatomy. All these factors, as we will discuss, may influence the end result of an ischemic episode. Such a comparison is necessary to formulate an overall concept of the mechanism of ischemic arrhythmias. Even within one species, such as the dog, it may be difficult to compare the different studies in regard to incidence, severity, and mechanism of arrhythmias induced by acute ischemia because different experimental protocols have been used.

In an effort to introduce some sort of standardization, a set of guidelines for the study of arrhythmias caused by ischemia, infarction, and reperfusion, known as the Lambeth Conventions, was published by Walker et al. in 1988.

The Lambeth Conventions addresses statistical problems, uniformity of animals, classification and detection of arrhythmias, definition and detection of ischemia and infarction. It does not particularly focus on arrhythmia mechanisms. The guidelines are especially useful when large numbers of animals (usually small animals such as rats) are used and their response to antiarrhythmic drugs is studied.

A great many factors related to the experimental procedures determine whether arrhythmias will occur and why they occur during the imposition of acute ischemia on the heart. Among the factors are (1) the method used to occlude the coronary artery; (2) the number of successive coronary artery occlusions because sometimes an artery may be occluded transiently; (3) the size of the ischemic area, which is dependent on the location of the occlusion and the number of preexisting collaterals; (4) the kind of anesthetic agents that are used or whether any have been used at all; (5) the presence of previous infarction or cardiac hypertrophy; (6) the heart rate; (7) whether the arrhythmias studied are during occlusion or after reperfusion, and (8) the activity of the autonomic nervous system. The following is a brief description of the main experimental variables.

Mode of Coronary Artery Occlusion

In studies on acute arrhythmias caused by ischemia, complete sudden occlusion of a coronary artery is often performed. In the anesthetized animal with the heart exposed, this may be done by tying a ligature around the vessel, or by clamping it with a broad clamp. This last method has the advantage that it permits release of the obstruction by release of the clamp, resulting in sudden reperfusion that can cause arrhythmias as well. In anesthetized animals with the chest closed, a coronary artery can be occluded with a balloon on the end of a catheter positioned in a coronary ostium. In conscious animals, complete occlusion can be performed by suddenly tightening a previously placed snare around the vessel, or by inflating a balloon occluder positioned around a coronary artery during a previous operation.

With any of these techniques there may still be some residual coronary blood flow to the ischemic regions through anastomoses of the occluded artery with nonoccluded arteries. The level of residual flow may determine the severity of the resulting ischemic arrhythmias. Coronary occlusion may also be implemented by injection of small diameter microspheres or latex into a coronary artery. This procedure also occludes the anastomosing vessels or collaterals and eliminates flow almost entirely, increasing the severity of ischemia. For the study of arrhythmias in later phases of ischemia and infarction, Harris (1950) introduced a technique by which a coronary artery is occluded in two stages: initially, a stenosis is produced resulting in a flow reduction in the order of 50%, and 30 minutes later the artery is completely occluded (described in more detail in Chapter III). The incidence of severe acute arrhythmias is considerably less following this procedure than after abrupt complete coronary occlusion (Harris 1950; Clark and Cummings 1956; Kabell et al. 1982). Hence the mode of occlusion may influence the experimental results.

Investigators using these techniques realize that the experimental occlusion of a coronary artery is significantly different from what happens in human hearts where often long standing atherosclerotic changes in the coronary arteries precede the final occlusive event, which is often the formation of a thrombus, possibly accompanied by vasospasm. These differences in mode of occlusion might certainly influence the nature and time course of electrophysiological changes. Therefore, one always has to be aware that the experimental situation cannot totally mimic what is happening in humans. As an example, the following case is shown in Figure 2.1. The patient from whom these recordings were obtained visited his cardiologist because in previous days he had experienced brief episodes of chest pain. In the office, an exercise test was performed, which was negative; that is, no changes in the ST segment of the electrocardiogram were noted, nor did pain appear. Upon leaving the office, intensive chest pain suddenly occurred and persisted. Within minutes an ambulance arrived and the electrocardiograms shown in Figure 2.1 were recorded on a Lown Trendscriber during transport of the patient to the hospital. Each line is a 30-second recording. Note the development of ST segment elevation in strips 3 to 8, and the return to a isoelectric ST segment in subsequent strips. A second period of ST segment elevation is seen in the lower strips, and in the next to last strip ventricular fibrillation suddenly develops. In the lowest strip the artifact produced by the defibrillator and the subsequent QRS complexes, indicating successful defibrillation, are seen. The fact that the ST segment was waxing and waning, suggests the occurrence of brief phases of total coronary occlusion separated by periods during which flow was temporarily restored. This "stuttering" ischemia alters the time course of events: instead of fibrillation occurring within 10 minutes, as would be expected from animal experiments in which total abrupt coronary ligation is performed, this arrhythmia only appeared about 1 hour after the onset of symptoms.

Location of Coronary Artery Occlusion

The size of the ischemic region that results from an experimental coronary occlusion and the severity of the ventricular arrhythmias that occur are related to the particular coronary artery that is occluded and the distance of the occlusion from the origin of the coronary artery. Stephenson and coworkers (1960) completely occluded the left anterior descending coronary artery at the highest level possible, an average distance of 10 mm from the ostium of the sinus of Valsalva, in 330 anesthetized dogs. During the first 30 minutes, 28% developed ventricular fibrillation. Of the 239 dogs that survived this 30-minute period, 71% developed ventricular fibrillation upon release of the occlusion. As already mentioned, reperfusion arrhythmias may occur in man upon cessation of coro-

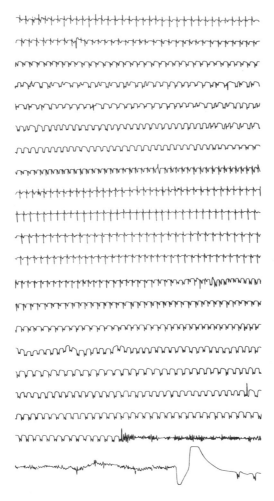

Figure 2.1: Selected strips of a continuous recording of the electrocardiogram of a patient in the very early phase of myocardial infarction. ST segment elevation is seen in the 3rd to 8th trace and in the 15th to 20th strip. Fibrillation occurred during the 20th trace. (Unpublished observations of R.W. Koster.)

nary artery spasm and animal experiments on reperfusion arrhythmias will be discussed separately. Occlusion of the circumflex at its origin has an even greater arrhythmogenic effect. The incidence of ventricular fibrillation was 58% in the study of Allen and Laadt (1950). The difference in the incidence of arrhythmias between left anterior descending coronary artery and circumflex occlusion is at least partly related to the size of the ischemic area that results because the circumflex supplies a greater area of the left ventricle than the left anterior descending coronary artery.

In studies in which the occlusion of the circumflex was several millimeters from the origin, the incidence of fibrillation decreased to around 20%, because the size of the ischemic region was greatly reduced. It was also found that the number of nonoccluded branches proximal to the ligature influenced the occurrence of arrhythmias; more branches result in greater sparing of myocardium from ischemic damage and hence fewer arrhythmias (Allen and Laadt 1950; Skelton et al. 1962). Still, even when the site of occlusion is taken into account, different studies report a different incidence of fibrillation. For example, when the circumflex artery was occluded at its origin in conscious dogs by McEachern et al. (1940) ventricular fibrillation occurred in 75% of the experiments compared to the 58% described above. Perhaps not only the location of the occlusion and size of the ischemic area, but also the size of the heart must be taken into account, since it is well known that heart size can influence the occurrence of ventricular fibrillation (McWilliam 1887). Data about heart weight have nearly always been lacking in the published reports of experimental results.

The incidence of ventricular fibrillation in these experiments is much higher than in the reports from clinical studies. There may be a number of reasons for these differences although they have not yet been precisely defined. For example, the abruptness of the occlusion in experimental studies may be greater than what happens clinically as illustrated by the records in Figure 2.1. Also the severity of ischemia, duration of the ischemic period, or size of the ischemic area may be different in the experimental studies than what occurs in humans. It is also likely that the activity of the autonomic nervous system, which has important influences on arrhythmogenesis is not comparable in the clinical and experimental situations.

The Role of Preexisting Collaterals

According to Meesmann and coworkers (1970; 1982), mortality due to primary ventricular fibrillation following coronary artery occlusion in dogs can vary from 0% to 100%, and this variability is related to whether or not preexisting collaterals are present. Following ligation of the left anterior descending coronary artery near its origin in their experiments, primary ventricular fibrillation did not occur when collaterals were present and occurred in 58% of hearts without collaterals. For occlusions of the circumflex branch these figures were 3.7% and 100%, respectively. There is also considerable variability in collaterals among different species of experimental animals, which may influence the effects of coronary occlusion. The coronary circulation of the pig is almost devoid of collaterals so that occlusion of a major coronary near its origin always produces a sizeable transmural zone without any coronary flow (Schaper 1971). As described above, this is not the case for the canine heart.

Anesthesia

Electrophysiological studies on ischemic arrhythmias are done on both anesthetized and unanesthetized animals. The presence or absence of anesthesia and the particular anesthetic agent used influences the incidence of arrhythmias caused by coronary occlusion but it is uncertain whether the mechanism causing the arrhythmias is also influenced. Anesthesia sometimes decreases the incidence of severe ventricular arrhythmias after coronary artery occlusion in dogs (Manning et al. 1939; Olichney and Modell 1958). On the other hand, the incidence of reperfusion arrhythmias after a 15-minute period of coronary occlusion was markedly lower in conscious dogs adapted to the laboratory conditions than in anesthetized dogs, and this was attributed to a lower level of adrenergic stimulation in the conscious animals (Bolli et al. 1986). In anesthetized pigs, ischemia-induced arrhythmias occurred more frequently during α-chloralose anesthesia than during barbiturate anesthesia (Bardaji et al. 1990). In contrast, ventricular fibrillation, produced by reperfusion following a 20-minute period of coronary artery occlusion occurred less often in animals anesthetized with α-chloralose than with pentobarbital (Wenger et al. 1984). In dogs with a 2-week-old infarct, programmed electrical stimulation in the conscious animal resulted in the induction of ventricular tachycardia. When the dogs were anesthetized with pentobarbital, induction of the tachycardia was abolished in 4 out of 10 dogs; when halothane was the anesthetic, the arrhythmia could no longer be induced in 5 out of 10 animals. The combination of fentanyl-droperidol plus nitrous oxide was most successful (9 out of 10 could still be induced) (Hunt and Ross 1988). It is unknown what the direct electrophysiological effects of the anesthetics are that provide an antiarrhythmic effect. One explanation for the lower severity of arrhythmias caused by coronary occlusion in anesthetized rats may be the fact that in these animals serum K^+ levels are higher than in conscious animals. An inverse relationship between K^+ concentration and ischemia-induced arrhythmias exists, at least in rats (Curtis et al. 1987).

The depth of anesthesia is also important because of its influence on the effects of the autonomic nervous system on the occurrence of arrhythmias. Autonomic nerve activity can either potentiate or obtund ischemic arrhythmias and the amount of nerve activity is diminished as the depth of anesthesia is increased. Therefore, the different levels of autonomic nerve activity between unanesthetized and anesthetized animals may also account for different effects of the coronary occlusion.

Successive Coronary Artery Occlusions

Brief successive periods of coronary artery occlusion and reperfusion have been induced in the same heart to cause ischemia, rather than a single long period of occlusion. When this is done, the electrophysiological changes during the first occlusion may be different from those during the second occlusion. Changes in the second, and any subsequent occlusions, however, have usually been reproducible (Ruffy et al. 1979; Cardinal et al. 1981; Fleet et al. 1985). These differences may be related to differences in extracellular K^+ and H^+

during the first and subsequent occlusions. (Both participate in the occurrence of ischemic arrhythmias as described later.) These studies suggest that whenever interventions are evaluated on the incidence of arrhythmias during successive periods of transient ischemia in the same heart, control values should not be obtained during the first coronary artery occlusion, but only after the response has stabilized during the second or third occlusion.

The incidence of reperfusion-induced arrhythmias is much lower after a second brief period of ischemia than after the first ischemic period (Shiki and Hearse 1987). The reasons for this preconditioning effect are unknown.

Presence of a Previous Infarction or Cardiac Hypertrophy

Patients may survive an acute myocardial infarction, but then the presence of a healed infarction is subsequently associated with an increased incidence of sudden arrhythmic death (Kannel and Thomas 1982). The arrhythmias may result from the effects of subsequent periods of acute ischemia on the heart with a healed infarct. Possible mechanisms are described later. Animal models have been developed to imitate the clinical situation. In the model described by Patterson et al. (1982), an anteroseptal infarct is produced by occluding the left anterior descending coronary artery for 90 minutes, and then reperfusing the ischemic region. During reperfusion, an area of stenosis is maintained to reduce flow and prevent severe arrhythmias. At the same time, a wire is inserted into the lumen of the circumflex artery. Several days later, in the conscious dog, current is applied through this wire, which results in platelet aggregation and transient reductions in blood flow through the circumflex branch. Ventricular fibrillation occurs more often after the current application in dogs with a previous infarction than in animals without an infarct. Studies in canine and feline hearts have shown that both spontaneous arrhythmias and arrhythmias produced by programmed electrical stimulation of the heart occur more frequently when acute ischemia is superimposed on a healed infarct compared to either acute ischemia or chronic infarction alone (Myerburg et al. 1982b; Garan et al. 1988; Sakai et al. 1989a).

In another model (Billman et al. 1982; Schwartz and Stone 1982) complete two-stage occlusion of the left anterior descending coronary artery produces an anteroseptal infarction, and a balloon occluder is placed around the circumflex artery. Two weeks later, the dogs are exercised, and during the last minutes of exercise, the balloon is inflated for 2 minutes. Whereas such a brief occlusion produces no arrhythmias in resting animals, it results in the occurrence of ventricular fibrillation when coupled with exercise, particularly after cessation of exercise.

Epidemiological studies have shown that hypertension and left ventricular hypertrophy are associated with increased incidences of sudden death in patients with coronary artery disease (Kannel et al. 1975). In dogs with left ventricular hypertrophy, caused by hypertension produced by unilateral nephrectomy and contralateral stenosis of the renal artery, ventricular fibrillation occurred much more frequently after coronary occlusion than in control dogs (Koyanagi et al. 1982a). This is most likely due to the increased size of myocardial infarction, relative to the area at risk, in dogs with hypertension. Hypertension also increases the rate of development of the infarction, and after 1 hour of coronary artery occlusion, more than twice as much midwall and epicardial muscle is infarcted in hypertensive dogs compared to control dogs. Treatment of hypertensive dogs with nitroprusside reduces infarct size and decreases the incidence of sudden death (Koyanagi et al. 1982b; Inou et al. 1987; Dellsperger et al. 1988). It is therefore likely that electrophysiological changes associated with left ventricular hypertrophy in itself are not responsible for arrhythmogenesis and that the increased incidence of ventricular fibrillation in hypertensive animals is secondary to the increased size of the ischemic area.

Isolated Langendorff-Perfused Hearts

Hearts isolated from dogs and pigs, and perfused through the coronary arteries by the Langendorff technique with mixtures of blood and artificial solutions have been utilized to study arrhythmias caused by sudden coronary occlusion (Downar et al. 1977a; Janse et al. 1980c). Advantages of this technique include the absence of extracardiac factors such as neural influences that complicate interpretation of the experimental results. Disadvantages are that in the absence of external work, changes caused by ischemia may develop somewhat slower than in the heart *in situ* and not be as severe. Isolated Langendorff-perfused hearts of small mammals (rabbits, rats, guinea pigs), in which global ischemia is induced by stopping perfusion, have also been used to study arrhythmias (Hondeghem and Cotner 1978; Penny and Sheridan 1983). In such models the effects of ischemia are more homogeneously distributed compared to models of regional ischemia. The incidence and mechanisms of arrhythmias in hearts with homogeneous ischemia versus those with localized regions of ischemia may be very different since the presence of boundaries between ischemic and nonischemic regions are probably important for the generation of arrhythmias. In addition, the choice of a medium with which the heart is perfused, has consequences for the electrophysiological properties of the perfused heart. Blood is the best choice, but it is not always available in sufficient quantities. The second best choice is a mixture of blood and an appropriate electrolyte solution. Hearts of small mammals are almost without exception perfused with electrolyte solutions alone. This alters the extracellular compartment. In blood-perfused cardiac muscle the ratio of extracellular and intracellular resistance is almost 1:1; when the tissue is perfused with Tyrode's solution this ratio becomes 1:7 (Riegger et al. 1989) because of a large increase in the volume of the extracellular space. The decrease in extracellular resistance has an influence on conduction velocity, namely an increase, and this may influence arrhythmogenesis.

In Vitro Models

Because of the difficulties in obtaining reliable microelectrode recordings from vigorously beating intact hearts, isolated cardiac preparations have often been used to elucidate transmembrane potential changes or changes in intracellular ion concentrations caused by ischemia. To this end, the preparations are placed in a tissue bath where they are superfused with solutions that are altered in such a way as to mimic ischemic conditions. The alterations include hypoxia, acidosis, absence of substrate for glycolysis, and an elevated K^+ concentration. Unfortunately, there is a great variety of "ischemic solutions"; ischemia has been mimicked by hypoxia alone, or by elevated K^+ concentrations alone; hypoxia has been studied in the presence and in the absence of glucose, in the presence and absence of acidosis, and in the presence and absence of high K^+ levels. Another category of "ischemic" solutions contains cyanide to prevent both oxidative phosphorylation and anaerobic glycolysis (Smith and Allen 1988). This makes a comparison of the different studies difficult and an extrapolation to the intact heart with regional ischemia even more difficult. As we shall see later, exposure to a severely hypoxic, acidic, high K^+ solution containing no substrate can induce similar changes in transmembrane potentials in isolated preparations as those found in intact hearts after coronary artery occlusion. This is not to say that a host of other factors (lysophosphoglycerides, catecholamines, prostacyclins, thromboxanes, leukotrienes, free oxygen radicals, platelet aggregating factors, etc.) may not have electrophysiological effects as well.

The Choice of a Model

There are a variety of experimental methods and models used to study arrhythmias caused by acute myocardial ischemia. We have mentioned only a few examples. Among the models, the many factors that determine incidence and severity of ischemia-induced arrhythmias may differ making a comparison of arrhythmia mechanisms in various studies difficult. Ideally, at least the following parameters should be controlled or if not controlled, at least taken into account: heart size, size of the ischemic area, number of collaterals, heart rate, level of anesthesia (or in conscious animals, level of stress), neural input to the heart, and, especially for small hearts, the gaseous environment (Fiolet et al. 1985).

Given all these different models, one is confronted with making a choice of which one to use. Different considerations lead to different choices. For example, the Langendorff-Tyrode's-perfused rat heart made globally ischemic is traditionally used for metabolic studies, the reasons being that rats are relatively cheap, a large number of experiments can be performed in a short period of time, and results can be compared with other rat studies. However, we would not choose the rat model for the study of mechanisms of ischemia-induced arrhythmias. On the one hand, action potential characteristics of the rat ventricle are much different from those of larger mammals such as dogs, pigs, or humans. Ventricular action potential duration is much shorter and there is no plateau phase. This might be related to the higher intrinsic metabolic rate of small mammals. Thus, the action potential of the shrew ventricle may be as short as 2 msec (Binah et al. 1989). When metabolic rate of small mammals is reduced by making them hypothyroid, action potential duration increases to values encountered in larger mammals (Binah et al. 1989). Not only are action potentials different, the time course of changes during ischemia may be much faster in small hearts than in larger hearts, further hampering comparison with events in humans. Another reason why we do not use small hearts is that many techniques for defining arrhythmia mechanisms require extracellular recording from a number of sites in the ischemic and normal regions, and this is very difficult to accomplish in small hearts. Finally, since regional ischemia is the most likely cause for the spontaneous arrhythmias encountered in humans with coronary artery disease, and the interaction between ischemic and nonischemic myocardium plays an essential role in arrhythmogenesis, global ischemic models are not our choice. This is not to say that globally ischemic hearts of small mammals should not be used; they can be very useful to study particular problems, for example to investigate the relationship between extracellular K^+ accumulation and resting membrane potential, or to study the time course of release of endogenous catecholamines. There are no "correct" or "incorrect" experimental models; the choice is governed by the problem one wishes to investigate.

Our own studies on the electrophysiology of ischemia- and infarct-induced arrhythmias have been primarily performed on hearts of larger animals, i.e., the dog and the pig. The hearts of both species are large enough to allow extracellular recordings from a large number of sites, and regional ischemia is easily produced by occluding a larger or smaller coronary artery. A comparison with the human heart presents some problems: the coronary anatomy of the pig heart can be compared to that of a healthy human heart in the sense that no (or very few) collateral connection between the coronary arteries exists. The dog heart, with its often abundant collaterals, may be compared to the human heart with long-standing coronary artery disease in which collateral connections have been formed. The specialized conduction system of the dog is very similar to that of humans as it is confined to the subendocardium. Thus, changes in ventricular activation caused by regional ischemia may be similar to those in the human heart. In contrast, the Purkinje system in the pig heart extends from endocardium, almost to the epicardium, resulting in an almost simultaneous activation of subendocardial and subepicardial muscle (Hamlin et al. 1975; Holland and Brooks 1976). Thus, changes in ventricular activation caused by ischemia will be different in the pig and in the human.

In hearts of large animals such as the dog or pig, coronary artery occlusion rapidly results in the kinds of arrhythmias shown in Figure 2.2. In this figure, 60 DC extracellular electrograms are shown, which were simultaneously recorded from the anterior surface of the left ventricle of an isolated Langerdor-

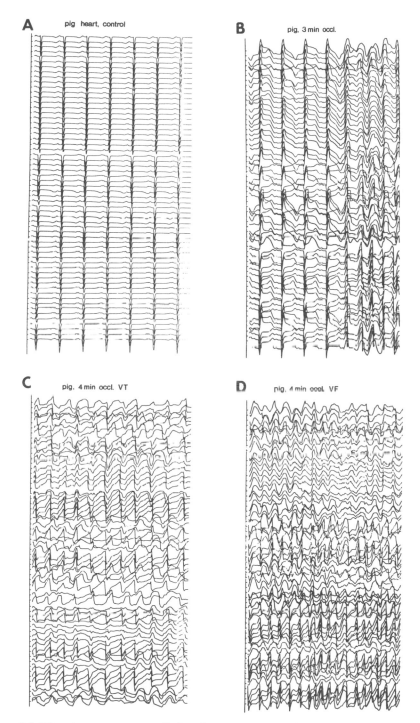

Figure 2.2: Direct current extracellular electrograms simultaneously recorded from the epicardial surface of the left ventricle of a pig heart before (panel A) and 3 to 4 minutes after (panels B-D) occlusion of the left anterior descending coronary artery. (Reproduced from Janse (1982a) with permission.)

ff-perfused pig heart before occlusion of the left anterior descending coronary artery (control panel A) and 3 to 4 minutes after occlusion (panels B, C, and D). We show these recordings to illustrate how quickly and dramatically the electrical behavior of a heart is altered when a region is made ischemic. In control conditions (panel A), the area under the electrodes is almost synchronously excited, and on the time scale shown, no differences in timing of the (negative) intrinsic deflections can be distinguished (in reality the difference between earliest and latest activated electrode sites is 15 msec). Three minutes after coronary occlusion (panel B), there is TQ depression and ST elevation in many of the complexes, and the configuration of the electrograms is drastically altered. Initially there still is sinus rhythm (left side of panel B), but at the end of the tracing spontaneous premature beats appear (right side of panel B) that form the beginning of a period of ventricular tachycardia, which eventually degenerates into ventricular fibrillation. The ventricular tachycardia is shown in panel C and the fibrillation in panel D. The last panel gives a visual impression of the electrical activity that causes, in MacWilliams' words (1923) " . . . violent and prolonged turmoil of fruitless activity". The next sections of this chapter are devoted to the electrophysiological changes that lead to these dramatic disturbances of the cardiac rhythm.

Electrophysiological Effects of Acute Myocardial Ischemia

Myocardial ischemia that results from coronary artery occlusion has a profound effect on the electrophysiological properties of cardiac cells. Changes in resting membrane potential and inward and outward currents during the action potential lead to alterations in conduction, refractoriness and automaticity, all of which contribute to the occurrence of ventricular arrhythmias. In addition to changes in active membrane properties, passive electrical properties are changed as well, and these changes also influence propagation in ischemic myocardium and contribute to arrhythmogenesis.

Resting Membrane Potential

Resting membrane potential has been measured with intracellular glass microelectrodes in whole hearts during ischemia. When we (MJJ) initially undertook to obtain such recordings, the prospect of trying to keep a microelectrode tip for any length of time inside a single cell in an intact beating heart was terrifying. Initially, we attempted to counteract the movements of the heart with a device suggested to us by B. Lewartowski from the University of Warsaw. This was a ring filled with agar that could be sutured onto the surface of the left ventricle. It was proposed that fixing this ring would diminish the movements of the tissue within the ring; the agar would prevent breaking of the microelectrode tip when lowering the electrode onto the heart. We tried unsuccessfully to obtain recordings from open-chest anesthetized animals with this technique. Therefore, we used isolated hearts perfused through their coronary arteries with a 1:1 mixture of blood and modified Tyrode's solution, where the prospect of immobilizing a region for microelectrode recording was better. In addition, we could reduce the force of contraction by adding calcium channel blockers to the perfusion fluid. After a year-and-a-half without success, it finally turned out that rings filled with agar were not needed. Using small microelectrode tips mounted on thin spiralled wires, and locally removing the epicardium to prevent breaking of the tips, it was possible to obtain reliable recordings from both isolated and *in situ* hearts that were beating vigorously (Downar et al. 1977a; Kléber et al. 1978).

It has been found that cells in the ischemic region depolarize within minutes following experimental coronary artery occlusion (Kardesch et al. 1958; Samson and Scher 1960; Prinzmetal et al. 1961; Czarnecka et al. 1973; Downar et al. 1977a; Russell et al. 1977; Kléber et al. 1978; Kléber 1983). In the isolated porcine heart, membrane potential decreased from normal values of around -80 mV to between -65 and -60 mV within 7 to 10 minutes following left anterior descending coronary artery occlusion (Kléber et al. 1978). During global ischemia in the isolated guinea pig heart caused by stopping total perfusion, resting membrane potential in the left ventricle decreased with a sigmoidal time course from -82 mV to -49 mV during 15 minutes of ischemia (Kléber 1983). Similarly, resting potential of isolated, superfused ventricular muscle declined when exposed to solutions designed to mimic the *in vivo* ischemic environment (Kodama et al. 1984).

The Role of K^+

The fall in resting potential in whole hearts has been linked at least partly to alterations in distribution of K^+ across the cell membrane. Increases in extracellular K^+ have been measured with ion selective electrodes soon after coronary occlusion both in hearts *in vivo* during regional ischemia and in isolated perfused hearts during global ischemia (Wiegand et al. 1979; Hill and Gettes 1980; Hirche et al. 1980; Weiss and Shine 1981; 1982a; 1982b; 1986; Kléber 1983; 1984; Coronel et al. 1988). A close association between the rise in extracellular K^+ and the decrease of resting membrane potential has been described. Extracellular K^+ activity in the isolated guinea pig heart increased from 4 mmol to 14.7 mmol within 15 minutes in the experiments of Kléber (1983). The calculated K^+ equilibrium potential was 7 mV more negative than the resting membrane potential in control conditions, but approached the resting potential during a 15-minute period of global ischemia (Kléber 1983). The accumulation of extracellular K^+ occurs in two phases. The first phase is rapidly reversible when reperfusion occurs within 15 minutes (Wiegand et al.

1979; Hill and Gettes 1980; Hirche et al. 1980), and resting potential also quickly returns to normal (Downar et al. 1977a). Following this first phase of increased extracellular K^+ during maintained occlusion, the K^+ concentration remains nearly constant, and sometimes even decreases somewhat for 10 to 20 minutes before a second increase in extracellular K^+ begins that is not reversed by reperfusion (Hill and Gettes 1980; Hirche et al. 1980). This phase is most likely due to irreversible cell damage.

An example of the triphasic change in extracellular K^+ in isolated guinea pig hearts made globally ischemic is shown in the top panel of Figure 2.3 where extracellular K^+ concentration in millimoles per liter is plotted versus time after onset of ischemia. Extracellular K^+ rises during the first 6–8 minutes, then falls slightly before rising again after 13–14 minutes. In the lower panel,

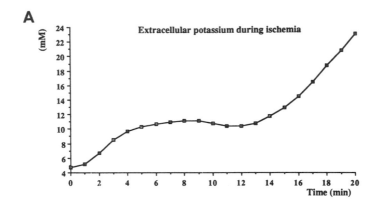

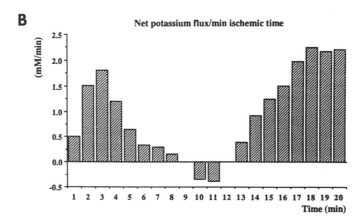

Figure 2.3: Panel A shows the extracellular K^+ concentration (ordinate) as a function of time elapsed after arrest of coronary flow (abscissa) in an isolated guinea pig heart. Panel B shows the net K^+ transfer out of the cells (ordinate) plotted in time windows of 1 minute (abscissa). (Reproduced from Wilde (1988) with permission.)

changes in net K^+ transfer in millimoles per minute on the ordinate are depicted in time windows of 1 minute on the abscissa. During the first 8 minutes of global ischemia there is a net transfer of K^+ from the intracellular to the extracellular space. In the period of the "dip" in the extracellular K^+ curve above, there is a net inward movement of K^+. After 18 to 20 minutes, the final phase of intracellular K^+ loss begins with an additional transfer of K^+ from the intracellular to extracellular space. There may be several reasons for the net inward movement of K^+ during the "dip" phase. As we shall see later, this phase coincides with the period during which ischemic cells produce no action potentials. Moreover (see below), there is evidence that at this stage of ischemia Na/K pumping can still be activated. A decrease in K^+ efflux from unexcited cells combined with an unaltered active K^+ influx caused by the pump would reduce extracellular K^+. Also, during this period there is a release of endogenous catecholamines (Carlsson 1987; Wilde et al. 1988) that may result in stimulation of the Na/K pump, enhancing active K^+ influx (Désilets and Baumgarten 1986). Adrenergic blockade prevents the "dip" in extracellular K^+ in the globally ischemic heart (Wilde 1988), as does application of a cardiotonic steroid (Weiss and Shine 1982a).

The increase in extracellular K^+ in the first 10 minutes is substantial; measurements have shown an average rate of increase of 1.5 mmol/min (Wiegand et al. 1979; Hill and Gettes 1980; Kléber 1983). However, it represents only a relatively small decline in intracellular K^+ concentration (from about 140 to 135 mmol) because the ions are transferred from an intracellular space that is three times larger than the extracellular space (Polimeni 1974). Also, an increase of 1.5 mmol/min corresponds to a transmembrane flux of less than 7% of the unidirectional steady state fluxes (Johnson 1976). However, eventually there may also be a significant loss of intracellular K^+ that contributes to a decrease in the K^+ equilibrium potential and resting potential. In isolated tissues made hypoxic, which is one component of the ischemic environment, intracellular K^+ measured with ion selective microelectrodes was reduced (Baumgarten et al. 1981; Guarnieri and Strauss 1982). Also, in Purkinje fibers surviving on the endocardial surface of infarcts, intracellular K^+ was reduced after 1–3 hours of coronary occlusion (Dresdner et al. 1987; Kline et al. 1992).

Mechanisms for Intracellular K^+ Loss   The net loss of intracellular K^+ reflects an imbalance between K^+ influx and efflux. Influx occurs mainly through the Na/K pump, an active energy consuming mechanism, whereas efflux may occur passively down concentration gradients through membrane channels. Studies in rabbit interventricular septum with radiolabeled K^+ have revealed that hypoxia-induced K^+ loss is caused by an increase in K^+ efflux, whereas (active) influx resulting from Na/K pump activity is unaffected (Rau et al. 1977). The maintenance of active Na/K pumping in early ischemic myocardium has also been demonstrated qualitatively by measuring changes in extracellular K^+ in guinea pig and rabbit hearts during induced alterations in heart rate (Weiss and Shine 1982a; 1986; Kléber 1983). The normal response to an increase in rate is an increase in Na^+ influx and K^+ efflux. The increase in intracellular Na^+ stimulates an increase in pump activity and active K^+ influx and Na^+ efflux reach a new steady state after only several minutes. Consequently, when rate increases, extracellular K^+ concentrations slowly rise until a plateau level is reached and then may begin to decline because of increased Na/K pump activity; when heart rate decreases extracellular K^+ decreases, even to levels below control because pump activity declines with a slow time course (Kunze 1977; Kline and Kupersmith 1982). When the Na/K pump is inhibited such as by cardiac glycosides, extracellular K^+ continues to rise after an increase in rate, without reaching a plateau, and does not "undershoot" control when rate is slowed (Kunze 1977). In ischemic myocardium this pattern of rise and fall in extracellular K^+ in response to rate changes is essentially normal, indicating that the Na/K pump is still functioning (Weiss and Shine 1982a; Kléber 1983). However, since the rate of pumping was not quantified some decrease in pump activity may not have been detected.

The finding that the Na/K pump is still functioning within the first 10 to 15 minutes of ischemia might be surprising in view of the experimental evidence that energy-rich phosphate compounds rapidly decline during the early phases of hypoxia and ischemia (Janse et al. 1979; Jennings et al. 1981). The cytoplasmic free energy generated by adenosine triphosphate (ATP) hydrolysis has been shown to decline during ischemia in a biphasic fashion; a rapid initial decrease from about 55 to 46 kJ/mol within the first 4 minutes followed by a plateau phase and then a secondary decrease after 10 to 15 minutes (Kammermeier et al. 1982; Fiolet et al. 1984). In addition, Bersohn et al. (1982) showed a small inhibition of enzymatic Na^+/K^+ ATPase activity in sarcolemmal vesicles isolated from ischemic rabbit hearts. Taken together with the data on the effects of rate on extracellular K^+ in ischemic muscle, it appears that a moderate decrease in Na^+/K^+ ATPase activity is compatible with maintenance of at least some active Na/K pumping.

Intracellular Na^+ concentration has also been measured during hypoxia and ischemia with conflicting results. In the rat heart, intracellular Na^+ concentration measured with a washout method during hypoxic perfusion (Fiolet et al. 1984) or with nuclear magnetic resonance during ischemia (Balschi et al. 1985), substantially increased (i.e., threefold). In contrast, measurements of intracellular Na^+ activity with ion-selective microelectrodes showed no change in the hypoxic dog heart (Nakaya et al. 1985), or only a moderate increase of 3 mmol (50%) in the hypoxic guinea pig heart (Wilde and Kléber 1986). In the ischemic guinea pig heart no change was observed during the first 15 minutes (Kléber 1983). It is possible that species differences exist between the rat on the one hand and the dog and guinea pig on the other hand, or differences in methodology may account for the different results. Rat hearts have a significantly higher metabolic rate than hearts from larger species (Loiselle 1985), and during ischemia, energy sources in the rat heart may be exhausted earlier than in hearts of rabbits or guinea pigs.

The measurements of intracellular Na^+ do not help determine the functional state of the Na/K pump. If inhibition of the pump did occur during acute ischemia it might not lead to a significant increase in intracellular Na^+ for several reasons. In early ischemia the rise in intracellular Na^+ expected from inhibition of the Na/K pump by 25% to 30% due to lack of oxygen in the ischemic environment (Kléber and Wilde 1986; Wilde and Kléber 1986) might be counteracted by the reduced Na^+ influx that undoubtedly occurs because of the depolarization of the membrane. The depolarization reduces the electrochemical gradient for Na^+, and causes ischemic myocardium to quickly become inexcitable, both limiting Na^+ influx (Janse and Kléber 1981). Thus, superfusion of isolated guinea pig ventricular muscle with a solution that mimics conditions in ischemia (hypoxia, acidosis, glucose-free, elevated K^+) and that causes depolarization, does not result in a significant increase in intracellular Na^+ activity, whereas intracellular Na^+ increases in a hypoxic solution with normal K^+ that causes no depolarization (Wilde and Kléber 1986). Since the increase of intracellular Na^+ appears to be small, the net cellular loss of K^+ is not compensated by an equivalent gain of intracellular Na^+. It has been suggested that, in order to maintain intracellular electroneutrality, K^+ loss is coupled to cellular anion loss (Mathur and Case 1973; Kléber 1983; Gaspardone et al. 1986).

Our discussion so far has suggested a possible mild depression of the Na/K pump that might contribute to some of the decrease in intracellular K^+ during acute ischemia via a decrease in K^+ influx. However, to account for the K^+ loss from the cells there must also be an increase in K^+ efflux as well. There are several possible mechanisms for this efflux. One involves an increase in membrane permeability to anions caused by ischemia. If this occurred, the membrane would then depolarize and K^+ would be passively redistributed. This possibility is suggested by experimental results that show that in low-flow ischemia, the loss of the anions, inorganic phosphate, and lactate follows the same time course as the loss of K^+ (Mathur and Case 1973). However, K^+ loss may also be the primary event, leading to depolarization and a secondary redistribution of anions. Vleugels et al. (1980) have shown that hypoxia induces an increase in K^+ conductance of the membrane at potentials remote from electrochemical equilibrium (loss of rectifier properties of the time-independent K^+ current). Weiss et al. (1989) concluded that during ischemia part of the cellular K^+ loss is not related to anion efflux and suggested that an increase in membrane conductance for K^+ was the most likely cause for the "nonanion-linked K^+ efflux." An increased conductance of K^+ channels might result from the effects of ATP depletion on ATP-sensitive K^+ channels (Noma 1983; Kakei et al. 1985; Noma and Shibasaki 1985). An ischemia-induced opening of these K^+ channels would only result in an increased K^+ efflux when membrane potential significantly deviates from the equilibrium potential for K^+. In globally ischemic rabbit and guinea pig hearts, glibenclamide, a drug that blocks the ATP-sensitive K^+ channel, had no effect on extracellular K^+ accumulation in quiescent hearts (Fosset et al. 1988). In beating hearts, glibenclamide slowed the increase of extracellular K^+ during the first 5 minutes of ischemia but the concentrations at 13–30 minutes were not influenced. It was therefore concluded that open ATP-sensitive channels contribute to extracellular K^+ increase only during the first 5 minutes of ischemia and only in hearts where, during repetitive action potentials, membrane potential deviates from the K^+ equilibrium potential (Wilde et al. 1989; 1990). Blockade of the ATP-sensitive K^+ channel has an antiarrhythmic effect in Langendorff-perfused rat hearts that are ischemic (Wolleben et al. 1989; Kantor et al. 1990) and this may be related to a reduced K^+ accumulation in the very early phase of ischemia.

It has been proposed that K^+ loss from cells and accumulation in the extracellular space during ischemia might be linked to the development of intracellular acidosis (Kléber 1983; 1984; Kléber et al. 1987b). It was shown that by changing CO_2 pressure in the atmosphere surrounding a globally ischemic guinea pig heart, and thereby inducing stepwise changes in the extracellular and intracellular pH of the subepicardial layers, fluctuations in extracellular K^+ activity immediately occurred. Acidification was immediately followed by K^+ accumulation, and alkalinization by transient K^+ depletion (Kléber et al. 1987b). Net K^+ efflux might then be secondary to electrogenic lactate efflux at a low extracellular pH, similar to that occurring in fatigued skeletal muscle (Mainwood and Lucier 1972). Intracellular acidification caused by internal dialysis increases a K^+ time-independent outward current supporting the proposal that K^+ loss is linked to acidosis (Sato et al. 1985). Finally, a reduction of extracellular water as a result of osmotic cell swelling may also contribute to an increase in extracellular K^+ concentration (Tranum-Jensen et al. 1981).

The Role of Ca^{2+}

Other causes for depolarization besides extracellular K^+ accumulation might also occur concomitantly. For example, when successive coronary occlusions of very short duration were performed in Langendorff-perfused canine hearts in which heart rate was alternatively normal (92 beats/min) or rapid (180 beats/min), the rise in extracellular K^+ was almost identical during each occlusion. However, the depression of the TQ segment in the direct current extracellular electrogram, a measure of depolarization of resting membrane potential, was markedly greater during the occlusion at the rapid heart rate (Blake et al. 1986; 1988). It has been proposed that some of the depolarization occurs as a direct consequence of intracellular calcium overload in ischemic myocardium (Clusin et al. 1983; 1984). In favor of this hypothesis is the finding that the Ca^{2+} entry blocker diltiazem produces a flow-independent reduction in TQ segment depression, which was interpreted as being due to a reduction of cellular depolarization during ischemia (Clusin et al. 1984). As yet, however, there is limited information to support the concept that during the first minutes of ischemia, intracellular calcium does indeed increase (Opie and Coetzee 1987). Measurements of intracellular Ca^{2+} in intact hearts have been made using nuclear magnetic resonance (NMR) spectroscopy after loading the hearts with calcium chelating agents such as 5,5'-difluoro BAPTA. Time-averaged measurements during 5-minute periods indicated that intracellular Ca^{2+} increases only after ischemic periods of 10 minutes, which is longer than the time for the initial depolarization of the membrane potential (Marban et al. 1987; Steenbergen et al. 1987; 1990). There is a three- to fivefold increase in cytosolic Ca^{2+} between 10 and 20 minutes after onset of ischemia that is reversible upon reperfusion. The use of indo-1, which shifts its fluorescence spectrum upon binding calcium, allows determination of intracellular Ca^{2+} on a beat-to-beat basis. An elevation of both systolic and diastolic Ca^{2+} was found using this technique, reaching a maximum within 90 seconds and declining thereafter (Clusin et al. 1989).

Therefore, on the basis of data available at present, the evidence to implicate an increase in intracellular calcium as a factor causing early depolarization is inconclusive. After ischemic periods longer than 10 to 15 minutes, an increase in intracellular calcium may play an important role in causing cellular uncoupling, which may have important effects on conduction and arrhythmogenesis (described later).

In Figures 2.4 and 2.5, schematic representations are given of the major changes in intra- and extracellular ion concentrations during the first 20 to 30 minutes of ischemia and their relationship to the depolarization of the resting membrane potential. Caution must be exercised when adhering too strictly to

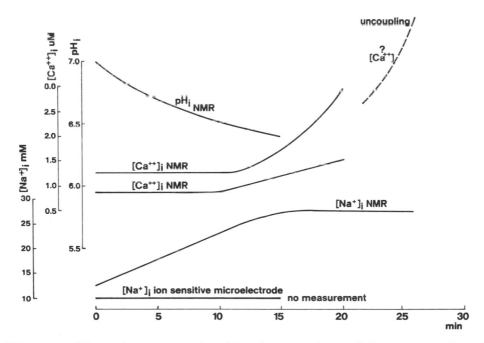

Figure 2.4: Schematic representation of the changes in intracellular concentrations of Ca^{2+} and Na^+ ions, and of intracellular pH during the early phase of ischemia. The concentrations of the ions and the pH are indicated on the ordinate and the time of ischemia on the abscissa. Data are taken from various studies, using different techniques (NMR = nuclear magnetic resonance.)

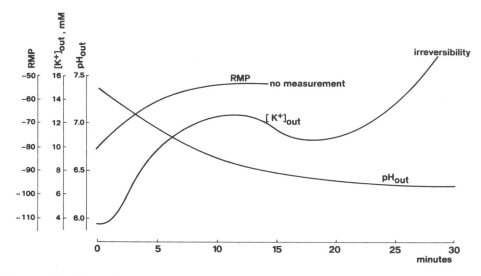

Figure 2.5: Schematic representation of changes in extracellular K$^+$ concentration, ([K$^+$] out), extracellular pH (pH out) and resting membrane potential (RMP) during the first 30 minutes of ischemia. Values for these parameters are on the ordinate and the time of ischemia is on the abscissa.

numbers. Data were obtained from various sources; not only do animal species differ, so do methods (for example NMR techniques and measurements with ion sensitive microelectrodes). Furthermore, animal models are different (global ischemia in isolated hearts of small mammals, regional ischemia in open- chest large mammals) and variables that may substantially alter the time course of events (heart rate, temperature) are not the same. To give just one example, extracellular pH after 10 minutes of ischemia may vary from 6.1 (Fiolet et al. 1984) to 6.7 (Kléber and Weber, unpublished observations). Despite many uncertainties, one may conclude that during the first 10 to 15 minutes intracellular Na$^+$ and Ca^{2+} concentrations remain relatively constant while intracellular pH falls as shown in Figure 2.4. There are clearly more experimental data required to establish what happens to these ions in the period between 15 and 30 minutes, when cellular uncoupling and irreversible cell damage occurs but some of the data indicate that intracellular Na$^+$ and Ca^{2+} may rise during this time period (Figure 2.4). During the initial 10 minutes, while Na$^+$ and Ca^{2+} are unchanging, there is a depolarization of the membrane potential, a significant increase in extracellular K$^+$ and a fall in extracellular pH as shown in Figure 2.5.

Free intracellular Mg^{2+} increases threefold or more after 15 min of ischemia (Kirkels et al. 1989; Murphy et al. 1989). This increase may modulate Ca^{2+} and K$^+$ channels and suppress Ca^{2+} inward current and K$^+$ outward current (Agus and Morad 1991). The importance of the change in intracellular Mg^{2+} during the early period of ischemia is uncertain.

The Role of Products of Lipid Metabolism

Other factors associated with the ischemic environment might also contribute to the depolarization of the membrane potential but identifying their contribution is a difficult problem. As pointed out by Corr et al. (1982), a set of "Koch's postulates" should be applied when determining the importance of a substance in the ischemic environment in causing electrophysiological changes. These postulates include: (1) a temporal relationship between the occurrence of the abnormal membrane potentials and a change in concentration of the substance in the ischemic environment must be demonstrated; (2) comparable effects as those occurring during ischemia should be found when normal cells are exposed to the substance administered exogenously in the same concentration as it is found in ischemic tissue if it is proposed that manifestation of the effects of the substance does not require a second substance to be present; (3) changes in the concentration of the substance must lead to exacerbation or amelioration of the electrophysiological change. It is far from easy to meet all the criteria, and much of the evidence for involvement of certain metabolites in the genesis of the electrophysiological alterations that cause arrhythmias is circumstantial.

A class of metabolites of phospholipids that accumulates in ischemic myocardium and that has been implicated as a cause of early electrical changes during ischemia, including the depolarization of the membrane potential, are the lysophosphoglycerides, among which lysophosphatidylcholine and lysophosphatidylethanolamine are the most important (Sobel et al. 1978). These substances, when added to the superfusate, produce electrical changes in isolated normal cardiac muscle and Purkinje fibers that are similar to those that occur in ischemic myocardium *in vivo* and *in vitro*, such as depolarization of the resting membrane potential, separation of the action potential upstroke into two components, and prolongation of postrepolarization refractoriness (Corr et al. 1979; Arnsdorf and Sawicki 1981; Clarkson and Ten Eick 1983). In the initial studies, levels of lysophosphoglycerides thought to exist in ischemic myocardium were probably overestimated because of artifacts introduced by the extraction procedure (Shaikh and Downar 1981). Also, in contrast to the quick return to normal of depressed ischemic action potentials *in vivo* following reperfusion of the occluded coronary artery, the effects of lysophosphoglycerides on *in vitro* preparations take a long time to disappear when the preparation is superfused with solution containing no lysophosphoglycerides (Corr et al. 1979). Still, it appears that when lysophosphoglycerides are bound to albumin, much lower concentrations are needed to produce membrane depolarization *in vitro* (Corr et al. 1981a). Moreover, the effects of small amounts of lysophosphoglycerides are additive to the effects of hypoxia and high K^+, and are intensified by concomitant acidosis (Corr et al. 1981a). More recent data indicate that lysophosphatidylcholine accumulates in ischemic myocardium within 3 minutes to levels sufficient to induce deleterious electrophysiological effects *in vitro*. The accumulation is most marked in hearts that develop ventricular fibrillation (Corr et al. 1987). It has been proposed that lysophosphoglycerides interact both with the hydrophobic and hydrophilic components of cell membranes and in low concentration are incorporated into the membrane, changing its functional properties. Clarkson and Ten Eick (1983) and Kiyosue and Arita (1986) found that lysophosphatidylcholine caused membrane depolarization by reducing K^+ conductance and postulated that it may act as a nonspecific depressant of membrane channels. At higher concentrations, lysophosphoglycerides cause loss of membrane phospholipids, and eventually the membrane is disrupted. Massive calcium entry then leads to cell death (Corr and Sobel 1982; Katz 1982). Therefore, low concentrations of lysophosphoglycerides may, in addition to the effects of high K^+ and low pO_2, influence the electrical changes of early ischemia, and higher concentrations may play an important role in causing irreversible cellular injury. Endogenous long-chain acylcarnitine, with a similar structure as lysophosphoglycerides, has recently been found to increase 70-fold in the sarcolemma during hypoxia and to induce similar electrophysiological changes as lysophosphoglycerides in neonatal rat myocytes (Knabb et al. 1986). Moreover, inhibition of acylcarnitine accumulation reduced the incidence of ventricular tachycardia and fibrillation during 5-minute periods of ischemia in cat hearts (Corr et al. 1989).

It is therefore obvious that many important questions remain to be explored concerning the mechanism of depolarization that occurs in the face of acute ischemia. Why is K^+ lost from the cell and what are the depolarizing membrane currents of primary interest? What is the role of lysophosphoglycerides and to what extent is calcium overload involved?

Changes in Intracellular and Extracellular Potentials

In 1879, Burdon-Sanderson and Page described the effects of injury to the surface of the frog heart on the electrocardiogram (recorded with a capillary electrometer) and noted that during activity the injured site became positive with respect to the uninjured surface. Many authors have subsequently studied the effects of injury, including those of ischemia on local extracellular electrograms (De Waart et al. 1936; Blumgart et al. 1937; Eyster et al. 1938; Sugarman et al. 1940; Nahum et al. 1943; Katcher et al. 1960; Cohen and Kaufman 1975; Bruyneel 1975). It became established that elevation of the ST segment caused by injury, as recorded with condenser-coupled amplifiers, could be due to both diastolic (TQ segment) depression and true (systolic) ST elevation. The earliest studies using microelectrodes in acutely ischemic myocardium provided evidence that the diastolic baseline depression was caused by localized loss of resting membrane potential resulting in a diastolic "current of injury" between healthy and ischemic cells (Samson and Scher 1960; Prinzmetal et al. 1961). Later studies established the mechanism for ST elevation caused by acute ischemia more clearly (Kléber et al. 1978).

In the following paragraphs we will describe in detail the changes in transmembrane action potentials during ischemia and discuss the relationship between these changes and those in the TQ and ST segments of the extracellular electrograms. Microelectrode recordings from the epicardial surface of intact hearts, either in open-chest animals or in Langendorff-perfused hearts, have shown that within a few minutes after coronary artery occlusion, the amplitude, upstroke velocity, and duration of ventricular muscle action potentials decrease along with the depolarization of resting membrane potential that we described previously. After depolarization to resting membrane potentials of around -60 to -65 mV, the cells become unresponsive (Czarnecka et al. 1973; Downar et al. 1977a; Russell et al. 1977; Kléber et al. 1978). However, before ischemic cells become unresponsive, the amplitude and duration of the action potentials often alternate and sometimes 2:1 responses occur during normal sinus rhythm. During the phase of alternation, action potentials with larger amplitudes and longer durations have upstrokes consisting of two components: the first has a more rapid rate of rise and depolarizes the cell to around -40 mV, the second has a slow rate of rise and depolarizes the cell to more positive levels. The upstrokes of the small action potentials that occur after each large one show only the first component (Downar et al. 1977a; Kléber et al. 1978; Cinca et al. 1980). We will illustrate these changes in the following figures and at the same time describe the relationships to changes in extracellular potentials, which determine the changes in the electrocardiogram. Figure 2.6 shows recordings made in an isolated pig heart, perfused with a 1:1 mixture of blood and Tyrode's solution. The upper tracings in each panel are transmembrane potentials recorded with a microelectrode. Zero potential level is indicated by a straight line and was obtained by withdrawing the intracellular microelectrode into the extracellular space (the differential electrode was located in the extracellular space as close as possible to the microelectrode). The lower tracings in each panel are unipolar direct current extracellular electrograms recorded from the same site as the microelectrode on the anterior aspect of the left ventricle. The "recording" probe used to obtain the extracellular electrogram was a cotton wick soaked in Tyrode's solution within a thin polyethylene tube that could be positioned within 1 mm from the microelectrode; the "indifferent" electrode was another wick attached to the root of the aorta. The straight line running through the extracellular electrogram was obtained by moving the extracellular recording probe to the aortic root; it serves as "0" potential for the extracellular recordings. In the control situation, resting membrane potential is -97 mV, and action potential amplitude 118 mV. The TQ and ST segments of the extracellular electrograms are isoelectric. The intrinsic deflection (rapid negative deflection) corresponds to the upstroke of the transmembrane action potential. Following coronary artery occlusion, the first change is a decrease in resting membrane potential without much change in action potential configuration, except for a reduction in upstroke velocity (top right panel, 2 1/2 min occl.). The loss of resting membrane potential is reflected in the direct current electrogram by a negative displacement of the TQ segment (TQ depression). Between 2 and 4 minutes following onset of ischemia, resting membrane potential further decreased from -86 to -75

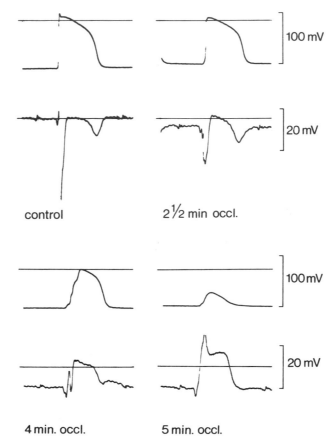

control   2½ min occl.

4 min. occl.   5 min. occl.

Figure 2.6: Transmembrane potentials (top traces) and local direct current (DC) extracellular electrograms (lower traces) from an isolated, perfused pig heart before (control), and 2 1/2, 4, and 5 minutes after occlusion of the left anterior descending coronary artery. (Reproduced from Janse (1986b) with permission.)

mV, with a concomitant increase in TQ depression from -2 to -11 mV (lower left panel, 4 min occl.). After 4 minutes, the action potential upstroke became slow and slurred, and the two components mentioned above are evident. Action potential amplitude decreased, and the moment of activation of the ischemic cell was delayed. After 5 minutes, the action potential was reduced to a very small amplitude response, which was probably unable to propagate (bottom right panel, 5 min occl.). At this stage, it is impossible to tell which part of the cellular response is an electrotonic potential reflecting activity in adjacent tissue, and which part is caused by regenerative inward current across the cell membrane. In the extracellular electrograms, true ST segment elevation has now become apparent. There still is a small negative deflection ("intrinsic deflection") that coincides with the transmembrane depolarization. Again, it is impossible to decide from such a recording whether this indicates local activation, or is merely the result of electrotonic current flow. The difficulties in defining local activation on the basis of extracellular electrograms and its consequences for the construction of activation maps, will be further discussed later. In the isolated pig heart, TQ depression begins on the average 1.5 minutes after coronary occlusion, true ST elevation after 4 minutes. In the *in situ* working heart, these changes occur much more rapidly. Figure 2.7 shows the rapid time course of these changes in a DC electrogram recorded from an intramural ischemic site in an *in situ* canine heart. Occlusion of the left anterior descending coronary artery was done at the arrow under the top trace at the left. Following occlusion, the signals are displayed at a slow paper speed so that the time course of change of the TQ and ST potentials (indicated by the thick black segment on the recording) can be seen. At the end of the top trace the paper speed was increased back to the original. In the lower trace, the TQ and ST segment changes that occur near the end of the 5-minute period of occlusion are at the left. It can be seen how quickly they return to their preocclusion state after the occlusion was released at the arrow. The speed of return is shown by the change in the thick black segment of the recording at slow paper speed.

After 5 to 8 minutes of ischemia, cells in the center of the ischemic zone fail to produce action potentials. This phenomenon is shown in the recordings in Figure 2.8 obtained from the pig heart, where again the transmembrane potentials are shown above and the DC extracellular electrograms below. The typical changes described in Figure 2.6 can be seen at 6 minutes of occlusion (upper right panel), while after 8 minutes (lower left panel) the cell is unresponsive. At this time, resting membrane potential is in the order of -65 mV. The extracellular complex is "monophasic", displaying a TQ segment depression of

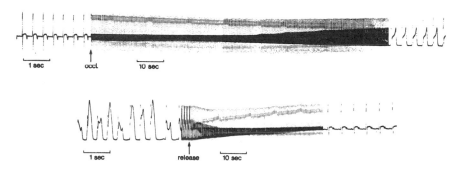

Figure 2.7: Intramural DC electrogram from a canine heart *in situ*. Following occlusion of the left anterior descending coronary artery (arrow, top panel), the signals are displayed at a slow paper speed (10 seconds) to show the time course of change of TQ and ST segment potentials indicated by the black region of the trace. In the lower trace, it can be seen how quickly TQ and ST segment potentials return to preocclusion values when, after a 5-minute period of ischemia, reperfusion is allowed by releasing the clamp on the coronary artery (arrow, release). The time scale during different segments of the recording are shown below the records. (Reproduced from Janse (1986b) with permission.)

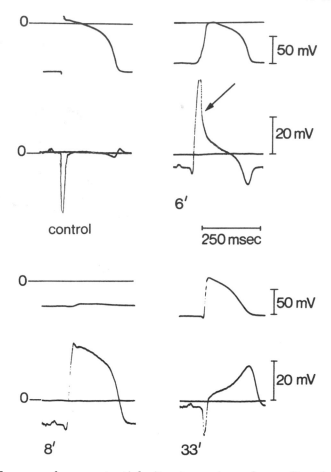

Figure 2.8: Transmembrane potentials (top traces in each panel) and extracellular electrograms (bottom traces in each panel) during the early phase of ischemia in an isolated perfused pig heart. The time after coronary occlusion is indicated beneath each panel. Electrical activity disappeared after 8 minutes (lower left) but improved after 33 minutes. (Reproduced from Janse and Durrer (1978) with permission.)

about −15 mV and an ST segment elevation in the order of +25 mV. This phase of unresponsiveness is transient. With maintained coronary occlusion, transmembrane potentials can again be recorded in previously unresponsive cells after about 15 to 30 minutes as is shown in the bottom right panel of Figure 2.8. These recordings were made 33 minutes after coronary occlusion. The action potentials at that time are abnormal in that they have a short duration, a low amplitude, and a reduced upstroke velocity, yet they are able to propagate. After 40 to 60 minutes, these action potentials disappear and the cells in the center of the ischemic zone become inexcitable and remain so.

Depending on the duration of the occlusion, these dramatic changes in electrical activity are rapidly reversible. Figure 2.9 shows the almost immedi-

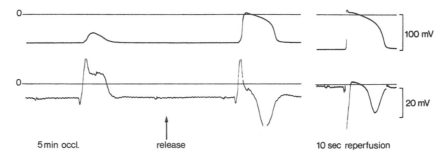

Figure 2.9: Reperfusion after 5 minutes of coronary occlusion (at the arrow) in the isolated pig heart immediately results in reappearance of action potentials (top traces) without a change in resting potential. Within 10 seconds (at the right), electrical activity is normalized. The simultaneous changes in the DC electrogram are shown in the bottom trace. (Reproduced from Janse (1986b) with permission.)

ate appearance of action potentials in an isolated pig heart when reperfusion was allowed after a 5-minute period of ischemia; within 10 seconds intra- and extracellular potentials were back to normal. This rapid reversal was also shown in the bottom trace in Figure 2.7. It is remarkable how quickly the TQ depression and ST elevation are reversed following restoration of flow. On the one hand, this is due to readmission of oxygen and nutrients, but perhaps more important is the washout of substances accumulated in the extracellular space, among which are K^+ ions. A similar return of action potentials and normalization of extracellular potentials was observed when 20 mL of anoxic saline was injected distal to the occlusion in the coronary artery without releasing the occlusion (Downar et al. 1977a). Rapid reversal of electrical changes cannot occur after prolonged periods of occlusion beyond 20–30 minutes.

Electrical Alternans

A characteristic feature of ischemic cells is that some time before they become completely unresponsive, they undergo a period when the amplitude and duration of the action potentials alternate from beat to beat. This produces alternation in the ST-T segment of the extracellular signals as well. Examples are shown in Figures 2.10 and 2.11. In both figures the transmembrane action potentials are shown in the top traces and the extracellular electrograms in the bottom traces. In Figure 2.10, the alternation in action potentials occurred after a 5-minute period of occlusion (bottom panel). In Figure 2.11, the alternation occurred after nearly 7 minutes of occlusion (bottom right panel). The upstroke of the larger action potentials is divided into two components and only the first component remains during the small response. Theoretically, two mechanisms may be involved. Electrotonic interactions in an area of inhomogeneous conduction may give rise to double-component action potentials. One

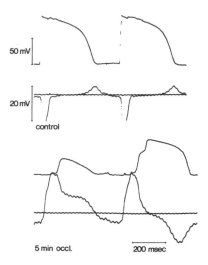

Figure 2.10: Alternation in action potential configuration 5 minutes after coronary occlusion in the pig heart. Action potentials are in the top traces of each panel, DC electrograms in the bottom traces. Control recordings are in the top panel, recordings 5 minutes after occlusion in the bottom panel. Note separation of action potential upstroke into two components in lower right potential. (Reproduced from Kléber et al. (1978) with permission.)

may also speculate that in this phase of ischemia, a separation between the fast Na^+ inward current and the L-type Ca^{2+} inward current has occurred. The fast Na^+ inward current, although depressed (partly as a consequence of the reduced membrane potential) is responsible for the first component of depolarization and carries the membrane potential to a level where the L-type Ca^{2+} current can be activated. The inward Ca^{2+} current would then be responsible for the second phase of the upstroke and for the long plateau phase. It apparently fails to be activated in every second beat, and the small amplitude response of short duration would be due to activation of the depressed Na^+ inward current only. It is difficult to furnish proof for this hypothesis, but in agreement with this speculation is the observation that the Ca^{2+} entry blocker verapamil abolishes alternation (Janse 1982b).

In experimental models, the phase of alternation is transient and brief. In humans, a similar transient alternation in the ST-T segment of precordial electrocardiograms is seen in the very early stages (3 to 5 minutes) of ischemia (Kléber et al. 1977; Cinca et al. 1980). Both in the experimental animal (Downar et al. 1977a; Carson et al. 1986; Abe et al. 1989) and in patients dying suddenly during ambulant ECG recording (Bayés de Luna et al. 1985), such alternans often precedes the onset of ventricular arrhythmias. In the pig, two periods of alternans have been observed, one at 2 to 7 minutes, the other at 15 to 40 minutes after coronary ligation, corresponding to the phases when so called 1A and 1B arrhythmias occur (Dilly and Lab 1988). These phases are described later. In particular, complexes with deep negative "T waves" seem

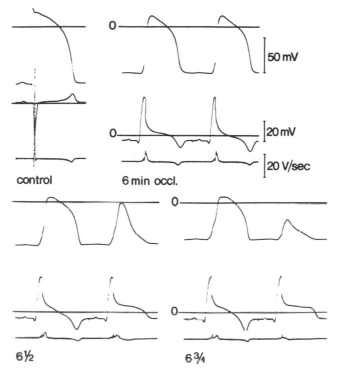

Figure 2.11: Transmembrane potentials (upper traces), local DC electrograms (middle traces) and dV/dt (V_{max}) of the upstroke of the transmembrane action potentials (lowest traces) recorded in the pig heart. The top left panel shows control recordings, the top right 6 minutes after occlusion, the lower left 6 1/2 minutes after occlusion and the lower right 6 3/4 minutes after occlusion. Alternation in action potentials and electrograms occurred at 6 3/4 minutes. (Reproduced from Janse (1982c) with permission.)

to herald the beginning of arrhythmias. A clinical example is shown in Figure 2.12, that shows precordial electrocardiograms of a patient with variant angina during a transient episode of ischemia. Recordings were taken continuously and stored on a tape recorder. Time 0 was arbitrarily chosen as 2 minutes before the patient woke up because of the chest pain. Note the rapid development of ST elevations (which are the sum of TQ depression and ST elevation) by 3 1/2 minutes and the occurrence of premature ventricular depolarizations following deep negative deflections after 5 1/2 minutes. The ST elevation and premature ventricular depolarizations then subsided quickly.

Mechanisms of Changes in the ST-T Segment

For a quantitative analysis of the relationship between changes in intra- and extracellular potentials produced by acute regional ischemia, detailed

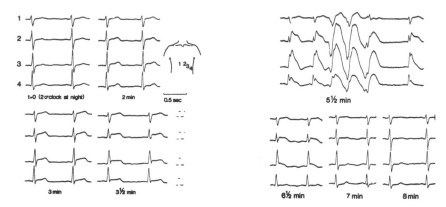

Figure 2.12: Precordial electrocardiograms recorded from a patient with variant angina during a transient episode of ischemia. The times of recording after onset of ischemia are indicated below each panel. (Unpublished observations of F.J.L. Van Capelle and M.J. Janse.)

knowledge of these potentials at multiple sites, of the geometry of the myocardial fibers, and of intra- and extracellular resistances in the various directions relative to fiber orientation is required. On a qualitative basis, these relationships can be understood by using the diagrams shown in Figures 2.13 to 2.16. Figure 2.13 uses the actual recordings of Figure 2.6. Potentials recorded before coronary occlusion are superimposed over the potentials recorded from the same cell and the same extracellular site, 4 and 5 minutes after coronary occlusion. In the diagrams it is also assumed that the intracellular potentials recorded before occlusion are representative of potentials in nonischemic myocardium at the time when recordings from ischemic cells were made. (This is not quite correct, because transmembrane potentials from the nonischemic side of the border will be influenced by electrotonic current flow across the border between ischemic and nonischemic tissue.) In Figure 2.13A, the potential gradients between intra- and extracellular compartments on both sides of the border between ischemic and nonischemic cells during diastole (at the time indicated by the vertical dashed line) are shown. The intracellular potential of the ischemic cell (solid trace at the top left) is more positive than the intracellular potential of the normal cell (dashed trace). Consequently, an intracellular current flows from ischemic towards normal cells. The direction of current flow is defined as relative movement of positive charges and is indicated by the long arrow from -64 mV (ischemic (I) resting potential) to -97 mV (normal (N) resting potential) at the right. This current crosses the cell membrane and flows in an opposite direction in the extracellular space (long arrow pointing from normal (N) to ischemic (I)). The presence of current sinks in the extracellular space of the ischemic tissue (indicated by the arrow pointing inward from -11 to -64) accounts for the TQ segment depression; current sources in the extracellular space of the much larger mass of normal myocardium (arrow pointing outward in N from -97 to $+1$) account for the "reciprocal" TQ seg-

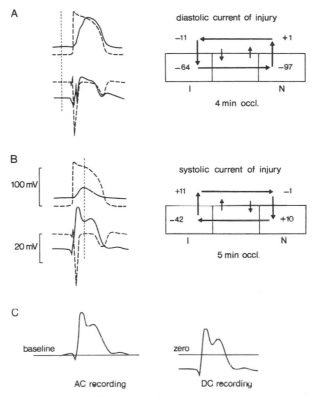

Figure 2.13: Mechanism of TQ and ST segment changes. Intra- and extracellular potentials of normal myocardium (dashed lines) are superimposed over potentials recorded after 4 and 5 minutes of coronary artery occlusion (solid lines) at the left in panels A and B. Potentials shown in Figure 2.6 were redrawn in this Figure. In the diagrams the local current circuits in diastole and systole are depicted (during the moments in the cardiac cycle indicated by a vertical dashed line through the redrawn potentials). Intra- and extracellular potentials are given in millivolts (mV) at the right. I = ischemic area, N = normal myocardium, each represented as one cell. In C, extracellular potentials are shown, recorded from the ischemic zone after 5 minutes of ischemia with both alternating current (AC) and direct current (DC) amplifiers.

ment elevation. These effects on the electrogram are indicated below the transmembrane recording by the solid trace (ischemic) superimposed on the dashed trace (normal). In Figure 2.13B, current flow during systole is illustrated. The moment in the cardiac cycle is indicated by a vertical dashed line through the potentials recorded before and 5 minutes after coronary occlusion. Now the intracellular compartment of the normal zone is positive ($+10$, N at the right) with respect to that of the ischemic area (-42, I at the left). Therefore the current circuit has an opposite direction to that in diastole, resulting in a positive extracellular space in the ischemic region ($+11$) (ST segment elevation) and a negative space in the normal part of the heart (-1) (reciprocal ST segment depression). The arrows show the opposite directions of intracellular

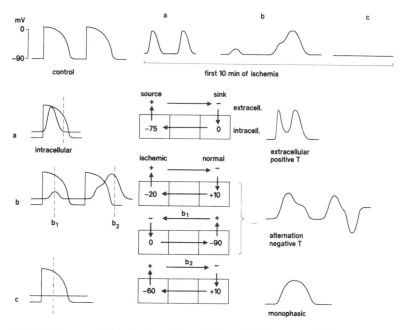

Figure 2.14: Diagrams illustrating the relationship between different transmembrane potentials recorded in an ischemic region and extracellular waveforms. At the top control action potential recordings and recordings during the first 10 minutes of ischemia (a, b, and c) are shown. Below at the left are action potentials recorded during the different periods of ischemia (a, b, c) superimposed on a control, normal action potential. At the right are diagrams indicating patterns of intracellular and extracellular current flow between ischemic and normal regions at the times indicated by the vertical dashed lines drawn through the action potentials. The arrows show the direction of current flow.

and extracellular current flow. In Figure 2.13C, the difference between AC and DC recordings is schematically shown. It should be emphasized that ST elevation as recorded by conventional electrocardiographic amplifiers (condenser-coupled AC amplifiers) can in fact be caused by a diastolic current, resulting primarily from a loss of resting membrane potential of ischemic cells. It can also be caused by a combination of diastolic and systolic current, where the latter is primarily due to a reduction of the amplitude of the action potentials of ischemic cells. Similar diagrams are used to illustrate changes in T waves, in Figure 2.14. At the top of the figure are shown action potentials recorded during control (prior to coronary occlusion) and during the first 10 minutes of ischemia after occlusion. The resting potential, upstroke and amplitude first are depressed (a) before alternation (b) and inexcitability (c) occur. Below this top trace, the current flow between normal and ischemic zones is diagrammed for each of these time periods. In Figure 2.14a, it is shown how shortening of the action potential in the ischemic zone is responsible for a large, positive T wave in the local extracellular electrogram. The ischemic action

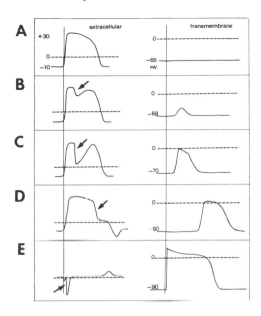

Figure 2.15: Schematic representation of a variety of extracellular waveforms that can be recorded from ischemic myocardium during the first 10 minutes after coronary occlusion at the left, together with the corresponding transmembrane potentials at the right. (Reproduced from Janse (1986b) with permission.)

potential is shown to have a much shorter duration than the normal action potential. At the time indicated by the dashed vertical line at the left, intracellular current flows from normal to ischemic regions because the normal is relatively positive. Extracellular current flows in the opposite direction. The ischemic region, therefore, acts as a source and the normal region as a sink. At the right is shown the positive extracellular T wave that results. In (b), during the period of alternation, the pattern of current flow is dependent on the type of ischemic action potential. This pattern at the times indicated by the dashed lines in the superimposed ischemic and normal action potentials at the left, is diagrammed at the right. During the low-amplitude response, (b_1), intracellular current flows from normal to ischemic regions and extracellular current from ischemic to normal. The ischemic region is the source and the normal region is the sink. During the large amplitude ischemic response (b_2), the direction of current flow is reversed as is the source and sink. This is responsible for the alternation in the T wave shown at the right. When inexcitability in the ischemic region occurs (c), intracellular current flows from normal to ischemic and extracellular current flows from ischemic to normal (at the time indicated by the dashed vertical line) giving rise to the monophasic extracellular recording at the right. It can be seen from the diagrams that it is an oversimplification to equate action potential shortening with positive T waves, or for that matter action potential lengthening with negative T waves. The changes in T waves are determined by differences in repolarization in ischemic and

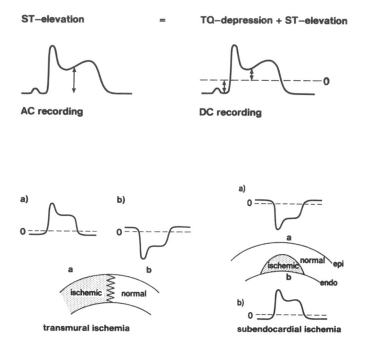

Figure 2.16: The upper panel shows how ST elevation as recorded with a normal condenser-coupled AC amplifier is in reality the sum of TQ depression and ST elevation as recorded with a DC amplifier. Lower panel shows diagrams of extracellular signals in transmural and subendocardial ischemia.

normal myocardium. In nonischemic hearts, such differences are largely caused by differences in action potential duration. In hearts with regional ischemia, both differences in action potential duration and activation delays contribute to differences in repolarization. Activation delays may be so large that, despite a shortened action potential, repolarization of the ischemic zone occurs later than in the normal zone as shown in Figure 2.14b(b_2). In such a situation, T waves in the ischemic zone become negative. Figure 2.15 catalogs the different extracellular waveforms that can be recorded from acutely ischemic myocardium (left column), together with the corresponding transmembrane potentials that give rise to these waveforms (right column). Normal extra- and intracellular potentials are shown in the bottom panel (E). In the panel above this (panel D), the ischemic cell has depolarized to −80 mV (causing the TQ depression shown in the electrogram at the left). The moment of activation of the ischemic region is considerably delayed, so that, despite action potential shortening, repolarization occurs later than in the normal area. Therefore, the extracellular complex shows a delayed intrinsic deflection (arrow), followed by a negative T wave. In the panel above this (C), an action potential from an ischemic cell (resting potential −70 mV) with less delay is shown; the T wave of the electrogram at the left is positive because repolarization of the ischemic cell now occurs earlier than in normal tissue and the intrinsic deflection (arrow) comes earlier. When resting membrane potential is − 68 mV (panel B), the very small response recorded with the microelectrode (at the right) still produces a negative deflection in the extracellular complex at the left. As stated earlier, from such a recording it is impossible to say whether this is an electrotonic depolarization or whether it still represents an active response. The top panel (A) shows the intra- and extracellular manifestations of conduction block; unresponsiveness in the ischemic zone (right) causes a monophasic extracellular complex at the left.

Figure 2.16 shows in a diagrammatic form that complexes with ST elevation (= TQ depression + ST elevation) are recorded from the epicardium of the ischemic zone in the case of transmural ischemia, whereas in subendocardial ischemia, epicardial electrograms show ST depression. In the lower panel at the left it is schematically depicted how in the case of transmural ischemia, complexes with TQ depression and ST elevation ("ST elevation" with AC recordings) are recorded from the epicardial surface of the ischemic zone (a), and "reciprocal" TQ elevation and ST depression ("ST depression") (b) are seen in DC electrograms recorded from adjacent myocardium. Similarly, in the case of subendocardial ischemia (at the right), complexes with ST depression (a) are recorded from the epicardium, signals with ST elevation (b) from the endocardium.

It must be emphasized that the relationship between transmembrane and extracellular potentials described above is only qualitative. For example, the amount of TQ depression at a certain site cannot be used as an index of local resting membrane depolarization (Johnson et al. 1987). In addition to the change in local resting membrane potential, the magnitude of TQ depression is also determined by the resistances encountered by the diastolic current flowing between ischemic and normal cells, and these will change with time during ischemia as we describe later.

Factors Causing the Changes in Action Potentials

The decrease in amplitude and upstroke velocity of action potentials of ischemic cells cannot be solely attributed to inactivation of Na^+ channels resulting from the decreased resting potential (Moréna et al. 1980; Nguyen-Thi et al. 1981). This was demonstrated in porcine hearts that were regionally perfused through a coronary artery with a normoxic, high K^+ solution. In these experiments subepicardial action potentials recorded in the presence of the high K^+ solution had larger amplitudes and faster upstrokes than action potentials recorded at the same site during coronary artery occlusion even though the action potentials under both conditions arose from similar levels of resting membrane potential (Moréna et al. 1980). Therefore, in addition to an increase in extracellular K^+ and the resulting decrease in resting potential other factors in the ischemic environment probably contribute to the decrease in depolarizing inward current, perhaps by acting on the Na^+ channels.

The ischemic environment of cardiac muscle has a special composition that results from the deprivation of blood flow. Not only is extracellular K^+ elevated but there is hypoxia, a low pH, no substrates, high pCO_2, and accumulation of substances such as lysophosphoglycerides, and catecholamines. Each may have an influence on membrane conductances and the various combinations may exert effects that are not predictable from the action of each substance alone. It is therefore impossible to elucidate the single contributions of these components to changes in the action potential by studies on the *in vivo* or arterially-perfused heart. Another approach then is to utilize solutions designed to mimic the ischemic milieu to perfuse hearts or to superfuse isolated preparations. However, these solutions can be only an approximate representation since all the components of the ischemic environment are not yet known, nor is the amount in which each component is present. In any case, individual components of ischemia can be added or deleted to determine their contributions to the changes in the action potentials.

Action potentials with the same characteristics as those recorded during ischemia in the *in situ* heart have been recorded from isolated preparations of ventricular muscle superfused with solutions containing several of the major ischemic components, such as hypoxia, low pH, high K^+ concentration, and no substrates for metabolism (Senges et al. 1979; Gilmour and Zipes 1980; Kagiyama et al. 1982; Weiss and Shine 1982b; Ruiz-Ceretti et al. 1983; Kodama et al. 1984; Nakaya et al. 1985; Wilde 1988; Rouet et al. 1989; Kimura et al. 1990). However, the combination of ischemic factors is often incomplete in studies on the effects of "ischemia" in superfused cardiac tissue. Thus, ischemia is often mimicked by hypoxia alone or by high K^+ alone (Senges et al. 1979), or by a combination of high K^+ and acidosis (Kagiyama et al. 1982), with or without the addition of catecholamines (Weiss and Shine 1982b) in substrate-containing solutions that are well oxygenated. In addition to the various compositions of the ischemic solutions, the source of the muscle that is studied in experiments using isolated superfused tissues may also influence the results. Action potential amplitudes and upstroke velocities were more reduced in sub-epicardial preparations than in subendocardial preparations exposed to the same "ischemic milieu" or to arrest of coronary flow in perfused preparations, indicating an intrinsic difference in "sensitivity" between both tissues (Gilmour and Zipes 1980; Kimura et al. 1986b; 1990). Studies using monophasic action potential recordings in intact dog hearts also reported on greater effects of ischemia in the subepicardium, where a more marked decrease in monophasic action potential duration was observed than in the subendocardium (Taggart et al. 1988).

The same changes in action potentials as those observed during coronary occlusion occur in isolated porcine hearts regionally perfused through a coronary artery with an hypoxic solution, containing no glucose, a high K^+ concentration, and made acidotic by the addition of lactate and hydrochloric acid. The time course for these action potential changes was the same as during coronary artery occlusion in the same heart (Moréna et al. 1980). Other studies in the canine heart, using recordings of monophasic potentials also have indicated that the combination of high K^+ and hypoxia imitates the changes caused by ischemia quite well (Donaldson et al. 1984). Thus, these several ischemic components seem to be the most important determinants of changes in the action potential. Figure 2.17 shows action potentials (top traces) and local direct current electrograms (bottom traces) recorded from the region perfused by the left anterior descending coronary artery in an isolated perfused pig heart. Records are shown during control, after 7 minutes of left anterior descending coronary artery occlusion, and 15, 20, and 25 minutes after perfusion of the left anterior descending coronary artery (LAD) distal to the occlusion. Both intra- and extracellular potentials were very similar either during occlusion of this artery (top middle panel), or when following a sufficiently long reperfusion period, the same artery was selectively perfused with a high K^+ acidic solution made hypoxic (top right panel). The similarities emphasize that hypoxia, low pH, and high K^+ are crucial components of the ischemic environment. The degree of hypoxia seems fairly critical. In the upper right panel, "ischemic" potentials were recorded when pO_2 of the perfusate was 33 mm Hg. In the lower

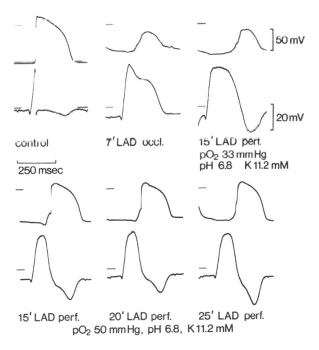

Figure 2.17: The upper panel shows the similarity between transmembrane potentials (upper tracings) and extracellular potentials (lower tracings) after a 7-minute occlusion of the left anterior descending coronary artery and, following 15 minutes of perfusion of the left anterior descending coronary artery with an hypoxic (pO_2 33 mm Hg), high K^+ (11.2 mmol), acidic solution (pH 6.8). In the lower panels, after a suitable normal reperfusion period, the left anterior descending coronary artery was again perfused with the same acidic, high K^+ solution, but pO_2 was now increased from 33 to 50 mm Hg. Potentials are now far less depressed. (Reproduced from Janse et al. (1980a) with permission.)

panels it is shown that a slight increase in pO_2 to 50 mm Hg improved the resting potential and action potential upstroke and preserved action potential configuration for a long time (15, 20, and 25 minutes of left anterior descending coronary artery (LAD) perfusion), while the effects of elevated K^+ concentration (reduction of resting membrane potential, shorter action potential duration, slight reduction of upstroke velocity) were still apparent. In addition, it has been found that partial recovery of the depressed action potentials occurs, both in isolated perfused hearts and in the isolated superfused preparations during maintained exposure to the "ischemic solution" (Gilmour and Zipes 1980; Moréna et al. 1980; Kimura et al. 1982; Nakaya et al. 1985). This recovery is shown in Figure 2.18. The control action potential and electrogram are shown at the top left. Perfusion with a high K^+, acidic, severely hypoxic solution produced the same changes as seen during ischemia: loss of resting membrane potential and alternation at 3 1/2 minutes (top right), the appearance of very small amplitude responses at 6 minutes (bottom left), and an improvement at 24 minutes despite maintained perfusion with the hypoxic solution (bottom right). This recovery is similar to that described in intact hearts with regional ischemia (Scherlag et al. 1974; Kléber et al. 1978; Kaplinsky et al. 1979; Janse

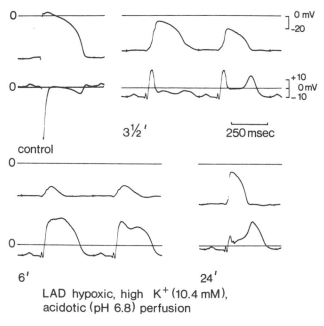

Figure 2.18: Imitation of potential changes during ischemia by left anterior descending coronary artery perfusion with hypoxic, high K^+ acidic solution. Recordings of the action potentials (top traces) and DC electrograms (bottom traces) are shown during control conditions (top left) and 3.5, 6, and 24 minutes after beginning of left anterior descending coronary artery perfusion. Note improvement in action potentials after 24 minutes of continuous perfusion. (Reproduced from Moréna et al. (1980) with permission.)

and Kléber 1981; Russell et al. 1984; Fleet et al. 1985), or in isolated guinea pig hearts with global ischemia (Penny 1984). In the latter, the spontaneous improvement in action potential amplitude and $\dot{V}_{max}$ of the upstroke did not occur after the hearts were depleted of their catecholamines or were treated with propranolol (Penny 1984). Therefore, the improvement may be due to ischemia-induced release of noradrenaline from local nerve endings, which has been shown to occur around 15 to 20 minutes after the beginning of ischemia (Schömig et al. 1984; Carlsson 1987), the time during which the improvement was observed (Wilde 1988). The hypothesis is that catecholamines stimulate the Na/K pump, resulting in a net uptake of K^+ by the ischemic cells (see "dip" in the K^+ curve of Figure 2.3). The cells thereby slightly hyperpolarize and this can lead to the appearance of action potentials in previously unresponsive cells. Another reason for the temporal improvement in electrical activity may be the fact that extracellular K^+ "diffuses" from the ischemic region towards the normal part of the left ventricle, leading to a reduction of extracellular K^+ in the ischemic zone after some 10 to 20 minutes (Coronel et al. 1988). The reduction in extracellular K^+ may be substantial, especially in ischemic tissue close to the boundary with normal myocardium, as is the restoration of electrical activity (Coronel 1988). Figure 2.19 shows this relationship between reduc-

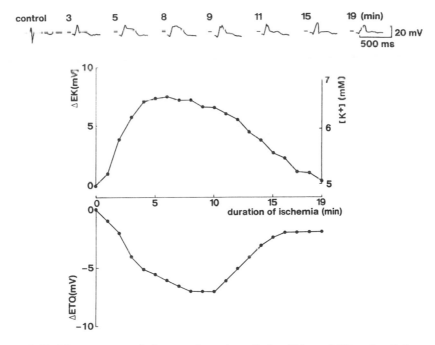

Figure 2.19: Time course of changes in extracellular K^+ and TQ potential recorded close to the border between ischemic and normal myocardium. Extracellular potentials during control and after coronary occlusion are at the top with the time of ischemia in minutes indicated above the recordings. The graphs below show changes in K^+ and TQ potentials. (Reproduced from Coronel et al. (1988) with permission.)

tion in extracellular K^+ and improvement in electrical activity. The time course is shown of changes in extracellular K^+ concentration (E_K(mV)) and TQ potential (ETQ(mV)) during a 19-minute period of regional ischemia recorded by an electrode close to the border with normal tissues. Changes in extracellular K^+ are here expressed as the change in millivolts recorded by the K^+-sensitive electrode. A tenfold change in E_K corresponds to a doubling of the K^+ concentration (shown on the right ordinate). In other words, 0 is 4.7 mmol K^+ while 10 mV is 9.4 mmol K^+. Electrograms recorded by the same electrode are shown in the upper panels. Note that after 8 minutes a monophasic potential and maximum change in TQ is recorded at a relatively low value of extracellular K^+ and that the subsequent decrease in extracellular K^+ (by diffusion into normal myocardium) and TQ potential is associated with recovery of electrical activity.

The exact changes in intracellular and extracellular pH that are caused by coronary artery occlusion are difficult to reproduce using ischemic solutions. In ischemia in the *in situ* heart, intracellular acidosis precedes extracellular acidosis. Extracellular pH then decreases after 15 seconds of ischemia (Benzing et al. 1971/1972) and is accompanied by an equally fast elevation of extracellular pCO_2 (Case et al. 1979). Both metabolic acidosis (Senges et al. 1979; Gilmour and Zipes 1980; Moréna et al. 1980) and respiratory acidosis (Kagiyama et al. 1982; Kodama et al. 1984) have been used in ischemic solutions in attempts to imitate these conditions. It has been proposed that respiratory acidosis approaches an ischemic situation more accurately, since intracellular pH is reduced more quickly in comparison to metabolic acidosis (Poole-Wilson and Cameron 1975; Kodama et al. 1984). The results of the various studies are somewhat confusing. Senges et al. (1979) found that lactate acidosis in combination with hypoxia and increased catecholamine levels prolonged the action potential but had no effect on resting potential, action potential upstroke velocity and conduction but in this study the solution did not contain an elevated K^+ concentration. In a study by Kagiyama et al. (1982), metabolic acidosis also lengthened the action potential, respiratory acidosis did not. At elevated extracellular K^+ concentrations, both forms of acidosis, but in particular respiratory acidosis, reduced maximum upstroke velocity secondary to a decrease in resting potential. Hypoxia was not induced in this study. In a series of experiments in which combinations of the three ischemic components (hypoxia, high K^+, and respiratory acidosis) were examined, the effects of hypoxia, at either normal or high extracellular K^+ levels were little influenced by acidosis (Kodama et al. 1984). Acidosis had no influence on upstroke velocity and on the recovery kinetics of maximal upstroke velocity after an action potential during hypoxia. However, action potential shortening in the presence of hypoxia and acidosis was less than when hypoxia was induced in the absence of acidosis. Therefore, it may be concluded that elevated extracellular K^+ and hypoxia are two major determinants of the changes in the action potential during acute ischemia and that in their presence the additional effects of acidosis are minimal. This is, however, an oversimplification because hypoxia itself produces intracellular acidosis, albeit to a considerably smaller extent than during ischemia (Allen and Orchard 1983; 1987; Ellis and Noireaud 1987). Moreover, cellular K^+ loss and ischemic acidosis might be interrelated as well (Cascio et al. 1989).

Depressed Fast Responses or Slow Responses?

The depressed upstrokes (decreased amplitude and velocity of depolarization) of action potentials with partially depolarized membrane potentials in ischemic regions after coronary occlusion may be caused by either a reduced fast Na^+ current (depressed fast response) or by the slow inward L-type Ca^{2+} current (slow response) (Cranefield 1975). The latter may occur if the level of resting potential is reduced enough to inactivate the Na^+ current. Cranefield et al. (1972) suggested that action potentials in acutely ischemic regions might be slow responses because action potentials caused by slow inward Ca^{2+} current were shown to occur in isolated cardiac fibers superfused with solutions containing elevated K^+ and catecholamines (Carmeliet and Vereecke 1969). Ischemic regions, as described above, also contain elevated K^+ and there may be a high norepinephrine level because the catecholamine is released from sympathetic nerve endings after coronary occlusion (Schömig et al. 1984; Carlsson 1987). At present, it is not possible to give a definite answer to the question of whether the depolarization phase of depressed ischemic action potentials is caused by partially inactivated rapid Na^+ inward current, or by slow inward Ca^{2+} current, or by some combination of the two. However, some observations indicate that, at least during the first 10 to 15 minutes of ischemia, the reduced upstroke of the action potential is caused by inward Na^+ current flowing through partially inactivated Na^+ channels. Attempts have been made to measure resting membrane potentials accurately in intact beating hearts during acute ischemia, although it must be emphasized that accurate measurement under these conditions is very difficult and not as reliable as in isolated superfused preparations. In isolated blood-perfused hearts after coronary occlusion, the depressed action potentials arose from membrane potentials more negative than about -60 mV, levels at which normally, the Na^+ channels are not expected to be completely inactivated. Upon further depolarization of the membrane to less than -60 mV, levels at which most rapid sodium channels are inactivated (Weidmann 1955; Beeler and Reuter 1970), the ischemic fibers were unresponsive during activation of surrounding nonischemic myocardium (Kléber et al. 1978; Kléber 1983). Ischemia abolishes catecholamine-induced slow responses in 27 mmol K^+ (Schneider and Sperelakis 1974), and the slow inward Ca^{2+} current is reduced by external acidification (Chesnais et al. 1975; Kohlhardt et al. 1976), and particularly by intracellular acidosis (Irisawa and Sato 1986). It is therefore quite possible that ischemia preferentially suppresses activation of the L-type Ca^{2+} channels. Average resting potentials at which ischemic cells became unresponsive in one study was -60.3 ± 1.45 mV (Kléber et al. 1986). In the same hearts, after excitability was restored by reperfusion with normoxic solution, slow responses could be induced by raising the K^+ concentration of the perfusate to 19.3 mmol (at which level the hearts became inexcitable) and adding adrenaline. Average resting potential at which slow responses occurred was -48.5 ± 2.8 mV (Kléber et al. 1986).

Although one interpretation of these results is that slow Ca^{2+}-dependent responses do not occur in the ischemic zone because of the failure of action potentials to occur at membrane potentials at which Na^+ channels are inactivated, another interpretation is also possible. The cells in the center of the ischemic zone that are depolarized to membrane potentials of -60 mV or less during ischemia might be excitable, but the excitatory currents provided by activation fronts invading the ischemic tissue may not be strong enough to excite them (Coronel et al. 1988). It also cannot be excluded that local release of noradrenaline in an ischemic region might prevent ischemic cells from becoming inexcitable at resting membrane potentials more positive than -60 mV, and that such release did not occur to a sufficient extent in the experiments discussed above, particularly since many of them were done in isolated perfused hearts.

No measurements of resting membrane potentials have been made from ischemic myocardium *in vivo*, between 15 to 30 minutes after coronary occlusion. Arrhythmias may still occur during this time (type 1b arrhythmias described later). This phase is associated with the reappearance of action potentials in cells that previously become unresponsive during the early minutes of ischemia (Downar et al. 1977a; Kléber et al. 1978; Janse and Kléber 1981). It is not possible to conclude whether slow Ca^{2+}-dependent responses occur during this phase of ischemia or whether depressed fast responses reappear. As described earlier, extracellular K^+ often decreases around this time (Hill and Gettes 1980; Hirche et al. 1980; Coronel et al. 1988) suggesting that the Na/K pump might succeed in decreasing the K^+ gradient across the cell membrane. This might be possible since the K^+ efflux is reduced because of the absence of action potentials. This could lead to a slight hyperpolarization that partly reactivates the rapid Na^+ channels. In the absence of reliable data on resting membrane potentials this explanation remains purely speculative. On the other hand, as mentioned above, there is some evidence linking the reappearance of action potentials to the local release of norepinephrine (Penny 1984), which might either hyperpolarize the membrane potential (Boyden et al. 1983; Wilde 1988), reactivating fast channels, or cause slow responses to appear (Cranefield 1975).

Even if the L-type Ca^{2+} inward current is not responsible for the entire action potential upstroke during ischemia, it may assume a greater role in causing phase 0 depolarization than in normal myocardial cells. As we described, in the first 10 minutes following coronary occlusion, the depressed upstroke of the action potential often shows two well-defined components (Downar et al. 1977a; Russell et al. 1977; Kléber et al. 1978). This phenomenon might result from a temporal separation of fast and slow inward currents (Niedergerke and Orkand 1966). Similar action potentials have been found in isolated preparations exposed to elevated K^+ concentrations. It has been shown that the first component is due to the depressed fast Na^+ inward current. This current brings the membrane potential into the range of potentials at which activation of the inward Ca^{2+} current occurs. The Ca^{2+} current is responsible for both the second component of the upstroke and the plateau (Mascher 1970; Windisch and Tritthart 1982; Arita and Kiyosue 1983). During the phase of electrical alternation, so often seen in the acute phase of ischemia (Hellerstein and Liebow 1950; Downar et al. 1977a; Kleinfeld and Rozanski 1977; Kléber et al. 1978; Cinca et al. 1980), the upstroke of the large action potential has two components, that of the small action potential only one. Activation of the inward Ca^{2+} current might occur only during every second beat.

Studies on the effect of putative Na^+ and Ca^{2+} channel blocking agents also throw some light on the role of fast and slow inward currents in the generation of the action potential upstroke in ischemic cells. Lidocaine, which interacts with Na^+ channels, has been shown to decrease the amplitude of, or abolish depressed fast responses in isolated Purkinje fibers, whereas in the usual therapeutic concentrations it has little effect on slow calcium-dependent responses in the presence of elevated extracellular K^+ and noradrenaline (Brennan et al. 1978). Lidocaine depressed or abolished the transmembrane action potentials recorded from the center of the ischemic zone in isolated porcine hearts, making it very likely that the upstrokes were initiated by the rapid Na^+ inward current (Cardinal et al. 1981). In a model where neonatal myocardial cells were transplanted to the adult hamster cheek pouch and became vascularized, ischemia was introduced by interrupting flow to these cells. The depressed action potentials recorded in the presence of ischemia resembled those recorded from other ischemic preparations and were suppressed by the Na^+ channel blocker tetrodotoxin and not by the L-type calcium channel blocker verapamil (Gilmour and Zipes 1982). This study provides additional evidence that depressed action potentials in ischemia may be due to "depressed fast responses"; that is, action potentials resulting from depolarizing current flowing through partially inactivated Na^+ channels.

Unfortunately, there is little information available on the effect of calcium channel blocking drugs on transmembrane action potentials recorded from ischemic cells in intact hearts. In isolated perfused porcine hearts, verapamil abolishes electrical alternans that is clearly present in the absence of the drug. In the presence of verapamil, action potentials shorten, have no plateau, and the upstroke has only one component. The second component that may be caused by slow inward current is abolished. At similar times after coronary occlusion, depolarization of resting membrane potential is less and action potential upstroke is faster in the presence of verapamil than in its absence. Figure 2.20 shows the effects of different concentrations of verapamil on action potentials recorded from the ischemic zone of an isolated porcine heart. A control coronary occlusion lasted 5 minutes, and was followed by a 20-minute reperfusion period. The effects of this period of occlusion on the action potentials are shown in the top trace and are typical of what we have described. Verapamil (0.25 mg/L) was added 20 minutes prior to another occlusion and the effects on action potentials are shown in the second trace. There is disap-

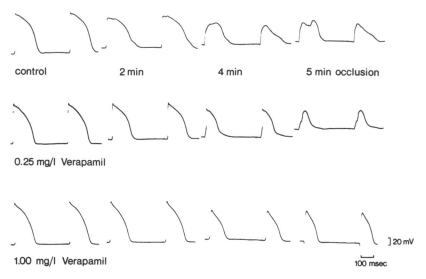

Figure 2.20: Effects of verapamil on action potentials recorded from the ischemic zone of an isolated porcine heart. A coronary artery was occluded for 5 minutes, three times in succession followed by 20 minutes of reperfusion. Verapamil was administered in two different concentrations following the first and second occlusion. (Unpublished results of M.J. Janse, A.A.M. Wilde and I. Kodama.)

pearance of alternans, less depolarization and preservation of a faster action potential upstroke in the presence of verapamil. These effects are even more marked in the third trace where a higher concentration of verapamil was added prior to a third occlusion. In experiments on the globally ischemic rabbit heart, verapamil also caused considerably less slowing of conduction, slightly less depolarization of resting membrane potential, and preservation of upstroke velocity (Kabell 1988). In an *in vitro* study where action potential characteristics were measured in an ischemic perfusate consisting of hypoxia, high K^+, and acidosis, it was found that pretreatment with verapamil prevented much of the reduction of action potential amplitude, upstroke velocity, and conduction velocity that is normally caused by ischemia (Kimura et al. 1982). It is uncertain how verapamil exerts these effects and there are a number of possibilities: (1) verapamil may cause the time course of ischemic changes in electrophysiology to slow because of the decreased energy utilization accompanying the decreased contractility that it causes; (2) verapamil may diminish a depolarizing inward Ca current (Clusin et al. 1984) thus maintaining membrane potential at a more hyperpolarized level; (3) a reduction in intracellular Ca^{2+} concentration caused by verapamil blockade of calcium channels might prevent an increase in K^+ conductance (Bassingthwaighte et al. 1976) and consequently prevent to some degree the loss of intracellular K^+. In fact, in the presence of verapamil extracellular K^+ does not rise to the same high levels that occur in its absence (Fleet et al. 1986). However, the negative inotropic effect would also be expected to prevent some of the rise in extracellular K^+.

Action Potential Duration and Recovery of Excitability

The duration of the ventricular muscle action potential has been shown to undergo a biphasic change after coronary artery occlusion in experiments in which action potentials have been recorded from the epicardial surface of whole hearts. Initially, it lengthens slightly. This lengthening, which is as much as 30 msec in isolated perfused hearts or hearts in animals with the chest open (Daniel et al. 1978; Downar et al. 1977a), is likely due to a slight reduction in the temperature in the subepicardial muscle layers. Subepicardial temperature also decreases after a coronary occlusion even when the chest is closed since the normal blood flow serves to warm the muscle. The duration of the refractory period during the first 2 minutes following coronary artery occlusion increases concomitantly with the lengthening of the action potential (Reynolds et al. 1960; Han et al. 1970; Downar et al. 1977a). Subsequently, action potential duration shortens mainly because of a shortening of the plateau phase. The shortening of the action potential duration is a result of the combined effects of a number of the components of the ischemic environment. Hypoxia has been shown to shorten action potential duration in the absence of the other components of ischemia and undoubtedly contributes to this effect of ischemia (Trautwein et al. 1954). Likely causes for action potential shortening during hypoxia are a decrease in the inward L-type calcium current and an increase in a time-independent outward K^+ current, mediated by an increase in intracellular Ca^{2+} activity, or increase in K^+ conductance. The increase in K^+ conductance results from the effects of ATP depletion on ATP-sensitive K^+ channels (Carmeliet 1978; Vleugels et al. 1980; Isenberg et al. 1983; Noma 1983). However, the effects of hypoxia alone are not the same as the effects of ischemia. Although hypoxia shortens the action potential similar to coronary occlusion, there is only a slight decrease in resting membrane potential and maximum upstroke velocity unlike the effects of coronary occlusion (McDonald and MacLeod 1973; Carmeliet 1978). Action potentials with large amplitudes and fast upstrokes, but of short duration, as seen during hypoxia alone (Trautwein et al. 1954; McDonald and MacLeod 1973; Carmeliet 1978; Moréna et al. 1980) have not been recorded from ischemic hearts. After coronary occlusion, shortening of action potential duration parallels the decrease in resting potential and action potential amplitude. Therefore, the decrease in resting potential may also contribute to the shortening of the action potential duration. Other components of the ischemic environment (high K^+, metabolic products, etc.) may shorten action potential duration as well.

Experimental evidence from *in vivo* hearts showing that refractory periods of ischemic myocardium shorten along with the action potential duration, after the first 2 minutes following complete coronary artery occlusion, is abundant (Brooks et al. 1960; Reynolds et al. 1960; Han and Moe 1964; Tsuchida 1965; Kupersmith et al. 1975; Elharrar et al. 1977; Russell and Oliver 1978). In studies where the effects of partial coronary occlusion were investigated, it was found that refractory periods shortened when flow was reduced to less than

50% to 70% of normal (Ramanathan et al. 1977; Batsford et al. 1978). However, some of the technical difficulties related to determining refractory periods in ischemic regions of the *in situ* heart sometimes make results of these experiments difficult to interpret. Refractory periods have been determined by using premature stimuli of a fixed duration, applied after a number of beats of a regularly driven rhythm. The coupling interval of the premature stimulus to the previous basic drive stimulus is decreased in steps until a propagated response is no longer obtained. Under ideal conditions, the threshold strength required to evoke a propagated response at the various coupling intervals during the cardiac cycle should be measured and so-called strength-interval curves should be obtained (Brooks et al. 1955). However, to determine a complete strength-interval curve is a time-consuming procedure. Since electrophysiological changes in ischemic myocardium occur rapidly, investigators usually have chosen a fixed stimulus strength and determined the shortest coupling interval at which a premature stimulus of that strength initiated a propagated response. That coupling interval was defined as the effective refractory period. The premature stimuli used to determine these refractory periods usually have had an intensity of 2 to 4 times diastolic threshold, but sometimes stimuli intensities of 10 to 15 times diastolic threshold were used (Batsford et al. 1978). The problem is that diastolic thresholds increase several-fold in acutely ischemic myocardium (Janse et al. 1985a), and therefore, the intensity of the premature stimuli necessary to elicit a response must be continuously increased during the development of ischemia. The very high current intensities that may be required to determine refractory period duration in ischemic myocardium may therefore excite myocardium at a distance from the local stimulation site. If the distant myocardium has a shorter refractory period than the local myocardium, the stimulus might elicit a response at the distant site at a time that the local myocardium is still refractory. This is illustrated in Figure 2.21 where two action potentials are shown that were recorded 5 minutes after coronary occlusion from ischemic sites in the pig heart that were 5 mm apart, (A)

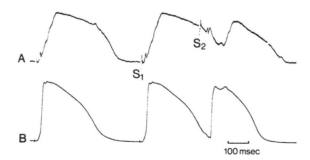

Figure 2.21: Action potentials recorded from a central ischemic site (A) in the porcine heart after coronary occlusion and from a site (B) recorded close to the border during measurement of refractory periods at site A using premature stimulation. S_1 is the response evoked by the basic drive stimulus and S_2 is the response evoked by the premature stimulus. (Reproduced from Janse et al. (1985a) with permission.)

recorded from a more central ischemic site and (B) from a less ischemic site near the infarct border. A strong premature stimulus S_2 following a basic stimulus S_1 and delivered as close as possible to the upper cell elicited a response. However, it first excited cells with a lower threshold and a shorter refractory period far away from the stimulus site, since the premature action potential of cell (B) close to the border occurred at least 60 msec earlier than the premature response at the site of stimulation. Refractory periods of tissue very close to the visual border between cyanotic, ischemic myocardium, and normally perfused tissue may shorten during ischemia (Janse et al. 1985a). Diastolic threshold in this region remains constant, at its preocclusion value, and therefore the use of high intensity stimuli to evoke a response is not necessary. Yet the results shown in Figure 2.21 might be interpreted to indicate that the local site (A) has a short refractory period, especially since in most experiments no means have been used to locate the exact site of origin of the premature responses (to determine that it did or did not originate locally). The finding that, by stimulating ischemic myocardium with strong premature stimuli, the ventricles may respond at shorter coupling intervals after coronary occlusion than during the preocclusion period, therefore, does not necessarily mean that refractory periods of ischemic cells shorten. Cells at the border, where refractory periods do shorten, may be excited from a distant stimulation site.

The refractory period of ischemic ventricular cells is not simply determined by the action potential duration as it is in normally polarized myocardium and Purkinje cells. In normal cells, the recovery of excitability is primarily voltage-dependent, and excitability is restored as the cells repolarize (Weidmann 1955; Hoffman and Cranefield 1960). On the other hand, ischemic fibers may remain inexcitable even after completely repolarizing (El-Sherif et al. 1974; Downar et al. 1977a; Lazzara et al. 1978a). This "postrepolarization refractoriness" is probably related to depolarization of the myocardial cell. In partially depolarized fibers, recovery from inactivation of both fast Na^+ and slow Ca^{2+} inward currents has been shown to be markedly delayed until many milliseconds after completion of repolarization. This was shown in experiments utilizing elevation of extracellular K^+ (which occurs in the ischemic environment) to reduce the membrane potential (Schütz 1936; Cranefield et al. 1972; Gettes and Reuter 1974). Stimuli delivered at completion of repolarization do not elicit normal action potentials, but instead, graded responses of increasing amplitude and upstroke velocities occur as the stimuli are applied later and later in diastole until a normal propagated response results (Schütz 1936; Gettes and Reuter 1974). Postrepolarization refractoriness that occurs in ischemic cells is unlike the response to hypoxia alone where refractory periods shorten along with action potential duration and the upstroke of stimulated premature action potentials is already maximal following complete repolarization (Kodama et al. 1984). In muscle fibers exposed to both high extracellular K^+ and hypoxia, recovery from inactivation is even more delayed than in fibers exposed to high K^+ alone or in fibers superfused with normal solutions in which membrane potentials are depolarized to the same level by electrical current (Kodama et al. 1984), showing the special interaction between these two major components

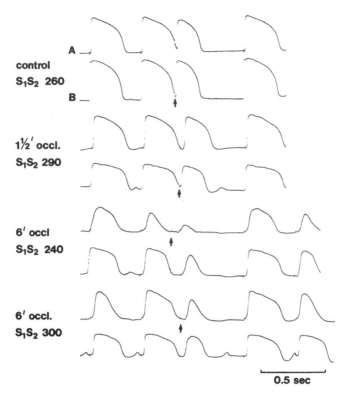

Figure 2.22: Changes in local excitability following coronary artery occlusion. In each panel simultaneous recordings of two action potentials from the epicardial surface of the pig heart are shown during control and after coronary occlusion. The arrows show the earliest coupling interval of S_2 that elicited a response. (Reproduced from Downar et al. (1977a) with permission.)

of the ischemic environment. Therefore, the refractory period actually can prolong in the central ischemic zone. Figure 2.22 shows some of the changes in action potential duration and refractory period described above. Two simultaneously recorded action potentials from sites 2.5 cm apart in the isolated perfused pig heart are displayed. Premature stimuli were applied to the ischemic region as indicated by arrows. The top panel shows the control effective refractory period, which was determined to be 260 msec. There is initial lengthening of the action potential duration and refractory period to 290 msec by 1 1/2 minutes after the coronary occlusion. At 6 minutes, marked alternation developed in the upper cell, with a 60-msec difference in refractory period between the short (240 msec) and the long (300 msec) action potential. There is also a long latency between premature stimulus and response, which is evident in the records. There is some baseline distortion due to movement artifacts.

Inhomogeneity   Harris and coworkers (1954) were the first to earmark the increase in extracellular K^+ during ischemia as a major factor causing arrhythmias. We believe that inhomogeneities in electrophysiological properties within the ischemic zone, largely caused by differences in extracellular K^+ are crucial in setting the stage for reentrant arrhythmias. There is general agreement that following coronary occlusion, there does not exist a lateral "border zone" of the ischemic region, in the sense of a continuous transition from ischemic to normal cells (Hearse and Yellon 1984). Cells are either ischemic, that is, they resort to an anaerobic metabolism, or they are not and function aerobically. There is no in-between state. Yet, although the ischemic cells are sharply demarcated from nonischemic cells, the boundary is irregular, with interdigitating peninsulae of ischemic and nonischemic tissue (Janse et al. 1979). Between the interdigitating regions, there is an important electrical and ionic cross talk. Direct current electrograms taken from the epicardial surface show a gradual increase of the diastolic and systolic extracellular fields (TQ depression and ST elevation) over a distance of approximately 1 cm (Kléber et al. 1978). Over similar distances, gradients in extracellular K^+ have been found, which may amount to 8 mmol (Coronel 1988). Thus, in the "border zone" differences in extracellular K^+ of 8 mmol between recording sites were found, whereas in the central ischemic zone these differences were in the order of only 2 mmol (Coronel et al. 1988). In these experiments extracellular K^+ was determined at multiple recording sites (up to 64 per heart). The ischemic zone was defined as the area where extracellular K^+ rose following coronary occlusion, the normal zone as the tissue where K^+ remained constant. The border was the line separating both zones. A "border zone" was arbitrarily defined as a zone of 1-cm width extending from the border line into the ischemic zone. The "central ischemic zone" was the ischemic tissue further than 1 cm from the border line. One of the reasons for the inhomogeneity in extracellular K^+ is that K^+ moves from the ischemic zone towards the normal zone. The movement of K^+ is probably caused by a combination of diffusion and mixing of the extracellular space because of the contractions of the heart. The movement of K^+ from ischemic to normal myocardium does not depend on collateral circulation (Coronel et al. 1988). Movement of K^+ can be reversed by perfusion of the normal myocardium with a high K^+ solution: under these conditions the gradient in extracellular K^+ is now such that the K^+ concentration is higher in the border zone than in the central ischemic zone. As described earlier, the movement of K^+ from ischemic to normal tissue is one of the reasons for the "dip" in the extracellular K^+ curve (see Figure 2.19). Another reason that we described may be a catecholamine-induced stimulation of the Na/K pump.

The mixing of extracellular K^+ and the flow of injury current between ischemic and nonischemic zones alters membrane potential in a relatively broad area interposed between the center of the ischemic zone and the normally perfused area, and this affects conduction and refractoriness within this broad area. We have already seen that recovery of excitability of acutely ischemic myocardium is delayed ("postrepolarization refractoriness") and this results in a lengthening rather than a shortening of the refractory period. However, in regions toward the border, refractory periods may not be prolonged as much as in the central ischemic region or they may even be shorter, resulting in significant inhomogeneities. The distribution of extracellular K^+ plays an important role in causing the inhomogeneities. When ischemic conditions are imitated *in vitro* by exposing cardiac preparations to hypoxic, acidic, high K^+ solutions, the recovery from inexcitability can be studied in greater detail than in intact hearts with regional ischemia and also, the effects of small differences in extracellular K^+ can be assessed. In these *in vitro* studies (Kodama et al. 1984; Wilde 1988), the recovery kinetics of the action potential upstroke were determined by measuring maximum upstroke velocity (dV/dt_{max}) of premature action potentials elicited at progressively longer intervals after a basic action potential. The time constant with which dV/dt_{max} of the premature action potential regains the values of the basic action potential was used as an index for recovery of excitability. It was found that in the presence of elevated K^+ concentrations (either with or without acidosis) hypoxia causes a significant prolongation of this time constant, and that in the presence of hypoxia, small differences in extracellular K^+ concentrations produced marked changes in the recovery kinetics of dV/dt_{max}. The increased recovery time was not solely due to the reduction in membrane potential by the elevated K^+ concentration: in partially depolarized cells hypoxia exerted a marked extra depressant effect (Kodama et al. 1984; Wilde 1988). Therefore, it is expected that these small differences in extracellular K^+ *in situ* would cause similar differences in refractoriness. Figure 2.23 shows in a schematic way the changes in action potential configuration, resting membrane potential, dV/dt_{max} of the basic action potential, and the recovery of dV/dt_{max} of premature responses following the basic action potential in simulated ischemia. The dV/dt_{max} is indicated by the height

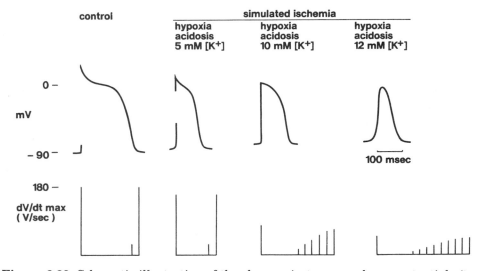

Figure 2.23: Schematic illustration of the changes in transmembrane potentials (top trace) and the recovery of maximal upstroke velocity, dV/dt_{max} (bottom trace), following an action potential in normal ventricular myocardium (control) and in three different conditions of simulated ischemia in which the extracellular K^+ is increased. This scheme is based on results obtained by Kodama et al. (1984) and Wilde (1988).

of the vertical bar in the bottom trace. The control (normal) action potential is at the top left. Below it is shown that the rate (dV/dt_{max}) of phase 0 depolarization is high (180 V/sec) and that complete recovery of the upstroke occurs upon complete repolarization, that is, an action potential stimulated at this time would have a normal dV/dt_{max}. The action potential shown next is the kind recorded in hypoxia and acidosis with only a slight elevation in extracellular K^+ (to 5 mmol) as might occur near the ischemic border zone. Action potential duration is shortened and so is the time course for recovery of the upstroke that occurs upon repolarization. Moving further into the ischemic region where extracellular K^+ is more elevated (10–12 mmol), the action potential upstroke becomes more depressed and the time course for recovery of the upstroke prolongs. The dV/dt_{max} of premature action potentials does not return until long after complete repolarization.

Of particular importance for the generation of arrhythmias is the duration and position of the period of "graded responses" following the basic action potential. These graded responses are indicated in Figure 2.23 by the submaximal upstroke velocities following repolarization. Impulses elicited during this period either do not propagate, because they are of low amplitude and do not produce enough local excitatory current, or they conduct at reduced speed. The duration of this period of "graded responses" is markedly prolonged when in the presence of hypoxia extracellular K^+ is raised from 10 to 12 mmol as shown in Figure 2.23. Therefore, a premature response that is initiated for instance 200 msec after the beginning of a basic action potential will be blocked in the tissue with an extracellular K^+ concentration of 12 mmol and still slowly conduct in the tissue with a K^+ concentration of 10 mmol. Differences in extracellular K^+ of this magnitude, and greater, are present in ischemic myocardium and thus are likely to play an important role in the formation of unidirectional block and reentry.

On the basis of the changes described above, it can be understood why conduction in ischemic myocardium becomes rate-dependent; that is, conduction characteristics vary with rate. Because of the strong time-dependence of recovery of excitability, the interval between successive depolarizations markedly influences amplitude and upstroke velocity of the action potentials. During regular rhythms that are relatively rapid, full recovery time may exceed the basic cycle length. A mere increase in sinus rate, for example caused by enhanced sympathetic activity, may unmask the inhomogeneity in recovery of excitability in the ischemic zone and produce unidirectional block and reentry even in the absence of an initiating premature impulse. An example is given in Figure 2.24, where four transmembrane potentials that were simultaneously recorded from the ischemic zone of the pig heart are shown. Initially, the atria are regularly driven at a basic cycle length of 400 msec. At this rate, activation of the four ischemic cells is fairly synchronous, and action potential configuration is relatively uniform. Upon a sudden increase in driving rate (cycle length 300 msec), this synchronicity becomes lost: cell 2 shows marked alternation, delayed activation (beat 5) and conduction block (beat 6). Within seconds, the ventricles were fibrillating.

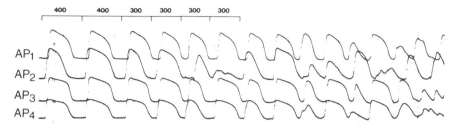

Figure 2.24: An increase in heart rate unmasks inhomogeneity within the ischemic zone and leads to ventricular fibrillation as shown in these recordings of action potentials from the pig heart. Note delayed activity (beat 5) and block (beat 6) in cell 2. (Reproduced from Janse et al. (1977) with permission.)

Spatial inhomogeneity in refractory periods is further enhanced by the fact that at the border between ischemic and normal myocardium, refractory periods may actually become shorter than normal as we discussed before (Janse and Downar 1977; Capucci et al. 1984; Janse et al. 1985a). An explanation for the shortening is given in the diagram in Figure 2.25, where in a schematic fashion the lateral "border zones" for extracellular K^+ concentration, pH and pO_2 are depicted. As mentioned earlier, the transition from normoxic to se-

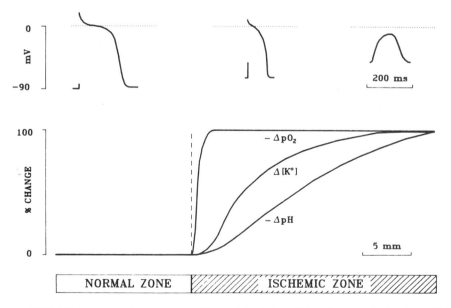

Figure 2.25: Diagrammatic representation of the lateral "border zone" of extracellular K^+ concentration, pH, and pO_2 (lower panel) and their relation to action potential characteristics (upper panel). At the border zone between normal and ischemic myocardium pO_2 may be reduced but extracellular K^+ and pH may be normal. (Reproduced from Coronel (1988) with permission.)

verely hypoxic tissue is sharp, that of tissue with normal extracellular K^+ to elevated extracellular K^+ gradual. Therefore, a rim of ischemic tissue exists with an extracellular K^+ concentration that is only minimally elevated, but where pO_2 is very low. Action potentials in this region are shortened, but time course of recovery of dV/dt_{max} in relation to full repolarization is hardly altered; that is, recovery is more rapid because of the accelerated repolarization as was also shown in Figure 2.23 (Kodama et al. 1984; Wilde 1988).

Several studies in which refractory periods at different sites have been determined with the premature stimulus techniques have reported that the dispersion in refractory periods (i.e., difference between longest and shortest refractory period) is increased in ischemic myocardium (Han and Moe 1964; Levites et al. 1976; Naimi et al. 1977). The limitations of the technique related to the use of high stimulation currents, as discussed previously, must be taken into account when interpreting these results. In addition, the rapid changes in refractoriness which occur during the first minutes of ischemia make it impossible to accurately determine refractoriness at a large number of sites at the same time, a prerequisite for demonstrating inhomogeneities. One way to determine inhomogeneities in excitability over a large area during a very short time period is to measure intervals between local activations during ventricular fibrillation. Lammers et al. (1986) have shown that there is a good correlation between the median interval between successive activations during atrial fibrillation at several sites in the atria and the refractory periods at these sites, determined in the classical way with the extrastimulus technique. The underlying hypothesis is that during fibrillation chances are that cells will be reexcited as soon as their refractory period is over. The advantage of this way of analysis is that one can record many electrograms simultaneously during ventricular fibrillation for a period of several seconds, and by determining the average cycle length at each site, obtain an estimate of local refractoriness. Such experiments have been performed in isolated perfused hearts, where ventricular fibrillation was induced by the application of a constant current via a 4-volt battery. Since coronary perfusion is maintained, the hearts can remain in fibrillation for a long period. Stable values for the average interval are reached after several minutes of fibrillation and these values remain stable for periods longer than 30 minutes (Ramdat Misier et al. 1988; Opthof et al. 1991). During "control" (before coronary occlusion), there was a very good correlation between the average fibrillation interval and refractory period duration measured in the conventional way; that is, sites with the shortest fibrillation interval had the shortest refractory periods, sites with the longest interval had the longest refractory periods. A plot of fibrillation interval versus refractory period at multiple sites produced a straight line with a correlation coefficient of 0.95. Figure 2.26 shows a graphic representation of the average fibrillation interval measured at 99 sites on the surface of the left ventricle. The electrodes were separated by 3-mm distances, and arranged in a grid of 9×11 electrodes. The multiple electrodes were positioned in such a way that, following occlusion of the left anterior descending coronary artery, the majority of electrodes were on ischemic myocardium, only those on the right-hand side being in contact

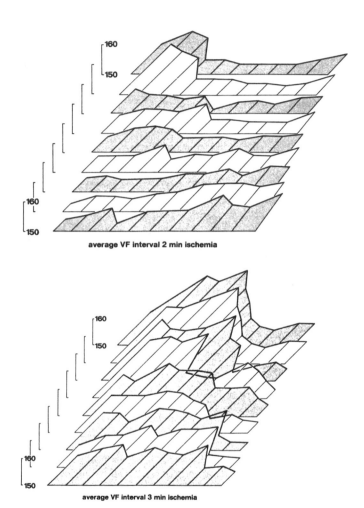

average VF interval 2 min ischemia

average VF interval 3 min ischemia

Figure 2.26: Average intervals between local depolarizations during ventricular fibrillation (ordinate) at 99 sites on the left ventricular surface of a perfused pig heart, 2 minutes and 3 minutes after left anterior descending coronary artery occlusion. The electrode array consisted of a regular grid of 9 × 11 electrodes, each 3 mm apart. Each line represents the local value of the ventricular fibrillation interval, which is equivalent to the local refractory period. For the sake of clarity, alternate rows of electrodes are shaded and unshaded. In each row, the two right-hand electrodes are on normal myocardium, all other electrodes are on ischemic tissue. After 2 minutes of ischemia, most ventricular fibrillation intervals are in the same range, except for 8 electrode sites in the upper left corner, that are longer. Note how after 3 minutes of ischemia (lower panel), there is a marked increase in ventricular fibrillation interval at all ischemic sites, and also that large differences between adjacent sites exist.

with normal tissue. After 2 minutes of coronary occlusion (top panel), most intervals fall in the same range, with the exception of several sites in the upper left corner where intervals are longer. After 3 minutes (bottom panel), the situation has drastically changed. Not only are intervals in the ischemic region much longer than on the normal side of the border, there are also large differences between adjacent sites within the ischemic border zone. In an attempt to quantify the degree of inhomogeneity, the largest difference in fibrillation interval between adjacent electrode sites during "control" fibrillation was determined in several experiments. This turned out to be 12 msec. A difference larger than 12 msec between adjacent sites was considered to be an index of inhomogeneity. After 1 minute of ischemia 5% of sites showed inhomogeneity, after 2 minutes 8%, and after 3 minutes 30%.

Conduction Velocity

The changes in the resting membrane potential, the depolarization phase of the action potential, the action potential duration, and time course of recovery of excitability have important effects on conduction in the ischemic region. During the first 2 minutes after coronary artery occlusion, an increase in conduction velocity has been measured (Gambetta and Childers 1969; Holland and Brooks 1976) as well as a decrease in diastolic threshold for stimulation (Elharrar et al. 1977). A moderate decrease in resting potential from its normal value of -90 mV to around -80 mV caused by a small increase in extracellular K^+ at this time could lead to the increase in conduction velocity, even though maximum upstroke velocity (one of the determinants of conduction velocity) may be slightly reduced, by depolarizing the membrane closer to the threshold potential (Dominguez and Fozzard 1970; Peon et al. 1978). Although such an increase in velocity has only been shown experimentally to occur in Purkinje fibers, it should also occur in ventricular muscle. After 2 minutes of coronary occlusion, delays in activation of ischemic myocardium on the order of 200 to 300 msec after the onset of ventricular activation, caused by slowing of conduction have been found (normally the ventricles are activated within 80 to 100 msec) (Conrad et al. 1959; Durrer et al. 1961; Boineau and Cox 1973; Waldo and Kaiser 1973; Scherlag et al. 1974; Williams et al. 1974; Elharrar et al. 1977; Rosenfeld et al. 1978; Kaplinsky et al. 1979). Delayed activation is especially prominent in ischemic subepicardium, whereas activation of subendocardial layers is relatively unaffected (Ruffy et al. 1979; Honjo et al. 1986). As expected, epicardial conduction delay increases when the heart rate is increased because the time course for recovery of excitability after an action potential is prolonged (Hope et al. 1974). Slowing of conduction in epicardial and intramural regions has been related to the degree of reduction in blood flow. No changes in conduction were observed with flows higher than 25% of normal, and conduction disturbances occurred only in areas with flows between 0.05 and 0.3 mL per gram tissue per minute (Russell et al. 1982). Slowing of conduction may be absent in subendocardial Purkinje layers despite a significant decrease in coronary blood flow. Resting membrane potential may not decrease too precipitously in this region due to the diffusion of oxygen from the cavitary blood into the subendocardium to a depth of 40–60 cells (Wilensky et al. 1986). After 10 to 30 minutes of coronary occlusion, activation delay in the subepicardium diminishes and the amplitude of bipolar extracellular complexes increases (Scherlag et al. 1974; Kaplinsky et al. 1979). This improvement of conduction is related to the appearance of transmembrane potentials in previously unresponsive cells that we described previously (Kléber et al. 1978; Janse and Kléber 1981).

Quantitative measurements of conduction velocity in the region of conduction delay during ischemia have been difficult to obtain. To measure conduction velocity accurately, detailed determinations of the sequence of activation is also necessary. Conduction velocity can most easily be estimated in regions where isochrones are parallel and conduction proceeds uniformly. In studies where simultaneous recording from 60 epicardial or intramural sites were made, values in the order of 20 cm/sec were calculated for the slowest conduction observed during a ventricular tachycardia caused by ischemia (Janse et al. 1980c; Janse and Kléber 1981). More precise determinations utilizing simultaneous recordings from 96 epicardial electrodes separated by 1-mm distances during stimulation of a centrally located electrode, showed that conduction velocity in the direction parallel to the fiber orientation decreased from a normal value of 50.08 ± 2.13 (SE) cm/sec to 33.3 ± 3.86 cm/sec after onset of ischemia before fibrillation or conduction block occurred in the isolated porcine heart. Conduction velocity in the transverse direction, which is normally slower than in the parallel direction, decreased from 21.08 ± 0.94 cm/sec to 13.0 ± 1.15 cm/sec (Kléber et al. 1986). Figure 2.27 shows the activation pattern of 1 cm^2 of the epicardial surface of the left ventricle of an isolated pig heart. The heart was paced from the center of the square and local electrograms were simultaneously recorded from 96 electrodes within the square. Numbers on the isochrones are in milliseconds, time 0 being the stimulus artifact. Conduction is faster in the horizontal direction (longitudinal conduction) than in the vertical direction (transverse conduction) during the control measurement shown in the upper left panel. In the upper right panel, the activation sequence is shown during global ischemia, when extracellular K$^+$ had risen to 6.5 mmol, just before the ventricle became inexcitable. The conduction delays are indicated by the closer spacing and increased number of isochrones. In the lower left panel, a similar activation pattern is seen when in the same heart during coronary perfusion, the K$^+$ level in the normoxic perfusion fluid was raised to 11.6 mmol. Conduction is not as slow (isochrones are not as closely spaced) indicating that during ischemia conduction slowing is not only caused by the rise in extracellular K$^+$. These values for conduction velocity during ischemia can be compared with the conduction velocity of slow response (calcium-dependent) action potentials to provide some indication if slow responses are present in the ischemic region. Conduction velocity in ischemic myocardium is distinctly higher than conduction velocities obtained in isolated Purkinje fibers

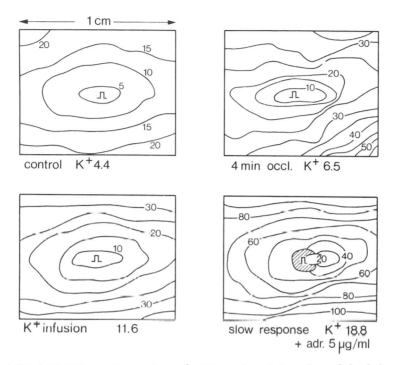

Figure 2.27: Activation pattern of 1 cm² of the epicardial surface of the left ventricle of an isolated pig heart. The heart was paced from the center of the square (pulse symbol) and local electrograms were simultaneously recorded from 96 electrodes within the square. Isochrones were drawn at 10-msec intervals. Activation maps are shown during normal coronary flow (upper left) during which extracellular K⁺ was 4.4 mmol/L, after 4 minutes of coronary occlusion when K⁺ was 6.5 mmol/L (upper right), during infusion of a solution through the coronary with a K⁺ of 11.6 mmol/L (lower left) and during an infusion of a solution with 18.8 mmol/L K⁺ and 5 μg/mL adrenaline to cause slow responses (lower right). (Reproduced from Janse et al. (1986) with permission.)

exposed to 15 to 18 mmol/L K⁺ and noradrenaline to make slow responses (Cranefield et al. 1972). It is also higher than conduction velocities in isolated hearts made inexcitable by perfusion with solutions containing 18.8 mmol/L K⁺, in which the subsequent addition of adrenaline resulted in the appearance of the slow response. Under these conditions activation occurred with a velocity of 12.3 ± 1.23 cm/sec in the longitudinal direction, and 5.0 ± 0.26 cm/sec in the transverse direction (Kléber et al. 1986). The lower right panel of Figure 2.27 shows the very slow conduction of the slow response, initiated by adding adrenaline to a normoxic solution containing 18.8 mmol/L K⁺. Thus, conduction velocity in ischemic myocardium is higher than the usual values reported for conduction of the slow response. The large delays in epicardial activation cannot be accounted for only by these measured decreases in conduction velocity. In addition, they are caused by irregular conduction from endocardium to epicardium at reduced speed around multiple sites of intramural conduction block.

Passive electrical properties

So far, we have concentrated on changes in active membrane responses and their importance in determining refractoriness, conduction, and arrhythmogenesis. Changes in passive electrical properties may, however, be equally important. By decreasing membrane conductance for Na^+, conduction velocity can only be reduced to about one third of its normal value, whereas by increasing the degree of cellular uncoupling it can be reduced by a factor of 20 before block occurs (Quan and Rudy 1990). Normally, the gap junctional connections between cardiac cells provide the pathways for electrical current flow and the low electrical resistance of the gap junctions in combination with the large amount and high speed of transmembrane ionic current flow during depolarization assures homogeneous conduction of the impulse, despite irregular branching patterns of cell bundles on a microscopic scale. Homogeneous conduction in the longitudinal direction of ventricular muscle fibers may be approximated to conduction in a linear cable consisting of excitable elements. However, the amount of local current flowing in a propagating wave front is not only determined by the resistance between and within the cells, but also by the resistance of the narrow extracellular clefts which make up approximately 20% of fiber volume. Recent measurements of cable properties of densely packed, arterially-perfused ventricular myocardium have shown that the lumped intracellular and extracellular resistive elements are of the same magnitude (Kléber and Riegger 1987). This means that both changes in intracellular and extracellular resistance have to be equally considered when assessing the role of the passive electrical properties on conduction during ischemia.

Engelmann, as early as 1875, described that myocardial cells became disconnected during the development of myocardial necrosis: "Solche Zellen, die waehrend des Lebens mit Verlust ihrer eigenen physiologischen Individualitaet mit anderen zu einem Individuum hoeherer Ordnung verschmolzen sind, erhalten beim Absterben ihre Individualitaet zurueck. . . . Die Zellen leben zusammen, aber sterben einzeln." (Such cells, which during life, at the expense of their own identity, are joined with other cells to form an entity of a higher order, regain their individuality when dying. The cells live together, but die alone. (Engelmann 1875). The property of injured cardiac cells to seal themselves off from neighboring cells ("healing over") is due to an increase in nexal (gap junctional) resistance (Délèze 1970; DeMello 1975). Exposure of isolated cardiac muscle preparations to hypoxia leads to a twofold increase in coupling resistance between cells (determined to a large part by an increase in gap junctional resistance) after 30 minutes and the effects of lowering pO_2 on coupling resistance are enhanced in the presence of elevated extracellular K^+ concentrations and a low extracellular pH (Wojtczak 1979; Ikeda and Hiraoka 1982; Gettes et al. 1985). Quantitative measurements of changes in coupling resistance, and of extracellular resistance, during the early stages of ischemia have been accomplished in an experimental model that enables the application of electrical cable theory for analysis. This preparation is the arterially, blood-perfused rabbit papillary muscle suspended in an artificial gaseous atmosphere developed by Kléber and Riegger (1987) in which transmembrane action potentials can be recorded and intra- and extracellular resistances can be accurately measured. Following arrest of arterial flow in this preparation, and changing the gaseous atmosphere to 95% N_2 and 5% CO_2 to cause ischemia, extracellular resistance (comprising both intravascular and interstitial resistance) immediately increases by about 30%. This increase is related to collapse of the vascular bed. Thereafter, there is a slow further increase in extracellular resistance most likely caused by osmotic cell swelling (Tranum- Jensen et al. 1981) and the consequent reduction of the extracellular space. The intracellular resistance remains unchanged during the initial phase of ischemia; this phase may vary from 12 to 23 minutes. Afterwards, rapid cellular uncoupling occurs to cause an increase in intracellular resistance (Kléber et al. 1987a). Figure 2.28 shows the results of one experiment in which the decrease in longitudinal conduction velocity (solid circles) and action potential amplitude (Vm, unfilled circles) and the changes in intracellular (r_i; filled triangles) and extracellular resistance (r_o, unfilled triangles) are plotted as a function of time elapsed after arrest of coronary flow (on the abscissa). During the initial minutes of ischemia

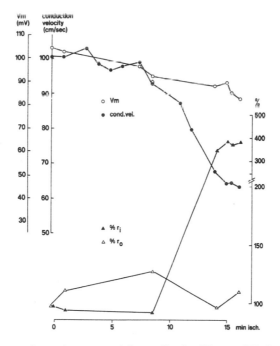

Figure 2.28: Changes in action potential amplitude (Vm, unfilled circles), conduction velocity (cond. vel., solid circles), intracellular resistance (r_i, solid triangles) and extracellular resistance (r_o, unfilled triangles) in a blood-perfused rabbit papillary muscle following arrest of coronary flow (min isch., on abscissa). The changes in Vm and conduction velocity are shown by the ordinate at the left, the changes in r_i and r_o by the ordinate on the right. (Unpublished results of A.G. Kléber, C. Riegger and M.J. Janse.)

conduction velocity falls in concert with a decrease in action potential amplitude and an increase in extracellular resistance. However, after 10 minutes of ischemia intracellular resistance increases to 400% of its initial value and conduction velocity falls more steeply than action potential amplitude. This sudden increase in intracellular resistance is in agreement with the results of a morphological study in which it was found that after 24 minutes of ischemia the majority of gap junctions became dissociated (McCallister et al. 1979). Focal pathological separation of intercalated disc membranes has been observed after 30 minutes of hypoxia, whereas after 1 hour of hypoxia gap junction surface density was reduced by 45% (Hoyt et al. 1990). Cellular uncoupling heralds the onset of irreversible damage. It always coincides with the second phase of extracellular K^+ accumulation (Kléber and Cascio 1989; Cascio et al. 1990).

Therefore, the changes in intra- and extracellular resistance have an influence on conduction velocity. During the initial phase, when intracellular coupling resistance remains unaltered, a small decrease in conduction velocity of about 15% can be expected as a consequence of the increase in extracellular resistance, assuming that the action potential upstroke remains unchanged (which it does not). The rapid cellular uncoupling that occurs later causes conduction to become slow and discontinuous and eventually leads to complete conduction block. Actual conduction velocity measured in acutely ischemic papillary muscles is lower than predicted by cable theory and this is due to the changes in action potential upstroke characteristics and excitability. So far, no precise quantitative assessment has been made of the relative contributions of the changes in both passive and "active" electrical properties to conduction velocity.

The reasons for electrical uncoupling have not been completely established. It is more than likely that the increase in intracellular calcium that occurs after 15 to 20 minutes of ischemia (Marban et al. 1987; Steenbergen et al. 1987; 1990) plays a major role, as well as intracellular acidosis since it is known that both factors increase coupling resistance (DeMello 1975; Hess and Weingart 1980; Reber and Weingart 1982).

Mechanisms of Arrhythmias During Acute Ischemia

Determination of Activation Sequences in the Heart: "Mapping"

The elucidation of the mechanisms causing arrhythmias in the acutely ischemic heart is the result of studies in which extracellular electrical recordings have been utilized. Before describing these studies in detail, we provide a brief background description of some of the methods that have been used.

Sequential and Simultaneous Mapping

In order to understand how and why an arrhythmia occurs, it is important to locate the site of origin and follow the spread of activation from that site.

Investigators in the early part of the century could do this visually. For example, Mayer (1906) followed contraction waves in rings excised from jellyfish with the naked eye, thus laying the foundations for understanding the physiology of circulating excitation. Unfortunately this cannot be done in the mammalian heart. When accurate recording of the extracellular potentials generated by cardiac muscle became possible by the construction of Einthoven's string galvanometer (Einthoven 1901), Lewis and Wybauw were the first to use these recordings to locate the site of origin of the normal heartbeat in the region of the sinus node and to follow the spread of excitation in the atria (Lewis et al. 1910; Wybauw 1910). The methods used can in essence be described as follows: A fixed "indifferent" electrode connected to the anode of the amplifier was positioned somewhere in the body of the animal, another electrode which could be moved from one site to the other on the surface of the atria (what is now called a "roving probe") was connected to the cathode of the amplifier. The extracellular potentials thus obtained are called unipolar recordings. Lewis introduced the term "intrinsic deflection" as that part of the unipolar signal indicating the arrival of the excitation process in the myocardium immediately beneath the exploring electrode. Nowadays, the most rapid negative deflection in the unipolar complex is defined as the moment of local activation. Lewis used the beginning of the negative deflection. The timing of activation of each of several recording sites of the roving probe was measured with respect to the timing of the intrinsic deflection of a fixed reference electrode; the time reference could be derived either from an electrode attached to some part of the heart or from a specific moment in the body surface electrocardiogram. The way to depict the sequence of activation was, on the one hand, to draw a diagram of the atrial surface and to indicate times of activation at the appropriate locations or else to draw isochrones separating areas activated within the same, arbitrarily chosen, time intervals. This technique, which may be called sequential mapping, was also used by Lewis and coworkers (Lewis 1920; Lewis et al. 1920) to determine spread of activation during arrhythmias such as atrial flutter. In Figure 2.29, a drawing of the right and left atria of the dog from Lewis' publication in 1920 is shown with activation times at various sites during a period of atrial flutter. The intrinsic deflection of a reference electrode in the inferior caval vein was chosen as the time reference. Activation times are in seconds relative to this time reference. S marks the point originally stimulated to induce flutter. During one cycle of the arrhythmia (cycle length 0.160 msec) the wave of activation travels from the inferior caval vein (time 0.0000) up along the crista terminalis and towards the right atrial appendage. It turns around the orifice of the superior caval vein at time 0.0750 and passes along the interatrial band to the left atrium (time 0.0900). A little later a new wave appears behind the inferior caval vein at time 0.1370 and the same activation sequence is repeated. Although no recordings were made on the left side of the intercaval region, this activation sequence was suggestive for circus movement reentry, even though Lewis was aware of the limitations: " . . . it remains to ascertain if this new wave is a continuation of the old one; if so, then a circus movement is proven". This example demonstrates the technique

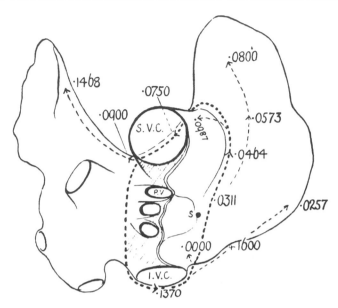

Figure 2.29: Lewis' diagram, showing the outline of a dog's left and right atria and the activation times he obtained during a period of atrial flutter. Numbers indicate activation times in seconds relative to a point at time 0. The broken lines and arrows indicate the course taken by the excitation wave. S.V.C = superior vena cava; I.V.C = inferior vena cava. (Reproduced from Lewis et al. (1920) with permission.)

of sequential mapping as it is still used today, and the difficulties in interpreting the data. To reiterate: the principles of sequential mapping are: (1) a fixed electrode on the heart is used as a time reference; (2) an electrode is moved from site to site; (3) activation times or isochrones are plotted on an anatomical representation of the region of study. Since each recording of the roving electrode is obtained during a different heartbeat, it follows that the impulse must spread in exactly the same way during each beat for accurate maps to be constructed. While this is the case for sinus rhythm, it is not the case for many arrhythmias. Furthermore, even for arrhythmias that have a stable origin and activation pattern, the initiating events cannot by analyzed by sequential mapping, nor can modes of termination of the arrhythmia be evaluated. These limitations of sequential mapping can be overcome by recording from a large number of sites simultaneously. The first to use these methods for determining the normal spread of activation in the ventricles were Durrer and van der Tweel (1953) and Scher and Young (1956). They used multiterminal plunge electrodes inserted into the left ventricular wall and displayed the electrical activity at each terminal simultaneously on different beams of specially constructed multichannel oscilloscopes (Figure 2.30). Initially, a limited number of signals (4 to 16) could be simultaneously recorded, using either multichannel oscilloscopes or instrumentation tape recorders (Durrer et al. 1970). Since the activation sequence of the ventricles was reconstructed using a number of sub-

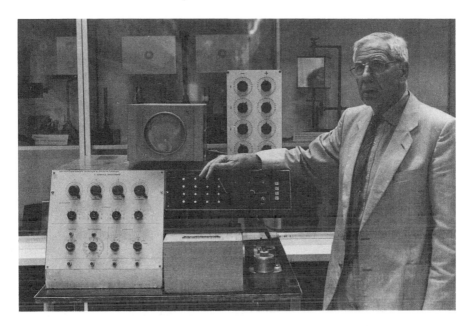

Figure 2.30: L.H. van der Tweel with the 4-channel oscilloscope that he built around 1950, that enabled D. Durrer and himself to record simultaneously from four intramural electrode terminals in the left ventricular wall of dogs and goats.

sequent simultaneous recordings from many intramural plunge electrodes, this technique was in essence a combination of sequential and simultaneous recording. The use of multiplexing systems in the late 1970s and early 1980s permitted recording of hundreds of signals simultaneously. The maximum number of recording electrodes is continuously being increased. It is not easy to determine the optimum number of simultaneous recordings to accurately depict activation sequences during a single cardiac beat. The main factors determining this number are the size of the tissue involved, the speed of conduction, and the complexity of the activation sequence. Thus, to depict the regular spread of activation from endocardium to epicardium in the human left ventricle during sinus rhythm, fewer recording sites are required than for the determination of the activation pattern during ventricular fibrillation. In the areas of the atrioventricular node, which may be no larger than a few cubic millimeters, even several hundred microelectrode recordings will not show the detailed sequence of activation because of the slow conduction and the complex three-dimensional activation pathways.

Extracellular Electrodes and Mode of Recording: Unipolar, Bipolar and Composite Electrograms

Electrodes that can be used for extracellular recording and mapping can differ not only in number but also in size and configuration. Electrode catheters often have recording terminals of several centimeters in width with a surface area of approximately 15 mm², whereas Spach and coworkers (1971) have used fine metal electrodes with tip diameters of 50 μm to record extracellular potentials. The use of very small electrodes guarantees that local events are recorded and the fine details of activation sequences can be analyzed on a microscopic scale. Thus, Spach et al. (1971; 1973; 1982) have shown patterns of activation of individual bundles of atrial cells, activation patterns of the atrioventricular node, and of small bundles of the ventricular specialized conduction system. Such details are missed when the average activity of a large area is sampled with a large electrode.

Another point to consider is the choice of DC or AC mode of recording. When measuring steady extracellular potential levels, or very slow changes, DC recordings are necessary. This requires the use of nonpolarizable electrodes. For this purpose, we used cotton wicks soaked in isotonic saline to measure changes in TQ and ST segments during acute ischemia (Janse et al. 1980c). The use of other types of nonpolarizable electrodes, such as chlorided silver wires, is fraught with difficulties because of shifts in DC potential caused by interaction of the tissue with the surface of the electrode. Another possibility is offered by the development of scintered electrodes that are much more stable. For the analysis of rapid potential changes during mapping of activation sequences, AC recordings are almost exclusively used because they are free from baseline drift and because steady potential changes are not important.

There are two modes of recording, unipolar or bipolar. Unipolar recording involves one electrode on the heart and another electrode, the "indifferent" one, as far away as possible, theoretically, beyond the zone of current flow that generates the electrical field. In bipolar recordings, both electrodes are on the heart, preferably as close together as possible. In Figures 2.31, 2.32, and 2.33,

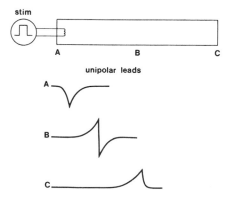

Figure 2.31: Schematic drawing of unipolar electrograms recorded from a strip of cardiac muscle (above), which is stimulated at site A. When activity is conducted away from the recording site, a negative complex is recorded (A). When the activation wave moves under the electrode, a biphasic complex results (B). When activity moves towards the recording site but stops at that site, the unipolar complex is positive (C).

5 min ischemia

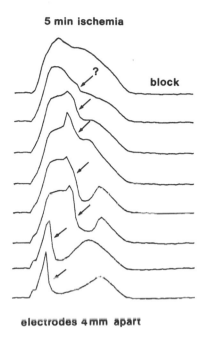

block

electrodes 4mm apart

Figure 2.32: Unipolar electrograms recorded from a row of electrodes, 4 mm apart on the epicardial surface of the left ventricle of a pig's heart, 5 minutes after coronary occlusion. Arrows point to intrinsic deflections indicating local activation. The upper tracing shows a monophasic potential, indicating absence of local activity (block). In the tracing below it, there is a small negative deflection of which it is impossible to say whether it represents local activity (that is, regenerative inward current across the cell membrane) or is merely the electrotonic reflection of activity at adjacent sites.

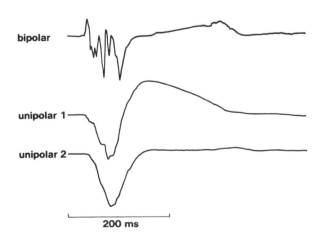

bipolar

unipolar 1

unipolar 2

200 ms

Figure 2.33: Bipolar and unipolar electrograms recorded during a ventricular tachycardia from the subendocardium of a dog heart following application of a strong DC shock. (Unpublished observations of J.M.T. De Bakker and R.N.W. Hauer.)

these different modes are schematically depicted. An advantage of unipolar recordings is that the presence of so-called extrinsic components, i.e., potentials generated by activity at a distance, gives some information about the direction of the spread of activation. Thus, it can be recognized from a single recording whether activity spreads away from the recording site (negative complex), towards it (positive deflection), passes underneath the electrode (biphasic complex), or stops at that site (only a positive deflection). These forms of the unipolar electrogram are shown in Figure 2.31. In unipolar recordings there is a well-defined moment indicating local excitation, the most rapid negative deflection, or intrinsic deflection. A disadvantage of unipolar recordings is that very small amplitude deflections might be obscured by larger potentials caused by remote activity. For example, Figure 2.32 shows unipolar electrograms recorded from a row of electrodes 4 mm apart on the epicardial surface of the left ventricle of a pig heart, 5 minutes after coronary occlusion. The recording in the bottom trace from near the border of the ischemic zone where cells still have rapid upstrokes has a prominent intrinsic deflection indicated by the arrow. Moving into the ischemic zone where the resting and action potentials are depressed (from bottom to top), the intrinsic deflections (arrows) become smaller and smaller until they are nearly lost in the large extrinsic waveform. The upper tracing does not have evidence of local activity, but there is a small negative deflection in the record below it (arrow and question mark) that might represent local activity. Another example is shown in Figure 2.33, where activity is recorded from small bundles of viable cells encased in the scarred subendocardium of a dog's left ventricle during a ventricular tachycardia. A bipolar electrogram is shown in the upper trace, which was recorded between electrodes 1 and 2, and the unipolar electrograms recorded from the same two electrodes are shown in the lower two tracings. The fact that the unipolar signals are negative, and the fact that the intrinsic deflections were the earliest found among a large number of recording sites, indicates that the recordings were very close to the site of origin of the arrhythmia. The amplification of the bipolar signal was eight times greater than that of the unipolar signals. Although multiple intrinsic deflections can be seen in the unipolar signals, they are partly obscured by the large extrinsic deflection; the presence of multiple deflections is much easier to detect in the bipolar signal.

Bipolar recordings have the advantage that the extrinsic potentials are canceled out, because they are common to both terminals and only local activity is recorded. In tissue where spread of activation is uniform, the polarity of the bipolar complex indicates direction of spread of excitation. The disadvantage is that no signals may be recorded when the wave front travels in a direction perpendicular to the line connecting both terminals. This feature is diagrammed in Figure 2.34. Bipolar recordings are shown at the left. At the top, the wave front (arrow) encounters first the positive pole and then the negative pole of the electrode giving rise to a positive deflection. In the bottom left diagram, the wave front first encounters the negative pole and then the positive pole giving rise to a negative deflection. However, in the middle left diagram the wave front encounters both poles simultaneously and no deflection is seen.

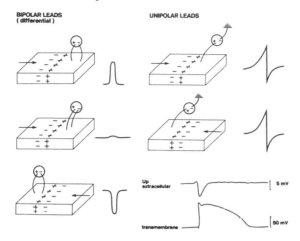

Figure 2.34: Differences between bipolar and unipolar electrograms. Bipolar recordings are shown in the column at the left. The polarity of the bipolar electrogram depends on the direction of the propagating wave (top and bottom diagrams). If the spread of activity is perpendicular to the line connecting both poles of the bipolar electrode as shown in the left, middle diagram, no deflection will be recorded. On the other hand, unipolar recordings shown in the diagrams at the right show activity no matter in what direction the wave front is moving. In the lower right panel, a unipolar extracellular electrogram and a transmembrane potential recorded at the same site are shown. The intrinsic deflection of the electrogram is coincident with the action potential upstroke.

The unipolar recordings at the right, however, show deflections no matter in which direction activation is spreading. Another disadvantage of the bipolar recording is that the shape of the bipolar complex, especially during complex activation patterns, is not easily interpreted.

A special electrode has been developed by El-Sherif and colleagues (El-Sherif et al. 1977a; 1977b) for recording electrical activity over large areas. This "composite electrode" consists of a long insulated wire, with multiple recording contacts along its length. Each recording pole is connected to the same amplifier so that the composite electrogram represents the sum of electrical activity occurring over a large area. The composite electrogram recorded from normal myocardium is a broad biphasic deflection, the duration of which depends on the area covered by the electrode. The composite electrogram has been used to locate reentrant circuits. The characteristic of the composite electrogram thought to be indicative of reentry is the phenomenon of continuous electrical activity. By this is meant that multiple deflections are present throughout the cardiac cycle, the baseline never being isoelectric. Sometimes, however, continuous electrical activity need not be indicative of a reentrant pathway (Janse et al. 1980c; Wit et al. 1982a; 1982b; Worley et al. 1982). Continuous electrical activity can occur in regions where activation maps have failed to demonstrate reentrant circuits and probably can occur at any site where there is slow, inhomogeneous activation that persists throughout the diastolic interval.

Identification of the Moment of Activation in Extracellular Electrograms

As mentioned earlier, the precise time the excitatory wave front passes underneath the recording electrode is provided by the intrinsic deflection in unipolar complexes. The intrinsic deflection is defined as the time of fastest negative displacement of the extracellular potential. This can often be identified by eye, or else by differentiating the signal to determine peak dV/dt. Difficulties in recognizing the intrinsic deflection arise when recordings are made from slowly conducting tissue such as in acutely ischemic myocardium as was shown in Figure 2.32. This is because action potential amplitude and the rate of rise of its upstroke progressively diminish following the onset of ischemia and extracellular current flow is small. Even in transmembrane potential recordings it is often impossible to distinguish which part of a slow, small depolarization is caused by electrotonic current flow from adjacent areas and which part is caused by local regenerative inward current. Such small depolarizations of the ischemic cells still give rise to slow negative deflections in the unipolar extracellular recordings, superimposed on an almost monophasic complex (second trace from the top in Figure 2.32). We (MJJ and colleagues) have arbitrarily chosen as time of activation the 50% level of such deflections. One could also arbitrarily set limits to the amplitude and rate of change of the intrinsic deflection, below which local activation is interpreted to be absent. It is not possible to define precisely what those limits are. At first glance this seems a serious limitation for the construction of activation maps for ischemic myocardium. However, it is not crucial to provide a precise definition of the limits. The construction of activation maps is not solely determined by the analysis of a single recording site. When at a particular recording site there is doubt as to whether there is local activation, examination of surrounding sites usually provides information that is helpful in reaching a decision. When there is a progressive reduction in size and slope of the "intrinsic deflection" in adjacent electrodes until completely monophasic potentials are recorded, there is no doubt about conduction block. Whether one investigator will still assign an activation time to the deflection marked by an arrow in Figure 2.32, where another might decide that there is no local activity, will only result in a slightly larger, or smaller, area of block. The total activation pattern is, in our experience, not seriously altered when two experienced investigators make activation maps from the same signals independently from each other.

The difficulty in analyzing a bipolar signal is that it has no single deflection. Theoretically, the bipolar signal is the difference of two unipolar complexes and thus has two moments of activation, one for each pole. It is not practical when constructing an activation map to assign two activation times to each recording site. Therefore, an intermediate value is selected as being representative of the time at which the tissue under both poles is activated. This is usually the peak of the deflection when it is a simple biphasic one. Problems arise when propagation between the two poles is so slow that the bipolar complex has a long duration, and thus, a wide peak. Other problems arise when there are multiple deflections that might be the result of inhomogeneous activation. This can occur in either bipolar or unipolar recordings. In the example shown in Figure 2.35, it would be difficult to assign a precise moment of activation at site B where there are multiple deflections. However, it is probably accurate to say that electrical activity remained at site B for the total duration of the electrogram. By looking at the recordings from sites A (above) and C (below), it can be seen that activity first occurred at A, then at B, and finally at C. For the construction of an activation map, it is permissible to assign a moment of activation at B that is intermediate between the earliest and latest deflection. Hence, the map shows that activation moved from A to B to C, although the precise pattern of activation at B is not evident.

The Construction of Activation Maps

When the activation times have been determined, they are plotted on a representation of the anatomical region from which they were recorded. The relative activation times at each recording site indicate how the wave fronts are moving. However, it is difficult to visualize spread of activation by looking at numbers, particularly when there may be hundreds of them. Therefore,

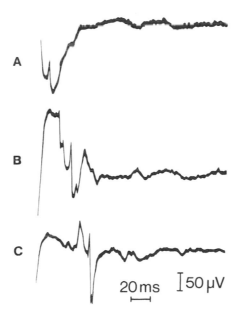

Figure 2.35: Three unipolar electrograms recorded from an isolated papillary muscle removed from a human, infarcted, left ventricle during surgery for medically intractable ventricular tachycardia and mitral valve replacement. Although activity spread from A, via B to C, the presence of multiple deflections in B make it impossible to assign one time of activation to site B. (Modified from De Bakker et al. 1988, with permission.)

isochronic maps are constructed in which those areas activated within the same time interval are separated by lines or isochrones. These intervals are arbitrary and are determined by the number of recording sites, the complexity of the activation pattern, and the total duration of the activation sequence. Ideally, one should have a number of recording sites in each isochronic area. Thus, when there are fewer recording sites, large intervals between isochrones are usually chosen. Widely spaced isochrones can show a general pattern of activation but fine details are often lost. Interpolation of isochrones, that is, drawing of isochrones at areas where there are no data points, is sometimes unavoidable when conduction is slow or inhomogeneous. A large number of isochrones interpolated in any one area may indicate either very slow conduction or conduction block. To distinguish slow conduction from block, limits for lowest values of conduction velocity have to be set. These limits depend on the experimental conditions. For example, in the atrioventricular node conduction velocity may be as low as 5 cm/sec, in acutely ischemic myocardium it will not be lower than 20 cm/sec (in the longitudinal direction) or 10 cm/sec (in the transverse direction). Isochrones in acutely ischemic myocardium that indicate conduction velocities of, for instance 2 cm/sec, are unrealistic on the basis of information available.

When larger numbers of recording sites are used, isochrones can be drawn at smaller intervals, thus revealing more details of the activation pattern. The following example shown in Figure 2.36 illustrates this. The data come from activation maps of the epicardial muscle overlying a canine infarct (the epicardial border zone). A monomorphic ventricular tachycardia was induced by programmed premature stimulation and simultaneous recordings were obtained from 192 bipolar electrodes with 3 mm between the bipolar pairs (distance between the two poles of a bipolar electrode was 1.5 mm). The top half of Figure 2.36 shows the isochronic map during one tachycardia cycle that would have been constructed if only relatively few electrodes had been used. There seems to exist a circulating excitatory wave, propagating around an area of block as pointed out by the arrows. The block is indicated by the thick shaded line. The isochrones are oriented perpendicular to this area of block. As shown in the lower half of the figure, where additional data points are added, the situation changes and is more complex. In particular, sites just below the "line of block" are excited almost simultaneously (125, 126, 121, 129 msec) and therefore isochrones have to be drawn parallel to the "line of block". This indicates that the excitation wave moved very slowly across the "line of block", which now becomes a region of very slow conduction. This example is used to show that as the number of electrodes is increased, the reconstructed pathways of excitation may change. We will discuss this particular example in more detail in Chapter IV on chronic myocardial infarction.

Two Phases of Early Ventricular Arrhythmias

MacWilliam wrote in 1923 that "after coronary ligation there is often a characteristic sequence of events. . . extrasystoles, first singly, then in irregular

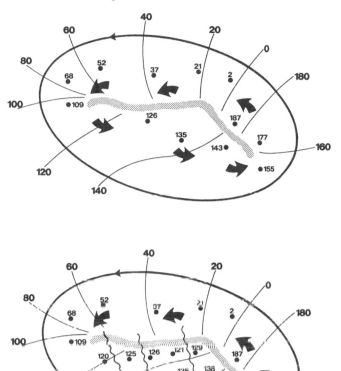

Figure 2.36: The influence of the number of recording sites on activation maps. Two isochronic maps of one cycle of a ventricular tachycardia are shown. Dots are electrode sites, numbers are local activation times in milliseconds. In the top map, activation times of a limited number of sites are shown. The activation sequence suggests the presence of an activation wave that circles around a line of conduction block (shaded area). Therefore, isochrones are drawn perpendicular to this line of block. In the lower half, activation times of a larger number of sites are shown. Because sites below the line of block are almost simultaneously activated, isochrones at 120 to 150 msec must be drawn more parallel to the line of block. The activation sequence now suggests that very slow conduction occurs across the "line of block".

runs, more or less continuous tachycardia, and finally fibrillation". During the first 30 minutes following experimental, complete coronary artery occlusion, ventricular arrhythmias (ventricular premature depolarizations, ventricular tachycardia and ventricular fibrillation) occur in two distinct phases. The first phase, called phase 1a or immediate ventricular arrhythmias, usually occurs between 2 and 10 minutes after occlusion, with the highest incidence of arrhythmias at around 5 to 6 minutes; the second phase called phase 1b or delayed ventricular arrhythmias occurs from approximately 12 to 30 minutes after occlusion, with a peak at 15 to 20 minutes. Sinus rhythm may be present between the two phases. The use of the word "delayed" to describe phase 1b arrhythmias may be confusing since this term is also used for the arrhythmias that occur 24 hours after coronary occlusion (Harris 1950) (see Chapter III). This bimodal distribution of early arrhythmias has been demonstrated in the dog (Haase and Schiller 1969; Kaplinsky et al. 1979; Ogawa et al. 1981; Kabell et al. 1982; Horacek et al 1984), in the pig (Frank et al. 1978; Hirche et al. 1980), in sheep (Euler et al. 1983), and in the rat (Parratt 1982). Individual animals may sometimes exhibit only 1a or 1b arrhythmias, but both phases may occur in the same animal (Kaplinsky et al. 1979; Meesmann 1982). There is no information available about whether arrhythmias also occur in humans with a similar bimodal distribution during the first 30 minutes of a developing myocardial infarction.

The experimental evidence suggests that the mechanism and/or site of origin of 1a and 1b arrhythmias is different. Phase 1a arrhythmias occur when there is a high degree of conduction slowing and delayed activation in the subepicardial muscle of the ischemic region. At this time, extracellular subepicardial electrograms are highly abnormal and consist of multiple components. They are fragmented similar to the electrogram shown in Figure 2.33. A change in the extracellular electrogram from a smooth high amplitude, biphasic deflection to a low amplitude, multicomponent deflection is often interpreted to be caused by membrane depolarization, and slow and inhomogeneous conduction. The phenomenon of "diastolic bridging" often precedes ventricular ectopic activity during the 1a phase (Kaplinsky et al. 1979). "Diastolic bridging" is continuous electrical activity in the form of multiple deflections (fragmented electrograms) that may persist for hundreds of msec from the QRS complex of a normally propagated beat originating in the sinus node to the beginning of the QRS complex of a premature ventricular depolarization, or between successive QRS complexes of a ventricular tachycardia. It is most easily recorded with a composite electrode. Continuous electrical activity recorded with a composite electrode after acute coronary artery occlusion in the canine heart is shown in Figure 2.37. In each panel, a lead II electrocardiogram and composite electrogram from the endocardial (endo) and epicardial (epi) surfaces of the ischemic zone are displayed. In panel A, which shows recordings obtained 5 minutes after the occlusion, the electrical activity in the epicardial recording during beat 3 bridges the diastolic interval to beat 4, which is a premature ventricular depolarization. There is, however, no diastolic bridging in the endocardial recording. Diastolic bridging has also been recorded from bipolar electrodes with interelectrode distances of 1 cm or less. On the basis of these electrogram characteristics, it was proposed that 1a arrhythmias are caused by reentry (Scherlag et al. 1970; Durrer et al. 1971; Boineau and Cox 1973; Waldo and Kaiser 1973; El-Sherif et al. 1975; 1977c; Kaplinsky et al. 1979). The reasoning is that during reentry, electrical activity persists within the reentrant circuit at all times during the cardiac cycle, since the impulse is continuously conducting around the circuit. Hence, an electrode located on the circuit should detect extracellular activity throughout the cycle as diastolic bridging

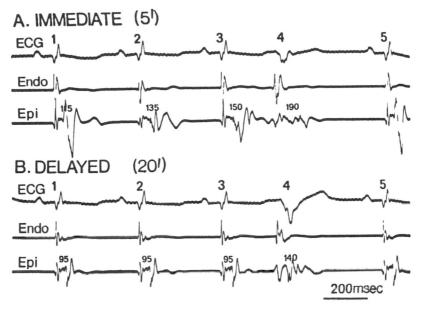

Figure 2.37: The electrocardiogram (ECG) and composite electrograms recorded from the endocardial (endo) and epicardial (epi) surfaces of the canine left ventricle 5 minutes (panel A; immediate) and 20 minutes (panel B; delayed) after coronary artery occlusion. (Reproduced from Kaplinsky et al. 1979, with permission).

or continuous electrical activity. If the circuit is relatively large, a large composite electrode is needed to cover it; if the circuit is small, a bipolar electrode with less than 1 cm interelectrode distance might be able to record from the entire circuit. Although the proposal derived from the electrogram characteristics that 1a arrhythmias are caused by reentry has been proven to be correct on the basis of mapping spread of activation by simultaneous recording from a number of sites, there are some flaws in the arguments that use diastolic bridging or continuous electrical activity as a proof for the occurrence of reentry. Continuous electrical activity can occur whenever or wherever there is slow, inhomogeneous activation. This characteristic may cause propagation to continue in some regions even after the rest of the heart has repolarized (during diastole) causing diastolic bridging in the absence of reentry (Janse et al. 1980c; Wit et al. 1982a).

Phase 1b arrhythmias often occur in the absence of evidence of abnormal epicardial conduction. Subepicardial electrograms recorded during the 1b phase are not as abnormal as during the 1a phase and there may be less spatial inhomogeneity of subepicardial activation delay during the 1b phase than during the 1a phase (Kaplinsky et al. 1979; Kabell et al. 1982; Euler et al. 1983; Russell et al. 1984). Panel B in Figure 2.37 shows epicardial and endocardial composite electrograms during this delayed arrhythmic phase, 20 minutes after coronary occlusion. Although the epicardial electrogram shows some fragmented components, continuous electrical activity throughout the diastolic interval does not occur with the ventricular premature depolarization (beat number 4). As during the immediate arrhythmias, endocardial electrograms are not highly abnormal during the delayed arrhythmias. Therefore, the arrhythmias of phase 1a are related to a marked increase in refractory period, conduction delay, and threshold for excitation, whereas during the 1b phase there is a partial recovery of these parameters (Horacek et al. 1984). In isolated guinea pig hearts with low-flow ischemia, 1b arrhythmias were always preceded by spontaneous improvement of action potential amplitude and upstroke velocity and by a shortening of the refractory period explaining why the electrograms may be less abnormal at this time. This improvement was absent when the hearts were treated with propranolol, or when they were depleted of catecholamines by pretreatment of the animals with 6-hydroxydopamine. β-Receptor blockade and catecholamine depletion also led to a reduction in the arrhythmias (Penny 1984). It is therefore quite likely that 1b arrhythmias may be related to release of endogenous catecholamines, which has been shown to occur between 15 and 20 minutes of ischemia (Schömig et al. 1984; Carlsson 1987; Wilde 1988). It therefore has been implied that mechanisms other than reentry (such as abnormal automaticity) might be the cause for 1b arrhythmias. However, it is still possible that electrophysiological abnormalities associated with reentry occur in regions of the ventricular wall other than the subepicardium and have not been detected.

Our own experiments (K. Koch, A. Schene, and M.J. Janse, unpublished results) suggest that there may be species differences in the mechanisms causing the 1b arrhythmias. Figure 2.38 shows data obtained during the occurrence of 1a and 1b arrhythmias in two open-chest pigs (left panels) and two open-chest dogs (right panels). In each animal activation times were measured from 60 intramural or epicardial electrodes, and the maximal activation delay is plotted (left ordinates) as a function of time elapsed after coronary occlusion (abscissa). Also indicated is the number of spontaneous ventricular premature depolarizations (shaded bars) or the occurrence of spontaneous ventricular fibrillation (VF). In all four animals, conduction delay rapidly increases and then declines after 8 to 10 minutes. In all four animals, the phase 1a arrhythmias (between 2 and 10 minutes) are associated with large activation delays. In the dogs, the phase 1b arrhythmias at 15 to 30 minutes after occlusion develop when activation delay has diminished. In the two pigs, however, a second phase of increased conduction delay precedes the phase of 1b arrhythmias. Therefore, the phase 1b arrhythmias in pigs may still be caused by reentry, although there is no evidence that this is the mechanism in dogs.

Reentry

Mapping experiments have demonstrated that circus movement reentry occurs during the 1a phase of ischemic arrhythmias (Janse et al. 1980c; Pog-

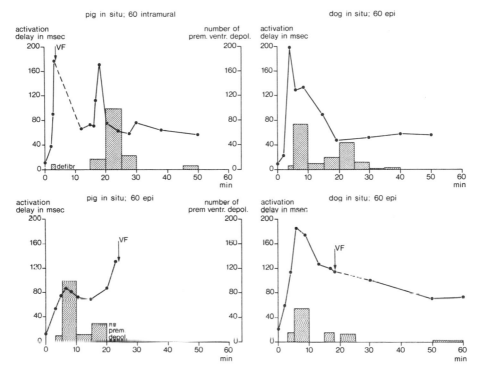

Figure 2.38: Activation delays associated with the occurrence of phase 1a and 1b arrhythmias in two open-chest pigs (left panels) and two open-chest dogs (right panels). The solid circles in each panel indicate the maximum activation delay plotted on the left ordinate versus time after coronary occlusion on the abscissa. Also indicated by the bars is the number of premature ventricular depolarizations (right ordinate) and the time of their occurrence. VF indicates the time of ventricular fibrillation. (Unpublished results of K. Koch, A. Schene, and M.J. Janse.)

wizd and Corr 1987b). Some examples from our own work are shown in Figure 2.39 to 2.41 (Janse et al. 1980c; Janse and Van Capelle, 1982b). The results were obtained by simultaneous recordings from 60 epicardial sites, or from 60 epicardial and intramural positions. The configuration of the multiple electrode array used for epicardial recording in Langendorff-perfused porcine hearts is shown in the upper right panel of Figure 2.39, where each dot is an electrode terminal and the dashed line indicates the border between ischemic and normal myocardium. Panels A and B in Figure 2.39 are activation maps of the first two spontaneous ectopic beats of a run of ventricular tachycardia that occurred 5 minutes after coronary occlusion. In A, earliest activity (time 0 was arbitrarily chosen) occurs at the border at the right. Although not shown, no electrical activity could be detected that filled the gap of 160 msec between latest recorded activity of the previous sinus beat and earliest activity during this ventricular premature beat. The premature impulse invades the ischemic subepicardium, but encounters a central area of temporary block (shaded zone).

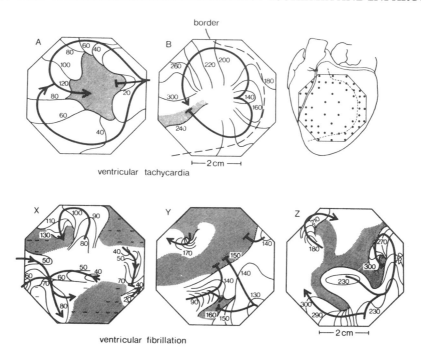

Figure 2.39: Activation patterns during a ventricular tachycardia that changed into ventricular fibrillation, 5 minutes following coronary occlusion in the isolated pig heart. Upper right panel shows the octagonal surface of the multiple electrode array on the anterior part of the ventricles. Each dot is an electrode terminal. Dotted line is the border of the ischemic zone. Panels A and B show the activation maps of the first two ectopic beats. Numbers at the isochrones are in msec, time 0 was arbitrarily chosen. Arrows indicate the general spread of excitation. Shaded areas are zones of block. Panels A and B show unidirectional block (T symbol indicates block), slow propagation around this zone and reexcitation of the zone proximal to the block after 140 msec. Panels X, Y and Z show presence of up to five independent wavelets traveling around multiple islets of temporary, functional block during fibrillation. (Reproduced from Janse and Van Capelle 1982b, with permission.)

Two semicircular wave fronts advance slowly through the ischemic myocardium around the area of block as indicated by the arrows, to merge after 120 msec distal to it. The zone of block is retrogradely invaded and traversed and the area proximal to the block (near the region where this wave front began) is reexcited in panel B after 140 msec. Again, in panel B, two semicircular wave fronts are set up, one of which is blocked after 240 msec (the one moving around the apex), the other continuing until 300 msec. At this point, the 2-second period of data storage ended, and it is therefore not known how this tachycardia continued. Nevertheless, reentrant excitation is clearly associated with these first two beats of the tachycardia. Somewhat later, when the tachycardia had degenerated into ventricular fibrillation, a second recording was made, and activation patterns of three successive "beats" are depicted in panels X, Y, and Z. In contrast to what appeared to be a large single circus movement

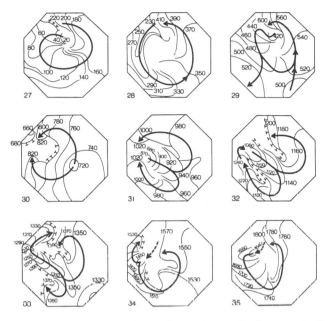

Figure 2.40: Patterns of activation during beats 27 to 35 of a ventricular tachycardia, of the area covered by the electrode shown in Figure 2.30. Note that basically one circus movement of fairly large dimensions is responsible for continuation of the tachycardia, although both dimension and position of the reentrant circuit changes from beat to beat. (Reproduced from Janse et al. 1980c, with permission.)

during the tachycardia phase (panels A, and B), multiple independent wavelets are now present as pointed out by the arrows. Wave fronts may collide, fuse, or describe a pretzel-like pathway (see wave front beginning at 80 msec in panel X in the upper part of the area covered by the electrode, continuing after 130 msec in panel Y, and after 180 msec in panel Z). At least five independent wave fronts are present in the area covered by the electrode. There are also large inexcitable regions at this time indicated by the shaded areas in panels X, Y, and Z.

Figure 2.40 demonstrates how the excitation pattern changed spontaneously from beat to beat during a ventricular tachycardia that ended after 30 seconds. Activation sequences are shown for beats 27 to 35 of the tachycardia. Most often, a single circus movement is responsible for continuation of this arrhythmia. During beat 27 (upper left panel), activation begins in the 20-msec isochrone and moves in a large circular pattern shown by the arrow, returning near to its origin after 220 msec. It continues from this point at 230 msec during beat 28 (upper middle panel) and follows a somewhat larger circular pathway (arrow), again returning to its origin at 410 msec. Once again, during beat 29 (upper right panel), it follows a similar circular pathway beginning at the 420 msec isochrone and ending at the 600 msec isochrone. However, additional wave fronts, possibly originating from reentrant circuits elsewhere, also occur

canine heart in situ

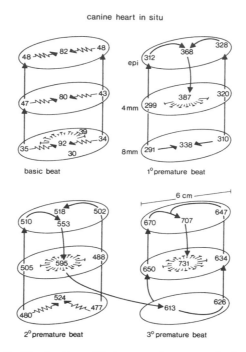

Figure 2.41: Schematic illustration of intramural reentry during the initial phase of an ischemia-induced ventricular tachycardia in a canine heart *in situ*. Simultaneous recordings were made from 20 intramural electrodes, each of which had an epicardial terminal and two intramural terminals, 4 mm and 8 mm below the epicardial surface. For the sake of clarity, only relevant activation times are indicated during the last sinus beat (basic beat), and the first three premature impulses. In each diagram subepicardial (top layer), intramural (middle layer) and subendocardial (bottom layer) activation is shown by the arrows. No reentrant activity could be detected between the basic beat and the first premature impulse, nor between first and second premature beats. Between premature beats 2 and 3, an intramural wave front reexcited the subendocardial (8 mm) layer at 613 msec (Unpublished results of K. Koch, A. Schene and M.J. Janse.)

(isochrone at 500 msec in the lower right part in beat 29). Furthermore, there is no continuity of activity between beats 29 and 30; a new wave front appears in a small area indicated by the 720 msec in beat 30 (middle left panel), 120 msec after activation during beat 29 ended. This could be an offspring of an intramurally located reentrant circuit, but also might be caused by some sort of focal activity. In beats 30 and 31, a figure-of-eight type of circus movement is present where two wave fronts propagate around an area of block, one clockwise, the other counterclockwise, and fuse in a final common pathway. To form this pattern, activity during beat 31 moves from the 870-msec isochrone to the 940-msec isochrone, the wave front splits with one moving upward around the base and the other downward around the apex. The two wave fronts merge after the 1020-msec isochrone. This figure-of-eight configuration is present also in beat 32 (middle right panel) beginning at the 1080 msec isochrone, but one wave front blocks at 1200 msec toward the base, the other toward the apex continues to complete a single reentrant loop after 1240 msec. The activation pattern in beat 33 (lower left panel) is rather complex, but it seems as if the wave front ending at 1390 msec continues in beat 34 (lower middle panel) at 1450 msec to create a new, single circus movement. Since relatively few electrodes were present in this area, we drew a dotted line connecting activity between 1390 and 1450 msec (beat 33 to 34) and between 1570 and 1640 (beat 34 to 35) to indicate our uncertainty.

The difference between ventricular tachycardia and ventricular fibrillation in these experiments was defined by the observation that fibrillation never terminated spontaneously, while tachycardia did, even though in the Langendorff-perfused hearts continuous coronary perfusion of the nonischemic myocardium was ensured. A second difference was the activation pattern, where during tachycardia a single reentrant circuit was often present, while during fibrillation there were multiple wavelets traveling independently around multiple islets of temporal (functional) block. Local electrograms often had a very irregular and chaotic appearance both during tachycardia and fibrillation. In one beat, they could show a fast, large intrinsic deflection indicating local activity, while in another beat, slow multiphasic, low-amplitude potentials indicating local block and electrotonic depolarization due to activity in adjacent tissue, could be present. A distinction between tachycardia and fibrillation could not be made from the characteristics of individual extracellular recordings.

Figures 2.39 and 2.40 show only epicardial activation patterns. Figure 2.41 shows schematically that intramural reentry might occur as well. In this experiment, 60 electrograms were simultaneously recorded from 20 intramural electrodes inserted into the ischemic part of the left ventricle of an *in situ* dog heart. Each electrode had a subepicardial recording terminal, and recording terminals 4 mm and 8 mm below the epicardial surface. The upper left panel shows the pattern of activation during a sinus (basic) beat. Activity begins in the subendocardium (35 and 34 msec) and moves toward the epicardium, reaching it after 48 msec. Subendocardial, intramural, and subepicardial activation is indicated by the zigzag arrows. Earliest activity during the first spontaneously occurring premature beat after coronary occlusion was found in the subendocardial (8 mm) layer at 291 msec (upper right panel). Activity again moved to the subepicardial layers, arriving there after 312 to 328 msec, and then headed back into intramural regions reaching the electrodes at a depth of 4 mm after 387 msec. No activity was found that connected latest activity during the last basic beat of the sinus rhythm (92 msec) to the earliest activated site during the first premature beat (291 msec), nor between latest activity of the first premature beat at 387 msec and earliest activity of the second premature beat at 477 msec (bottom left panel) so there is no case for intramural reentry here. Intramural reentry, however, seemed to occur between the second and third premature beats. During the second premature beat, activity moved from the subendocardium at 480 msec to the subepicardium; delayed epicardial activity at 553 msec excited a midmural layer at 595 msec, and from there the subendocardium was reexcited at 613 msec in the third beat (bottom right). As discussed in the section on "mapping", such activation maps, which are based on simultaneous recordings from a relatively small number of electrodes must be interpreted with caution.

The most complete activation maps during ischemia-induced arrhythmias available at present are provided by the studies of Pogwizd and Corr (1987b; 1990). They recorded simultaneously from 232 intramural sites in the relatively small feline heart. They calculated that this was equivalent to recording from 2800 sites in the larger canine heart. In their studies, tachycardia was usually maintained by intramural reentry within the ischemic myocardium, but nonreentrant mechanisms (during which no reentrant circuits were detected) also contributed. The transition from ventricular tachycardia to ventricular fibrillation was exclusively due to intramural reentry (Pogwizd and Corr 1990). The smallest reentrant pathways during ischemia were 1.8 cm (diameter 0.6 cm). Our mapping experiments, based on simultaneous recording from 60 sites (and later 128 sites), usually found slightly larger reentrant circuits in hearts of pigs and dogs; diameters were between 1 and 2 cm (Janse et al. 1980c). Since cycle lengths of the ventricular tachycardias in the feline heart were on the order of 200 msec (Pogwizd and Corr 1990) the impulse must have propagated with a conduction velocity of 9 cm/sec in the reentrant pathway of 1.8 cm. This is lower than the conduction velocity of 20 cm/sec, estimated from activation maps during tachycardia in experiments on canine and porcine hearts (Kléber et al. 1986). This difference may be due to species differences, and to the differences in spatial resolution of the activation maps.

Mapping experiments have fulfilled the first two of Mines' criteria: demonstration of unidirectional block and reconstruction of the pathways of activation. The final proof for reentry, cessation of the arrhythmia when the circuit is cut through, has not yet been accomplished during acute ischemia. In view of the continuously changing pattern of activation during tachycardia, fulfillment of Mines' third criterion seems an impossibility.

Whereas reentry is responsible for maintenance of tachycardia and fibrillation, there is some doubt whether the initiating premature beats are always caused by reentry. In some instances the very first ectopic impulse is certainly caused by reentrant excitation (Pogwizd and Corr 1987b), and an example is shown in Figures 2.42 and 2.43. Figure 2.42 shows 12 selected unipolar electrograms out of 125 simultaneously recorded electrograms from the epicardial surface of an isolated perfused dog heart, 7 minutes after occlusion of both the left anterior descending coronary artery branch and the circumflex artery. The electrode configuration is shown in the bottom panels of Figure 2.43, as are the positions of recording sites a to l. The first beat shown in Figure 2.42 is the last basic beat resulting from stimulation of the right ventricle. Arrows point to intrinsic deflections indicating local activation. The second complex is the first nonstimulated beat that initiates ventricular fibrillation. The activation patterns of last basic and first ectopic beats are shown in the isochronic maps in Figure 2.43. From the site of stimulation during the basic beat (upper left, pulse symbol), activity spreads in two directions. After exciting site j at

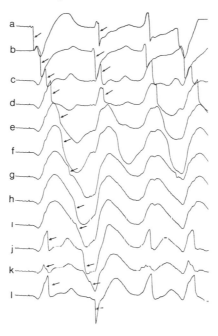

Figure 2.42: Selected unipolar electrograms from an isolated dog heart 7 minutes after occlusion of both the left anterior descending and circumflex arteries. The position of sites a to l are indicated in Figure 2.43. The first complex is the last basic beat resulting from stimulation of the right ventricle, the second complex is the first premature depolarization that initiates ventricular fibrillation. Arrows point to intrinsic deflections indicating time of local activation. (Reproduced from Janse et al. 1986, with permission.)

110 msec, the wave front on the anterior surface of the ventricles meets a zone of block around the 120-msec isochrone (note intrinsic deflection at j, and absence of intrinsic deflection in the initial part of the electrogram recorded at i in Figure 2.42). The wave front propagates via sites d, e, and f around the block, and turns back via sites g, h, and i to reexcite site j after 355 msec (see second intrinsic deflection in the electrogram recorded at j in Figure 2.42). The length of this reentrant circuit is in the order of 8 cm (since the electrodes were spaced at 5-mm distances, the length of the reentrant pathway could not be determined with greater accuracy). The impulse needed 235 msec to propagate in this pathway, indicating a conduction velocity on the order of 30 cm/sec, which fits well with measurements of conduction velocity in acutely ischemic myocardium. After reexciting the tissue in the neighborhood of site c, another attempt to follow the same circular pathway occurs, but this wave front is blocked close to 420 msec in the map of the first premature beat (Figure 2.43). It is noteworthy that another premature wave front emerged at about 380 msec close to the ischemic border (indicated by an asterisk in Figure 2.43, upper right panel) that was responsible for premature excitation of sites b and a. Thus, the premature activation of the ventricles was not caused by a single

7 min LAD + CIRC occlusion
subendocardium intact

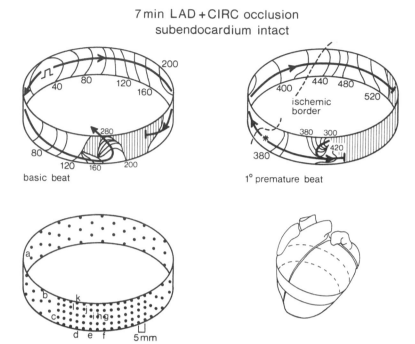

basic beat

1° premature beat

5 mm

Figure 2.43: The multipolar electrode, from which selected electrograms are shown in Figure 2.42, consisted of a 2-cm wide band containing 215 electrode terminals that was wrapped around both ventricles as shown in the bottom two panels. The electrode configuration in the lower left panel shows where each electrode terminal was located (at the dots). Interelectrode distances in the ischemic zone were 5 mm, elsewhere 15 mm. The site of stimulation is indicated by a square wave in the upper left panel. Isochronic maps and arrows show patterns of activation during the basic beat (top left) and first premature beat (top right). Time 0 was the stimulus artifact, numbers are in msec, arrows indicate general direction of activation fronts, shaded areas are zones of block, dotted line is the ischemic border. (Reproduced from Janse et al. 1986, with permission.)

event, but by at least two different sources of ectopic activity. One is classical circus movement reentry, the other is unknown.

Nonreentrant Mechanisms

Nonreentrant mechanisms may also be operative to cause arrhythmias during the acute ischemic period. The results of experiments suggesting the coexistence of a second arrhythmogenic mechanism are the following:

(1) Ventricular premature depolarizations can originate from the normal side of the ischemic border, which frequently is separated from the is-

chemic zone displaying delayed activity by an inexcitable zone (Janse et al. 1980c; Janse and Van Capelle 1982a).

(2) During recording from either epicardial or intramural regions, no evidence of continuously propagating activity bridging the gap between the latest activation attributed to the last impulse propagated from the atria and the earliest activity during the ectopic impulse has been found during single or multiple premature depolarizations or the initial beats of tachycardia (Janse et al. 1980c; Janse and Van Capelle 1982a). However, this is a point of controversy since, in a study utilizing 112 simultaneous intramural recordings, evidence was found for reentrant activity occurring at the ischemic border from epicardium to endocardium during single premature depolarizations or the first beat of tachycardia (Downar and Parson 1981). In the study on the feline heart by Pogwizd and Corr (1987b), the initiation of single ventricular premature beats, or the first beat of a ventricular tachycardia was caused by intramural reentry 76% of the time. Earliest ectopic activity almost invariably occurred in the subendocardium at the border of ischemic and nonischemic tissue. However, 24% of the time, the first beat of a tachycardia was initiated by a nonreentrant mechanism in either subendocardium or subepicardium at the boundary of the ischemic area. A nonreentrant mechanism was defined by the absence of intervening electrical activity between the last sinus beat and the beginning of the ectopic beat. Therefore, it seems that nonreentrant mechanisms are sometimes the cause of premature beats or the initial beats of tachycardia.

(3) When lidocaine was administered in high doses prior to coronary artery occlusion, electrical activity within the ischemic zone became more rapidly depressed than in the absence of the drug and within minutes myocardial fibers in the central ischemic region were inexcitable (Cardinal et al. 1981). The incidence of ventricular fibrillation was greatly reduced by lidocaine, possibly because multiple reentrant circuits could not occur in the inexcitable central ischemic zone. However, the incidence of single and multiple premature ventricular depolarizations was unaltered suggesting that they were not dependent on reentry.

(4) A difference can be seen in the canine heart between the effects of coronary artery ligation and coronary embolization with latex on the putative dual arrhythmogenic mechanisms, e.g., reentrant and nonreentrant. After coronary artery ligation, during which some collateral flow persists to ischemic myocardium, both premature ventricular depolarizations and ventricular tachycardia occur. After coronary embolization with latex, collateral flow does not persist. Although ischemic changes may be much more severe, ventricular tachycardia and fibrillation do not occur whereas ventricular premature depolarizations are still frequent (Euler et al. 1981). The depression in the ischemic zone may be homogeneous after embolization, preventing the formation of multiple reentrant circuits necessary for fibrillation. Yet, the second arrhythmogenic (nonreentrant) mechanism is not altered. In contrast to these findings are the observations of Cinca et al. (1984), that embolization of the left anterior descending coronary artery with latex in the pig heart results in a greater incidence of ventricular fibrillation than coronary occlusion. The difference in the experimental results are not yet explainable, although it may be related to the different experimental models.

On the basis of these results, the hypothesis has been proposed that during the first 10 minutes after coronary artery occlusion (phase 1a arrhythmias), two different arrhythmogenic mechanisms occur. One mechanism, reentrant excitation, causes ventricular premature beats, ventricular tachycardia, and ventricular fibrillation. The other nonreentrant mechanism causes premature ventricular depolarizations, which may initiate reentry. The exact mechanism underlying the nonreentrant ectopic activity is unknown. Abnormal automaticity in partially depolarized, ischemic myocardium is unlikely to occur since it should be suppressed by the elevated K^+ concentrations present in ischemic tissue (Katzung et al. 1975). Triggered activity, either induced by early or delayed afterdepolarizations is a possibility. Early afterdepolarizations have been recorded *in vitro* from ischemic papillary muscles (Ten Eick et al. 1976). They occur in Purkinje fibers, when acidosis is combined with slow heart rates (Coraboeuf and Boistel 1953; Coraboeuf et al. 1980) and have also been shown to occur when Purkinje fibers are exposed to lysophosphatidylcholine (Arnsdorf and Sawicki 1981). However, early afterdepolarizations are also suppressed at K^+ levels above 5 mmol/L. If the occurrence of early afterdepolarizations in ischemic myocardium is unlikely, in view of the elevated K^+ concentrations, the possibility exists that they may still occur in Purkinje fibers in the subendocardium adjacent to ischemic myocardium that are exposed to lysophosphoglycerides leaking out of the ischemic myocardium, as well as to protons but to lower concentrations of K^+ ions. One may speculate whether, at some critical level of these components, triggered activity based on early afterdepolarizations may arise from these Purkinje fibers especially when heart rate is slow. Another factor that may cause early afterdepolarizations during early ischemia is stretch, caused by the paradoxical movements of the ischemic part of the ventricular wall (Lab 1978; 1982).

The occurrence of delayed afterdepolarizations as the nonreentrant mechanism should require calcium "overload" of the ischemic cells. Delayed afterdepolarizations have not been recorded from ischemic myocardium, possibly because intracellular Ca^{2+} is not very high during the first 10 minutes (Marban et al. 1987; Steenbergen et al. 1987). In addition, severe hypoxia such as that which occurs in ischemic myocardium has been shown to suppress delayed afterdepolarizations that are induced by cathecholamines in isolated guinea pig papillary muscles (Coetzee and Opie 1987). Lysophosphoglycerides however, can induce delayed afterdepolarizations and triggered activity in isolated Purkinje fibers when combined with acidosis (pH 6.7) and a slightly elevated K^+ concentration of 7 mmol/L (Pogwizd et al. 1986). Prolonged mild hypoxia (pO_2 of 230 mm Hg) and acidosis produce delayed afterdepolarizations due to intracellular calcium overload (Adamantidis et al. 1986). Thus, whereas delayed afterdepolarizations are unlikely to occur in severely ischemic myocardium, it is possible that they might arise from Purkinje fibers in the vicinity of ischemic muscle, where pO_2 and extracellular K^+ are only moderately changed because of the exposure to oxygenated blood of the ventricular cavity, and where lysophosphoglycerides may become attached to the cell membrane.

Another possible nonreentrant mechanism for phase 1a arrhythmias is that the flow of injury current across the ischemic border may cause ectopic activity (Janse et al. 1980c; Janse and Kléber 1981; Janse and Van Capelle 1982a). We describe this mechanism next.

The Role of Injury Currents

The flow of current across the boundary between ischemic and normal myocardium has been implicated for many years as a possible factor that might contribute to the genesis of ectopic activity (Harris 1950; Harris et al. 1954; Hoffman 1966). Such current flow should, theoretically, be generated by the differences in membrane potential between closely adjacent regions either during diastole or during the action potential, the differences in membrane potential being caused by injury to the ischemic region. Ischemic cells have lower membrane potentials and a different time course of repolarization than normal cells. That current flowing between depolarized muscle fibers and polarized fibers may cause ectopic activity has been demonstrated in isolated guinea pig ventricular trabeculae, superfused in a two-compartment bath with one chamber containing 145 mm K^+ and the other 4 mm K^+. Current flowing from the compartment where the tissue was depolarized by the high K^+ towards the compartment superfused with normal solutions depolarized the fibers in the normal solution and induced abnormal automaticity (Katzung et al. 1975).

The presence and nature of the injury currents that occur during ischemia have been deduced by studies on changes of the TQ and ST segments of DC unipolar extracellular electrograms recorded on either side of the ischemic border. Analysis of the electrograms has indicated that both the magnitude and direction of flow of injury currents in acute ischemia change during the cardiac cycle. Depression of the TQ segment in DC extracellular electrograms recorded from the ischemic tissue indicates injury current flowing during diastole (Kléber et al. 1978). It is predicted from a theoretical analysis that, in diastole, when the intracellular compartments of partially depolarized ischemic cells are positive to the intracellular compartments of normal cells as we described in Figure 2.13, intracellular current flows from ischemic towards normal cells. This gives rise to transmembrane currents that result in current sources in the extracellular space on the nonischemic side of the border and current sinks on the ischemic side of the border (see Figure 2.13). It has been demonstrated that this diastolic current of injury causes a reduction of 20% in the diastolic stimulation threshold in a zone of several millimeters outside the ischemic border, presumably by bringing resting membrane potential of nonischemic cells closer to threshold potential (Coronel et al. 1991). The largest currents flow during markedly delayed activity of ischemic tissue because normal cells have already repolarized by the time ischemic cells are excited and depolarize as is shown by b_2 of Figure 2.14. At the moment the normal cells have repolarized, current sources exist in the normal tissue adjacent to the border, and have been estimated to be in the order of 2 μA/mm^3. This can be compared to current sources produced by a broad wave front propagating through normal myocardium in which the excitatory current has a large safety factor. These current sources are in the order of 5 μA/mm^3 (Janse et al. 1980c). It has been proposed that this current flowing between the ischemic cells with delayed activity and the normal cells which have repolarized or are repolarizing, through an inexcitable segment of depolarized cells interposed between the two, reexcites the normal cells to cause premature depolarizations (Janse et al. 1980c). This mechanism is schematically illustrated in Figures 2.44 and 2.45. Figure 2.44 shows a diagram of the flow of "injury current" between ischemic cells and nonischemic cells. In the bottom panels the upper tracings represent transmembrane potentials, the lower tracings the corresponding extracellular electrograms. From left to right are shown a site with delayed activation, a site where there is no action potential ("inexcitable") and a site showing normal electrical activity. At the moment indicated by the dashed line, when the ischemic site is activated and the normal myocardium is already repolarized, a current flows through the inexcitable segment from ischemic to normal myocardium in the intracellular space (diagram above). This current emerges as a current source in the normal myocardium, and could, when strong enough, depolarize the normal cells to threshold thus causing a premature depolarization. Figure 2.45 shows a schematic diagram of a possible mechanism for ventricular premature depolarizations originating in Purkinje fibers close to the ischemic border that also involves current flow between ischemic and

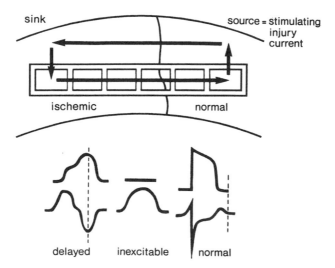

Figure 2.44: A schematic diagram showing flow of "injury current" between ischemic cells and nonischemic cells is at the top. The arrows indicate the direction of current flow. Below are shown drawings of transmembrane potentials (top traces) and electrograms (bottom traces) from the ischemic zone which was activated with delay (delayed), an inexcitable zone located between the ischemic and normal zone, and the normal zone.

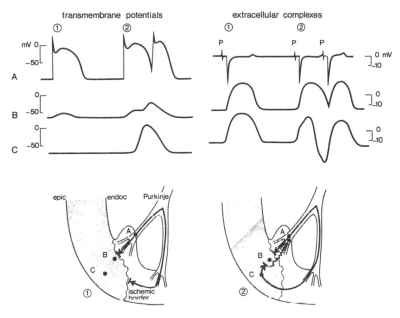

Figure 2.15: Possible mechanism of ventricular premature depolarizations originating in Purkinje fibers close to the ischemic border. Transmembrane potentials are shown in the top left panel and extracellular electrograms in the top right panel. The diagram at the lower left shows the location at which the transmembrane potentials were recorded. The arrows in the diagrams below show the pattern of activation. (Reproduced from Janse 1986c, with permission.)

normal regions. Hypothetical transmembrane potentials from normal Purkinje fibers (A), inexcitable cells in the ischemic area close to the border (B) and ischemic cells responding in a 2:1 fashion during normal sinus rhythm (C) are drawn in the upper left panel. These locations are shown in the diagram in the lower left panel. In the upper right panel, corresponding extracellular electrograms at these sites are redrawn. The ischemic myocardium is shaded in the drawings of the heart and the Purkinje strand (A) is in electrotonic contact with the ischemic myocardium. During beat 1, the impulse propagating from the atrium is blocked between A and B and conduction block also occurs elsewhere so that site C is not excited (upper left panel and lower left diagram). In beat 2, there is again block between A and B, but C is activated with great delay via another pathway (lower right diagram). Activity at C is not conducted via B to A, but electrotonic currents traverse the region of bidirectional block and reexcite A. The magnitude of the current may also be sufficient to induce early or delayed afterdepolarizations, possibly resulting in single or multiple premature beats. In a computer model imitating the proposed conditions at the ischemic border zone, subthreshold depolarizations caused by injury currents flowing through an inexcitable gap also increased spontaneous diastolic depolarization of latent pacemakers resulting in repetitive automatic activity (Janse and Van Capelle 1982a).

The hypothesis that ectopic activity is caused by injury current flow is supported by the studies on arrhythmias caused by embolization of a coronary artery with latex that we described before (Euler et al. 1981). Persistence of ventricular premature depolarizations and a decreased incidence of fibrillation under these conditions that cause inexcitability of the ischemic region is consistent with the expectation that injury currents are larger during embolization because of the sharper demarcation between ischemic and normal myocardium, while reentrant circuits are abolished by the more severe ischemic damage. In conclusion, it must be emphasized that the mechanisms responsible for the premature ventricular depolarizations in the first 10 minutes (as opposed to tachycardia and fibrillation) are not definitely known. Intramural reentry does not account for all the ectopic activations. They might alternatively be caused by a "focal" mechanism. Injury currents might play a role, either by reexciting normal cells across the border, or by inducing triggered activity.

The Role of the Purkinje System

Up to this point we have emphasized how the changes in electrical activity of the ventricular muscle cells after coronary occlusion may lead to the occurrence of arrhythmias either by reentrant excitation or by nonreentrant mechanisms involving the flow of injury currents. It has also been suggested that some ectopic activity in the early phase of ischemia might originate from Purkinje fibers because Purkinje activity sometimes may precede ventricular muscle activity during spontaneous premature ventricular depolarizations (Bagdonas et al. 1961; Janse et al. 1986). This is demonstrated in Figure 2.46, which shows four extracellular electrograms recorded from an isolated, perfused dog heart at two different time scales, a slow scale at the left and an expanded scale at the right. In A, two basic beats propagated from the atria are followed by two spontaneous ventricular premature beats ("extra"). These premature beats initiate ventricular tachycardia (B), which finally changes into ventricular fibrillation (C) after the 71st ectopic impulse. In the top trace, recorded from the nonischemic myocardium close to the ischemic border, activity caused by Purkinje fibers is pointed out by the arrows. In the second and third traces, myocardial activity from the nonischemic subendocardium (endo) and subepicardium (epi, normal zone) is shown; the lowest tracing was recorded from ischemic subepicardium (epi, ischemic zone). Note that both during normally propagated and ectopic beats during the tachycardia phase (panel B), Purkinje activity precedes myocardial activity indicating that the arrhythmias might originate in the Purkinje system.

It is not certain whether, or to what extent, the electrophysiological properties of subendocardial Purkinje fibers are changed during the initial phase of acute ischemia and what role these changes might play in the occurrence of the acute arrhythmias. Because of the location of the Purkinje fibers on the endocardial surface, it has not been possible to record intracellular potentials

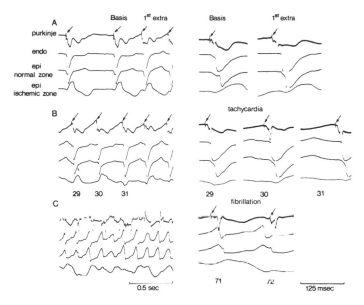

Figure 2.46: Four extracellular electrograms recorded from an isolated perfused dog heart at two different time scales. Panel A shows two basic (sinus beats) and two extra beats starting ventricular tachycardia. Panel B shows ventricular tachycardia and panel C shows ventricular fibrillation. Note that during normally propagated and ectopic beats Purkinje activity (arrows) precedes myocardial activity. (Reproduced from Janse and Van Capelle 1982b, with permission.)

during coronary occlusion in the intact heart. Therefore, possible ischemia-induced changes must be deduced from extracellular electrogram recordings. Conflicting data exist as to whether or not there are early changes in these extracellular electrograms. The deflections caused by activation of Purkinje fibers did not show appreciable changes after coronary occlusion in some studies in canine hearts (Bagdonas et al. 1961; Cox et al. 1973) and porcine hearts (Janse et al. 1980b) whereas a decrease in amplitude, and even a disappearance of Purkinje spikes within 15 seconds after coronary occlusion in the dog heart has also been reported (Lazzara et al. 1974; Scherlag et al. 1974). Figure 2.47 shows subendocardial (subendoc) and subepicardial (subepic) electrograms recorded from an *in situ* canine heart during a 5-minute ischemic period caused by coronary occlusion and 2 minutes after reperfusion (after release of the occlusion). Arrows indicate activity generated by subendocardial Purkinje fibers. The Purkinje spikes decreased in amplitude during ischemia, but remained present. Two to one block between Purkinje fibers and subendocardial muscle developed at 4 and 5 minutes of ischemia. After 5 minutes, subepicardial complexes were monophasic indicating absence of local activation, while subendocardial muscle still showed a delayed intrinsic deflection in every second beat. One possible reason for the apparently conflicting results may be that because of the change in dimension of the regionally ischemic ventricular wall, slight movement of the recording electrode sometimes causes a disappearance

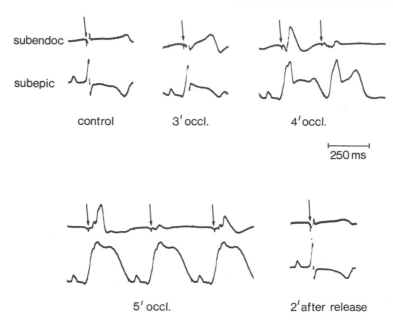

Figure 2.47: Subendocardial (subendoc) and subepicardial (subepi) electrograms from an *in situ* canine heart. Arrows point to activity generated by Purkinje fibers. Records are shown prior to (control) and at various times after occlusion (occl) of the coronary artery as well as after release of the occlusion. Note preservation of Purkinje spikes during ischemia. (Unpublished results of R. Cardinal and M.J. Janse.)

of Purkinje electrograms. Another more likely explanation is that Purkinje cells in different locations are affected differently by coronary occlusion. Superficial fibers located immediately beneath the endocardium probably receive adequate amounts of oxygen and substrate via diffusion from the cavitary blood to maintain normal electrophysiological properties for a while after they are deprived of their coronary arterial supply. This has been shown in experiments by Wilensky et al. (1986) in which isolated preparations of rabbit interventricular septum were perfused through a coronary artery and placed in a tissue bath where they were superfused as well so that transmembrane potentials could be recorded. During the first 10 minutes of ischemia, produced by coronary occlusion, action potential amplitude and upstroke velocity in the first 40 to 60 myocardial cell layers beneath the endocardium remained well preserved. Extracellular K^+ was less elevated and extracellular pH decreased less in this region than in deeper layers where severe electrophysiological alterations occurred (Wilensky et al. 1986). Purkinje fibers are also more resistant to hypoxia than muscle fibers (Goldenberg and Rothberger 1937; Bagdonas et al. 1961). Purkinje fibers that are more deeply embedded within the subendocardial muscle are more dependent on coronary artery blood supply and therefore, coronary occlusion probably affects them more. As yet, there is no precise information on the relationship between distance from the endocardium and changes in electrophysiological characteristics in Purkinje fibers in the acute phase of ischemia. Although it may therefore be expected that superficial Purkinje fibers might maintain normal electrophysiological characteristics in the acute phase of ischemia, they might still be influenced by substances leaking out from the subjacent ischemic muscle cells.

Some possible mechanisms by which premature ventricular depolarizations or tachycardia could originate from subendocardial Purkinje fibers overlying ischemic myocardium, or in close proximity to the ischemic border are: (1) micro-reentry or reflection in small parts of the Purkinje network, particularly when part of it is located more deeply within the ischemic myocardium and subjected to high extracellular K^+ concentrations (Schmitt and Erlanger 1928; Wit et al. 1972a; 1972b); (2) triggered activity, emerging from either early or delayed afterdepolarizations (see Wit and Rosen 1986). Subthreshold depolarizations caused by injury currents (Janse et al. 1980c; Janse and Van Capelle 1982a) and stretch caused by loss of contractility and systolic bulging of ischemic myocardium (Lab 1978; 1982) could both be factors that induce repetitive activity due to triggered activity. Delayed afterdepolarizations leading to premature depolarizations have been observed in bovine Purkinje fibers even in the presence of high extracellular K^+ concentrations, indicating that triggering can occur in Purkinje fibers in an "ischemic" milieu (Carmeliet 1980). Moreover, lysophosphoglycerides have been shown to induce triggered activity in Purkinje fibers exposed to high K^+ and acidosis (Pogwizd et al. 1986). It is therefore likely that Purkinje fibers that are not hypoxic because of their proximity to well-oxygenated cavitary blood, but that are exposed to substances that leak away from ischemic myocardium, can develop triggered activity. However, all these possibilities remain speculative, since there is as yet no solid evidence that these mechanisms occur in intact hearts with regional ischemia.

In view of the limited number of recording sites in those studies that showed early Purkinje fiber activity during ectopic beats, it is also uncertain whether the site of earliest recorded activity is truly the site of origin of the ectopic impulse. Rather than being the site of origin, the Purkinje network might be the exit route for excitation coming out of an intramural reentrant circuit in ischemic ventricular muscle. Thus, it has been shown that in isolated perfused canine hearts, destruction of the subendocardium, including the Purkinje system, by intracavitary application of phenol did not abolish ectopic activity during either ischemia or reperfusion as would be expected if ectopic activity originated in the subendocardial Purkinje system. Ventricular fibrillation, however, did not occur after destruction of the subendocardium. In these experiments, the presence of reentrant circuits within the ischemic region was documented. The revolution time of the impulse in these circuits was 340 to 400 msec, accounting for the slow tachycardias observed after subendocardial destruction (Janse et al. 1986). Fibrillation may not have occurred because impulses from these circuits were not rapidly conveyed throughout the ventricles due to the absence of the Purkinje system, but rather, activated the ventricles slowly through ventricular muscle. The extent of subendocardial necrosis in these experiments was not quantified and it can therefore not be excluded that a reduction in tissue mass played a role in the prevention of fibrillation. Selective destruction of subendocardial Purkinje fibers by application of lugol increased the ventricular fibrillation threshold in nonischemic hearts (Damiano et al. 1986), suggesting a possible role for the Purkinje network in the genesis of ventricular fibrillation.

The Role of Heart Rate

In patients, changes in heart rate often precede the onset of acute ischemic arrhythmias and, therefore, might be implicated to some extent as a cause of arrhythmias (Adgey 1982). In the early phase of myocardial ischemia, alterations in the activity of both the parasympathetic and sympathetic nervous systems occur and might cause the changes in rate. Enhanced parasympathetic activity, which causes bradycardia and hypotension, is most frequently associated with inferior wall infarction and was present in 48% of patients seen within 30 minutes after the onset of symptoms in the series studied by the Belfast group (Webb et al. 1972; Pantridge et al. 1974; 1981). In the very early phase of myocardial infarction, the sudden occurrence of severe bradycardia and hypotension has been associated with ventricular fibrillation (Pantridge et al. 1981) but it is uncertain whether the low heart rate or the hypotension is the more important arrhythmogenic factor. Enhanced sympathetic activity, which causes sinus tachycardia and/or hypertension, is most often associated with anterior wall infarction and was found in 35% of patients seen during the first 30 minutes (Webb et al. 1972; Pantridge et al. 1974). In a series of 48 patients who developed ventricular fibrillation in the early phase of myocardial infarction, there was a significant increase in heart rate immediately prior to ventricular fibrillation (Adgey 1982) suggesting that in the early phase of ischemia high heart rates may also be arrhythmogenic.

The experimental evidence that bradycardia in the early phase after coronary artery occlusion causes electrophysiological changes that are arrhythmogenic is, although often quoted, far from convincing. Han and coworkers (1966) reported that after about 5 minutes of ischemia, ventricular premature depolarizations occurred more frequently at low heart rates (during stimulation of the vagus), but whether ventricular tachycardia or fibrillation also occurred more frequently was not mentioned. Chadda and associates (1974) showed that ventricular premature depolarizations and ventricular fibrillation occurred predominantly at low heart rates, between 60 and 90 minutes, and at high heart rates, between 180 and 200 minutes after coronary artery occlusion, but not at intermediate rates between 90 and 180 minutes. On the basis of these results they proposed that there is an optimal heart rate at which arrhythmias are reduced as had previously been shown by Wit et al. (1972b). However, the time after coronary occlusion at which arrhythmias occurred was not specified in this study and results were shown covering the first 3 hours. This leads to difficulties in interpreting the data since arrhythmias occurring during the first minutes may have different mechanisms than arrhythmias occurring at 3 hours and the effects of rate on the different mechanisms may be different. In patients with acute myocardial infarction, ventricular fibrillation occurs at the so-called "optimal" heart rate (Adgey 1982; Lie et al. 1975). Other studies have failed to find an arrhythmogenic effect of bradycardia during the early phase of ischemia. Kerzner et al. (1973) found that vagal stimulation during the first 30 minutes after occlusion did not precipitate ventricular fibrillation. However, after 3 hours vagal stimulation caused ventricular premature depolarizations and between 4 and 9 hours, ventricular tachycardia was induced in all animals. At these later times, as we describe in Chapter III, arrhythmias are caused by automaticity and suppression of the sinus node pacemaker will enhance the ability of the ectopic pacemakers to control the ventricles. When complete atrioventricular dissociation was produced by injecting the AV node with procaine (another way of causing a slow ventricular rate), ligation of the left main coronary artery, causing ischemia of 80% of the left ventricle, induced ventricular fibrillation in only 3 of 14 dogs, whereas all animals with an intact AV node, normal sinus rhythm and a faster ventricular rate fibrillated within 3 minutes (Webb and Field 1958). In the studies of Scherlag et al. (1970; 1976; 1983) a slow heart rate protected against arrhythmias in the acute ischemic phase whereas bradycardia elicited arrhythmias 3 hours after occlusion.

One explanation usually given to support the idea that bradycardia should be arrhythmogenic is that in normal myocardium an increased dispersion in refractory periods in the order of 40 msec has been found after slowing of the heart rate (Han et al. 1966). Such a dispersion in refractory periods is thought to facilitate the establishment of unidirectional block of premature impulses, one of the prerequisites for reentry. In addition to the dispersion of refractory period hypothesis, slowing of rate below a critical level has also been shown to further depress conduction in partially depolarized Purkinje fibers and increase the number of reentrant impulses (Wit et al. 1972b). Although the mechanism for additional conduction slowing was not investigated, it may be related to additional depolarization caused by a decrease in activity of the rate-dependent electrogenic Na/K pump. However, it is questionable whether a dispersion of the refractory period as small as 40 msec, especially in the presence of the long refractory periods associated with slow heart rates, can lead to reentrant arrhythmias. Differences in refractory periods at multiple sites in the order of 40 msec are a normal finding in the nonischemic canine left ventricle and such a dispersion, even in the presence of short refractory periods caused by successive application of five premature stimuli, do not cause arrhythmias (Janse 1971). It has been shown that a dispersion of at least 100 to 130 msec is necessary for initiation of reentrant ventricular arrhythmias (Kuo et al. 1983). Furthermore, although the methodological problems inherent in the determination of refractory periods in ischemic myocardium must be taken into account, it has been found that the disparity between refractory periods of normal and ischemic myocardium increases as heart rate increases, and decreases when the heart beats slowly (Kent et al. 1973).

Bradycardia may actually decrease early reentrant arrhythmias because ischemic damage to myocardial fibers is decreased at slower heart rates. There also may be a difference between the effects of bradycardia and the effects of sudden changes in cycle length, from short to long. In the acute phase of ischemia, the sudden occurrence of long cycles may be followed by ventricular fibrillation as has been observed in patients with acute myocardial infarction (Pantridge et al. 1981) and in patients dying suddenly during ambulatory electrocardiographic recording (Gradman et al. 1977; Nikolic et al. 1982; Roelandt et al. 1984; Leclercq et al. 1988). The occurrence of ventricular fibrillation following sudden long cycle lengths in patients might be explained by some experimental results. It has been shown that sudden introduction of a long pause can result in the appearance of large action potentials with slow upstrokes in acutely ischemic cells showing no response when the heart is paced at a normal rate (Downar et al. 1977a). Also in ischemic cells that at a normal rate show small amplitude responses, a sudden prolongation of the RR interval will be followed by action potentials with marked alternations in amplitude, the first large amplitude action potentials have long durations and the small amplitude action potentials have short durations (Janse et al. 1985a). Thus, a long cycle length can result in the reappearance of electrical activity in previously unresponsive cells and can increase inhomogeneity by inducing alternation of action potential amplitude and duration. The increased inhomogeneity might increase the likelihood for reentry in acutely ischemic myocardium.

As already mentioned, there is evidence both from studies in humans (Adgey 1982) and from experiments in canine hearts (Scherlag et al. 1974) that an increase in heart rate exacerbates arrhythmias in acute ischemia. An increase in rate leads to more severe ischemic damage and an increase in the size of the ischemic area (Shell and Sobel 1973). Theoretically, this effect should increase the possibility for occurrence of reentrant circuits and the number of reentrant circuits that might coexist. An increased heart rate also increases the delay in recovery of excitability of ischemic cells, which is rate-dependent (Downar et al. 1977a; Janse 1982b). Slight differences in the time constants of recovery of maximum upstroke velocity between adjacent cell groups become evident as cycle lengths are shortened and lead to asynchronous activation (see Figure 2.24). In addition to the effects of increased heart rate, direct effects of noradrenaline on ischemic myocardium have to be considered when the increase in heart rate occurs reflexly. These effects of catecholamines are discussed next.

The Role of the Sympathetic Nervous System

The sympathetic nervous system plays a role in the genesis of ventricular arrhythmias in the early phase of myocardial ischemia. The evidence comes from a wide variety of clinical and experimental studies including: (1) demonstration that plasma catecholamine levels are elevated during the occurrence of ischemia-induced arrhythmias (Ceremuzynski et al. 1969; Strange et al. 1978); (2) documentation of increased release of catecholamines in ischemic tissue at the time arrhythmias are most frequent (Shabab et al. 1969; Schömig et al. 1984); (3) studies showing a decrease in incidence and severity of arrhythmias after cardiac denervation, adrenergic blockade or catecholamine depletion (Cox and Robertson 1936; Sheridan et al. 1980; Norwegian Multicenter Study Group 1981; Puddu et al. 1988); (4) direct correlations between the occurrence of emotional stress and severity of arrhythmias (Skinner et al. 1975; Randall and Hasson 1981; Skinner 1987); (5) demonstration of arrhythmogenic effects of increased sympathetic activity in the presence of ischemia (Verrier and Lown 1978; Schwartz and Stone 1982) and even in normal hearts (Armour et al. 1972; Cardinal et al. 1986), and (6) identification of subgroups of both dogs and patients with myocardial infarction that are at high risk for sudden death by the analysis of baroreflex sensitivity (Schwartz and Stone 1985; La Rovere et al. 1988). Baroreflex sensitivity is tested by noting the decrease in heart rate that occurs upon a rise in blood pressure following intravenous administration of phenylephrine. Plots of change in RR interval versus change in blood pressure reveal individuals with a steep slope (strong vagal reflexes) and individuals with less steep slopes ("depressed baroreflex sensitivity"). The lower the slope, the greater the susceptibility for subsequent sudden death. However, there is a large variability in the results of all these studies and many reports are conflicting. This is undoubtedly due, to a large extent, to the complex effects of the sympathetic nervous system on the heart and to the variability in animal models that have been used. Thus in the different reports, there is no standardization of animal species, number of animals studied, heart size, size of the ischemic area, degree of collateralization, heart rate, changes in blood pressure, whether or not the animals were conscious, depth of anesthesia when used for coronary artery occlusion, time of occurrence of arrhythmias, and type of arrhythmia.

Despite this variability, the general consensus is still that sympathetic activation enhances arrhythmogenesis and sometimes is even needed for the occurrence of acute ischemic arrhythmias. However, the mechanisms for this sympathetic effect are not understood. Sympathetic activation may be arrhythmogenic through indirect or direct effects on cardiac muscle electrophysiology. We categorize indirect effects as sympathetic-induced hypokalemia (Nordrehaug and von der Lippe 1983), sinus tachycardia (we have discussed the effects of heart rate on arrhythmia occurrence) or an increase in the size of an ischemic area that may lead to more reentrant circuits (Verrier et al. 1987). On the other hand, direct effects are exerted on the cardiac muscle fibers to influence the membrane currents. It is beyond the scope of this book to cover the vast literature on this subject. Corr et al. (1986) have recently reviewed it in detail. However, we briefly discuss some possible direct arrhythmogenic catecholamine effects.

There is evidence that ischemia causes an increased release of noradrenaline only after 10–20 minutes (Marshall and Parratt 1980; McGrath et al. 1981; Riemersma 1982; Abrahamsson et al. 1983; Forfar et al. 1983; Dart et al. 1984; Schömig et al. 1984). Increased overflow of noradrenaline into the venous effluent during reperfusion of either regionally or globally ischemic hearts has been detected only after ischemic periods longer than 7.5 to 10 minutes (McGrath et al. 1981; Forfar et al. 1984; Schömig et al. 1984; Carlsson 1987; Wilde 1988). Even in the presence of cardiac sympathetic stimulation, extra noradrenaline release is not evident in ischemic myocardium during the first 10 minutes in contrast to the marked increase in noradrenaline release in normal myocardium (Dart et al. 1984). The reason for this is that neuronal reuptake of noradrenaline is enhanced, and neurotransmission impaired during the first 10 minutes of ischemia (Dart et al. 1984; Schömig et al. 1984). In phases later than 10 minutes, progressive accumulation of noradrenaline in the extracellular space occurs. However, local increases in catecholamine turnover occur early in ischemia, and in addition to enhanced neuronal reuptake, an α-adrenoreceptor-mediated feedback mechanism initially prevents output into the coronary venous effluent (Forfar et al. 1985). Thus, spontaneous noradrenaline release could be detected as early as 3 minutes after ischemia when neuronal reuptake was blocked by desmethylimipramine and α_2 receptors were blocked by yohimbine (Forfar et al. 1985).

Thus, accumulation of catecholamines in the extracellular space of the ischemic region may play a role in the genesis of phase 1b arrhythmias or the reperfusion arrhythmias that follow 15–20 minute ischemic episodes (described later), but probably not the phase 1a arrhythmias. As we described, after 15 to 20 minutes of ischemia the depressed action potentials in the ischemic region are restored; resting membrane potential increases, action potential amplitude increases and action potentials occur in regions that were previously inexcitable. The return of electrical activity might lead to the formation of reentrant circuits. Penny (1984) has suggested that increased catecholamine levels at this time may be responsible for these changes in electrical activity. Catecholamines have been shown to hyperpolarize resting membrane potential in isolated depolarized cardiac muscle preparations (Trautwein and Schmidt 1960; Hoffman and Singer 1967) either by increasing Na/K pump activity (Désilets and Baumgarten 1986) or K^+ conductance (Boyden et al. 1983) and these effects may be the cause of hyperpolarization of the ischemic cells. In isolated cardiac muscle preparations exposed to "ischemic" solutions (high K^+, low pO_2, low pH, absence of glucose) the addition of noradrenaline does indeed cause a transient hyperpolarization accompanied by a transient increase in action potential amplitude and duration (Wilde 1988).

Other suggestions for possible mechanisms for the induction of arrhythmias by catecholamines come from studies on isolated superfused preparations of cardiac tissue. Catecholamines enhance phase 4 depolarization in normal Purkinje fibers through β-adrenergic stimulation (Wit et al. 1975) but there is no evidence that this effect contributes to the acute ischemic arrhythmias caused by occlusion alone. Idioventricular rates in the canine heart determined during vagal stimulation are unaltered during acute ischemia (Scherlag et al. 1974; Kaplinsky et al. 1978). The failure to demonstrate an increased idioventricular rate would also seem to eliminate enhanced abnormal automaticity caused by catecholamines in partially depolarized Purkinje or muscle cells as an arrhythmogenic mechanism (Katzung et al. 1975). A high extracellular K^+

concentration such as that found in the acute ischemic environment suppresses abnormal automaticity (Katzung et al. 1975; Imanishi and Surawicz 1976). Catecholamines have also been shown to decrease automatic firing in cells depolarized by mechanical trauma, anoxia, or toxic drug effects by hyperpolarizing the maximum diastolic potential (Trautwein and Schmidt 1960; Hoffman and Singer 1967).

Catecholamines may restore conduction in muscle fibers partly depolarized by high extracellular K^+ to membrane potentials less than about -60 mV (Cranefield 1975). The effect is a result of an increase in inward L-type calcium current and the induction of slow response action potentials (Carmeliet and Vereecke 1969). In the early phase of ischemia, stimulation of the stellate ganglia causes an increase in conduction velocity in the ischemic region (Millar et al. 1976; Janse et al. 1985c) and this would not be expected if slow response action potentials occurred. An increase in conduction velocity should tend to prevent reentry rather than promote it. We have already discussed other reasons why it is unlikely that slow responses are a major cause of arrhythmias during the first 10 to 15 minutes of ischemia. However, no information is available whether or not catecholamine-induced slow responses are involved in arrhythmogenesis at a later time (phase 1b arrhythmias). Catecholamines also induce early and delayed afterdepolarizations (Cranefield 1975; Hoffman 1978, Wit and Rosen 1986; Priori and Corr 1990); whether this effect occurs in the acutely ischemic environment because of the rise in extracellular K^+ is uncertain. Delayed afterdepolarizations were not induced in canine Purkinje fibers exposed to 12–15 mm K^+, although they did occur in bovine Purkinje fibers under the same conditions (Wit et al. 1972a; 1972b; Carmeliet 1980). In atrial fibers modest increases in K^+ have been shown to increase delayed afterdepolarization amplitude and cause triggered activity (Henning et al. 1987).

Role of Ventricular Dysfunction

There is abundant clinical evidence that impaired left ventricular function is an important factor identifying patients with coronary artery disease that are at high risk for sudden death (Weaver et al. 1976; Schulze et al. 1977; Cobb et al. 1980; Myerburg et al. 1980; Goldstein et al. 1981; Pitt 1982). The possibility that regional wall motion abnormalities resulting from acute ischemia may have an effect on the electrophysiological characteristics of ischemic myocardium was explored by Lab and colleagues (Lab 1978; Covell et al. 1981; Lab 1982; Lab et al. 1984; Lab 1987). They showed that in a lightly loaded isolated papillary muscle that shortened isotonically the duration of the intracellular calcium transient was increased. This in turn led to an increase in action potential duration and to the development of early afterdepolarizations. In regional ischemia the ischemic segment of the left ventricle shows out-of-phase movement, with lengthening of the ischemic segment during early systole followed by late shortening. Just as in the isolated muscle preparations, recordings of monophasic potentials with suction electrodes indicated that action potential duration was prolonged and that the terminal repolarization phase was distorted by a "hump" similar to an early afterdepolarization. This afterdepolarization could lead to a "triggered" extrasystole. Action potential prolongation and/or early afterdepolarizations have also been observed in normal hearts following local traction (Gornick et al. 1989), after release of stretched isolated muscle preparations (Kaufmann et al. 1971), during balloon valvuloplasty in patients with congenital pulmonary stenosis (Levine et al. 1988), or during sudden outflow obstruction late in diastole (Franz et al. 1989). In the last study, however, action potential duration was shortened. The suggested mechanism underlying this "mechano-electrical coupling" was that muscle shortening reduces the binding of calcium to the contractile proteins. This results in an increase in unbuffered intracellular calcium that in turn prolongs the action potential duration and leads to the development of early afterdepolarizations either by enhanced electrogenic Na/Ca exchange or by a calcium-activated inward current. In Chapter I, we also described stretch-activated channels that might also play a role here (Hansen et al. 1990). In addition to early afterdepolarizations, stretch of Purkinje fibers and cardiac muscle preparation can induce abnormal automaticity and delayed afterdepolarizations (Dudel and Trautwein 1954; Kaufmann and Theophile 1967; Wit et al. 1973).

Whereas these studies point to possible arrhythmogenic mechanisms based on disturbances in impulse formation caused by acute alterations in mechanical behavior during acute ischemia, other studies in nonischemic hearts have reported on electrophysiological alterations caused by chronic heart failure. In hypertrophied hearts of cats in which clinical signs of heart failure were present, resting membrane potential, action potential amplitude, and maximum upstroke velocity were markedly reduced (Gelband and Bassett 1973). These changes were related to heart failure per se since they were not found in ventricular muscle of cats with hypertrophy uncomplicated by failure. Another study on hypertrophied left ventricle of cats reported the presence of fibrotic areas on the endocardial surface with intermingling of viable muscle cells and connective tissue. In these areas relatively normal action potentials were interspersed with electrically silent zones and potentials of abnormal configuration, that is short duration, low amplitude, notched upstrokes and reduced membrane potentials (Cameron et al. 1983). Such findings indicate the presence of slow conduction and dispersion of refractoriness, which are factors predisposing to reentry.

Other factors associated with congestive heart failure which could play a role in arrhythmogenesis are hypokalemia, enhanced sympathetic activity, and increased levels of circulating catecholamines. As yet there is insufficient information from adequate animal models that could lead to a satisfactory explanation for the arrhythmogenic effects of heart failure.

Reperfusion Arrhythmias

The observation that ventricular fibrillation may occur within seconds after restoration of blood flow to myocardium made ischemic by a period of coronary occlusion (reperfusion) was originally made in the 19th century (Cohn-heim and Schulthess-Rechberg 1881) and later confirmed in the middle of the 20th (Tennant and Wiggers 1935; Blumgart et al. 1941). In fact, ventricular fibrillation may occur more frequently following reperfusion than after coro-nary artery ligation (Stephenson et al. 1960). There is a relationship between the length of the ischemic period during the coronary occlusion in experimental animals and the occurrence of reperfusion arrhythmias (Battle et al. 1974; Sheridan et at. 1980; Balke et al. 1981; Manning and Hearse 1984). At least a 3-minute ischemic period during occlusion is necessary before reperfusion arrhythmias occur (Corbalan et al. 1976). The incidence of reperfusion-induced ventricular fibrillation increases when occlusion periods are lengthened from 5 minutes to 20 or 30 minutes. Also, in dogs reperfusion-induced fibrillation tends to occur more often when severe arrhythmias develop during occlusion (Murdock et al. 1980; Balke et al. 1981). Reperfusion arrhythmias decrease when reperfusion is delayed beyond 30 to 60 minutes (Manning and Hearse 1984). A similar dependence on the time of the ischemic period has been found in other species. The onset of irreversible injury during ischemia is related to the decrease in reperfusion arrhythmias after 20–30 minutes (Penny and Sheridan 1983; Manning and Hearse 1984) since the arrhythmias must arise in viable cells (see below). Reperfusion arrhythmias have been prevented when reperfusion occurs gradually instead of abruptly (Sewell et al. 1955; Petro-poulos and Meijne 1964; Yamazaki et al. 1986), although prevention has not always been observed (Sheridan 1987).

Reperfusion after a 30-minute occlusion in dog hearts results in two dis-tinct periods of reperfusion arrhythmias (Kaplinsky et al. 1981). Immediately after reperfusion, ventricular fibrillation is the dominant arrhythmia. The likelihood of fibrillation occurring after reperfusion is greater if fibrillation occurs during the period of occlusion. If no fibrillation occurs immediately upon reperfusion, a delayed period of arrhythmias may occur 2 to 7 minutes later, characterized by ventricular premature depolarizations and ventricular tachy-cardia.

In humans with a developing myocardial infarction, reperfusion caused by administration of thrombolytic agents induces ventricular arrhythmias al-though ventricular fibrillation is rare. The most common arrhythmia is acceler-ated idioventricular rhythm with rates between 70 and 95 beats/min (Sclarov-sky et al. 1978; 1983; Rentrop et al. 1981; Goldberg et al. 1983). The absence of fibrillation may be because of the relatively long delay (hours) between occlusion of the coronary artery and the reperfusion, similar to that seen in the animal experiments. Thrombolysis of an occluded coronary artery, either spontaneously or by drug administration, within 30 minutes of occlusion might cause a higher incidence of fibrillation based on the results of the experimental studies.

The electrophysiological mechanisms causing the immediate and delayed reperfusion arrhythmias are most likely not the same. During relatively brief periods of ischemia (i.e., no longer than 20 minutes) there is marked depression of transmembrane action potentials, and even inexcitability as we have described. Sudden reperfusion results within seconds in a very rapid restoration of action potentials to this ischemic myocardium (Downar et al. 1977a; Penkoske et al. 1978; Murdock et al. 1980; Kaplinsky et al. 1981) although the return of electrical activity is not equally rapid for all cells (Downar et al. 1977a). These restored action potentials have reduced upstroke velocities and low amplitudes and the duration and amplitude often alternate between high amplitude and long duration and low amplitude and short duration. After 20 to 30 seconds of reperfusion, action potential configuration has returned to normal (Downar et al. 1977a). During the first 30 seconds of reperfusion, there is a marked inhomogeneity in the action potentials within the ischemic area and at the border with nonischemic myocardium. Action potentials of different cells within the ischemic zone often alternate out of phase, some showing relatively high amplitudes and long durations while at the same time others are little more than local responses as described above. Action potential duration of cells close to the ischemic border may shortened by as much as 60 to 100 msec during reperfusion (Janse and Downar 1977; Coronel et al. 1992). This effect on the transmembrane potentials recorded from an ischemic region of the pig heart after coronary occlusion and reperfusion is evident in Figure 2.48. At the top left is a control action potential and DC electrogram and at the top right the typical effects of a 5-minute period of coronary occlusion can be seen. Within 1 minute of reperfusion (bottom left), action potential duration is markedly shortened. On the one hand, this may be due to the fact that substances that accumulate in the extracellular space of the ischemic compartment such as K^+, lactate and other metabolites, transiently influence electrophysiological characteristics of normal cells close to the ischemic zone as they are washed out of the ischemic compartment (Nakata et al. 1990). On the other hand, action potential shortening of previously ischemic cells during reperfusion is accompanied by a rapid return of extracellular K^+ concentration to normal values, even with an "undershoot", during which extracellular K^+ concentration may reach values that are up to 1 mmol lower than preischemic (and control zone) values (Ilebekk et al. 1988; Aksnes et al. 1989a; 1989b; Tosaki et al. 1989; Coronel et al. 1992). The cellular uptake of K^+ and the shortening of the action potential in reperfused myocardium may be caused by an increased activity of the Na/K pump, which overshoots its mark and leads to depletion of extracellular K^+. The increased activity of the pump could be secondary to adrenergic stimulation (Penny et al. 1985). A moderate shortening of the action potential during reperfusion following a period of low-flow ischemia in the guinea pig heart has been reported by others (Penny and Sheridan 1983), and reoxygenation of hypoxic Purkinje fibers also induces action potential shortening (Abete et al. 1988). It is quite possible that the increased inhomogeneity in action potential duration in and around the previously ischemic zone immediately after abrupt reperfusion is a major factor contributing to the occurrence of fibrillation by enhancing the likelihood for reentry. In the cat, vagal stimulation initiated just prior to reperfusion markedly reduced the incidence of reperfusion arrhythmias, and this was caused by the reduction in heart rate (Zuanetti et al. 1987). This may be related to the fact that at long cycle lengths

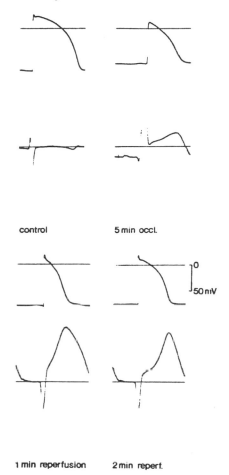

Figure 2.48: Transmembrane potentials (top trace) and DC electrograms (bottom trace) recorded prior to (control, top left) and during a brief period of ischemia (5 min occl., top right) followed by reperfusion (bottom panels) demonstrate marked shortening of the action potential during the early reperfusion phase (at 1 minute). This is accompanied by the appearance of peaked T waves in the electrogram as can be seen by comparing the lower left panel with the upper left panel. (Unpublished results of M.J. Janse and E. Downar.)

unidirectional block based on inhomogeneities in refractory periods, one of the prerequisites for reentry, is less likely to occur than at short cycle lengths. As suggested by Corr and Witkowski in their review (1983), the fact that the highest incidence of reperfusion-induced ventricular fibrillation occurs after a 20- to 30-minute period of ischemia (a time when some cells show irreversible injury) may be related to maximal heterogeneity when irreversibly and reversibly injured cells are juxtaposed.

Studies in which activation has been mapped with simultaneous extracellular recordings have demonstrated the presence of multiple reentrant circuits in the ischemic area during reperfusion-induced fibrillation (Janse 1982a). The origin of the initial ectopic impulses that induce fibrillation is close to the border and these impulses usually are not caused by reentry (Downar and Parson 1981; Ideker et al. 1981; Janse 1982a; Pogwizd and Corr 1987a). In the study of Pogwizd and Corr in the cat heart (1987a), 75% of the reperfusion arrhythmias that occurred were initiated by a nonreentrant mechanism and the ventricular tachycardia that followed was maintained by a mechanism other than reentry 61% of the time. During the initial phase of a ventricular tachycardia that degenerates into ventricular fibrillation, the activation fronts appear at a very rapid rate of 600 to 700 per minute and each activation spreads across the nonischemic myocardium in an organized single wave front. The body surface electrocardiogram during the initial period appears disorganized because of variable time intervals between successive wave fronts, where one wave front starts before the previous one ends (Ideker et al. 1981). No data are as yet available about detailed activation patterns of ischemic and nonischemic myocardium during the transitory phase between the occurrence of these initial ectopic beats and ventricular fibrillation.

There is no evidence for an increase in normal automaticity as a cause of the immediate reperfusion arrhythmias in the canine although such enhanced automaticity might contribute to the occurrence of the delayed reperfusion arrhythmias. Several studies have failed to demonstrate an increased idioventricular rate in the dog heart during vagal inhibition of the sinus rate immediately after reperfusion (Levites et al. 1975; Ramanathan et al. 1977; Murdock et al. 1980) and sometimes even a decrease in idioventricular rate has occurred (Levites et al. 1975). Idioventricular rate is an index of automaticity. Since the period of occlusion in these studies ranged from 10 to 15 minutes, and in one study reperfusion occurred after a period of partial coronary occlusion of 15 minutes (Ramanathan et al. 1977), the possibility exists that a longer ischemic period might cause increased idioventricular automaticity upon reperfusion. In the canine heart an increase in automaticity is evident during the delayed reperfusion arrhythmias and can be unmasked by vagal stimulation (Kaplinsky et al. 1981). As mentioned previously, accelerated idioventricular rhythm, an arrhythmia that may be caused by automaticity, often occurs after thrombolytic procedures designed to disrupt a coronary occlusion in patients, and in such patients ischemia obviously must have been present for some time (Goldberg et al. 1983). This may be comparable to the delayed reperfusion arrhythmic phase in the experiments on canine hearts. In the cat, vagal stimulation during occlusion showed a normal idioventricular rate, but immediately after reperfusion idioventricular rate was increased (Penkoske et al. 1978). Therefore, unlike in the dog, there may be an early increase in automaticity. The increased idioventricular rate could be prevented by α-adrenergic blockade, as could the occurrence of ventricular fibrillation (Sheridan et al. 1980) suggesting a relationship between the two.

There is reason to consider, however, that some reperfusion arrhythmias might be a result of enhanced abnormal automaticity based on the results of experiments on isolated, superfused tissues. Purkinje fibers, isolated from guinea pig hearts made globally ischemic for 20 minutes and then placed in normal, oxygenated, Tyrode's to mimic reperfusion, displayed rapid, sustained rhythmic activity at maximal diastolic potentials in the range of -65 to -50 mV. The mechanism for the rhythmic firing is abnormal automaticity related to the depolarization of the membrane potential. Within 15 minutes of superfusion (reperfusion), maximum diastolic potential increased to -90 mV, and the spontaneous rate slowed (Naumann d'Alnoncourt et al. 1982; 1983). Isolated canine Purkinje-papillary muscle preparations superfused with "ischemic" solutions (hypoxia, acidosis, elevated lactate, no substrate, normal [4 mmol/L] or elevated [10 mmol/L] K^+) for 40 minutes also showed arrhythmogenic activity when "reperfused" with oxygenated, "normal" Tyrode's solution. During the period in the ischemic solution membrane potential depolarized and action potential duration decreased (Ferrier et al. 1985). Return to normal superfusate resulted in immediate hyperpolarization, followed by a period during which the Purkinje fibers depolarized again. This period lasted for about 30 minutes, before the fibers repolarized to their normal maximum diastolic potential. During the period of depolarization following "reperfusion", delayed afterdepolarizations, leading to triggered activity occurred. The final repolarization phase was associated with repetitive activity caused by abnormal automaticity.

The use of an "ischemic" solution (hypoxia, lactate acidosis, and glucose depletion, but with normal K^+) causes an elevation of intracellular Na^+ activity. Following readmission of oxygen, washout of metabolites, and normalization of pH, there is a rapid fall in intracellular Na^+ activity associated with hyperpolarization. This is most likely due to stimulation of Na/K pump activity and of the Na/Ca exchanger (Strauss et al. 1989). The increase of intracellular Ca^{2+} (also probably occurring from calcium release from the sarcoplasmic reticulum) could then activate a nonselective cation channel, leading to an inward current and cause the membrane depolarization that enables abnormal automaticity to occur (Strauss et al. 1989).

As suggested above, the nonreentrant mechanism involved in reperfusion arrhythmias might sometimes be triggered activity caused by delayed afterdepolarizations, although this has not been demonstrated in vivo. Circumstantial evidence in support of this hypothesis is the fact that reperfusion arrhythmias may be suppressed by calcium entry blockers (Ribeiro et al. 1981) and by α-adrenergic blocking agents (Sheridan et al. 1980). These agents decrease cytosolic calcium during reperfusion (Sharma et al. 1983) and may thereby suppress delayed afterdepolarizations (Cranefield 1977; Kimura et al. 1984). Delayed afterdepolarizations have been shown to occur during reoxygenation of isolated, hypoxic papillary muscles. They were abolished by blocking calcium release from the sarcoplasmic reticulum by ryanodine (Hayashi et al. 1987). It has indeed been shown that reperfusion, or restarting of oxidative metabolism after a period of metabolic blockade, results in intracellular calcium overload (Smith and Allen 1988; Stern et al. 1989). This appears to be due to spontaneous release of calcium from the sarcoplasmic reticulum. When oscillations of intracellular calcium are synchronized to the preceding action potential, arrhythmias occur (Smith and Allen 1988; Mulder 1989; Mulder et al. 1989). Calcium overload seems to be a key factor in causing reperfusion-induced triggered activity based on delayed afterdepolarizations.

Recordings of monophasic action potentials from the endocardium of intact cat hearts during ischemia and reperfusion have shown frequent occurrence of deflections resembling early afterdepolarizations following reperfusion (Priori et al. 1990). Even though such findings must be interpreted with caution because of the difficulties in distinguishing deflections caused by mechanical motion of the heart from true oscillations of membrane potential in monophasic action potential recordings (Olsson et al. 1990), they suggest a possible role for early afterdepolarization-induced triggered activity. Early afterdepolarizations and the triggered activity that they cause have been described in isolated superfused rabbit Purkinje fibers when returned from an ischemic solution to normal Tyrode's solution, simulating reperfusion (Rozanski and Witt 1991).

The question has arisen whether reperfusion arrhythmias are primarily caused by readmission of oxygen, rather than by restoration of flow, since hypoxic reperfusion reduces the incidence of fibrillation (Yamada et al. 1988). The experiments with "ischemic" solutions with normal extracellular K^+ concentrations support this view. However, some caution must be used when interpreting the *in vitro* studies, in which the rise in intracellular Na^+ during exposure to the ischemic solution is a key factor explaining events following reoxygenation (Strauss et al. 1989). Intracellular Na^+ activity during ischemia is influenced by two mechanisms with opposing effects: (1) partial inhibition of the Na/K pump causes an increase of intracellular Na^+, and (2) decrease of passive Na^+ influx in ischemic myocardium depolarized by high extracellular K^+ will decrease intracellular Na^+. The net result may be an unchanged intracellular Na^+ during the initial phase of ischemia (Wilde and Kléber 1986; Kléber and Cascio 1989).

We do not discuss the possible role of free radicals in causing reperfusion arrhythmias since little is known about their electrophysiological effects and because much of the evidence that interventions against production of free radicals protects against reperfusion-induced ventricular fibrillation is circumstantial (Hearse 1989). There are also studies reporting on a lack of effect of free radical generating systems and of free radical scavengers on arrhythmogenesis following reperfusion (Coetzee et al. 1990).

Chapter III

Delayed Ventricular Arrhythmias in the Subacute Phase of Myocardial Infarction

Time Course of Occurrence and Characteristics of Delayed Ventricular Arrhythmias

In 1950, A. Sidney Harris published a paper in the first volume of *Circulation* on experimental ischemic ventricular arrhythmias in the canine heart that was destined to become a classic (it still is cited at least 40 times per year). Whereas, until that time the rhythm disturbances that occurred soon after a coronary artery occlusion were the main focus of laboratory investigation, Harris described the arrhythmias that occurred during the subsequent several days after occlusion in animals that did not die of ventricular fibrillation during the early and acute arrhythmic phase. In order to do this, he first had to enhance the possibility for survival beyond the early arrhythmic phase and he accomplished this goal by occluding the left anterior descending coronary artery near its origin in two stages. The first stage consisted of a 30-minute partial occlusion during which a ligature was tightened around the artery and a 20-gauge needle lying along side it that prevented complete constriction. The needle was then removed " . . . leaving the artery constricted, but still permitting some blood to pass" (Harris 1950). In fact, approximately 40% to 50% of normal coronary flow may remain after the first stage of occlusion (Kabell et al. 1982). In the second stage a complete and permanent occlusion was accomplished with a second ligature. Although not documented by statistical analysis of a large set of data until much later (Kabell et al. 1982), Harris reported that the severity of the early ventricular arrhythmias was reduced after this procedure and hence, survival after the two-stage ligation was enhanced. Despite the reduced incidence of death, an infarct does develop that is probably as large as the one that occurs after the single-stage complete occlusion (Harris 1950; Kabell et al. 1982).

Before we describe the characteristics and mechanisms of the arrhythmias that occur during the subsequent hours and days after coronary occlusion, we digress for a moment to mention two points. The first concerns possible reasons why early ventricular arrhythmias may be less severe after the two-stage occlu-

267

sion than a single-stage occlusion, although the final size of the infarct is similar after both procedures. Our discussion is to some extent speculative, since this interesting observation has not been completely investigated. The sinus rate is not affected differently by a one-stage or two-stage procedure, so differences in rate cannot account for the differences in the severity of the arrhythmias (Kabell et al. 1982). (Recall that acute ischemic arrhythmias may be more severe if there is a rapid sinus rate.) However, during a two-stage occlusion, a large part of the ischemic zone does become unresponsive (no electrical activity is detected) at an earlier point in time than after abrupt one-stage ligation and this may be the reason why lethal acute arrhythmias occur less frequently (Coronel et al. 1989). In Chapter II we described the time course of the increase in extracellular K^+ after a complete coronary occlusion and how conduction block occurs in the ischemic region when K^+ reaches a high level. During the two-stage occlusion procedure, the extracellular K^+ rises during the low-flow ischemia after the first stage of occlusion and reaches a level by the end of the first stage (after 30 minutes) that is normally reached after 6 minutes of total occlusion. Most electrograms recorded in the ischemic region during the first stage are not severely affected, possibly because of the patchy nature of the low-flow ischemia caused by residual blood flow and this might account for the absence of severe arrhythmias at this time (Coronel et al. 1989). After the second stage of occlusion, which is complete occlusion, extracellular K^+ rises from the elevated level that exists at the end of the first stage and quickly reaches the levels that cause large areas of conduction block and inexcitability. The extracellular K^+ level that causes large areas of inexcitability is reached much sooner after the second-stage occlusion than it is reached after a one-stage occlusion (Coronel et al. 1989). The consequence of the early development of a large area of inexcitable myocardium is a reduction in the area in which slow conduction can occur. Since ventricular fibrillation requires the presence of multiple reentrant wavelets, the probability for reentry and fibrillation is likely to be reduced when the greater part of the ischemic myocardium is unable to be excited. Hence, there is a lower incidence of continuous activity in composite electrogram recordings and fewer phase 1a acute arrhythmias that are caused by reentry after the two-stage technique (Kabell et al. 1982). The phase 1b arrhythmias that occur after about 10 minutes are not altered (Kabell et al. 1982). A similar mechanism was proposed to explain the antifibrillatory effect of lidocaine when this drug was administered prior to sudden coronary occlusion, e.g., it caused a larger area of inexcitable myocardium to develop more rapidly (Cardinal et al. 1981). The second point that we wish to mention is that the rhythm changes that occur over the next several days after the two-stage occlusion (described below) are similar to those that occur after an abrupt single-stage occlusion if early ventricular fibrillation does not occur. Thus, the electrophysiological changes responsible for the later phases of arrhythmias are probably not modified by the two-stage procedure; only survival of the early arrhythmic phase is enhanced. However, even though survival through the early arrhythmic phase is enhanced because of the reduction of the incidence of ventricular fibrillation within the first 10 minutes, sudden death can occur

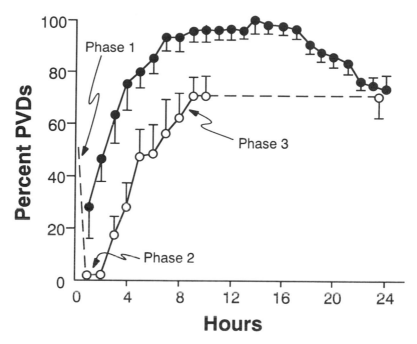

Figure 3.1: The time course of appearance of delayed spontaneous ventricular arrhythmias in a group of dogs with two-stage occlusion of the left anterior descending coronary artery (unfilled circles) and in a group of dogs with a 2-hour period of occlusion followed by reperfusion (filled circles). The ordinate indicates percent of total beats that were ventricular beats (PVDs), calculated at hourly intervals. Each point on the curves indicates mean ± SEM, obtained from four dogs in each group. (Unpublished data of H. Karagueuzian and A.L. Wit.)

later during the first 24-hour period, usually between 12 and 18 hours (Scherlag et al. 1989). We will discuss this further below.

Figure 3.1 (unfilled circles) shows the time course of appearance of ventricular arrhythmias over the 24-hour period that follows a two-stage occlusion of the left anterior descending coronary artery in the canine heart. The data were obtained by Holter monitoring after the complete occlusion and include the time period during which the animals were recovering from pentobarbital anesthesia (approximately the first 4–6 hours). The time course for the appearance of the delayed arrhythmias does not seem to be significantly influenced by the time it takes to awaken from the anesthesia as shown by Harris' experiments comparing pentothal and ether (Harris 1950). However, anesthesia does have some effects on the characteristics of the arrhythmias which are described later. In the figure, the percent of all beats that are ventricular in origin is plotted on the ordinate with time on the abscissa. The acute ischemic phase of arrhythmias indicated by the initial burst of ventricular activity (called phase 1 by Harris) is followed by a period of 3 to 6 hours, during which the predominant rhythm is sinus rhythm (phase 2) (Harris 1950; Scherlag et al. 1989).

Occasional ventricular premature depolarizations may occur during this time. After this period has elapsed, there is a gradual increase in the frequency of ventricular premature depolarizations, and by 8 hours, numerous ventricular ectopic beats coexist with sinus beats (phase 3). After 12–24 hours (the subacute phase of infarction) most or all beats can be of ventricular origin. The arrhythmias at this time are called the delayed spontaneous arrhythmias: delayed because of their time course of appearance and spontaneous both because they appear "spontaneously" and because they are mostly caused by spontaneous impulse initiation (described later).

The progressive increase in frequency of arrhythmias is also shown in Figure 3.2, which displays continuous ECG recordings taken at various time periods after the coronary artery occlusion. The recordings in panel A show only a single ectopic ventricular beat (arrow in trace 52) during the early time

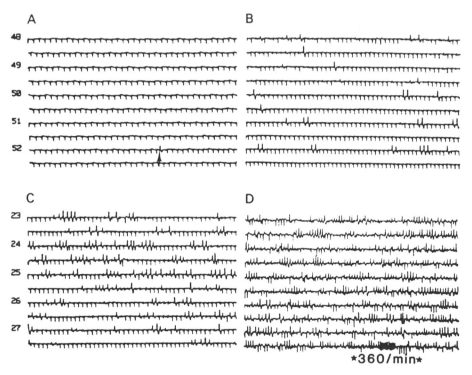

Figure 3.2: The time course of appearance of ventricular arrhythmias as seen in portions of the 24-hour ECG recordings from a dog with acute myocardial infarction 1–5 hours (A), 7 hours (B), 12 hours (C), and 18 hours (D) after left anterior descending coronary artery ligation. These recorded portions illustrate the typical times at which ectopic beats appear (within 5–7 hours of left anterior descending coronary artery ligation). The onset of multiform ventricular ectopic beats and tachycardia tended to be about 12 hours after coronary artery ligation and persisted throughout the remainder of the 24-hour recording period. Occasional runs of monomorphic ventricular tachycardia at rates between 300 and 400 per minute (D) were seen in those dogs that died suddenly. (Reproduced from Scherlag et al. (1989) with permission.)

period of 1–5 hours. A greater frequency of ventricular beats is seen at 7 hours (panel B); a still greater frequency at 12 hours (panel C); while at 18 hours (panel D) most beats are ventricular in origin.

During the progression of ventricular arrhythmias shown in Figures 3.1 and 3.2, approximately 25% to 35% of animals die (Harris 1950). Twenty-four hour Holter monitors have shown that death is caused by severe ventricular arrhythmias (Scherlag et al. 1989). Included among the ventricular ectopic beats that are increasing in frequency with time and preceding the onset of sudden death are short salvos of ventricular tachycardia with cycle lengths of 200 msec or less. They become quite prominent after 12–18 hours. In Figure 3.3, the top six traces of the Holter recording from a dog at 18 hours shows these salvos of ventricular tachycardia. The rapid repetitive ventricular beats were then followed by a long run of rapid monomorphic ventricular tachycardia at a rate of 350 per minute, which then degenerated into ventricular fibrillation after 90 seconds. Sustained polymorphic ventricular tachycardias at rates of 400–600 per minute, similarly degenerating into ventricular fibrillation, have

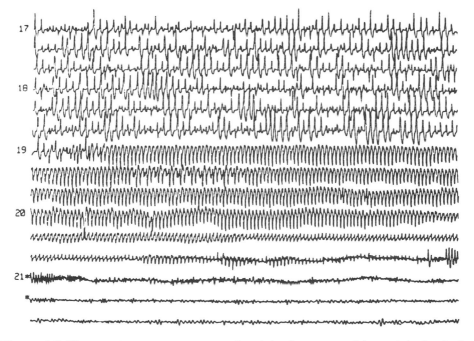

Figure 3.3: The spontaneous occurrence of sustained monomorphic ventricular tachycardia and ventricular fibrillation leading to sudden death 18 hours after left anterior descending coronary artery ligation in a dog. This portion of the recorded ECG shows that during multimorphic ventricular tachycardia (minutes 17 and 18), close-coupled beats led to sustained ventricular tachycardia at a rate of 350 per minute (minutes 19 and 20), which degenerated to ventricular fibrillation within 1.5 minutes (star at 21st minute). Each line represents 20 seconds of electrocardiographic data. (Reproduced from Scherlag et al. (1989) with permission.)

also been recorded (Scherlag et al. 1989). Ventricular fibrillation may also immediately follow a salvo of ventricular premature beats without a preceding sustained tachycardia (Scherlag et al. 1989). These rapid salvos of ventricular premature beats and tachycardias do not occur in dogs that survive; ventricular premature beats and tachycardias have longer cycle lengths (Scherlag et al. 1989). The high sympathetic tone in some of the dogs during recovery from surgery may precipitate the rapid salvos of ventricular beats that initiate the fatal arrhythmias since these salvos can be prevented by β-receptor blockade (Patterson et al. 1986) or left stellate ganglionectomy (Patterson et al. 1991).

Also plotted in Figure 3.1 (filled circles) is the time course for occurrence of ventricular arrhythmias that result if the left anterior descending coronary artery is not permanently occluded but reperfusion occurs 2 hours following the two-stage ligation. When the period of complete occlusion is so long, severe reperfusion arrhythmias culminating in ventricular fibrillation do not often occur. Rather, ventricular premature depolarizations appear soon after reperfusion begins and their frequency gradually increases during the next 8 hours. After this time there is persistent tachycardia, which then lasts for the next 1 to 2 days. These tachycardias have identical electrophysiological and electrocardiographic characteristics to the delayed tachycardias that occur after permanent occlusion and probably have the same underlying mechanisms. Reperfusion, however, causes them to occur sooner than the arrhythmias after permanent occlusion for reasons that are not understood (Mathur et al. 1975; Karagueuzian et al. 1979; Balke et al. 1981; Davis et al. 1982). Both experimental models are related to clinically occurring arrhythmias as we discuss later.

The gradual increase in the frequency of arrhythmic ventricular depolarizations with time after left anterior descending coronary artery occlusion reflects an increase in the propensity of the ventricles to initiate impulses, and is not a consequence of decreases in spontaneous sinus rate (which might under certain conditions lead to the appearance of ventricular arrhythmias). This is evident from experiments in which the sinus node firing has been inhibited by stimulation of the vagus nerves, or in which AV block has been produced, and the rate of spontaneous ventricular beating quantified. In the normal ventricle, spontaneous beating does not commence for 15 to 30 seconds or more, after the ventricles are not activated by atrial impulses, such as following vagal stimulation, as shown in the top trace of Figure 3.4. The quiescent period results from overdrive suppression of the normal ventricular pacemaker (Vassalle et al. 1967; Vassalle 1977). If prevention of ventricular activation by a supraventricular pacemaker is maintained, spontaneous ventricular rate then gradually increases to a final steady state level of about 30 to 45 per minute, representing normal intrinsic ventricular automaticity. After the two-stage occlusion of the left anterior descending coronary artery, ventricular rate after vagal inhibition of the sinus node is not greatly affected for about 2 hours (Scherlag et al. 1976). In Figure 3.4, panel b shows a single couplet of ventricular beats that occurred followed by some escape beats that may have a junctional origin during vagal stimulation after 1 hour. However, often the ventricular escape time and rate of the ventricular pacemaker are similar to those

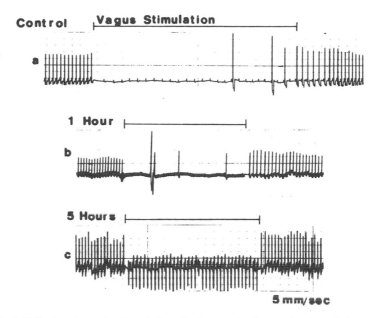

Figure 3.4: Effects of vagal stimulation before and after occlusion of the left anterior descending coronary artery. The period of vagal stimulation is indicated by the horizontal line above each panel. (a) Prior to occlusion, stimulation of the left vagus induced complete atrioventricular block with ventricular asystole for 17 seconds before the appearance of an idioventricular escape rhythm. Sinus rhythm immediately resumed upon cessation of vagal stimulation. (b) One hour after coronary occlusion, vagal stimulation induced asystole that was followed after 3 seconds by a couplet of ventricular beats. There is another pause after the couplet that was interrupted by single escape beats. Sinus rhythm resumes after cessation of vagal stimulation. (c) Five hours after occlusion, ventricular tachycardia appeared at a rate of 132 per minute, within 0.5 seconds of vagal stimulation, the concurrent sinus rate being 156 per minute. Ventricular tachycardia lasted the entire duration of vagal stimulation. (Reproduced from Kerzner et al. (1973) with permission.)

that occur during control measurements prior to occlusion. After 2 to 4 hours of coronary occlusion, the time for ventricular beats to appear after inhibiting the sinus node is greatly reduced to about 2 seconds and couplets and salvos of ventricular beats occur. By 4 to 9 hours after occlusion ventricular beating often begins at a rate of 80 to 130 per minute within less than 1 second after inhibiting the sinus node as is illustrated in Figure 3.4, panel c (Kerzner et al. 1973). Although this rate is still on average slower than the sinus rate, it is fast enough to cause periodic arrhythmias. In dogs that still have periods of sinus rhythm at 24 hours after occlusion, vagal inhibition of the sinus node causes the immediate appearance of ventricular beats at rates ranging from 140 to 200 per minute (Kerzner et al. 1973; Scherlag et al. 1976; Spinelli et al. 1991).

Some electrocardiograms recorded from dogs 1 day after coronary occlusion are shown in Figure 3.5 and illustrate the distinctive characteristics of the delayed arrhythmias. Often, there are periods of both sinus rhythm and ven-

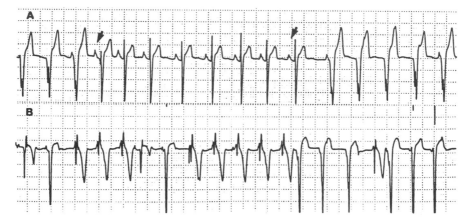

Figure 3.5: Monomorphic ventricular tachycardia in a dog 24 hours after occlusion of the left anterior descending coronary artery is shown in the lead II ECG in panel A. The arrows indicate a period of sinus rhythm. Multimorphic ventricular tachycardia in a dog 24 hours after occlusion of the left anterior descending coronary artery is shown in panel B. Each box represents a time period of 0.20 seconds.

tricular tachycardia. This may occur when the sinus rate is within 10–15 beats of the ventricular rate leading to atrioventricular dissociation. The spontaneous ventricular arrhythmias usually have rates of 160–200 per minute, similar to the ventricular rates determined during vagal stimulation. Occasionally, slower ventricular rhythms with rates around 120 per minute also occur if the sinus rate is also slow (Logic et al. 1969). When premature ventricular depolarizations follow sinus beats or during the onset of periods of ventricular tachycardia, the ventricular beats usually occur after the T wave of the preceding sinus beat, and are most apparent after long sinus cycles (Scherlag et al. 1974). The QRS complexes of the ectopic beats may be monomorphic or multiform. These electrocardiographic characteristics are those of an accelerated idioventricular rhythm or idioventricular tachycardia and are likely caused by arrhythmogenic mechanisms involving abnormal impulse initiation rather than abnormal conduction (described later). Strangely enough, in some instances when the ventricular rate (determined during periods of sinus inhibition by vagal stimulation) is clearly more rapid than the sinus rate, there may still be periods of sinus rhythm as well as ventricular rhythm (Spinelli et al. 1991). It is not understood how the sinus rhythm could dominate for periods of time under these circumstances, since any atrial capture occurring because of proper timing of an atrial impulse in the ventricular cycle should be promptly followed by a return of the ventricular rhythm. Spinelli et al. (1991) have proposed that periods of sinus rhythm might result if sinus impulses somehow can cause transient exit block of impulses from the arrhythmogenic focus in the ventricle. Exit block from these foci has been demonstrated in microelectrode studies on isolated tissues from 24-hour-old infarcts (Friedman et al. 1973b; Rosenthal 1986) and are described later. In other hearts, when ventricular rate is more rapid than the sinus rate, only ventricular tachycardia without sinus beats is evident as would be expected.

Early coupled ventricular premature depolarizations can also occur on occasion and may be followed by rapid runs of ventricular tachycardia (up to 300 per minute). An example of electrocardiograms showing this phenomenon is displayed in Figure 3.6. This kind of event is similar to the one that precedes sudden death occurring between 12 and 18 hours after coronary occlusion as discussed above, when the rapid tachycardias degenerate into ventricular fibrillation (Scherlag et al. 1989). These arrhythmias rarely seem to cause fibrillation after 24 hours. The rapid arrhythmias may be caused by reentry initiated by the premature beats (El-Sherif et al. 1982). The electrocardiographic characteristics of the delayed arrhythmias that occur after the 2-hour period of coronary occlusion followed by reperfusion are identical to those shown in Figures 3.5 and 3.6.

The delayed ventricular arrhythmias persist for 24 to 72 hours, after which time the rate decreases as does the frequency of ventricular premature depolarizations (Harris 1950). The basic electrocardiographic characteristics of the arrhythmias remain similar to those at 24 hours. Sinus rhythm is usually restored after 3 days, but inhibition of supraventricular activation of the ventricles (such as by stimulation of the vagus) may still reveal some enhanced ventricular automatic firing at this time.

Delayed ventricular arrhythmias also occur after occlusion of the left circumflex in the dog, but survival for long periods of time after this procedure is much less frequent than after left anterior descending coronary artery occlusion, probably because of the larger size of the ischemic region. A single-stage

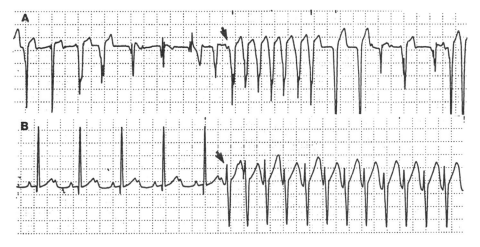

Figure 3.6: Examples of rapid ventricular tachycardias following early coupled ventricular premature depolarizations (arrows) in the dog 24 hours after permanent occlusion of the left anterior descending coronary artery. Each box represents a time period of 0.20 seconds.

occlusion of the septal artery in the canine, which is the first perforating branch of the left anterior descending artery, can also cause delayed arrhythmias with similar characteristics to those described above, except that the rate is slower (Spear et al. 1977). Whether the slower rate is a result of the smaller infarct that results from septal artery occlusion as compared to left anterior descending coronary artery occlusion or to a different site of origin of the arrhythmias is uncertain. Acute ischemic arrhythmias occur after septal artery occlusion, but they are not severe and the incidence of ventricular fibrillation is low. Therefore, there is no need for a two-stage occlusion to enhance survival. Atrioventricular conduction block does occur, but is transient and disappears after 6 to 8 hours when the delayed arrhythmias appear (Jackrel et al. 1970).

Delayed arrhythmias also occur after occlusion of the right coronary artery of the canine heart at its origin. Since, after right coronary occlusion there is no severe acute arrhythmic phase, it is not necessary to occlude the artery in two stages in order to prevent early fibrillation (Sugi et al. 1985). The time course of the appearance of these arrhythmias is similar to the time course after occlusion of the left anterior descending artery. Premature ventricular depolarizations do not appear with any consistency until about 6 hours after occlusion and then increase until 75% to 99% of the rhythm is ventricular after 17 hours (Sugi et al. 1985). Although in general, the characteristics of these arrhythmias are similar to those that occur after occlusion of coronary arteries that supply the left ventricle, the arrhythmias can be divided into two distinct subgroups according to their rates. One subgroup has rates of 160 to 245 per minute while the other subgroup is distinctly slower (120 to 145 per minute). The different subgroups may have different mechanisms as described later.

A similar period of delayed ventricular arrhythmias also occurs in the porcine heart 24 to 48 hours after coronary artery occlusion (Jagadeesh and Seth 1974); it does not occur in the feline heart (Reynolds et al. 1979). It is unknown whether spontaneous delayed arrhythmias occur in other experimental animals. Of primary importance is whether these arrhythmias occur in humans.

Effects of the Autonomic Nervous System on Delayed Ventricular Arrhythmias

Like the acute arrhythmias, the autonomic nervous system has influences on the delayed arrhythmic phase, both on the time course of its development and the frequency and characteristics of the arrhythmias. These influences are the result of a variety of mechanisms including: (1) influences on the development of the infarct after occlusion, and (2) modulation of the sinus rate and the rate of impulse initiation by the ventricles. However, some of the results of experiments on relationships between the autonomics and the delayed arrhythmic phase are not easily understood.

Sympathetic denervation of the heart causes a reduction in the incidence of delayed ventricular arrhythmias or even the total absence of delayed arrhythmias if the denervation is accomplished long enough before the coronary occlusion so that by the time of the occlusion the heart is mostly depleted of catecholamines (Schaal et al. 1969; Ebert et al. 1970). Dogs so denervated in the study of Schaal et al. (1969) (sympathetic and parasympathetic) died from progressive cardiac failure between 30 and 48 hours after coronary occlusion. Death was accompanied by progressive bradycardia and widening of the QRS, but no ventricular arrhythmias. If the heart is denervated shortly before the coronary occlusion, the delayed arrhythmias still occur as expected. In this situation the catecholamine content of the heart is not much reduced. However, there may be some modification of the characteristics of phase 2—the period between the early and the delayed arrhythmias. The cardiac rhythm during phase 2 is mostly sinus except in dogs anesthetized with pentothal, who show agitation upon waking from the anesthesia during this period. The agitation may be accompanied by the occurrence of ventricular ectopic beats whereas animals that are anesthetized with a longer-acting drug remain subdued during phase 2 and do not have arrhythmias (Harris et al. 1951). Sympathectomy just prior to the coronary occlusion reduces the phase 2 arrhythmias during awakening from the pentothal anesthesia indicating that these arrhythmias result from hyperactivity of the sympathetic nervous system. Sympathectomy just prior to the coronary occlusion does not noticeably alter the time period that elapses until the appearance of phase 3 (the delayed) arrhythmias. However, the rate of the arrhythmias may be reduced (see below).

The reason why the delayed arrhythmias did not occur after prior sympathectomy that resulted in catecholamine depletion in the two studies cited above is difficult to understand. Delayed arrhythmias have been reported to occur in dogs after myocardial catecholamine depletion with reserpine (Maling et al. 1959). One might suppose that the absence of arrhythmias could be a consequence of the effects of denervation on the size and distribution of the infarct. Reducing the effects of the sympathetic nervous system on the heart either by β-receptor blockade or by denervation may decrease the size of an infarct caused by a coronary artery occlusion (Bache 1984). It is known that in order for delayed arrhythmias to develop, the subendocardial Purkinje system must be affected by the occlusion and this requires that the infarct encroaches on the Purkinje system (Friedman et al. 1973a; 1973b). How this causes the arrhythmias is the subject of a later discussion. Therefore, if the limitation of infarct size by denervation precludes or limits the inclusion of the Purkinje system in the ischemic region, the delayed arrhythmias would be expected to be reduced or abolished. Both Schaal et al. (1969) and Ebert et al. (1970) indicate that the infarcts in their studies were of similar size after denervation compared to the infarcts in their nondenervated control group. However, the exact extent of the infarcts was not investigated by quantitative techniques that might have detected subtle changes. In particular, infarct size after denervation might grossly appear the same as without denervation although the subendocardial layers of Purkinje fibers might be involved only without denervation.

Sympathetic activity during the delayed arrhythmic phase (at 24 hours) may influence the severity (incidence and rate) of the arrhythmias by several mechanisms. The influences are partially the consequences of whether the sympathetic effects are directed predominantly at the sinus node, at the ventricles, or some combination of the two. Changes in sinus rate alone influence the frequency of ventricular beats. Unlike during the acute arrhythmic phase where an increase in sinus rate increases the severity of the arrhythmias, during the delayed phase an increase in sinus rate, which might result from sympathetic activation, decreases the arrhythmias. This is a characteristic expected of overdrive suppression of an automatic arrhythmia. Situations where the sympathetics to the sinus node might be selectively activated are uncertain but a specific sympathetic neural pathway to the sinus node does exist (Randall 1984). The sympathetic nervous system also influences the rate of impulse initiation by the ventricles during this arrhythmic phase. This influence is demonstrated by several kinds of data. First, anesthesia may decrease the frequency of ventricular beats and slow the rate of tachycardia. With pentobarbital, the decrease in frequency of ventricular beats is often a consequence of an increase in sinus rate caused by the vagolytic action of the barbiturate, but it can also result from a decrease in ventricular rate (Scherlag et al. 1989). A decrease in the arrhythmias also occurs after chloralose, which slows the sinus rate and presumably decreases general sympathetic activity to the ventricle (Constantin and Martins 1987). Other evidence is provided by the effect of sympathetic denervation after the delayed arrhythmias have already been established. When canine hearts were isolated 24 hours after left anterior descending coronary occlusion and perfused through the coronary arteries with blood from a donor dog, the isolated hearts remained arrhythmic and the electrophysiological characteristics of the arrhythmias were similar to the arrhythmias that occurred *in situ* (Dangman et al. 1977). The major effect of isolating the heart was a decrease in the firing rate of both the sinus node and the ventricles, which can be attributed mostly to sympathetic denervation. However, the ventricular rate was still accelerated over that of the sinus node showing that the effects of infarction on rhythm persisted without maintained sympathetic influence. Sympathetic denervation of the *in situ* infarcted heart 24 hours after occlusion also affects the arrhythmias (Harris et al. 1951). Sympathetic ganglionectomy reduces the heart rate and the frequency of arrhythmias (Martins 1985). A more local kind of sympathectomy produced by the application of phenol to the epicardial surface in regions near the origin of the arrhythmias also decreased the frequency of the ventricular beats presumably without affecting the sinus node (Martins 1985). The phenol destroys the sympathetic nerves that course through the epicardium and then transmurally (Barber et al. 1984) to the site of impulse origin, which is in the subendocardial Purkinje system. (A discussion on mechanisms and origins of these arrhythmias comes later.) The decrease in the ventricular beats caused by this local sympathectomy shows that the arrhythmogenic site remains innervated after infarction and that the nervous system exerts a tonic effect on the genesis of the ectopic impulses (Martins 1985). Other regions of infarcts are denervated because the ischemia also destroys the nerves (Martins and Zipes 1980; Barber et al. 1984; Martins et al. 1989). Another demonstration of the sympathetic control of the delayed ventricular arrhythmias is provided by the effects of β-receptor blocking drugs, which after intravenous administration, significantly reduce the ventricular rate (Hope et al. 1974; Constantin and Martins 1987). The β-blocker, metoprolol, administered into the left anterior descending coronary artery distal to the occlusion also decreased the rate of the ventricular arrhythmia without having any systemic effects on the blood pressure (Constantin and Martins 1987).

A corollary to the reduction of the arrhythmias by the removal of the tonic sympathetic effects is the increase in the severity of the arrhythmias that can occur if the activity of the sympathetic nervous system is intensified. As discussed above, this might result from a selective activation of sympathetic nerves to the ventricles over the sinus node or, if the sympathetic activity to both is increased, a greater sensitivity of the ventricles to catecholamines than the sinus node. Electrical stimulation of the sympathetic nerves, or stimulation through exercise, causes a precipitous increase in the frequency of ectopic impulses, or the rate of ventricular tachycardia. Ventricular rates of 200 to 250 per minute can be caused by sympathetic stimulation of hearts with 1- to 2-day-old infarcts. Sympathetic stimulation may also precipitate ventricular fibrillation (Harris et al. 1971). Otherwise, as we have mentioned, fibrillation during the period of delayed arrhythmias occurs very rarely. After spontaneous arrhythmias subside, 2 to 4 days after coronary occlusion, sympathetic stimulation can cause reappearance of premature ventricular depolarizations and tachycardia (Harris et al. 1971). Similarly, intravenous norepinephrine or epinephrine markedly exacerbate the ventricular arrhythmias at 24 hours and cause the reappearance of ventricular arrhythmias during the period between 4 and 12 days when the spontaneous arrhythmias have mostly disappeared. Sympathetic stimulation or catecholamine administration in the doses used do not usually cause ventricular arrhythmias in noninfarcted hearts. Although sympathetic stimulation does increase the idioventricular rate in noninfarcted hearts (by increasing the rate of spontaneous impulse formation of Purkinje fibers), the maximum rate is only in the range of 60 to 80 per minute, approximately twice the normal rate (Vassalle et al. 1968; Spear and Moore 1973), and not fast enough to escape the dominance of the sinus node to cause arrhythmias. Similarly, catecholamines had only a modest positive chronotropic effect on ventricular pacemakers when tested on the ventricular rate of noninfarcted hearts with experimental heart block (Roberts et al. 1963). The rapid arrhythmias that occur in infarcted hearts, therefore, suggest that the subendocardial Purkinje fibers, where the arrhythmias arise (see below), have an increased sensitivity to catecholamines, which has indeed been verified by microelectrode studies on isolated preparations (Cameron and Han 1982; Cameron et al. 1982).

Impulse initiation during the delayed arrhythmic phase is not enhanced by α-receptor stimulation with phenylephrine (Constantin and Martins 1987), nor is it prevented by α-receptor blockade with phenoxybenzamine (Maling et al. 1959). Although there is some evidence for α-receptor proliferation during acute ischemia and modulation of impulse initiation by α-receptor stimulation (Corr et al. 1981b; Hamra and Rosen 1988) it does not appear to be involved in the delayed arrhythmic phase.

The parasympathetic nervous system has not been shown to have an effect on impulse initiation by the ventricles during the delayed arrhythmic phase other than through effects exerted by slowing the rate of the sinus node (see our discussion on vagal escape). Although acetylcholine can slow the rate of Purkinje fiber firing at high concentrations (Bailey et al. 1972; Danilo et al. 1978; Gadsby et al. 1978) and can depress slow response action potentials (Bailey et al. 1979), vagal stimulation in dogs with infarcted hearts does not decrease the rate of firing of ventricular pacemakers during arrhythmias that occur 24 hours after left anterior descending coronary artery occlusion (Kerzner et al. 1973; Spinelli et al. 1991). Parasympathetic activation might also be expected to slow the rate of delayed ventricular tachycardias by its modulation of sympathetic discharge; enhanced vagal activity to the ventricles can inhibit norepinephrine release from sympathetic nerve endings (Levy 1971). So far, a reduction in rate of ventricular tachycardia has not been shown in experimental studies.

Mechanisms of Delayed Ventricular Arrhythmias

From the electrocardiographic characteristics of the delayed ventricular arrhythmias caused by either left anterior descending or right coronary artery occlusion, electrophysiological mechanisms that cause the arrhythmias can be deduced. The spontaneous occurrence of ventricular ectopic beats during long sinus cycle lengths and their appearance late in the diastolic interval suggests that abnormal impulse initiation is a prominent mechanism. The period of quiescence during the long cycle is sufficient to allow a pacemaker in the ventricle to depolarize to threshold and initiate a ventricular beat. Other arrhythmogenic mechanisms such as triggered activity caused by early afterdepolarizations or reentrant excitation often begin with a short diastolic interval although the proposed electrocardiographic differences associated with the different mechanisms are not an infallible way of determining the mechanism. That the frequency of ventricular ectopic beats increases when the sinus node is slowed by vagal stimulation, and that an abnormally rapid ventricular rate ensues when the sinus node is stopped (Scherlag et al. 1974; Horowitz et al. 1976; Moore et al. 1978; Spinelli et al. 1991) is also consistent with the expected characteristics of an automatic mechanism. When the dominance of the sinus node is removed, the pacemakers in the ventricles can fire uninhibited from overdrive by the more rapid supraventricular pacemaker. If triggered activity caused by delayed afterdepolarizations was the dominant mechanism causing the ventricular arrhythmias (El-Sherif et al. 1983b), inhibition of the atrial rhythm should also result in a significant decline in the rate of ventricular firing. This assumption is based on the likelihood that atrial beats would trigger cardiac fibers in the ventricles with delayed afterdepolarizations to fire at rapid rates (Spinelli et al. 1991). However, after sinus node inhibition by vagal stimulation, the ventricular rate remains the same as during periods of ventricular arrhythmia without inhibition of the sinus node (Spinelli et al. 1991). Atrioventricular dissociation and fusion beats are also consistent with a mechanism that involves automaticity in the ventricles competing with the sinus node pacemaker. Whenever the sinus cycle length decreases, perhaps during sinus arrhythmia, the sinus node can once again overdrive the ventricular pacemaker. This accounts for the observations that the idioventricular tachycardias terminate with sinus capture of the ventricles. Arrhythmias caused by triggered activity or reentry, on the other hand, sometimes terminate suddenly and are usually followed by a period of quiescence since the sinus node may be overdrive-suppressed during the tachycardia.

Normal automaticity (automaticity at normal levels of diastolic potentials), however, does not appear to be the primary cause of accelerated idioventricular tachycardia after left anterior descending coronary occlusion. Twenty-four hours after coronary occlusion, there is little or no evidence for overdrive suppression, which is characteristic of normal pacemakers. After vagal stimulation, for example, the ventricular rhythm appears almost immediately at a stable rate, as discussed above and shown in Figure 3.4 (Kerzner et al. 1973; Scherlag et al. 1974, Spinelli et al. 1991). This is a characteristic of abnormal automaticity, which occurs at reduced levels of membrane potentials. On the other hand, vagal arrest of supraventricular pacemakers in the normal heart is followed by a quiescent period that may last more than 30 seconds because the normal ventricular pacemakers are suppressed by the overdrive stimulation of the sinus node. Once they begin to fire, their rate gradually increases to a steady level of around 30 to 50 per minute. (Vassalle et al. 1968).

Abnormal automaticity can also be implied as the primary mechanism causing accelerated idioventricular tachycardia from the results of experiments showing the response of the ventricles during tachycardia to electrical stimulation (Le Marec et al. 1985; Spinelli et al. 1991). In normal ventricles driven by Purkinje fibers with normal automaticity (after experimentally induced heart block), pacing at a rate that is faster than the spontaneous rate is followed by a period of quiescence when pacing is terminated, before the ventricular pacemaker cells begin to fire again. When the ventricular pacemaker begins to fire, the firing rate is initially slow and then it gradually speeds up to its steady state level, a characteristic that is also seen after vagal arrest of the sinus node (Vassalle et al. 1968). The period of quiescence and the initial firing rate are related to both the frequency and the duration of the overdrive pacing. Overdrive pacing at a faster rate, or for a longer period of time, or both, prolongs the period of quiescence that follows, and the initial rate is slower. On the other hand, the different response of the arrhythmic ventricles 1 day after coronary occlusion is shown in Figure 3.7 (Le Marec et al. 1985). The recovery cycle length (time period between cessation of pacing and the first spontaneous beat) is plotted on the ordinate and the cycle length of overdrive pacing is on the abscissa. Curves are plotted for different periods

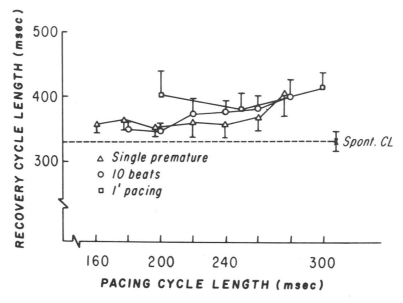

Figure 3.7: Effects of single premature stimuli, ten paced beats, and pacing for 1 minute on the recovery cycle length (vertical axis) of ventricular tachycardia in 15 dogs 24 hours after infarction caused by left anterior descending coronary artery occlusion. The horizontal axis is the pacing or extrastimulus cycle length. All the recovery beats were of ventricular origin. The broken line is the spontaneous cycle length of the ventricular tachycardia before pacing. The three curves do not differ significantly from one another. The recovery cycle lengths are longer than the cycle length of the spontaneous ventricular tachycardia ($p < 0.05$). (Reproduced from Le Marec et al. (1985) with permission.)

of pacing ranging from single premature beats to 1 minute. After 10 beats of pacing (unfilled circles), the recovery cycle length is not prolonged, but in fact is slightly shortened as the cycle length of overdrive is shortened from 300 to 160 msec. After 1 minute of overdrive pacing (unfilled squares), there is a small increase in the recovery cycle length that is much less than that which occurs in the normal ventricles (Le Marec et al. 1985). This lack of prominent overdrive suppression is characteristic of abnormal automaticity that occurs in cells with partially depolarized membrane potentials (Dangman and Hoffman 1983). Occasionally, some moderate overdrive suppression may occur suggesting that in those hearts, automaticity is arising at a more negative level of membrane potential (Spinelli et al. 1991). Other arrhythmogenic mechanisms are expected to respond differently to the overdrive pacing. Triggered arrhythmias caused by delayed afterdepolarizations might sometimes show a decrease in the return cycle length and even an acceleration of the rate after a period of overdrive (overdrive acceleration) but if the overdrive is sufficiently long or fast there may be transient slowing or even termination of the arrhythmia (Wit et al. 1981b). Reentrant activity may either be entrained or terminated by overdrive; termination usually occurs at a critical rate of stimulation. The ventricular arrhythmias in the 24-hour-old infarct are not usually stopped following rapid overdrive pacing. The absence of overdrive suppression is also characteristic of arrhythmias that occur 1 day after coronary occlusion and reperfusion (Davis et al. 1982) and also the ventricular arrhythmias with rates of 150 or more that occur after right coronary occlusion, leading to the same conclusion that they are caused by abnormal automaticity (Sugi et al. 1985). However, the subset of tachycardias with rates of less than 150 per minute that occur after a right coronary occlusion can be overdrive-suppressed by rapid ventricular stimulation. Therefore, enhanced normal automaticity may cause these arrhythmias that arise in the right ventricle (Sugi et al. 1985).

The response of the accelerated idioventricular tachycardias to some pharmacological agents also supports the conclusions derived from the electrocardiographic characteristics and pacing studies, that a primary mechanism causing these arrhythmias is abnormal automaticity (Le Marec et al. 1985; Karagueuzian et al. 1986b). The conclusions are based on a library of information that has been gathered concerning the effects of antiarrhythmic drugs on different arrhythmogenic mechanisms in isolated cardiac tissue preparations. Lidocaine, in therapeutic concentrations, suppresses delayed afterdepolarizations (caused by toxic amounts of digitalis or other inhibitors of the Na/K pump) (Sheu and Lederer 1985) and normal automaticity in isolated, superfused bundles of cardiac Purkinje fibers (Le Marec et al. 1985), but has little or no effect on abnormal automaticity (caused by depolarization with current passed through an intracellular microelectrode) (Brennan et al. 1978; Naumann d'Alnoncourt et al. 1981). Lidocaine has little suppressant effect on the ventricular ectopic rate in dogs 24 hours after left anterior descending coronary artery occlusion (Le Marec et al. 1985) and little effect on the faster arrhythmias caused by right coronary artery occlusion (Karagueuzian et al. 1986b). Ethmozine® (Du Pont Pharmaceuticals, Wilmington, DE, USA), which suppresses abnormal automaticity and delayed afterdepolarizations but not normal automaticity in experiments on isolated, superfused bundles of Purkinje fibers does suppress the ventricular ectopic rate after left anterior descending coronary artery occlusion (Le Marec et al. 1985). Therefore, an arrhythmogenic mechanism that is not suppressed by lidocaine but is suppressed by Ethmozine is abnormal automaticity (Table 1). Other antiarrhythmic drugs such as flecai-

Table 1
Effects of Several Antiarrhythmic Drugs on Different
Arrhythmogenic Mechanisms

Drug	Normal	Abnormal	DAD
Lidocaine	+ +	−	+ +
Ethmozin	+ (−)	+ +	+ +

+ = suppression.
− = no effect.
(Reproduced from Le Marec et al. 1985 with permission.)

nide and encainide do not significantly depress the rate of ventricular firing in hearts with 24-hour infarcts, consistent with the failure of most class I antiarrhythmic drugs to suppress abnormal automaticity in therapeutic concentrations (Spinelli et al. 1991). However, these drugs may sometimes prolong the period of overdrive suppression following vagal stimulation (Spinelli et al. 1991). The mechanism for this effect is not known.

Flunarizine is another drug that has been used as a tool to determine mechanisms of cardiac arrhythmias. It is a calcium antagonist that can decrease intracellular calcium in cells that are calcium-overloaded by a mechanism other than blocking the calcium channels (Borgers et al. 1984). It specifically prevents triggered arrhythmias caused by delayed afterdepolarizations because of this effect. In the experiments of Vos et al. (1990), flunarizine had little effect on the tachycardias that occurred 16–24 hours after occlusion of the left anterior descending coronary artery, indicating that the primary mechanism of these arrhythmias is not triggered activity. In contrast, flunarizine has been shown to terminate arrhythmias in the canine heart caused by digitalis toxicity, which are known to be caused by triggered activity dependent on delayed afterdepolariztions (Vos et al. 1990).

Since it had been proposed that triggered activity caused by delayed afterdepolarizations was the most important cause of the accelerated ventricular arrhythmias (El-Sherif et al. 1983b), Le Marec et al. (1986) determined the effects of doxorubicin on the delayed ventricular arrhythmias. Doxorubicin specifically depresses delayed afterdepolarizations and triggered activity without affecting automaticity or conduction properties that might lead to reentrant excitation. Doxorubicin does not affect the delayed arrhythmias, consistent with the conclusion that abnormal automaticity is the major arrhythmogenic mechanism in left ventricular infarction. The slow channel-blocking drug verapamil may also slow or convert to sinus rhythm some arrhythmias caused by left anterior descending coronary occlusion (Melville et al. 1964) and the rapid subgroup of tachycardias caused by right coronary occlusion (Karagueuzian et al. 1986b), an effect predicted for an abnormal automatic mechanism. However, the hypotensive effect of verapamil in the canine with an infarct often leads to a reflex increase in sympathetic activity to the ventricles that may overcome the suppressant effect of verapamil on ventricular pacemakers.

Although abnormal automaticity is the dominant arrhythmogenic mechanism, some of the arrhythmic beats are probably caused by triggered activity or reentrant excitation. If occasional beats or series of beats are caused by these mechanisms it would not be possible to distinguish them by the experimental approaches described above. There is some evidence that triggered activity caused by delayed afterdepolarizations may occur, especially 2–3 days after left anterior descending coronary occlusion (Le Marec et al. 1985). At this time ventricular arrhythmias are on the wane or have subsided, although ventricular automaticity as assessed by the vagal escape characteristics is still enhanced. Ventricular premature depolarizations and tachycardia can be induced by overdrive pacing of the sinus rhythm. The coupling interval between the ventricular premature beat and the last paced beat is directly related to the pacing cycle length as is expected of triggered activity (Le Marec et al. 1985).

The rapid tachycardias that occasionally begin with a closely coupled premature ventricular depolarization at 24 hours after coronary occlusion or those that cause sudden death at 12–18 hours are probably caused by reentry. Similar tachycardias can be induced by bursts of rapid stimuli applied to the ventricles or by premature stimulation of the ventricles at short coupling intervals. When these tachycardias are sustained, they can also be terminated by overdrive or premature stimulation of the ventricles (El-Sherif et al. 1982; Scherlag et al. 1983; 1989). Although initiation and termination of tachycardias by electrical stimuli does not prove that they are caused by reentry (because these characteristics also apply to triggered arrhythmias), mapping impulse propagation has shown that these arrhythmias are caused by reentry, usually in the epicardial border zone of surviving ventricular muscle cells (El-Sherif et al. 1982).

Relationship of Experimental Delayed Ventricular Arrhythmias to Clinical Arrhythmias

Are the delayed ventricular arrhythmias that occur in the canine heart related to clinical arrhythmias associated with myocardial ischemia and infarction? This is a difficult question to answer, but an extremely important one since we should know whether the interesting information that has been learned about the causes of the experimental arrhythmias will eventually help with the understanding of clinical arrhythmias. After all, this is a primary goal of the laboratory research. It is well known that ventricular arrhythmias occur in patients within the first 72 hours after the onset of symptoms indicating a myocardial infarction (Bigger et al. 1977). A comparison with the experimental arrhythmias of the time course of appearance of these clinical arrhythmias after onset of coronary occlusion, their electrocardiographic characteristics and their possible mechanisms determined by pacing and drug responses may help to answer the question.

First, let us consider the time course of the occurrence of ventricular arrhythmias after the onset of symptoms indicative of infarction in humans to see if there are any similarities to the laboratory model. The occurrence of early, "pre-hospital" arrhythmias in humans within the first hours after the onset of symptoms has already been discussed in Chapter II and are the clinical counterpart of the acute ischemic arrhythmias. There are very few studies in patients with acute myocardial infarction in which electrocardiographic recording was begun early after the onset of symptoms and then continued for long enough periods of time to determine what happens after this acute arrhythmic phase. Furthermore, to make a meaningful comparison with the experimental data it is necessary to have information from patients who have not received antiarrhythmic drug therapy since such therapy might influence the occurrence of any

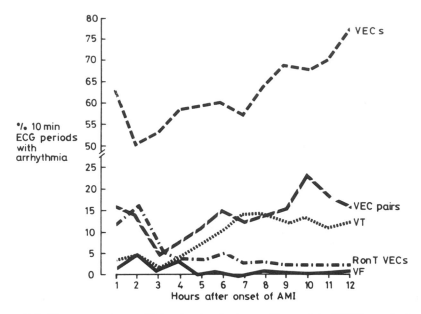

Figure 3.8: The percentage of 10-minute electrocardiographic (ECG) analysis periods containing specific ventricular arrhythmias is shown related to time from the onset of the symptoms of acute myocardial infarction (AMI) in a group of patients. VEC = ventricular ectopic complexes; VF = ventricular fibrillation; VT = ventricular tachycardia. (Reproduced from Campbell et al. (1981) with permission.)

later phase of arrhythmias. Given that it has become standard practice at many hospitals to administer antiarrhythmic drugs even in the absence of life-threatening arrhythmias, these kinds of data are also scarce.

Campbell et al. (1981) looked carefully at the first 12 hours after the onset of symptoms which, for lack of any better indicator, is assumed to coincide with the onset of the coronary occlusion. Their data are summarized in Figure 3.8. A bimodal distribution for the occurrence of arrhythmias similar to that in the canine heart was found. During the first 3 hours, ventricular ectopic complexes (dashed line, VECs) were common (65%), including singles, pairs (dashed line, VEC pairs) and ventricular premature impulses occurring on the T wave (R-on-T dashed-dotted line). Primary ventricular fibrillation (VF) occurred in a subset of the study group (solid line) during this time, usually initiated by an R-on-T premature ventricular depolarization. The incidence of early ventricular premature depolarizations (R-on-T ectopics) and ventricular fibrillation both declined around 3 hours after onset of symptoms (Figure 3.8). In the next 4–12-hour period, the incidence of primary ventricular fibrillation and R-on-T ventricular ectopic complexes was low. In addition the total number of ventricular ectopic complexes decreased by 3 hours. After 3 hours there was a progressive rise in the incidence of ventricular premature depolarizations and ventricular tachycardia, to 12 hours, after which no further data were obtained. Primary ventricular fibrillation and R-on-T ventricular ectopic complexes did not occur at the later time. The data suggests an early and a delayed phase of ventricular arrhythmias, separated by a period of decreased arrhythmias.

Northover (1982) also found that ventricular tachycardia, defined as three or more successive premature ventricular depolarizations at a rate of 100 per minute or more, reached a peak between 8 and 14 hours and declined thereafter in patients that did not have early ventricular fibrillation. In Figure 3.9, which shows data from this study, the ventricular tachycardia (VT) index, which is plotted on the ordinate, is a calculation based on the number of occurrences of paroxysms of tachycardia, the length of each paroxysm and the rate of the paroxysms. The 12-hour peak in the survivors is an indication of a maximum number of paroxysms per hour and a maximum number of ventricular beats in each paroxysm at this time. In support of the results of both Campbell et al. (1981) and Northover (1982) are the results of other studies in which electrocardiographic recording began 8 hours after the onset of symptoms. A high incidence (47%) of ventricular tachycardia or slow ventricular rhythms has been reported (Spann et al. 1964; Lichstein et al. 1975), whereas in studies in which electrocardiographic recordings have been made early after the onset of symptoms such as in mobile coronary care units, the frequency of occurrence of ventricular tachycardia has been low (for example 4% in the study of Pantridge et al. 1981). Therefore, there is clinical evidence that there is a "delayed" phase of ventricular tachycardia during which ventricular fibrillation does not occur often.

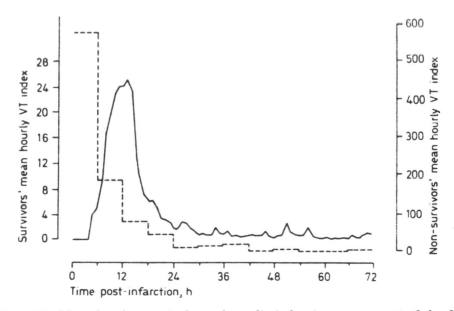

Figure 3.9: Mean hourly ventricular tachycardia index (a measurement of the frequency of occurrence of ventricular tachycardia) among survivors (solid line) and non-survivors (dashed line) during the first 72 hours after onset of symptoms of acute myocardial infarction. (Reproduced from Northover (1982) with permission.)

The time course of occurrence of the delayed arrhythmic phase in humans as shown in Figures 3.8 and 3.9 is similar to the time course of occurrence of the experimental arrhythmias depicted in Figure 3.1. One would expect such a similarity only in those patients who suffered from an abrupt occlusion of a coronary artery and not in those patients who have had repetitive periods of transient ischemia eventually leading to a more prolonged occlusion that resulted in infarction such as in those patients with unstable angina. Also, the time course for the appearance of arrhythmias is likely to be different in patients who have had a complete occlusion of a coronary artery followed by thrombolysis that may occur spontaneously. This phenomenon is analogous to the experimental canine model in which a coronary artery is occluded for several hours with a ligature and then reperfused by releasing the ligature (Karagueuzian et al. 1979). Information from clinical studies with thrombolytic agents such as streptokinase sheds some light on events that may happen during spontaneous thrombolysis. Electrocardiographic monitoring in patients during thrombolytic therapy has shown an onset of ventricular arrhythmias coincident with reperfusion that is documented angiographically (Goldberg et al. 1983; Gorgels et al. 1988). These arrhythmias then may persist for the following 24 to 48 hours before they subside. If this also happens after spontaneous reperfusion, then the phases of arrhythmias may not be the same as after abrupt occlusion without reperfusion. For example, there may be an early phase of acute arrhythmias soon after the occlusion and a second phase of arrhythmias after the thrombolysis, whenever this occurs. Interestingly, this is the exact pattern for the occurrence of ventricular arrhythmias in the canine heart after a prolonged period of complete occlusion (1 to 2 hours) followed by reperfusion. The remarkable similarities permit us to use the canine data to comment on possible mechanisms of these clinical "delayed" reperfusion arrhythmias later.

The second comparison that we need to make is between the electrocardiographic characteristics of the delayed arrhythmias in the canine infarction models and the clinical ventricular arrhythmias that occur during the 12–72-hour postocclusion period. Comparison of electrocardiographic characteristics is helpful in speculating whether similar arrhythmogenic mechanisms are involved. We described previously that many of the delayed tachycardias in the canine, both after occlusion and after occlusion plus reperfusion, have the characteristics of accelerated idioventricular rhythms or idioventricular tachycardia, although other ventricular arrhythmias (ventricular tachycardia) also occur. Accelerated idioventricular rhythms also occur in patients after either an anterior or posterior myocardial infarction (Figure 3.10, bottom trace) or they occur after thrombolysis (Goldberg et al. 1983; Cercek et al. 1987; Gorgels et al. 1988). This rhythm is usually defined by clinical electrocardiographers to have the following characteristics: (1) the arrhythmia begins with a long coupled ventricular beat that often occurs during a long sinus cycle length; (2) the arrhythmia is characterized by 3 to 20 widened or bizarre QRS complexes at a rate similar to the prevailing sinus rate and alternating with periods of sinus rhythm; (3) the rate is usually less than 100 beats/min and regular; and (4) fusion beats commonly occur (Norris and Mercer 1974). All of these

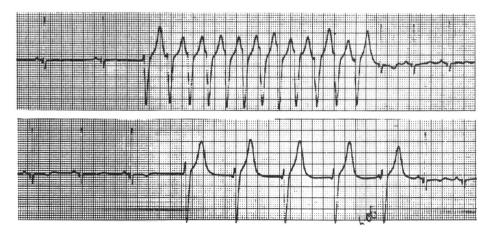

Figure 3.10: Accelerated idioventricular rhythm after myocardial infarction in humans. (Reproduced from de Soyza et al. (1974) with permission.)

characteristics, except for the fusion beats, are shown in the bottom ECG trace in Figure 3.10. These characteristics are expected of an arrhythmia caused by an accelerated ventricular pacemaker rather than reentry for reasons we have already discussed. On the other hand, ventricular tachycardia is usually defined as three or more successive beats of ventricular origin beginning with a short coupled premature ventricular depolarization, having a cycle length of less than 500–600 msec and terminating abruptly, not because of sinus capture. However, some clinical electrocardiographers believe that a clear distinction between accelerated idioventricular rhythms and ventricular tachycardia may be more difficult to make than originally proposed and that there may be mechanistic relationships between the two arrhythmias. Although accelerated idioventricular rhythm occurs in the presence of a long sinus cycle length, it may also occur when the sinus cycle length is not long, but when sinus rates are 70–90, similar to the onset of ventricular tachycardia (de Soyza et al. 1974). In these instances the initial cycle length of the arrhythmia may not be long and the occurrence of the ventricular beat is not dependent on sinus slowing. Accelerated idioventricular rhythms at fast rates of 120 or more have also been reported. Paroxysmal ventricular tachycardias occur in the same patients and within the same time period as accelerated idioventricular rhythms and often have the same QRS morphologies, suggesting a relationship between the two. In the study of de Soyza et al. (1974), 83% of patients with accelerated idioventricular rhythm also had paroxysmal ventricular tachycardia. Figure 3.10 shows recordings from one of these patients during paroxysmal tachycardia (top trace) and accelerated idioventricular rhythm (bottom trace). Ventricular extrasystoles with similarly shaped QRS complexes also occurred in these patients. Paroxysmal ventricular tachycardias sometimes have rates that are exact multiples of the rate of accelerated idioventricular rhythm in the same patient suggesting that the accelerated rhythm may be the same arrhythmia as tachycardia, but with exit block from the initiating focus. However, ventricular tachycardias with rates that are not exact multiples also seem to be common.

What can we conclude from this information? We venture the following. There is a delayed phase of ventricular arrhythmias in humans separated from an early phase by a period of decreased ventricular ectopic activity when there is abrupt occlusion of a coronary artery. The period of decreased ectopic activity may be shortened or absent if there is spontaneous thrombolysis. Arrhythmias during this delayed phase have electrocardiographic characteristics that are similar to those that occur in the experimental models. Accelerated idioventricular rhythm and paroxysmal ventricular tachycardia occur in both. There seems to be an association between the two kinds of arrhythmias, which suggests a mechanistic relationship.

From the similarities in the electrocardiographic characteristics of the clinical and the experimental arrhythmias, it might be concluded that the clinical arrhythmias are to a large extent caused by automaticity, but only fragments of the additional information needed to distinguish between normal and abnormal automaticity (as detailed for the experimental studies) is available. In an early report of Wellens et al. (1974) in which they stimulated the hearts of patients with acute myocardial infarction and ventricular tachycardia that developed within 24 hours of the onset of symptoms, it was indicated that the return cycle length after three successive premature beats was shorter than the tachycardia cycle length. Since these tachycardias could not be started nor stopped by stimulation they were probably caused by automaticity and not reentry. Since the application of several stimuli did not transiently suppress the tachycardia cycle length, they may not have been caused by normal automaticity. Shortening of the return cycle is consistent with an abnormal automatic mechanism or triggered activity caused by delayed afterdepolarizations that sometimes show overdrive acceleration. However, we need more pacing data of the kind obtained in the experimental study of Le Marec et al. (1985) to provide us with information necessary to assign an abnormal automatic mechanism to these arrhythmias.

The results of clinical trials or studies on the effects of antiarrhythmic drugs on ventricular tachycardias associated with acute myocardial infarction are also difficult to utilize for the purpose of assigning a mechanism to the accelerated ventricular rhythms and tachycardias. Many of the published results do not distinguish between the characteristics of the tachycardias being treated nor the time of the occurrence relative to the onset of symptoms. Lidocaine has been shown to effectively suppress some of the ventricular tachycardias and not others. We could find no report specifically describing the actions of lidocaine on the clinical accelerated idioventricular tachycardias that may be most analogous to the delayed ventricular tachycardias in the canine heart. However, there are data concerning the effects of the slow channel-blocking drug, verapamil. Verapamil does suppress the rate of accelerated idioventricular arrhythmias associated with myocardial infarction in humans and may restore sinus rhythm. These effects of verapamil are shown in Figure 3.11 (Sclarovsky et al. 1983). The top ECG strip shows an accelerated idioventricular rhythm and the middle strip

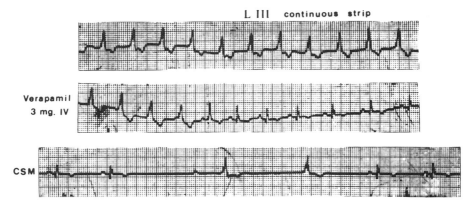

Figure 3.11: Administration of verapamil intravenously (IV) to a patient with sustained accelerated idioventricular rhythm results in termination of the arrhythmia. Carotid sinus massage (CSM) in the bottom trace fails to uncover the presence of accelerated idioventricular rhythm but shows two ventricular escape beats of morphology similar to the accelerated idioventricular rhythm. (Reproduced from Sclarovsky et al. (1983) with permission.)

shows conversion to sinus rhythm by verapamil. After restoration of sinus rhythm, carotid massage to slow the sinus rate may reveal either a markedly slowed ventricular rhythm with the same QRS morphology or the rhythm may no longer be present as shown in the bottom strip of Figure 3.11. These results strongly imply that the accelerated ventricular tachycardias are caused by abnormal automaticity but there is a possibility of triggered activity that is sensitive to verapamil as well.

The Development of an Infarct and Its Relationship to the Origin of the Delayed Ventricular Arrhythmias

After a coronary artery occlusion, many of the acutely ischemic myocardial cells that were involved in the generation of the acute ischemic arrhythmias eventually die and the infarct begins to form. Structural evidence for cell death becomes apparent only after 15 to 20 minutes of severe ischemia caused by complete coronary artery occlusion in the canine heart (Jennings et al. 1965). However, there are often areas within the infarcted region where, for a number of reasons, myocardial fibers survive the acute ischemic period; we will discuss these reasons later. Some of the surviving cells may also have participated in the generation of the acute ischemic arrhythmias since, as discussed in Chapter II, transmembrane potentials of some cells improve 10–15 minutes after the onset of ischemia, indicating recovery. When myocardial fibers survive in an area of ischemia, they may develop unusual electrophysiological properties because of continued ischemia and cause arrhythmias at a later time. Such surviving fibers are the cause of the delayed phase of ventricular arrhythmias, which is the subject of this discussion as well as the chronic arrhythmias that we will discuss in Chapter IV. We would suppose that the likelihood of delayed or chronic arrhythmias in hearts with infarcts that do not contain surviving myocardial fibers is greatly reduced. The structure of the developing infarct, therefore, has an important influence on arrhythmogenesis. Not just the size of the infarct, which has long been known to be linked to the severity of arrhythmias (Roberts et al. 1975; Geltman et al. 1979; Coromilas et al. 1985), but also the microanatomy as reflected in the occurrence and distribution of surviving myocardial fibers.

After a coronary occlusion it takes time for cells to die and infarct, and it takes time for the size of an infarcted region to reach its final limits, which are usually governed by the area of myocardium supplied by the occluded artery. The time course with which an infarct develops after an abrupt occlusion of a major coronary artery near its origin and the structural changes that occur in dying and viable fibers during infarct development helps explain why the delayed ventricular arrhythmias do not appear for 6 to 8 hours in the canine model. For the most part, the delayed arrhythmias arise in the Purkinje system that survives on the endocardial surface of transmural infarcts because ischemia eventually alters its electrophysiological properties; it takes many hours for these alterations to occur. Because the time course of infarct development is so instrumental in understanding the mechanisms causing the delayed arrhythmias, we will first describe it before discussing the arrhythmogenic mechanisms.

The Wave Front Phenomenon of Cell Death and Necrosis

Much of the data describing the time course of infarct development in the canine heart come from studies on the effects of circumflex occlusion. However, similar events likely accompany left anterior descending coronary occlusion as well. After complete occlusion of a major coronary artery supplying the left ventricle, there is a gradient of ischemia transmurally across the ventricular wall. The subendocardial zone is affected the greatest since coronary flow is reduced here to less than 15% of that in normal regions (Jennings et al. 1975). In the mid- and subepicardial regions coronary flow is initially higher, 15% to 30% of normal (Jennings et al. 1975). The gradient of coronary flow and ischemia after occlusion is thought to be a result of several factors, one of which is the effects of a transmural gradient of myocardial wall tension. During systole, transmural tension is normally greatest in the subendocardium and limits perfusion of this region more than in the midwall or subepicardium. This distribution of flow persists in the presence of the reduced flow caused by the coronary occlusion (Becker et al. 1973; Wüsten et al. 1974). A second and related factor in the canine is that most intercoronary arterial anastomoses are in the subepicardium and few if any are in the subendocardium. After occlusion of a major artery, some flow to the region supplied by that artery may persist through these interarterial anastomoses. Therefore, the first region of myocardium to die is in the subendocardium. A transmural gradient of metabolic rate may be a third factor that contributes to the initial cell death in the subendocardium, although its existence has been questioned (Van der Vusse et al. 1990). Some experimental evidence indicates that the subendocardial muscle has greater metabolic demands than other regions and is therefore more quickly affected by the period of ischemia (Dunn and Griggs 1975). However, despite the very low coronary flow, ischemic injury in these cells is reversible for as long as 20 minutes after occlusion and it is only after this time period that evidence of cell death becomes apparent (Jennings et al. 1960). This evidence is in the form of critical alterations in cell ultrastructure. If reperfusion is instituted before the 20 minutes, the cells recover their normal structure and function and an infarct does not develop. The acute ischemic arrhythmias discussed in Chapter II are occurring during this initial 20-minute period, many arising in the more mildly ischemic subepicardial region. However, despite the increased sensitivity of the subendocardium to ischemia for the reasons described above, the Purkinje system on the endocardial surface of the ventricles as well as several layers of ventricular muscle immediately beneath it are, for the most part, unaffected by this early ischemia, probably because they receive oxygen and nutrients directly from the ventricular cavity that bathes them.

Figure 3.12 diagrams how an infarct develops with time in the canine heart, based on the studies of Reimer and Jennings and coworkers (1977; 1979) with a circumflex occlusion but modified by the results of Fenoglio et al. (1979) using an occlusion of the left anterior descending coronary artery. Initially after about 30 minutes of coronary occlusion, death of ventricular muscle in the subendocardium occurs in an area that is at least several millimeters from the endocardial surface (Figure 3.12, black region in panel A). Muscle and Purkinje fibers in a zone of several millimeters, between the dead muscle and the endocardial surface, remain viable (arrows). Electrograms recorded from the subendocardial region of the normal left ventricle prior to coronary occlusion show both Purkinje and muscle deflections (Figure 3.13, control). In the experiments of Cox et al. (1973), 30 minutes after a coronary occlusion there was only a small decrease in muscle potential amplitude and Purkinje electrograms were not changed showing that this region remains viable and relatively unaffected (Figure 3.13, 30 minutes). Lazzara et al. (1973) did find a decrease in the amplitude of the Purkinje fiber electrograms soon after left anterior descending coronary occlusion, but electrical activity continued in the Purkinje system, showing the relative lack of effect of the acute ischemia. Although midmyocardial and subepicardial muscle are not irreversibly injured at this time a decrease in the amplitude of the bipolar extracellular electrograms recorded from both regions indicates that the ischemia has a transmural electrophysiological effect (Cox et al. 1973). Cell death then progresses as a "wave front" from the necrosing core in the subendocardium towards the subepicardium (Reimer et al. 1977) and towards the endocardial surface (Fenoglio et al. 1979; Reimer and Jennings 1979; Reimer et al. 1981), moving more slowly towards the endocardial surface than towards the epicardial surface. After 1 hour, the necrotic wave front moves into the midmyocardial wall (black area in panel B, Figure 3.12) where electrograms become smaller with time (Cox et al. 1973). At this time there still are several millimeters of viable muscle cells separating the necrotic region from the Purkinje fibers on the endocardial surface. In the electrograms recorded at the endocardial surface both ventricular muscle and Purkinje deflections still occur (Figure 3.13, 1 hour). The normal ultrastructure of the subendocardial muscle and Purkinje fibers 1 hour after coronary occlusion, illustrated in Figure 3.14, is added proof

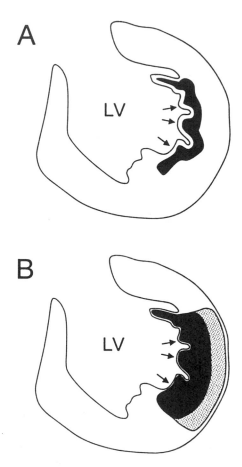

Figure 3.12: Diagram of wave front of necrosis phenomenon. Panel A shows an area of necrosis (shaded black) after approximately 30 minutes of coronary occlusion. The arrows show the unaffected subendocardial muscle and Purkinje fibers. Panel B shows the area of necrosis (shaded black) after 1–3 houses of occlusion. The stippled region shows the further progression of necrosis with time. The arrows indicate the surviving subendocardial Purkinje layer. LV = left ventricle.

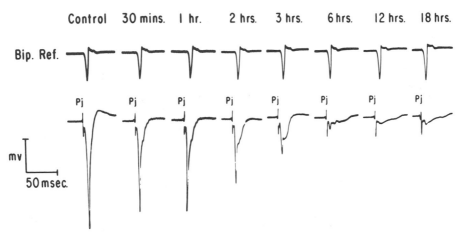

Figure 3.13: Electrograms recorded from ventricular muscle in a normal region (Bip. Ref. top traces) and from the subendocardium of the left ventricle in an infarcting region (bottom traces) in the canine heart. The times listed above the electrograms indicate the duration of coronary artery occlusion. No change in the amplitude of the Purkinje complex (Pj) occurred after coronary occlusion despite its immediate proximity to a severe localized subendocardial infarction. The progressive loss of the large negative bipolar electrogram following the Purkinje deflection in the bottom trace with time after the coronary artery occlusion indicates loss of ventricular muscle caused by the subendocardial infarction. (Reproduced from Cox et al. (1973) with permission.)

that the wave front of cell death has not yet reached the endocardial surface (Fenoglio et al. 1979). Positioned between these normal appearing fibers and the subendocardial core of dead cells is a region comprised of about 5 to 10 cell layers where the sarcolemma of the muscle fibers is still intact, but numerous alterations in intracellular structure have occurred. These alterations include a marked increase in the number of lipid droplets, a decrease in the glycogen content, and relaxation of the sarcomeres with wide I bands and L lines. Adjacent to this intermediate layer, muscle cells in the necrosing core have a disrupted sarcolemma. With the passage of time the wave front of ischemic injury also involves the subepicardium (stippled region in Figure 3.12B) while the rim of viable muscle cells on the endocardial surface is gradually lost. At 6 hours, only one to two layers of subendocardial ventricular muscle cells in most regions contain no or minimal ultrastructural alterations. The ultrastructure of the Purkinje fibers is mostly normal, but there is an increase in the number of lipid droplets in the fibers. The Purkinje fiber electrogram at 6 hours in Figure 3.13 is not altered. By 12 hours, only the Purkinje electrogram in Figure 3.13 remains. The disappearance of the muscle electrogram is caused by the wave front of ischemic injury moving into this subendocardial region. The majority of muscle cells immediately beneath the intact Purkinje fibers have extensive sarcolemmal breaks and other ultrastructural signs of cell death at this time. At 18–24 hours, mostly Purkinje fibers remain on the endocardial surface of the infarct and form an endocardial border zone (Fenoglio et al.

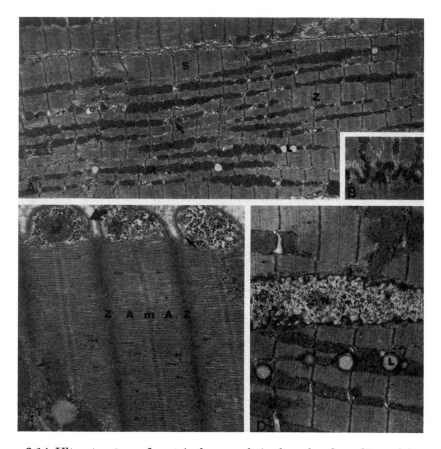

Figure 3.14: Ultrastructure of ventricular muscle in the subendocardium of the canine left ventricle 1 hour after coronary artery occlusion. Panel A shows the second and third muscle cells beneath the subendocardial Purkinje fibers. Sarcomeres (S) are uniformly contracted. Z bands (Z) are in register across the cells. Mitochondria (M) are normal, glycogen (arrow) is abundant and scattered lipid droplets (L) are present (× 6,300). Panel B shows the normal-appearing intercalated disks (arrows). Panel C shows the muscle cell at a higher magnification (× 24,500). The arrow indicates the scalloped sarcolemma. A bands (A), Z bands (Z), and M lines (m) are clear. I bands are not discernible. T indicates T tubules and small arrows show sarcoplasmic reticulum, both of which are normal. M indicates mitochondrial cristae that are distinct. Panel D shows focally abundant lipid droplets (L) in the third and fourth subendocardial ventricular muscle cells beneath the Purkinje fibers. N indicates the nucleus (× 9,450). (Reproduced from Fenoglio et al. (1979) with permission.)

1979). The surviving Purkinje fibers are pointed out by the arrows in panel A of Figure 3.15. The cells appear normal with centrally located nuclei, well-defined myofibrils and intercalated disks. They are separated from the infarcting muscle below by an expanded extracellular space that may result from edema. The survival of the subendocardial Purkinje fibers is seen more clearly in panel B, which is a photomicrograph of a section through a 2-week-old in-

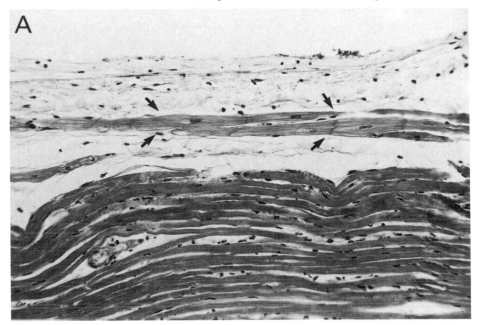

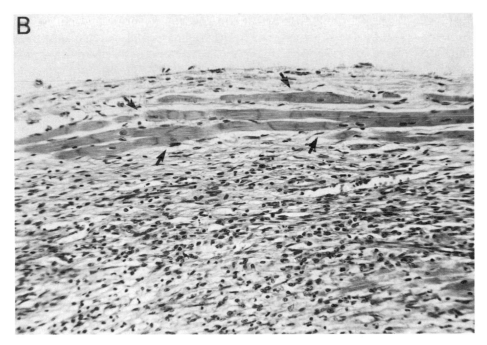

Figure 3.15: Purkinje fibers in the endocardial border zone. Panel A is a histologic section from a 24-hour-old canine infarct caused by left anterior descending coronary artery occlusion. At the top is the endocardial surface and left ventricular cavity. The first two cell layers beneath the surface (arrows) are surviving Purkinje fibers characterized by centrally located nuclei, well-defined myofibrils, and intercalated disks. Beneath the Purkinje fibers and the expanded extracellular space caused by edema is the infarcted ventricular muscle characterized by a lack of well-defined myofibrils and eccentrically located nuclei. Panel B shows the surviving Purkinje fibers (arrows) trapped in the developing subendocardial scar of a 2-week-old infarct. The endocardial surface is at the top.

farct. At this time, the infarcted myocardium is being replaced by a connective tissue scar. Electrical activity can still be recorded from the Purkinje fibers 18 hours after coronary occlusion (Figure 3.13) (Cox et al. 1973). They are the initiators of most of the delayed arrhythmias.

The accumulation of large numbers of lipid droplets in the surviving sub-endocardial Purkinje fibers between 6 and 24 hours after occlusion indicates that they are affected by the ischemia and this is related to the changes in their transmembrane potentials that cause the arrhythmias (discussed later). The "wave front" of cell death that proceeds towards the epicardial region also stops short of the epicardial surface (Reimer and Jennings 1979; Ursell et al. 1985). In transmural canine infarcts caused by occlusion of the left anterior descending coronary artery, anywhere from 1 to 30 layers of subepicardial muscle fibers survive forming the epicardial border zone where arrhythmias may also arise.

The wave front of ischemic injury encroaches on more and more of the ventricle during the second phase described by Harris (1950), between 1 and 8 hours after occlusion, when ventricular arrhythmias are usually not present. The lack of arrhythmias during this time period is puzzling. One would think that as the wave front caused new ventricular muscle to become more and more ischemic and then go on to die, the electrical changes in these dying muscle cells would resemble those that occur in subepicardial cells during the first minutes of ischemia that are related to the occurrence of the acute ischemic arrhythmic phase. Although increased ventricular firing rates can be revealed by vagal stimulation beginning at about 4 hours after occlusion, the rapid tachycardias and fibrillation characteristic of the acute phase do not occur despite the progressive muscle cell ischemia and death.

The time course and pattern of the progression of ischemic damage, and the occurrence and location of surviving myocardial fibers is expected to vary in different animal species. One reason is the interspecies variability in coronary artery anatomy. For example, in the porcine heart a similar "wave front" of cell death occurs. However, after only 2 hours, a layer of cells as small as about 200-μm thick immediately beneath the endocardial and epicardial surfaces are free of, or only show minimal ischemic injury. All other cells in the ventricular wall show maximal ischemic damage (Fujiwara et al. 1982). The pig heart does not have any significant collateral circulation accounting for the more rapid progression of ischemic cell death (Schaper 1971). The occurrence of a wave front of ischemic injury in the porcine heart cannot be ascribed to the same mechanism as in the canine heart, that is, a gradient of collateral flow from subendocardium to subepicardium. The regional arterial blood flow throughout the center of the infarcted region has been measured to be less than 0.05 mL/min (Fujiwara et al. 1982) and there is no gradient of flow from subendocardium to subepicardium. There may be a few epicardial collaterals responsible for some epicardial cell survival and endocardial cells may survive because of diffusion from the ventricular cavity. Fujiwara et al. (1982) have suggested several possible mechanisms to account for the early wave front phenomenon of cellular injury in the porcine heart. They postulated that it results from a transmural gradient of wall stress and intramyocardial pressure along with a more intense acidosis in the inner third of the wall because of a high glycogen content. No information is available about survival of myocardial fibers in transmural infarcts in porcine hearts in later stages of ischemia and infarction and the relationship of surviving fibers to delayed arrhythmias that do occur in this species. In the cat, an animal in which the delayed arrhythmias do not occur, one would think that there would be no surviving subendocardial Purkinje fibers, but this is not the case (Myerburg et al. 1977).

But what occurs in humans? Since the time course of the movement of the wave front is related to the occurrence of the delayed ventricular arrhythmias, does a similar wave front phenomenon occur? If it does, it would be expected to be related to the location of the coronary occlusion and the rapidity of the events causing the occlusion. That is, a rapidly occurring occlusion near the origin of a major artery might most closely resemble the experimental models. In humans, the subendocardial region is also the most vulnerable to ischemia as in the canine and is the first area to undergo necrosis associated with ischemia (Lee et al. 1981). Thus, the wave front should start out in the same region. A transmural gradient of collateral flow might not be expected because, unlike in the dog, in humans there are intramural and subendocardial anastomoses in addition to the subepicardial anastomoses (Lee et al. 1981). However, despite these anastomoses, nonhuman primates do show a gradient of collateral blood flow with the greatest flow in the subepicardial region (Weisse et al. 1976), another similarity to the canine model. As a final argument for a similar wave front in humans, myocardial cells do survive in the subepicardium (Lee et al. 1981; Bolick et al. 1986; Littmann et al. 1991) and subendocardium (Fenoglio et al. 1976; 1983; De Bakker et al. 1988; 1990) of human infarcts. In the subendocardium, structurally intact Purkinje fibers remain that are alive since electrograms can be recorded from them (see Chapter IV). These Purkinje fibers are indicated by the arrows in Figure 3.16, which is a photomicrograph of a histological section of the endocardial surface of a healed infarct. Thus, there are many similarities between the pathological development of human and canine infarcts. Taken together with the information on the electrocardiographic characteristics of the human arrhythmias, we suggest that the mechanisms for occurrence of the delayed arrhythmias are similar in humans and the experimental models.

Myocardial infarction still occurs when a coronary occlusion is followed by reperfusion if the period of occlusion lasts for more than 20 to 30 minutes. Thus, as we have discussed, spontaneous thrombolysis is associated with infarction arrhythmias. Reperfusion, however, influences the anatomy of the infarct, including its size and, perhaps more importantly, the amount and location of the surviving myocardial fibers. The wave front of cell death probably still occurs in the canine model in which the left anterior descending coronary artery is occluded for several hours followed by reperfusion. Initial cell death is still expected to occur in a similar subendocardial region as after permanent occlusion of the same artery and begin spreading towards the endocardium and subepicardium during the period of occlusion. This spread is then probably

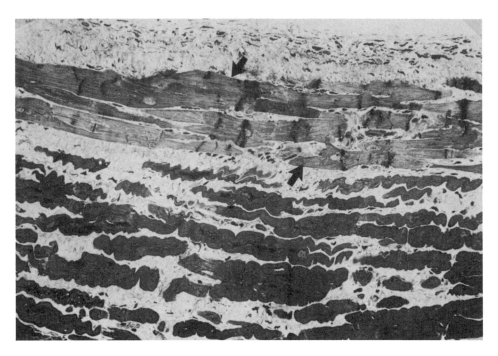

Figure 3.16: Subendocardial muscle bundles in an endocardial resection from a patient with a healed myocardial infarction. The bundles contain large, pale-staining Purkinje fibers (arrows). The Purkinje fibers are located immediately beneath the thickened endocardium and separated from underlying ventricular myocardium by connective tissue. (Magnified × 325.) (Reproduced from Fenoglio et al. (1983) with permission.)

modified by the reperfusion, during which there is a return of coronary flow to those regions in which the microvasculature has remained intact during the period of occlusion. In regions where the vascular wall is severely ischemic, it becomes fragile and breaks during the reperfusion causing hemorrhage into the myocardium. However, the subendocardial and subepicardial myocardial cell layers are usually reperfused since these areas remain viable along with the vascular cells during the period of occlusion. Blood flow to the subendocardial cell layers is restored almost to normal values (Karagueuzian et al. 1980). The effect of the reperfusion is to limit the movement of the wave front towards the endocardial surface, resulting in a wider surviving endocardial border zone consisting of muscle fibers as well as the Purkinje fibers. In Figure 3.17, the

Figure 3.17: Structure of the endocardial surface of a reperfused infarct (A) and an infarct caused by permanent occlusion (B) after 72 hours. In the reperfused infarct (A) a zone of 15–20 intact myocardial cells (M) persists beneath the subendocardial Purkinje fibers (P). These cells have distinct nuclei and well-preserved cell borders as contrasted with the deeper infarcted myocardium (H). In the infarct caused by permanent occlusion (B), no zone of viable ventricular myocardium is present beneath the subendocardial

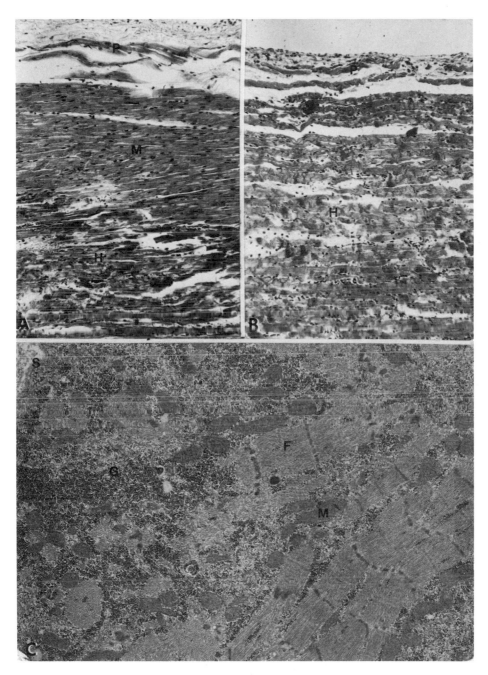

Purkinje fibers (P). The infarcted myocardium (H) is characterized by extensive contraction bands, loss of distinct myocardial nuclei, lysis of individual myocardial cells, and an inflammatory infiltrate. Panel C at bottom shows an electron micrograph of a subendocardial Purkinje fiber in a 24-hour reperfused infarct. The structure of the fiber is entirely normal and there is no accumulation of lipid. S = sarcolemma; G = glycogen; M = mitochondria; F = myofilaments. (Reproduced from Karagueuzian et al. (1980) with permission.)

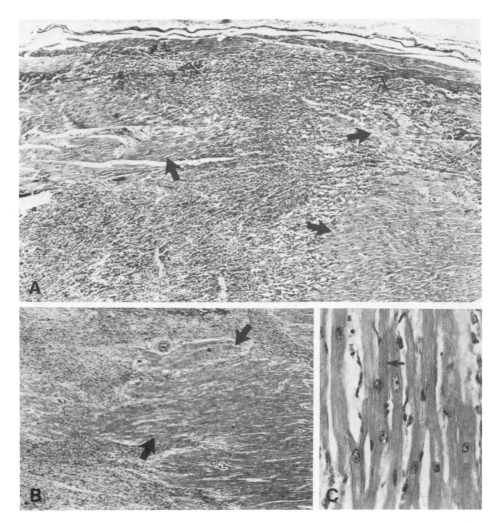

Figure 3.18: Photomicrographs of infarcted regions in hearts 3 days (panel A) and 5 days (panel B) after occlusion and reperfusion of the left anterior descending coronary artery. In panel A, the infarcted area contains numerous groupings of apparently intact muscle fibers (arrows). At higher magnification (panel C) these fibers show distinct cross-striations (arrow) and nuclei. On the endocardial surface (top of panel A), an increased number of normal-appearing muscle cells are present (unfilled arrow). In the central zone of the infarct in panel B, groups of myocardial cells with normal staining characteristics (arrows) are surrounded by granulation tissue. The presence of such presumably viable myocardial cells within the infarcted area is characteristic of the reperfused infarct. (Panels A and B are magnified × 38, panel C × 375.) (Reproduced from Karagueuzian et al. (1979) with permission.)

region of myocardial cell survival in the subendocardium of a reperfused infarct is compared to the region of cell survival in the subendocardium of an infarct caused by permanent coronary occlusion. In the reperfused infarct (panel A), 15–20 intact muscle cells (M) persist beneath the surviving subendocardial Purkinje fibers (P), whereas in the permanent occlusion infarct (panel B), only two layers of subendocardial Purkinje fibers (P) survive and the rest of the subendocardium is infarcted (H). The ultrastructure of the surviving Purkinje fibers in the reperfused infarct (panel C) is normal; the fibers do not have the accumulation of lipid droplets found in Purkinje fibers after permanent occlusion (Karagueuzian et al. 1980). These cells still develop abnormal electrophysiology that causes delayed arrhythmias (see below). Similarly, movement of the wave front of necrosis towards the epicardium is retarded by the restoration of blood flow to subepicardial muscle after reperfusion, and in general, the extent of the surviving epicardial rim of muscle (the epicardial border zone) is increased. Reperfusion may also prevent death of some intramural muscle fibers and the infarct takes on a "mottled" structure; that is, there are regions of viable muscle scattered among the necrotic regions (Karagueuzian et al. 1979; Michelson et al. 1980). The surviving intramural muscle fibers can be seen in Figure 3.18, panels A and B where they are indicated by the arrows. Panel C shows these fibers at a higher magnification; their structure appears normal. The intramural surviving muscle is likely to be important in arrhythmogenesis. Surviving subendocardial and intramural muscle is also apparent in some human infarcts (see Chapter IV) and in some instances might be the result of spontaneous reperfusion.

Origin of Delayed Ventricular Arrhythmias

At the time the delayed arrhythmias appear between 8 and 10 hours after coronary occlusion in the canine heart, there are only a few surviving layers of ventricular muscle cells adjacent to surviving subendocardial Purkinje cells. At the time delayed arrhythmias reach their maximum intensity, at around 24 hours after occlusion, electrical activity is not evident in most of the infarcted ventricular wall (Friedman et al. 1973a; 1973b; Lazzara et al. 1973; Horowitz et al. 1976). Figure 3.19 shows recordings obtained at intramural sites in the center of the infarcted region of the anterior left ventricle with a transmural needle electrode as well as recordings obtained from the adjacent noninfarcted ventricular wall. In the infarcted region (panels 2 and 3) the most distal recording pole of the electrode is in the ventricular cavity and shows the broad QS form of the cavity potential (trace C). The potential is generated by distant electrical activity and is devoid of any local signals. The next trace is a recording from the electrode in the subendocardium (trace SE) and also shows the QS form, similar to the recordings from the ventricular cavity (Durrer et al. 1961; 1964). However, in the subendocardial region, a rapid deflection with an amplitude of about 400 μV can also be seen (arrows, trace SE), indicating the pres-

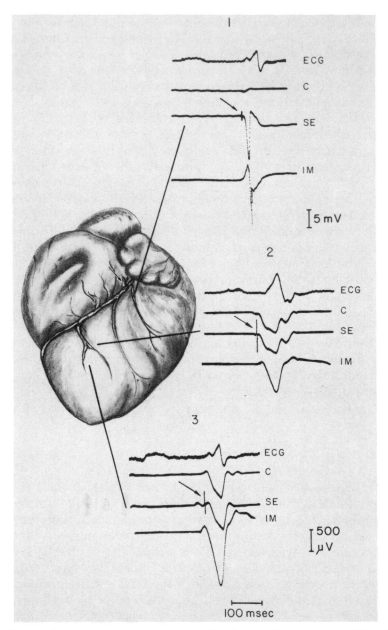

Figure 3.19: Bipolar recordings from infarcted and noninfarcted myocardium in the *in situ* canine heart 24 hours after coronary artery ligation. The extensive left ventricular infarct is depicted as the unshaded area adjacent to the anterior descending coronary artery. Noninfarcted regions are shaded. In each panel on the right, the top trace is a lead II electrocardiogram (ECG). The second trace (C) shows the potential recorded within the left ventricular cavity with bipolar electrodes; the third and fourth traces are subendocardial (SE) and intramural (IM) bipolar electrograms recorded from the designated areas. Calibrations at the right apply only to the electrograms and not the ECG. The 5-mV calibration is for panel 1 only. The 500-μV calibration is for panels 2

ence of viable cardiac fibers surviving on the endocardial surface of the infarct (Durrer et al. 1964; Friedman et al. 1973a; Scherlag et al. 1974; Horowitz et al. 1976; Sugi et al. 1985). This electrogram has the same characteristics as those recorded from Purkinje fibers in normal regions (trace SE in panel 1) (Durrer et al. 1961) and in fact verifies the anatomical studies showing that the Purkinje fibers remain alive. Recordings from within the depths of the infarcted ventricular wall as exemplified by the trace labeled "IM" in panels 2 and 3, only show a slow broad deflection that is similar in its time course and shape to the cavity potential and likewise is only a reflection of distant electrical activity. These recordings should be compared to the intramural recording from the noninfarcted region (IM in panel 1) where there is a large sharp spike generated by local activity. Subendocardial Purkinje electrograms can be recorded from many regions within the infarct but not from every region. This leaves open the possibility that some of the Purkinje system may not survive after the coronary occlusion. An alternative explanation is that the Purkinje system may not be originally present in some of these regions.

During sinus rhythm, the electrical activity of the Purkinje fibers within the infarcted region occurs after depolarization of the His bundle and bundle branches and slightly before the onset of the QRS complex (Figure 3.19, panel 3). This activity is from the peripheral Purkinje fibers. This part of the conducting system survives the transmural infarction that extensively involves the left side of the septum and is the site of origin of ventricular arrhythmias. The localization of the origin of the delayed arrhythmias to the surviving peripheral Purkinje fibers in the *in situ* heart comes from studies in which multiple recordings have been obtained from endocardial, intramural and epicardial regions in and around the infarct during the ventricular arrhythmias (Friedman et al. 1973a; 1973b; Scherlag et al. 1974; Horowitz et al. 1976; Spielman et al. 1978; El-Sherif et al. 1982). In these studies the earliest detectable electrical activity in the ventricles was sought as well as some indication of how the impulses spread from the arrhythmogenic focus to the rest of the heart. Earliest activity

---

and 3. Panel 1 is recordings from a noninfarcted region of the left ventricle. A low-amplitude wave was recorded from within the left ventricular cavity (C); this wave occurred simultaneously with the QRS complex of the surface ECG. An early, rapid deflection signifying Purkinje fiber activation is seen in the subendocardial electrogram (arrow, trace SE) and is followed by a deflection of greater amplitude and duration coincident with the QRS complex, denoting activation of ventricular muscle. A large amplitude deflection, signifying ventricular muscle activity, is seen in the intramural electrogram (IM). Panel 2 is recordings from sites within the infarct during a ventricular premature depolarization and Panel 3 is recordings from sites within the infarct during a sinus beat. Amplification of electrograms in panels 2 and 3 is ten times that shown for noninfarcted area in panel 1. Again, a slow wave lasting the duration of the QRS complex of the ECG was recorded within the left ventricular cavity (C). Similar slow deflections are seen in the subendocardial (SE) and intramural (IM) recordings. However, in the subendocardial recordings a rapid deflection that signifies subendocardial Purkinje fiber activity (arrows) is seen prior to the slow deflection. (Reproduced from Friedman et al. (1973a) with permission.)

often occurs in these subendocardial Purkinje fibers (Friedman et al. 1973a; Horowitz et al. 1976; Spear et al. 1977; El-Sherif et al. 1982), which become the most highly automatic region of the ventricular specialized conducting system by 18–24 hours after coronary occlusion (Hope et al. 1976). (In the noninfarcted left ventricle, the His bundle or bundle branches are usually the most highly automatic and the source of escape ventricular rhythms after sinus node arrest or atrioventricular block (Hope et al. 1976)). Thus, in Figure 3.20,

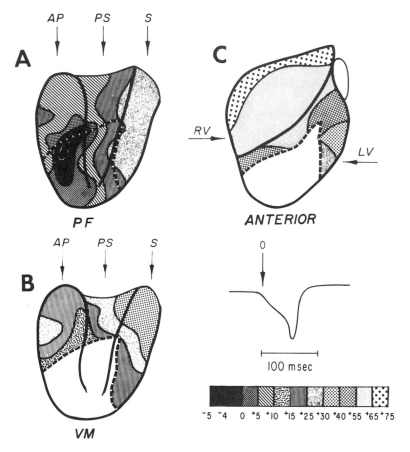

Figure 3.20: Activation map of a ventricular beat originating from subendocardial Purkinje fibers in an infarcted canine heart 24 hours after coronary occlusion. The sequence of activation is indicated by shading according to the scale at the bottom right (relative to the onset of the QRS). Panel A shows the sequence of activation in the surviving Purkinje network in the infarcted region. The site of earliest activation is indicated by the darkest shaded area. Panel B shows the sequence of activation in the subendocardial muscle of the infarct. The large unshaded region is the dead zone. The muscle surrounding this zone is activated well after the Purkinje system. Panel C shows the activation of the epicardial surface. The large unshaded region in the anterior left ventricle (LV) is the infarcted region. Epicardial activation occurs well after the onset of the QRS. (Reproduced from Dangman et al. (1988) with permission.)

which shows maps of endocardial and epicardial activation of a single beat of a ventricular tachycardia, the subendocardial Purkinje system in the infarcted region is activated the earliest, within the first 20 msec (panel A), while the epicardium is activated the latest (panel C). For this beat, earliest activity was detected in a focus of approximately 10-mm diameter towards the base of the infarcted anterior papillary muscle and left ventricular apex (darkest shaded region in panel A). Only Purkinje fiber activity was detected on the endocardial surface of this infarct and the activation map in panel A shows spread in the Purkinje system. From the focus of early activity, excitation may spread retrogradely into the left bundle branch on the septum and up to the His bundle (Horowitz et al 1976). Activity also can spread towards the margins of the infarct where it invades ventricular muscle. Panel B in Figure 3.20 shows the activation pattern of the subendocardial ventricular muscle bordering the infarcted region, which is activated after earliest activity appeared in the Purkinje system (panel A). Once entering this muscle, activation proceeded transmurally towards the epicardial surface of the left ventricle where, in this example, it emerged at the border of the infarct on the lateral left ventricle, posteriorly and inferiorly (panel C). From here activation of the rest of the noninfarcted left ventricle occurred. During tachycardia right ventricular activation occurs after the initiation of left ventricular activation and right ventricular epicardial breakthrough occurs after left ventricular epicardial breakthrough. Activation may proceed from the site of arrhythmia origin, retrograde to the His bundle and then antegrade through the right bundle branch to activate the right ventricle or activation might cross the ventricular septum to enter the subendocardial Purkinje system on the right side. Sometimes the tachycardia is characterized by multiform QRS complexes on the surface ECG. Such multiform complexes can be generated either by shifting foci of impulse initiation from one site to another, resulting in changing activation patterns (El-Sherif et al. 1982) or by changing pathways of propagation of impulses exiting from a single focus.

In summary, therefore, after left anterior descending coronary occlusion in the canine heart, it is the subendocardial Purkinje fibers of the left ventricle that are usually activated earliest during the accelerated idioventricular tachycardias. Earliest epicardial excitation occurs along the margin of the infarcted region 10 to 20 msec after earliest activity in the Purkinje system. Impulse conduction occurs in the subendocardial Purkinje fibers to the margins of the infarct where there is surviving ventricular muscle, and then proceeds towards the epicardial surface (Horowitz et al. 1976; Spielman et al. 1978; El-Sherif et al. 1982). In addition to this activation pattern, which is evidence that the subendocardial Purkinje fibers are the source of arrhythmias, Horowitz et al. (1976) stimulated the left ventricle through the electrodes from which they recorded earliest Purkinje fiber activity and observed that the QRS complex of the ECG was nearly identical to the one that occurred during the arrhythmia. Activation of the ventricles was also similar during stimulation from these sites and during the spontaneous arrhythmia. This provides important confirmation of the conclusions derived from the mapping studies.

Because it is very difficult to insert large numbers of electrodes into the subendocardium in the *in situ* heart, the activation maps of this region have a low spatial resolution and do not show detailed patterns of endocardial activation, although they are adequate to show the general site of origin of the arrhythmias. Another approach to locate the origin has been to map endocardial activation in the isolated perfused or superfused left ventricle. In these preparations, transmembrane potentials can also be recorded from the cardiac fibers at the sites where the rhythms originate. Some of these data are described in the section on the electrophysiological properties of the arrhythmogenic foci, but they also show a subendocardial Purkinje fiber origin for the ectopic impulses (Friedman et al. 1973a; 1973b; Lazzara et al. 1973; 1974; Ohta et al. 1986).

Earliest activity during accelerated idioventricular tachycardia, occurring on the epicardial surface overlying the infarct rather than the endocardial surface, has been found occasionally, raising the possibility that in some instances ventricular impulses may originate in surviving muscle of the epicardial border zone (Scherlag et al. 1974; Dangman et al. 1988). In an activation map published by Dangman et al. (1988) from an isolated canine heart with a 24-hour-old infarct supported by perfusion from a donor dog, the earliest site of activation was in the epicardial border zone from which there was a concentric spread of excitation away from this site. Earliest endocardial activation occurred about 10 msec after the earliest epicardial activation. However, as we have emphasized, the majority of tachycardias arise in the subendocardium.

In addition to the accelerated idioventricular tachycardias, we described that there may be occasional runs of more rapid tachycardia 1 day after occlusion of the left anterior descending coronary artery that begin with a short coupled premature impulse. The origin of these spontaneously occurring rapid rhythms has not been determined because of their infrequent occurrence and their transient nature. However, similar tachycardias are sometimes induced by applying premature stimuli or rapid trains of stimuli to the ventricles during the accelerated idioventricular rhythms (El-Sherif et al. 1982; Scherlag et al. 1983). Excitation of the heart has been mapped during these induced arrhythmias, which may be similar to the spontaneously occurring rapid arrhythmias. The origin appears to be mostly in the subepicardial rim of ventricular muscle that also survives in a transmural myocardial infarct (the epicardial border zone) and the mechanism is reentrant excitation. These arrhythmias closely resemble those that occur in more chronically infarcted hearts. Excitation maps of reentrant tachycardias in the epicardial border zone are described in Chapter IV.

Delayed ventricular tachycardias also occur in several other experimental canine models. The origin of the delayed arrhythmias in the occlusion-reperfusion model has not been investigated in the *in situ* heart using mapping techniques. We would guess that it is also in the endocardial border zone of surviving cardiac fibers, on the basis of the microelectrode studies on the cellular electrophysiology of this region (described later). After septal artery occlusion, which also causes delayed arrhythmias, the extent of the infarction is mostly confined to the septum, and may extend to both the right and left septal surfaces (Spear et al. 1977). The infarction, therefore, occurs where the bundle of

His and bundle branches are located along with some subendocardial Purkinje fibers of the more distal Purkinje system. These conducting tissues survive the infarction in the same way that Purkinje fibers survive occlusion of the left anterior descending coronary artery. Earliest activity during ventricular tachycardia occurs in the more peripheral Purkinje system near the margins of the infarct either on the left or right side of the septum, as shown in Figure 3.21. In panel B, the x's show the early time of occurrence of activity in the

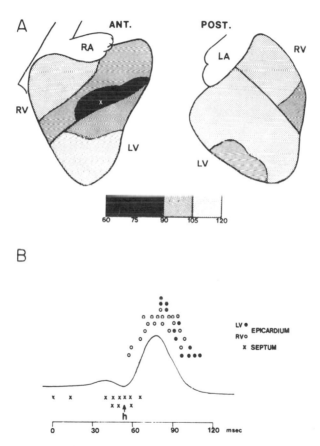

Figure 3.21: The sequence of epicardial activation and septal activation during spontaneous ventricular tachycardia 24 hours after septal coronary occlusion. In A, anterior and posterior views of the epicardial surface of the heart are shown. The sequence of epicardial activation is indicated by the gradation in shading. The scale below in A indicates the epicardial activation time interval in milliseconds for each of the gradations in shading. In B, the epicardial activation times indicated by the circles and the subendocardial septal activation times indicated by the x's are plotted on a common time axis relative to the electrocardiographic tracing of the lead II QRS configuration during the tachycardia. Time 0 for this graph is the earliest septal activation site. The epicardial activation times in A are also referred to the earliest septal activation site at time 0. The filled circles in panel B are left ventricular epicardial sites, the unfilled circles are right ventricular epicardial sites. The arrow indicated by h defines the time of retrograde His bundle activation. (Reproduced from Spear et al. (1977) with permission.)

septal Purkinje system relative to activation of the left ventricular epicardium (filled circles), right ventricular epicardium (unfilled circles), and the QRS complex. Strangely, earliest activity never seems to arise in the His bundle or the bundle branches (Spear et al. 1977). The septal peripheral Purkinje activity often precedes His bundle activation by more than 50 msec; the time of His bundle activation is indicated by the "h" in panel B. In this example, earliest epicardial activation occurred more than 60 msec after earliest septal activity, along the interventricular septum on the right ventricle as shown by the black area in panel A. When earliest Purkinje activity occurs on the left side of the septum, earliest epicardial activity might appear on the left ventricle adjacent to the interventricular septum or activation of the ventricle contralateral to the site of earliest activation might occur via retrograde propagation to the His bundle and then antegrade propagation through the conducting system (Spear et al. 1977). Stimulation of the septum through electrodes recording earliest activity during tachycardia resulted in a similar QRS morphology and a similar activation pattern in the experiments of Spear et al. (1977), further confirming the validity of the conclusions derived from the limited activation maps.

Right coronary artery occlusion and the resulting right ventricular infarction also result in a delayed phase of tachycardia. Earliest activity during tachycardia has been found to occur mostly in the subendocardial Purkinje fibers of the right ventricle that are, therefore, usually the source of the arrhythmias (Sugi et al. 1985).

There are no electrophysiological studies locating the origin of delayed spontaneous arrhythmias in humans. As we have discussed, pathological anatomy studies show that Purkinje fibers on the endocardial surface of transmural human infarcts often remain structurally intact and therefore, are viable (Fenoglio et al. 1976). They therefore may be the site of origin of some ventricular tachycardias.

Electrophysiological Properties of Surviving Myocardial Fibers in the Endocardial Border Zone

Experimental Methods

The delayed ventricular arrhythmias are caused, for the most part, by abnormal impulse initiation and they arise in Purkinje fibers that survive on the endocardial surface of the infarcts in the endocardial border zone. A more complete understanding of the mechanisms causing these arrhythmias requires detailed information on what happens to the transmembrane potentials of the arrhythmogenic fibers during the course of ischemia, since alterations of the action potentials cause the arrhythmias. In our discussion of the acute ischemic arrhythmias, we pointed out that much of the description of the effects of ischemia on the transmembrane potentials of myocardial fibers in regions where acute arrhythmias originate was obtained from microelectrode recordings from the intact heart, sometimes *in situ*. This approach was made possible by the origin of many of the arrhythmias in muscle near the epicardial surface. These arrhythmogenic muscle fibers could be reached with a microelectrode. These experiments provided information pertinent to understanding the mechanisms of the arrhythmias. However, this approach has not been possible for the study of the Purkinje fibers that give rise to the delayed spontaneous arrhythmias because it has not been possible to insert a fragile glass microelectrode into the ventricular cavity of a beating heart and obtain membrane potential recordings with it. Instead, information pertinent to the mechanism of the delayed arrhythmias has been obtained by recording transmembrane potentials from the subendocardium in isolated pieces of tissue removed from the infarcted canine heart at various times after coronary occlusion and superfused in a tissue chamber with physiological solutions (Friedman et al. 1973a; 1973b; Lazzara et al. 1973; 1974; Friedman et al. 1975; Allen et al. 1978; Cardinal and Sasyniuk 1978; Sasyniuk 1978). This experimental approach to the study of ischemic arrhythmias was suggested to one of us (ALW) in 1971 by Brian Hoffman during the 1-hour car trip we sometimes took together to our homes on Long Island. In this way, not only have the action potentials been characterized at the time arrhythmias occur, but also the time course of electrophysiological changes during the first 24 hours after occlusion has been followed.

However, one must be aware of possible limitations in studying pathological tissues removed from the pathological environment. For many years a debate occurred as to whether the electrical activity of even normal cardiac tissue that was superfused with a physiological solution in a tissue chamber was truly representative of the electrical activity that occurs in the *in situ* heart. There is now general agreement that it is, provided the tissue is thin enough to prevent the development of an anoxic core (Cranefield and Greenspan 1960; Janse et al. 1978). The most important differences between isolated tissue superfused with physiological solutions, and arterially, blood-perfused muscle relate to differences in the extracellular space. Thus, in blood-perfused muscle, the extracellular space comprises 19% of total volume, while in superfused tissue it comprises 30%. This has important consequences for conduction velocity and amplitude and configuration of the extracellular electrogram. In experiments by André G. Kléber at the University of Berne, conduction velocity increased from 56 to 60 cm/sec, the amplitude of the extracellular electrogram decreased from 49 to 38 mV and the steepness of the intrinsic deflection of the electrogram decreased from 57 to 24 V/sec when an arterially, blood-perfused papillary muscle placed in a gaseous environment was suddenly superfused with a thin (20 μm) layer of Tyrode's solution (A.G. Kléber, personal communication). Transmembrane potentials, however, are essentially unchanged when changing from blood perfusion to superfusion with a physiological saline solution (Rosen et al. 1972). The same argument for pathological tissue has not been settled. With regard to the studies on isolated tissues from infarcts, these tissues are removed from an ischemic environment in the heart where they may be exposed to a variety of products of ischemia. They are then superfused with solutions that have ion compositions and oxygen content that are usually considered to be normal, although the pO_2 of oxygenated Tyrode's solution is higher than normal. Any alterations in transmembrane potentials that are an immediate result of the abnormal external environment *in situ* (for example, elevated extracellular potassium) would probably be reversed by exposing the tissue to a normal environment provided by the superfusate. However, an important question to consider is, are the subendocardial Purkinje fibers exposed to an abnormal environment *in situ* 18–24 hours after coronary occlusion? We do not think so because their subendocardial location insures that they are bathed by ventricular cavity blood that should be normally oxygenated and contain the usual supply of nutrients. Nevertheless, as described later, the transmembrane potentials do begin to change as soon as the tissue is put into the superfusion chamber. For the purpose of interpreting the data from these tissues isolated from the heart, we assume that changes in the transmembrane potentials that are not readily reversible by superfusing the fibers with normal solutions represent changes caused by the long exposure to the abnormal environment *in situ*, abnormalities in the transmembrane potentials that are not dependent on the external environment.

A picture of the isolated preparation from the left ventricle of the canine heart that we used to investigate the transmembrane potentials of the myocardial fibers in the endocardial border zone of infarcts is shown in Figure 3.22 (Friedman et al. 1973a; 1973b). A similar preparation was utilized by Lazzara and Scherlag and colleagues who were conducting identical experiments at the same time (Lazzara et al. 1973; 1974). The preparation consists of the anterior papillary muscle (PM) and the interventricular septum (VS) extending from near the base of the ventricle to the apex. The pale color of the infarct is readily discernible on the endocardial surface. In most of these preparations the basal septum and the portion of the papillary muscle above the insertion of the false tendon were not infarcted. The border between infarcted and noninfarcted myocardium is distinct and easily recognized. The outer (epicardial and midmyocardial) two thirds of the ventricular wall were removed to make the preparation thin enough to mount in the tissue chamber. Microelectrodes were used to probe the endocardial surface of this tissue and to record the transmembrane potentials.

Electrophysiological Properties of Purkinje Fibers in One-Day-Old Infarcts

Rather than sequentially follow the cellular electrophysiological changes that occur after coronary occlusion in the Purkinje and muscle fibers that comprise the endocardial border zone, we will first look at the cellular activity in this region during the period of maximum arrhythmias at around 24 hours after coronary occlusion and identify the abnormalities associated with the arrhythmias. Later we will trace how these electrophysiological abnormalities

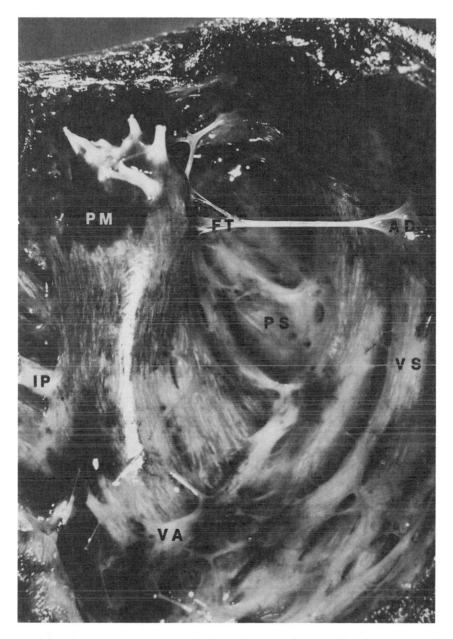

Figure 3.22: Isolated preparation of infarcted myocardium and bordering noninfarcted regions removed from the canine heart 24 hours after coronary occlusion. Photograph was taken immediately after completing the dissection of the freshly excised heart and before beginning *in vitro* superfusion; the endocardial surface is shown. VS = interventricular septum; PS = paraseptal free wall; IP = interpapillary free wall; PM = anterior papillary muscle; VA = left ventricular apex; AD = anterior division of left bundle branch; FT = free-running false tendon. The infarcted region consisting approximately of the apical two thirds of the papillary muscle, paraseptal free wall, and ventricular septum appears pale and the noninfarcted tip of the papillary muscle and basal paraseptal free wall and ventricular septum are darker. (Reproduced from Friedman et al. (1973a) with permission.)

develop from the moment of the coronary occlusion. When, after 24 hours of left anterior descending coronary occlusion, tissue from the infarct region of the canine heart is superfused in a tissue chamber, transmembrane potentials can be recorded from several layers of Purkinje fibers on the endocardial surface. This further confirms the results of the pathological studies and extracellular recordings from the *in situ* hearts showing that subendocardial cells remain viable in the infarct. After the microelectrode is pushed through these surface layers (approximately 1 to 5 layers of Purkinje fibers), no further transmembrane potentials can be recorded because the muscle beneath is dead. In noninfarcted left ventricular preparations, transmembrane potentials can be recorded from ventricular muscle for depths of 20 cell layers or more beneath the subendocardial Purkinje fibers (Friedman et al. 1973a). Rapid, repetitive activity (200 to 400 beats/min) occurs in most regions of the isolated preparations as shown in Figure 3.23. Transmembrane potential recordings obtained from the Purkinje fibers in an isolated preparation similar to the one in Figure 3.22 are shown. Action potentials in traces 1 and 2 are from the infarcted areas

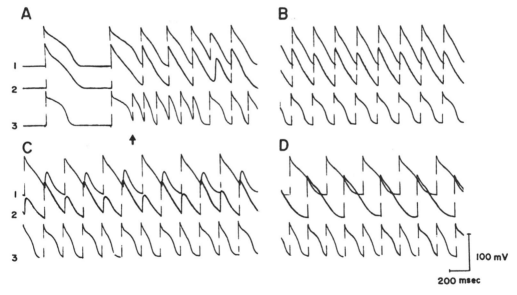

Figure 3.23: Spontaneously occurring rapid activity in subendocardial Purkinje fibers isolated from a canine heart subjected to anterior descending coronary artery ligation 24 hours before study. The *in situ* heart prior to excision demonstrated sustained ventricular tachycardia. The records shown were obtained 30–40 minutes after the preparation had been mounted in the perfusion chamber. Action potentials shown in traces 1 and 2 were recorded from subendocardial Purkinje fibers at the base of the anterior papillary muscle and the apex of the paraseptal free wall, respectively; both areas were located in the infarcted zone. Action potential durations of both these fibers were markedly prolonged (see text). Action potentials shown in trace 3 were recorded from a subendocardial Purkinje fiber in the noninfarcted tip of the anterior papillary muscle. (Reproduced from Friedman et al. (1973b) with permission.)

and the action potential in trace 3 is from the noninfarcted tip of the papillary muscle. In panel A, during electrical stimulation of the isolated tissue (first two action potentials in each trace) rapid, nonstimulated activity begins at the arrow. The repetitive activity is initially irregular and more rapid in the noninfarcted zone than the infarcted zone. Panel B shows this rapid activity after it became regular at a cycle length of 200 msec in both noninfarcted and infarcted regions. Panels C and D show two other instances of tachycardia in the same preparation. Such rapid activity does not occur in preparations isolated in the same way from noninfarcted hearts; normal left ventricular preparations beat spontaneously at rates of 4–10 per minute (Friedman et al 1973b; 1975; Lazzara et al. 1973). It appears that the factors causing arrhythmias *in situ* are still present in the isolated preparations resulting in this rapid activity. Microelectrode recordings obtained within 10 to 20 minutes after isolation of the preparations show that Purkinje fiber transmembrane potentials towards the center and apex of the infarcted region may be very depressed, maximum diastolic potential of many fibers may be more positive than -60 mV, and the upstrokes are very slow (less than 50 V/sec). An example of recordings from these subendocardial Purkinje fibers is shown in Figure 3.24. In this experiment, the action potentials that are shown were recorded by moving the micro-

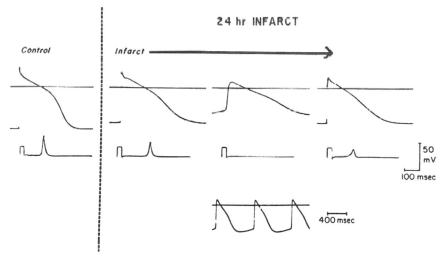

Figure 3.24: Depression of transmembrane potentials of subendocardial Purkinje fibers within an infarct. Action potentials shown were recorded by moving the microelectrode laterally from the noninfarcted tip of the papillary muscle (control) across the border of the infarct represented by the broken line into the infarcted region. The Purkinje fiber transmembrane action potentials are shown with a horizontal line denoting the zero reference potential. The trace beneath the action potential records is the differentiated signal of a 100-mV sawtoothed pulse with a 200-V/sec slope of depolarization (square pulse) and the depolarization phase of the action potential. The record at the bottom for the infarct data shows action potentials from the fiber in the middle section recorded at a slower sweep speed. (Reproduced from Friedman et al. (1973a) with permission.)

electrode laterally from the noninfarcted tip of the papillary muscle (control), across the border of the infarct (represented by the dashed line), into the infarcted region. The control action potential is normal, whereas the maximum diastolic potential and action potential upstroke and amplitude diminish as the recording site moves further into the infarct. Spontaneous diastolic depolarization is also a prominent characteristic of the Purkinje cells in the infarct as is illustrated in the records at the bottom in Figure 3.24. The most severe alterations in membrane potentials appear to exist in the most severely ischemic regions.

Changes occur in the electrical characteristics of these isolated preparations with time during the superfusion in Tyrode's solution. The very rapid activity present immediately after isolation from the heart usually disappears after 30 to 40 minutes. There may be a substantial increase in the maximum diastolic potential and action potential upstroke with time, and the number of cells exhibiting spontaneous diastolic depolarization decreases as does the slope of spontaneous diastolic depolarization (Friedman et al. 1973b; Lazzara et al. 1973; Dresdner et al. 1987). The reasons for these changes have not been elucidated, but their occurrence is intriguing. Lazzara et al. (1973) considered the possibility that the Purkinje fibers are moved from an hypoxic environment to a well-oxygenated environment when taken from the heart and placed in the superfusion chamber and that the increased availability of oxygen might lead to recovery of the membrane potential. However, superfusion of the fibers with an hypoxic Tyrode's solution in their studies did not prevent the time-dependent recovery process. It seems unlikely that the blood in the left ventricular cavity of the *in situ* heart 24 hours after coronary occlusion is hypoxic. However, the pO_2 of Tyrode's solution gassed with the usual 95% O_2-CO_2 mixture is around 700 mm Hg, which is much greater than the pO_2 of arterial blood, which is around 100 mm Hg. The possibility that the increased availability of oxygen because of the extra high pO_2 *in vitro* can overcome depressed oxidative enzyme function in these cells cannot yet be eliminated. Another possible reason for the increase in the transmembrane potentials of the Purkinje fibers during superfusion is that "arrhythmogenic substances" are being washed out of the tissue (Lazzara et al. 1973; Downar et al. 1977b). If such substances exist and could be identified, this would seem to be an important discovery. But what could such substances be? One day after coronary occlusion most of the ions and enzymes from the underlying necrotic ventricular muscle should be gone and we do not know what else might be left behind. An unanswered question is why the unknown arrhythmogenic substances, if they exist, are not washed away from the infarcted region in the *in situ* heart leading to the disappearance of the arrhythmias earlier than after several days, which is the usual time course of disappearance (Lazzara et al. 1973).

Despite the early improvement after 1 to 2 hours of superfusion, the transmembrane potentials of the Purkinje fibers surviving in infarcts still remain abnormal. The persistence of abnormal electrophysiological properties, even after several hours of superfusion, indicates that electrophysiological changes caused by the long previous period of ischemia *in situ* are not readily reversible and not totally dependent on the extracellular environment. The abnormalities that persist in surviving Purkinje fibers even after a prolonged period (2 hours or more) of superfusion with normal Tyrode's solution consist of the following.

(1) The Purkinje fibers have reduced resting membrane potentials, which may vary from values that are less than −60 mV to values only a few millivolts less than the normal of −90 mV. This range of membrane potentials is shown in the top panel of Figure 3.25. Maximum diastolic potential is plotted on the abscissa and the percent of the sampled fibers in both infarcts (stippled bars) and normal regions (solid bars) having the different values of maximum diastolic potential are on the ordinate.

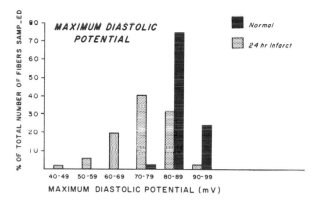

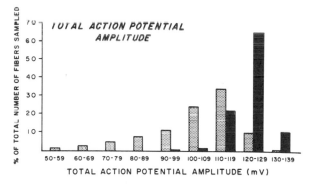

Figure 3.25: Frequency distribution of pooled values for maximum diastolic potential and action potential amplitude of superficial subendocardial Purkinje fibers (first cell layer) in six normal noninfarcted preparations (solid columns) and in the infarcted regions of seven infarcted preparations (stippled columns). Ordinate is the percent of the total number of fibers impaled having values within the defined intervals indicated on the abscissa. Top: Note that the largest percent of sampled fibers in normal, noninfarcted preparations had maximum diastolic potentials of −80 to −90 mV. In contrast, most of the sampled action potentials from infarcted preparations had maximum diastolic potentials positive to −80 mV. Bottom: Note that most of the action potentials recorded in normal, noninfarcted preparations had total amplitudes greater than 120 mV; most of the action potentials recorded in infarcted preparations had lower amplitudes. (Reproduced from Friedman et al. (1973a) with permission.)

NORMAL   24 hr INFARCT

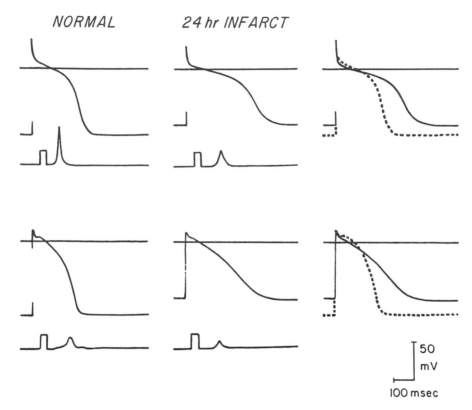

Figure 3.26: Action potentials recorded from a Purkinje (top panel) and muscle fiber (bottom panel) at the apex of a noninfarcted left ventricle of the canine heart are shown at the left (normal). Action potentials recorded from a Purkinje (top panel) and muscle fiber (bottom panel) surviving in the endocardial border zone at the apex of an infarcted canine ventricle 24 hours after coronary occlusion are shown in the middle. At the right, these action potentials from the normal (dashed trace) and infarcted hearts (solid trace) are superimposed. (Reproduced from Friedman et al. (1973a) with permission.)

Forty percent of the fibers sampled in infarcts after 1 hour of superfusion had membrane potentials between -70 mV and -79 mV, while less than 5% of normal fibers had these membrane potentials. A recording from a fiber in this group is shown in the top traces of Figure 3.26, where the transmembrane potential recorded from a Purkinje fiber in an infarct is compared to one recorded from a noninfarcted ventricle. At the top right, the two transmembrane potentials are superimposed, with the one from the normal heart indicated by the dashed trace. A substantial number (35%) of cells in the infarct also have lower membrane potentials of -40 mV to -70 mV, whereas cells in normal hearts do not have such low membrane potentials. A transmembrane potential recorded from a fiber in this group is shown in Figure 3.24. The lowest membrane potentials occur towards the center and apex although membrane potentials from one small region to another may still be quite different. The reduction in membrane potential may have several important consequences. It is at least partly the cause of the reduced amplitude and upstroke velocity of the action potential by causing partial inactivation of the sodium channels. The action potential amplitudes are plotted in the bottom panel of Figure 3.25. Many fibers have amplitudes of less than 100 mV that, which does not occur in normal Purkinje fibers. The reduction in maximum diastolic potential also may be linked to the occurrence of automaticity and triggered activity (described in (4) and (5) below).

(2) The upstroke velocity (V_{max}) of some Purkinje cells surviving in infarcts is as low as 20 V/sec, (such as the one shown in Figure 3.24), but there is a wide range of values, including normal ones (about 500 V/sec). The V_{max} in the population of Purkinje fibers sampled in the study of Friedman et al. (1973a) shown in Figure 3.27 demonstrates this distribution. The percent of cells sampled with different upstroke velocities in the infarcted regions are plotted (stippled bars) and compared to noninfarcted hearts (solid bars). Most of the Purkinje fibers in the infarcts have significantly lower upstroke velocities than normal fibers. The decreased upstroke has some effects on the activation of the surviving Purkinje network. Activation of the subendocardial Purkinje network during the early period of superfusion *in vitro* occurs much more slowly than normal because of the generalized marked reduction in maximum diastolic po-

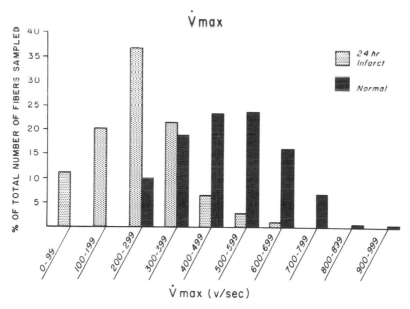

Figure 3.27: Frequency distribution of the maximum upstroke velocity ($\dot{V}_{max}$) of subendocardial Purkinje fiber action potentials. Ordinate is the percent of the total number of fibers impaled having values of V_{max} within the defined intervals indicated on the abscissa. Note that 70% of the action potentials of Purkinje fibers in infarcted regions (stippled columns) had $\dot{V}_{max}$ of less than 300 V/sec; these low values were found in only 10% of fibers in noninfarcted preparations (solid columns). (Reproduced from Friedman et al. (1973a) with permission.)

tential and upstroke velocity of the action potential. After longer periods of superfusion, when resting potential has increased, activation of the surviving Purkinje fibers generally occurs with a normal conduction velocity (Kienzle et al. 1987), except in localized regions where severely depressed upstroke velocities persist. *In situ*, subendocardial activation does not appear to be substantially delayed during the 24-hour period after a coronary occlusion (Lazzara et al. 1978a). This would not be expected if the Purkinje cells were as depolarized *in situ* as they are *in vitro* during the early period of superfusion. Therefore, in addition to possible washout of substances *in vitro* leading to recovery of these cells as discussed before, it is also possible that placing them in the highly oxygenated Tyrode's temporarily depresses the transmembrane potentials. At the borders of the infarct where some underlying ventricular muscle may survive surrounded by dead or dying muscle, there may be marked conduction delays between Purkinje and muscle activation and between activation of adjacent groups of muscle cells. Such marked delays and asynchrony may result from high-resistance coupling between cell groups as a result of the prolonged ischemia and infarction. Evidence of electrotonic interactions between these groups of muscle cells consistent with high-resistance coupling is seen as prepotentials and distortions in the time course of repolarization (Kienzle et al. 1987). The relation of these conduction delays to the genesis of arrhythmias is uncertain.

(3) Action potential duration of Purkinje fibers surviving in infarcts 24 hours after coronary occlusion is prolonged (Friedman et al. 1973a; Lazzara et al. 1973). Prolongation results both from an increase in the duration of the plateau phase (2) and the final phase (3) of repolarization. The prolongation of the action potential duration is totally unexpected since acute ischemia causes shortening of the action potential duration. Figure 3.28 shows plots of the frequency distribution of action potential duration measured to both 50% (APD_{50}) and 100% (APD_{100}) repolarization of normal Purkinje fibers (solid black bars) and Purkinje fibers in infarcts (stippled bars) in the experiments of Friedman et al. (1973a). The distribution of action potential durations of Purkinje fibers in infarcts is shifted significantly to the right, in the direction of increased duration (for example, the mean APD_{100} in this study was 418 ± 35 msec for infarcts versus 296 ± 23 msec for normals). This prolongation in action potential duration is particularly striking when Purkinje cells from the apical region of the infarct are compared with Purkinje cells in the apical region of noninfarcted left ventricle as is shown in Figure 3.26. Normally the action potential duration at the apex is about 250 msec as shown by the recording at the top left (normal). This is the region where the shortest duration action potentials in the normal peripheral Purkinje system are located. In the infarcted apex, action potential durations of more than 450 msec may occur (top middle, 24-hour infarct). The apex, therefore, becomes the region where the longest action potential durations in the peripheral Purkinje system are located 24 hours after coronary occlusion. The occasional muscle cells that survive in the subendocardial border zone also have a prolonged action potential duration as is illustrated in the bottom traces of Figure 3.26. The action potential of a muscle fiber in a 24-hour infarct (solid trace) is superimposed on that of a normal

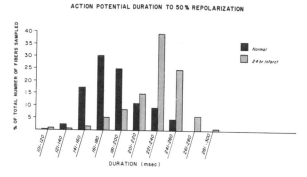

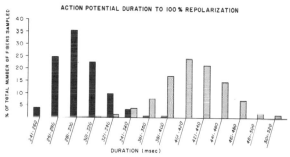

Figure 3.28: At the top is the frequency distribution of time to 50% repolarization in subendocardial Purkinje fibers. At the bottom is the frequency distribution of time to 100% repolarization in subendocardial Purkinje fibers. Pooled results from the first subendocardial cell layer of six normal preparations (solid columns) and the infarcted region of seven infarcted preparations (stippled columns) are presented. The ordinate represents the percent of the total number of fibers impaled having values within the defined intervals indicated on the abscissa. Note that most of the action potentials recorded from noninfarcted preparations had durations to 50% repolarization of 101–220 msec and that most of the Purkinje fiber action potentials recorded in infarcted regions had durations to 50% repolarization of 201–300 msec. Note also that most of the action potentials recorded from noninfarcted preparations had durations to 100% repolarization of 241–340 msec and that 95% of the action potentials recorded from Purkinje fibers in infarcted preparations had durations of 340–520 msec. (Reproduced from Friedman et al. (1973a) with permission.)

fiber (dashed trace) at the right. That action potential durations in the subendocardium of the infarcts become longer than those in the surrounding noninfarcted myocardium contributes to conduction abnormalities of premature beats. Reentrant excitation can be easily induced by premature beats in subendocardial Purkinje fibers in isolated and superfused infarct preparations because of the prolonged duration (Friedman et al. 1973b; Lazzara et al. 1973; Cardinal and Sasyniuk 1978). In regions of extensive anteroseptal myocardial infarction, the action potential duration of the subendocardial Purkinje fibers is extremely prolonged as are the relative and effective refractory periods compared to the Purkinje fibers in the surrounding noninfarcted regions. Action potential duration and refractory period increase from the base of the left ventricle to the apex of the heart. When premature impulses arising at the borders of the infarct propagate into these areas with long action potential durations and refractory periods before complete recovery of responsiveness, conduction is markedly slowed. In addition, the action potential durations of adjacent fibers in the infarct are not homogeneous; action potential duration and refractoriness are prolonged more in some fibers than in others. This leads to conduction block in some regions and not others, the appropriate conditions for reentry to occur. An illustration of this is shown in Figure 3.29. A schematic representation of the endocardial

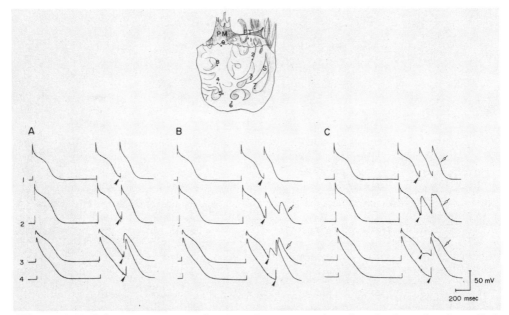

Figure 3.29: Inhomogeneous conduction of premature impulses in the subendocardial Purkinje fiber network of a canine infarcted preparation 24 hours after coronary occlusion. Top: schematic representation of the preparation. Light area indicates infarcted region. PM = papillary muscle; FT = false tendon; S = septum. The numbers in this drawing denote the locations of sites from which subendocardial Purkinje fiber action potentials were recorded during premature stimulation. Two stationary microelectrodes were utilized to record action potentials from sites 1 and 4 throughout the experiment. Premature stimuli (at variable coupling intervals with the basic stimulus) were applied through the intracellular microelectrode at site 1. The response resulting directly from this premature stimulus is indicated by the solid arrows on each trace in A, B, and C. At each coupling interval a third (roving) microelectrode was utilized to record action potentials from sites 2, 3, and 5–9. These action potentials were displayed simultaneously with those recorded from sites 1 and 4. By this method, the relative sequence of activation of these nine recording sites by the premature impulse was determined. For the records shown in A, B, and C, action potentials were recorded from sites 1, 2 and 4 during premature stimulation at three given coupling intervals and then from sites 1, 3, and 4 at the same coupling intervals. The records shown are a composite of the recordings obtained at these four sites. In each of these sections, the numbered traces were recorded from the correspondingly numbered sites on the accompanying diagram of the preparation. (Reproduced from Friedman et al. (1973b) with permission.)

surface of the left ventricle is shown at the top of the figure. The light area indicates the region that is infarcted. Action potential recordings shown below were from some of the sites numbered on this diagram. Panels A, B, and C show the Purkinje fiber action potentials recorded from site 1 in normal myocardium, and sites 2, 3, and 4 in the infarcted region, during premature stimulation at site 1. The action potential durations of the Purkinje fibers in the infarcted region are longer than in the normal region. In panel A, the premature impulse (arrow) was stimulated 320 msec after a basic paced impulse and it conducted into the infarct to sites 2, 3, and 4 and depolarized the Purkinje fibers at these sites nearly simultaneously. In panel B, the premature impulse was stimulated at a coupling interval of 300 msec and blocked near recording site 3 as indicated by the low amplitude depolarization at this site (black arrow on trace 3). This same premature impulse, however, conducted slowly to site 4 without blocking (black arrow on trace 4) because this site recovered excitability earlier than site 3. Additional depolarizations at sites 3 and 2 (unfilled arrows), which follow the response at site 4 are reentrant impulses from site 4, which block before reaching site 1. In panel C, the premature coupling interval was decreased to 280 msec. The premature impulse blocked before reaching site 3 (low amplitude deflection indicated by black arrow on trace 3), conducted slowly to site 4 without blocking (black arrow on trace 4), and returned to activate sites 3, 2, and 1 as a reentrant impulse (unfilled arrows). Continuous reentry might also be caused by this mechanism giving rise to tachycardias. Reentrant excitation in the endocardial border zone has been mapped *in vivo* (El-Sherif et al. 1982) during rapid tachycardia 1 day after coronary occlusion. However, it does not appear to be a common occurrence. Nevertheless, occasional reentrant beats may be interspersed among the automatic beats that predominate during periods of tachycardia.

At rapid heart rates, slow activation also occurs in the subendocardial Purkinje system of the infarcts because of the prolonged action potential duration. Impulses continuously enter the Purkinje system before it is completely repolarized from a previous impulse and can lead to aberrant QRS complexes. Records obtained from a normal Purkinje fiber (control column) and a Purkinje fiber in the endocardial border zone of a 1-day-old infarct at different rates of stimulation are shown in Figure 3.30. The rate of phase 0 depolarization is indicated by the differentiated signal below the action potentials. In normal controls, decreasing the stimulus cycle length from 600 to 230 msec did not significantly affect the rate of rise of the upstroke since each action potential arose from a fully repolarized membrane potential. This was possible since the action potential duration shortened significantly at the rapid rate. In the infarct, as cycle length decreased from 600 to 250 msec, each action potential arose from an incompletely repolarized membrane potential, causing a decrease in the rate of upstroke depolarization and slowing of conduction.

(4) Spontaneous diastolic depolarization, which is so prominent soon after infarcted tissue is placed in the superfusion chamber, remains in some Purkinje cells even after a long period of superfusion and causes automatic impulse initiation, although the rate of firing is slower compared

Control   Infarct

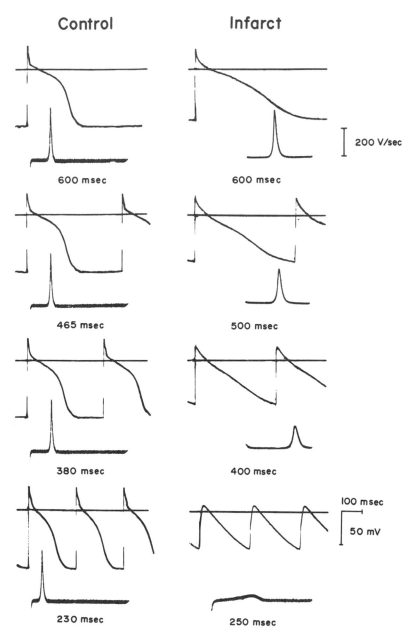

Figure 3.30: The effects of decreasing stimulus cycle length on Purkinje fiber action potentials. The left column shows action potentials recorded from a subendocardial Purkinje fiber in a noninfarcted canine heart. The right column shows action potentials recorded from a Purkinje fiber with a long action potential duration, in the endocardial border zone of a 24-hour-old canine infarct. Below each action potential recording is the differentiated rate of rise (V_{max}) of the upstroke. The cycle length of stimulation is also indicated. (Unpublished results of A.L. Wit.)

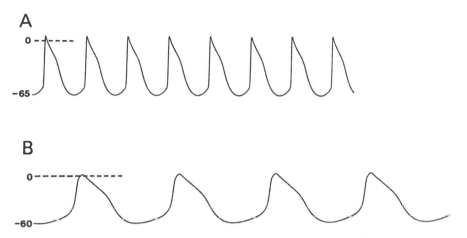

Figure 3.31: Action potentials from Purkinje fibers in the endocardial border zone of a 24-hour-old canine infarct, recorded at slow (panel A) and fast (panel B) oscilloscopic sweep speeds. The cycle length in panel A is 420 msec, the cycle length in panel B is 480 msec. (Unpublished records of K. Dresdner and A.L. Wit.)

to the first 20 minutes. Figure 3.31 shows action potentials recorded from a Purkinje fiber in the infarcted region with spontaneous diastolic depolarization. Because of the enhanced automaticity of these peripheral Purkinje fibers, they act as the pacemakers for the isolated preparations, even when the His bundle or bundle branches remain (Hope et al. 1976). Normally the more proximal conducting system has the faster automatic rate (Hope et al. 1976). Automaticity in Purkinje cells that have low maximum diastolic potentials (about − 60 mV) such as the one shown in Figure 3.31, is classified as abnormal automaticity. Overdrive stimulation of abnormal automaticity does not cause much overdrive suppression. The effects of overdrive stimulation on an automatic Purkinje fiber in a 1-day-old infarct is shown in Figure 3.32. The spontaneous cycle length of the fiber in the top trace (Auto CL) is 740 msec just prior to the 1-minute period of overdrive stimulation at a cycle length of 600 msec. Upon termination of the overdrive, the first spontaneous cycle length (RCL) is 760 msec, an insignificant increase compared to the preoverdrive value. The bottom trace of the figure shows that a 1-minute period of overdrive stimulation at a shorter cycle length of 400 msec results in more suppression of the first spontaneous cycle length (to 860 msec), but this is still much less than the overdrive suppression of normal automaticity (Le Marec et al. 1985). Automaticity in subendocardial Purkinje fibers in infarcts is also not very sensitive to the antiarrhythmic drug lidocaine; spontaneous diastolic depolarization is minimally suppressed in the usual therapeutic concentrations (Allen et al. 1978; Le Marec et al. 1985). It has been shown that lidocaine has little effect on the membrane currents responsible for the abnormal automatic mechanism. On the other hand, the antiarrhythmic drug Ethmozine, which has been shown

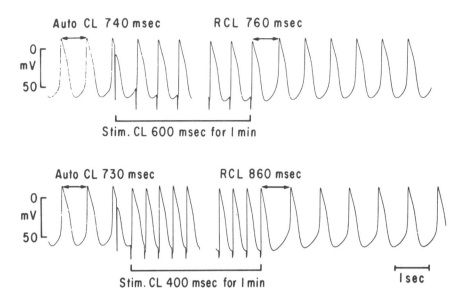

Figure 3.32: Effects of pacing on a Purkinje fiber in a 24-hour infarcted canine preparation 3 hours after excision from the heart. Top: spontaneous cycle length (Auto CL) = 740 msec; stimulation at a basic cycle length of 600 msec for 1 minute (underlined) minimally prolonged the recovery cycle (RCL) to 760 msec. Bottom: stimulation at a basic cycle length of 400 msec for 1 minute induced hyperpolarization (−5 mV) and a longer recovery cycle of 860 msec. There was modest overdrive suppression, followed by a gradual decrease of the spontaneous cycle length over 20 beats, at which time it had returned to its previous cycle length. (Reproduced from Le Marec et al. (1985) with permission.)

to suppress abnormal automaticity in several laboratory models, does suppress the spontaneous activity of the depolarized Purkinje fibers (Le Marec et al. 1985). Automaticity has also been observed in Purkinje fibers in infarcts with maximum diastolic potentials in the more normal range of −75 to −85 mV (Allen et al. 1978), indicating that different automatic mechanisms (abnormal and normal) exist 24 hours after coronary occlusion, related to differences in membrane potential.

Automatic Purkinje fibers with low maximum diastolic potentials sometime show various degrees of entrance and exit block (Friedman et al. 1973b; Lazzara et al. 1973; Rosenthal 1986). Both entrance and exit block are related to the low membrane potentials of cells in and around the automatic focus which decrease the stimulating efficacy of the depolarizing inward current. Figure 3.33 shows variable entrance and exit block from an automatic focus in an isolated superfused infarct preparation. In each panel, the action potentials in trace 1 were recorded from a subendocardial Purkinje fiber in the infarct with a prolonged action potential duration, while the action potentials in trace 2 were from a Purkinje fiber in the noninfarcted tip of the anterior papillary muscle. Action potentials in trace 3 were recorded from an automatic Purkinje

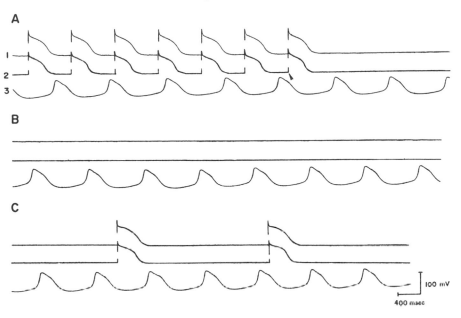

Figure 3.33: Entrance and exit block in a severely depressed subendocardial Purkinje fiber in the infarcted area of a canine heart. Action potentials in trace 1 were recorded from a subendocardial Purkinje fiber with a markedly prolonged action potential duration at the base of the anterior papillary muscle in the infarcted area. Action potentials in trace 2 were recorded from a Purkinje fiber in the noninfarcted tip of the anterior papillary muscle. Action potentials in trace 3 were recorded from a region of depressed potentials at the apex of the paraseptal free wall in the infarct. A: The false tendon was stimulated at a cycle length of 700 msec, resulting in depolarization at sites 1 and 2. However, action potentials in trace 3 did not have a fixed temporal relationship to the stimulated action potentials in traces 1 and 2, indicating some degree of entrance block. The action potentials in trace 3 were spontaneously occurring, since, after electrical stimulation was terminated (arrow), spontaneous activity continued in the bottom trace but was not conducted to the rest of the preparation (exit block). B: Records are a continuation of those in A, illustrating that exit block from this spontaneously depolarizing fiber was both complete and sustained. The cycle length of this spontaneous activity after termination of electrical stimulation was identical to its cycle length immediately preceding termination. C: Spontaneous depolarization continued in the bottom trace 5 minutes after termination of electrical stimulation. In addition, occasional depolarizations were seen in traces 1 and 2. (Reproduced from Friedman et al. (1973b), with permission.)

fiber in the infarct at the apex of the paraseptal free wall. In panel A, the false tendon was electrically stimulated at a cycle length of 700 msec resulting in depolarization at sites 1 and 2. However, the stimulated activation did not influence the automatic firing rate of the fiber in trace 3 since there was a high grade of entrance block into this region. After stimulation was stopped (records at end of panel A and in panel B) automatic activity continued in the region where trace 3 was recorded but activity did not propagate out to the surrounding myocardium (exit block). In panel C, spontaneous depolarization continued in the bottom trace and activity occasionally conducted out to activate surrounding regions. These kinds of phenomena in the superfused infarct preparations are predicted to be the cause of parasystole in the *in situ* heart.

(5) Delayed afterdepolarizations occur in some Purkinje fibers in isolated superfused infarcts and can cause triggered activity (Allen and Wit 1976; Dangman and Hoffman 1980; El-Sherif et al. 1982; Le Marec et al. 1985; Gough and El-Sherif 1989; Boutjdir et al. 1990). The occurrence of delayed afterdepolarizations suggests that intracellular calcium levels in the Purkinje fibers are elevated. There is a controversy, however, concerning the importance of the triggered activity in the genesis of the tachycardias that occur in the *in situ* heart with a 24-hour-old infarct. Le Marec et al. (1985) have shown that the occurrence of delayed afterdepolarizations is dependent on the level of the maximum diastolic potential and the temperature of the Tyrode's superfusate. In cells with low membrane potentials, generally less than -70 mV, abnormal automaticity and not delayed afterdepolarizations were prevalent in their experiments when the superfusate temperature was 38°C to 39°C, the rectal temperature of the dog with a 1-day-old infarct. Therefore, they proposed that this was the most important mechanism of arrhythmogenesis. Although membrane potential recordings obtained during a triggered rhythm may not appear any different from the recordings obtained during an automatic rhythm, both being characterized by spontaneous depolarization during diastole, the response of the Purkinje fibers to overdrive stimulation and to drugs can assist in determining the mechanism of impulse initiation. As we discussed above, overdrive stimulation is not followed by a change in the cycle length of the rhythm, a hallmark characteristic of abnormal automaticity (Le Marec et al. 1985). Triggered rhythms are predicted to be accelerated or terminated by overdrive. Lidocaine does not terminate rhythms caused by abnormal automaticity but can stop triggered activity and lidocaine does not usually stop the rhythms in the infarcted tissue. Le Marec et al. (1986) also found that the anthracycline antibiotic doxorubicin suppresses delayed afterdepolarizations and triggered activity fairly specifically and does not greatly influence abnormal automaticity in several different laboratory models. Doxorubicin also does not suppress the spontaneous firing of the Purkinje fibers in the infarcts suggesting that triggered activity is not the mechanism for impulse initiation (Le Marec et al. 1986). According to Le Marec et al. (1985), at low superfusion temperatures (36°C to 37°C), delayed afterdepolarizations may assume a more important role in impulse initiation *in vitro* even though this does not appear to be the major arrhythmogenic mechanism operating *in situ*. As the membrane potential hyperpolarizes during the course of prolonged superfusion *in vitro*, the rate of automaticity slows and spontaneous activity may cease. The Purkinje fibers with the higher levels of maximum diastolic potential may show delayed afterdepolarizations when they are stimulated. A recording obtained from a fiber with delayed afterdepolarizations is shown in Figure 3.34. These delayed afterdepolarizations have the same characteristics as delayed afterdepolarizations caused by other factors such as digitalis or catecholamines (Ferrier 1977; Wit and Rosen 1986). The amplitude of the delayed afterdepolarizations increases as the basic rate increases

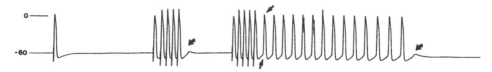

Figure 3.34: Delayed afterdepolarizations in a subendocardial Purkinje fiber surviving in a canine infarct 24 hours after coronary occlusion. At the far left, a single stimulus was applied, resulting in an action potential without an afterdepolarization. In the middle, five stimulated action potentials were followed by a small delayed afterdepolarization (curved arrow). At the right, five stimulated action potentials are followed by triggered activity beginning at the arrows and terminating with a delayed afterdepolarization (curved arrow).

until they reach threshold and initiate triggered activity. Premature activation can have a similar effect. Catecholamines and elevated extracellular Ca^{2+} can increase their amplitude and also cause triggering (El-Sherif et al. 1983b; Le Marec et al. 1985). Caffeine and ryanodine can stop the triggered activity by interfering with the process of calcium uptake and release by the sarcoplasmic reticulum (Boutjdir et al. 1990). Purkinje cells in infarcts, with membrane potentials negative to -70 mV are more likely to be found at the margins of the infarcted region and normal region and in smaller infarcts. Triggered activity is, therefore, likely to contribute to the tachycardias in 1-day-old infarcts but is not the primary mechanism of impulse initiation at this time. As time progresses beyond 1 day after infarction, membrane potential of the Purkinje fibers throughout the infarct increases and afterdepolarizations may assume a more important role.

Cellular Electrophysiological Mechanisms Causing Ischemic Arrhythmias

The conclusions we can make about the mechanisms of the ventricular arrhythmias from the studies on transmembrane potentials of Purkinje fibers in the 1-day-old infarcts are similar to those conclusions that were arrived at from the investigations of the *in situ* heart. Both the *in vitro* studies and the studies on the *in situ* canine heart support the hypothesis that abnormal automaticity in the subendocardial Purkinje fibers is an important cause of the delayed arrhythmias occurring spontaneously some 24 hours after coronary artery occlusion. The abnormal automaticity results because the Purkinje cells are partially depolarized. Depolarization alone is sufficient to result in abnormal automaticity without the necessity to postulate the occurrence of additional electrophysiological changes. Two major factors cause pacemaker shifts from the sinus node to the Purkinje fibers in the infarcted region: first, the enhanced spontaneous diastolic depolarization which increases automaticity in the Purkinje fibers to levels close to or more rapid than that in the sinus node, and second, the diminution or disappearance of overdrive suppression of the subendocardial Purkinje fibers, which is a characteristic of abnormal automaticity (Dangman and Hoffman 1983). Because of the lack of overdrive suppression, pacemaker shifts to the ventricles can occur during transient increases in the sinus cycle length. This does not happen in the normal heart because the normal automaticity of the Purkinje fibers is suppressed by the rheogenic Na/K pump and long periods of quiescence are required for the suppression to be removed. Entrance block into sites where pacemakers are located, caused by the reduction in the membrane potential, also prevents supraventricular pacemakers from capturing the ventricular ones and facilitates the appearance of ventricular beats during transient increases in the sinus cycle length as during a sinus arrhythmia. Automaticity at higher levels of membrane potential (normal automaticity) also can occur in some fibers and probably causes some of the arrhythmic beats. Arrhythmias caused by abnormal automaticity are clearly separated from those caused by normal automaticity by their different rates after right ventricular infarction (Sugi et al. 1985).

Other potential arrhythmogenic mechanisms were also identified in the studies on the transmembrane potentials. The relative roles of triggered activity caused by delayed afterdepolarizations and reentry in causing ventricular tachycardia are more difficult to assess. They do not appear to be the primary mechanisms causing the arrhythmias but they probably do cause some of the arrhythmic ventricular impulses. Rapid runs of ventricular tachycardia that begin with a short coupling interval and terminate spontaneously sometimes occur during an accelerated idioventricular rhythm. These tachycardias might be reentrant (arising either in the epicardial border zone or in the endocardial Purkinje system) or they might be caused by triggered activity. Either reentry or triggered activity can be initiated by a premature automatic impulse. Since delayed afterdepolarizations are more likely to occur in Purkinje fibers with higher levels of membrane potentials and such fibers are more likely to be found in small than in large infarcts, triggered activity might play a larger role in causing arrhythmias when the infarcts are small.

Early and Late Cellular Electrophysiological Changes

To determine how long it takes for the cellular electrophysiological changes in the Purkinje system that cause arrhythmias to develop, preparations of infarcted canine left ventricle were removed from the heart at different times after the coronary occlusion, ranging from about 20 minutes to 14 hours, and transmembrane potentials recorded from subendocardial fibers during superfusion in a tissue chamber (Lazzara et al. 1974; Fenoglio et al. 1979). The microelectrode recordings from the endocardial surface of preparations of the left ventricle removed from the ischemic region 20–30 minutes after coronary occlusion have shown the presence of both ventricular muscle and Purkinje

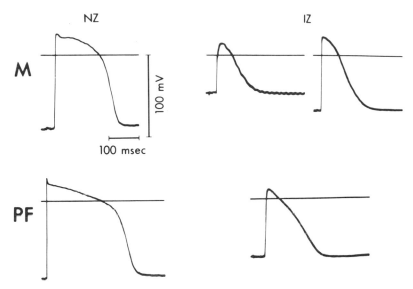

Figure 3.35: Intracellular potentials of myocardial cells (M) and Purkinje fibers (PF) in ischemic zones (IZ, at the right) and normal zones (NZ, at the left) of a preparation from a canine heart excised 20 minutes after occlusion of the left anterior descending coronary artery. The recordings from the ischemic zone were initially made 13 minutes after excision. An M action potential was recorded from the ischemic zone 28 minutes after excision and is shown on the far right. (Reproduced from Lazzara et al. (1974) with permission.)

fibers since the wave front of cell death has not yet arrived. Figure 3.35 shows that there is a marked reduction in resting membrane potential, action potential amplitude and upstroke velocity, and action potential duration of both the Purkinje (PF, bottom trace at the right) and muscle cells (M, top trace at the right) at this time (Lazzara et al. 1974). Maximum diastolic potential is reduced to around -60 to -70 mV during the first 60 minutes of superfusion (Lazzara et al. 1974). No spontaneous diastolic depolarization occurs in the Purkinje fibers (Lazzara et al. 1974). The changes in the ventricular muscle action potentials are similar to those that occur in the subepicardial fibers during acute ischemia and the changes in the Purkinje fiber action potentials are similar to those that have been shown to occur *in vitro* during simulated acute ischemia. However, electrical activity in subendocardial muscle may not be as depressed as in subepicardial muscle during this initial period of ischemia because subendocardial muscle still receives some nutrients and oxygen by diffusion from cavity blood. There also may be an intrinsic difference in membrane responsiveness between the two types of ventricular muscle. The upstroke velocity of epicardial muscle cells is decreased more than in endocardial muscle cells after depolarization to similar levels of membrane potential (Gilmour and Zipes 1980). It has been proposed that the greater resistance of the Purkinje fibers to ischemia contributes to the preservation of endocardial muscle electrical activity through electrotonic interactions (Gilmour et al 1984). That is, hyperpolarizing current flow may occur from the more polarized Purkinje fibers to the depolarizing ventricular muscle fibers opposing the depolarization of the muscle fibers caused by the metabolic changes of ischemia. The depression of the Purkinje fiber membrane potentials recorded in the *in vitro* preparations correlate with the observations that the amplitude of Purkinje electrograms recorded from the *in situ* heart may decrease, in some regions, immediately after coronary occlusion (Lazzara et al. 1974). Conduction velocity in the Purkinje system is moderately reduced *in vitro* (to about 0.70 m/sec) but not to the extent that might be necessary to cause reentry (Lazzara et al. 1974). This is also consistent with measurements in the *in situ* heart that show that activation of the subendocardium is only slightly prolonged during acute ischemia caused by ligation of the left anterior descending coronary artery (Lazzara et al. 1974). Transmembrane potentials return to normal after 1 or 2 hours of superfusion with normal Tyrode's solution, suggesting that either substances that depress the transmembrane potentials, such as elevated extracellular K^+, are washed out of the subendocardium or ischemic changes are reversed by the availability of oxygen in the superfusate.

At later times after coronary occlusion, subendocardial muscle and Purkinje fibers begin to manifest abnormal electrical activity that is not caused only by alterations in the extracellular environment and reversible ischemic metabolic effects, but that probably results from ischemia-induced alterations in cell metabolism and membrane function that are not readily reversible (Fenoglio et al. 1979). Already after one hour of occlusion, both muscle and Purkinje fibers have a reduced membrane resting potential, action potential amplitude and upstroke velocity, and an abnormal action potential duration (muscle fibers have a prolonged duration, Purkinje fibers have a shortened duration), which remain during several hours of superfusion with normal solution (Fenoglio et al. 1979). These changes are illustrated in Figure 3.36 by the recordings labeled "1 hr". The occurrence of electrophysiological changes that are not readily reversible appear to be related to the time course of infarct growth (or movement of the wave front of cell death) towards the endocardial surface. At 1 hour, 10–12 ventricular muscle cell layers still separate the necrotic core from the subendocardial Purkinje fibers at most sites, but the wave front is near enough to the endocardium to cause the ischemic changes in the action potential. Between 1 and 14 hours, resting membrane potential, and action potential amplitude and upstroke velocity of the Purkinje fibers remain fairly constant while action potential duration prolongs progressively with time. The time-dependent changes are shown in Figures 3.37 and 3.38 where maximum diastolic potential (MDP), action potential amplitude (APA), and action potential duration (APD) are plotted versus time after coronary occlusion. After 6 hours, only 2 to 4 layers of intact, viable, ventricular muscle cells remain in many regions between the necrotic muscle and the several layers of Purkinje fibers (Fenoglio et al. 1979). The surviving muscle cells have reduced maximum diastolic potentials, action potential amplitudes and upstroke velocities, and the action potential durations are prolonged (Figure 3.36, ventricular muscle

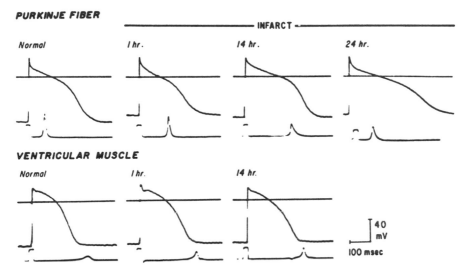

Figure 3.36: Changes in duration of Purkinje fiber and ventricular muscle action potentials with time after coronary artery occlusion. Top row of panels are Purkinje fiber action potentials and bottom row are ventricular muscle action potentials. Action potentials in far left panels were recorded from a Purkinje fiber and muscle fiber at the base of the anterior papillary muscle in a noninfarcted preparation (normal). Action potentials in right panels were recorded from Purkinje fibers and muscle fibers at the base of the anterior papillary muscle in infarcts isolated 1, 14, and 24 hours after coronary occlusion. Action potential duration of Purkinje fibers and ventricular muscle cells in infarcted areas were significantly longer than normal by 14 hours. (Reproduced from Fenoglio et al. (1979) with permission.)

action potential at 14 hours) (Fenoglio et al. 1979). The surviving muscle and Purkinje cells form the endocardial border zone at the time when ventricular premature depolarizations become apparent (Wit et al. 1981a). However, spontaneous diastolic depolarization is usually not seen in Purkinje fibers between 6 and 14 hours after coronary occlusion (Fenoglio et al. 1979). During the next 6 hours, when the frequency of ventricular premature depolarizations and tachycardia increases, most of the muscle cells on the endocardial surface die, but the Purkinje cells remain viable and begin to exhibit spontaneous diastolic depolarization (Friedman et al. 1973a; 1973b; Lazzara et al. 1973). Between 14 and 24 hours, another large decrease in resting potential of the Purkinje fibers occurs, as well as a further decrease in action potential amplitude and upstroke velocity (Figure 3.37). Action potential duration further increases (Figure 3.38). The prolonged duration of the Purkinje fiber action potentials is shown in the 14-hour and 24-hour recordings in Figure 3.36. In addition, passive electrical properties change; by 24 hours, input resistance, membrane resistance, and axial resistance of subendocardial Purkinje fibers overlying the infarct have increased, perhaps indicating partial cellular uncoupling (Argentieri et al. 1990).

The absence of spontaneous diastolic depolarization and automaticity in

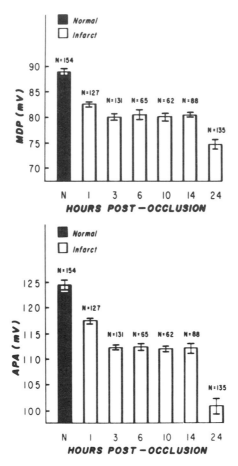

Figure 3.37: Changes in maximum diastolic potential (MDP) (top) and total action potential amplitude (APA) (bottom) of Purkinje fibers surviving in canine infarcts with increasing time after coronary artery occlusion. Column heights represent mean values for first Purkinje cell layer in five normal noninfarcted preparations (solid columns) and in infarcted regions of each group of infarcted preparations (unfilled columns) studied at times indicated on abscissa. Brackets indicate ± SE; N is number of impalements from which mean values were calculated. (Reproduced from Fenoglio et al. (1979) with permission.)

the subendocardial Purkinje system between 6 and 14 hours after coronary occlusion, a time when ventricular arrhythmias are usually prominent, is quite puzzling. Many of the characteristics of the arrhythmias at these times are similar to those of the 24-hour arrhythmias and lead to the conclusion that they are caused by an automatic mechanism. However, it appears that the automatic foci might not be in the Purkinje system. In a few of our experiments (Fenoglio et al. 1979) we found cells with prominent spontaneous diastolic depolarization 7–8 cell layers beneath the endocardial surface in 6–14-hour-old infarcts. A recording from one of these cells is shown in Figure 3.39. The

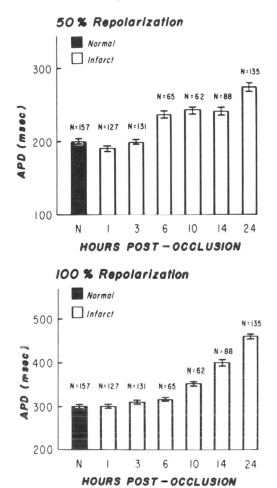

Figure 3.38: Changes in action potential duration (APD) measured to 50% repolarization (top) and 100% repolarization (bottom) of surviving subendocardial Purkinje fibers with increasing time after coronary artery ligation. Column heights represent mean values for the first Purkinje cell layer in five noninfarcted preparations (solid columns) and in infarcted regions of each group of infarcted preparations (unfilled columns) studied at times indicated on abscissa. Brackets indicate ± SE; N is number of impalements from which mean values were calculated. (Reproduced from Fenoglio et al. (1979) with permission.)

middle trace shows action potentials recorded from a cell in the seventh layer. Maximum diastolic potential is low and there is prominent spontaneous diastolic depolarization. Although, because of the low membrane potential, the action potential configuration cannot be assigned to either Purkinje cells or muscle, because the cells are located deep in the subendocardium, we would venture to say that it is a muscle fiber. Normally, Purkinje fibers are not found this deep. The bottom trace in the figure was recorded simultaneously from a

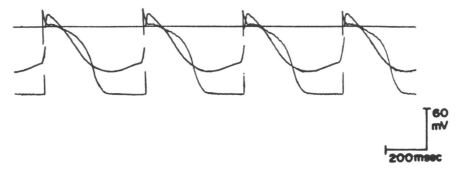

60
mV

200 msec

Figure 3.39: Spontaneous diastolic depolarization in a subendocardial fiber. Action potentials recorded simultaneously from a Purkinje fiber in first cell layer (bottom trace) and from a fiber seven cell layers beneath the endocardium (middle trace) are shown. The preparation was not being stimulated. The fiber with spontaneous diastolic depolarization may be a muscle fiber. Top trace is the reference 0 for both action potentials. (Reproduced from Fenoglio et al. (1979) with permission.)

subendocardial Purkinje fiber in the infarct. Therefore, the automatic foci causing arrhythmias at 6–14 hours after coronary occlusion may be in some of the ventricular muscle cells that are surviving in the endocardial border zone. Depolarized ventricular muscle cells can develop abnormal automaticity (Katzung et al. 1975; Imanishi and Surawicz 1976). The origin of the spontaneous arrhythmias may be at the interface of the infarcted dead myocardium and the ischemic but viable myocardium in the endocardial border zone. During the first 14 hours, the ischemic but viable myocardium at this interface is ventricular muscle. However, it may take 4–6 hours of ischemia for automaticity to develop in the muscle fibers. After 14 hours when most of the muscle has died, the interface is between the dead muscle and the Purkinje fibers. Then, spontaneous diastolic depolarization develops in the Purkinje system, which becomes the source of the arrhythmias.

The spontaneously occurring ventricular tachycardias in the canine model of infarction diminish in frequency by 48 hours, and by 72 hours sinus rhythm is usually restored. The abatement of arrhythmias can be correlated with the gradual return towards normal of the transmembrane potential of the surviving Purkinje cells although the ventricular muscle has vanished. There is a significant increase in the resting membrane potential, action potential amplitude and $\dot{V}_{max}$ by 3 days after coronary artery occlusion and spontaneous diastolic depolarization is no longer prominent (Lazzara et al. 1974; Friedman et al. 1975). Delayed afterdepolarizations can sometimes be induced by stimulating the cells at rapid rates. Action potential duration remains prolonged. The prolonged action potential of a Purkinje fiber in a 3-day-old infarct is illustrated in Figure 3.40; below, the recording (solid trace) is superimposed on a normal action potential indicated by the dashed line. Reentrant excitation can still be induced at this time by the same mechanism that we described in the Purkinje

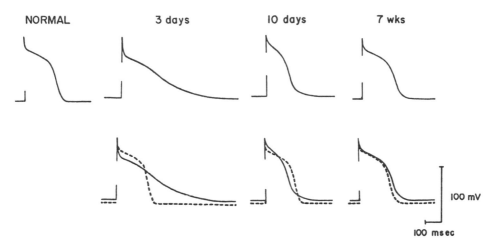

NORMAL   3 days   10 days   7 wks

100 mV

100 msec

Figure 3.40: The change in action potential duration of Purkinje fibers in the subendo-cardial border zone of canine infarcts with time after coronary occlusion. At the top left is the action potential of a Purkinje fiber in a noninfarcted (normal) heart. To the right of this record are action potentials of Purkinje fibers in infarcts of the ages shown above each recording. Below each of these traces the action potential of the Purkinje fiber in the infarct (solid trace) is superimposed on the action potential of the normal Purkinje fiber (dashed trace). (Unpublished records of D.L. Friedman and A.L. Wit.)

system at 24 hours. After 3 days, there is also a progressive decline in action potential duration, and reentrant activity can no longer be easily induced in isolated preparations by premature impulses. Although the resting potential and the upstroke of the action potential are normal by about 10 days after the coronary occlusion, the action potential duration decreases to less than normal before it finally returns to normal during the next few weeks (Figure 3.40).

Effects of Reperfusion After Coronary Occlusion On Cellular Electrophysiology

Although the origin of the delayed ventricular arrhythmias that occur after a several-hour period of coronary occlusion followed by reperfusion of the ischemic myocardium in the canine has not been located by the kinds of mapping techniques used to study infarcts caused by permanent occlusion, we suspect that they also arise in the endocardial border zone. The cellular electrophysiological characteristics of the muscle and Purkinje fibers that survive there have been defined from studies on the same kinds of isolated and superfused tissue preparations that were used to study permanent occlusion infarcts (Karagueuzian et al. 1980). Some of the changes in the Purkinje fiber action potentials at 24 hours after reperfusion are similar to those after permanent occlusion but are not as severe. Resting membrane potential is reduced by 10 mV (to around -80 mV) and there are corresponding moderate reductions in action potential amplitude and the rate of phase 0 depolarization. Action potential duration is only slightly prolonged. Although spontaneous diastolic depolarization and automaticity occur, it does not seem to be as prominent as in the permanent occlusion infarcts. This leads to the question of whether the arrhythmias arise in the Purkinje system. The surviving ventricular muscle also has similar action potential changes as the Purkinje fibers but pacemaker activity has not been detected in muscle. It is hard to relate the abnormal muscle action potentials to possible mechanisms causing the arrhythmias.

The resting potential, action potential amplitude, and upstroke velocity of the Purkinje cells recover with time. The action potential duration does not prolong more at 3 days as it does in permanent occlusion infarcts before returning to normal values. After 9–10 days, the action potentials are the same as in the permanent occlusion infarcts (Karagueuzian et al. 1980). Therefore, even though normal blood flow is restored to these cells by the reperfusion, a 2-hour period of occlusion is sufficient to cause long-lasting changes in the cellular electrophysiology. We suspect that such long-lasting changes may also occur in other regions made ischemic by short periods of occlusion and may lead to electrophysiologically "stunned" myocardium.

Mechanisms for the Survival of Subendocardial Purkinje Fibers After Coronary Artery Occlusion

There are several possible reasons that might explain why subendocardial Purkinje fibers survive within the infarcted region and go on to develop abnormal electrical activity that lasts for several days while the ventricular muscle only survives for short periods of time. The region of the subendocardium within several millimeters of the left ventricular cavity has multiple sources of blood supply. The peripheral ramifications of the left anterior descending coronary arterial tree is one important source. Fine capillaries from these ramifications are interspersed among the subendocardial Purkinje fibers and ventricular muscle. These capillaries eventually connect with venules and veins that drain the coronary blood into several conduits; blood returns in the great cardiac veins to the coronary sinus and the right atrial cavity, and some blood may drain directly into the left ventricular cavity through arterioluminal or arteriosinusoidal vessels (Prinzmetal et al. 1947; Wiggers 1952; Myers and Honig 1966; Moir 1969). In addition to the normal coronary flow bringing oxygen and nutrients to the subendocardial fibers through these capillaries, it has been proposed that some retrograde flow from the cavity into subendocardial layers might occur offering an additional or alternative source of oxygen and nutrients (Myers and Honig 1966). The functional significance (Wiggers 1952) or even the existence of such flow is controversial (Moir 1969). A third possible source of oxygen and nutrients is by physical diffusion from the ventricular cavity into the subendocardial layers.

Of importance, then, in determining why myocardial fibers in the endocardial border zone survive a coronary occlusion are the effects of the occlusion on these various sources of nutrients and oxygen. Occlusion of the left anterior descending coronary artery does decrease the coronary blood supply in the subendocardial capillary system to very low levels (Dangman et al. 1979; Karagueuzian et al. 1980). Blood flow, estimated from microsphere studies, is reduced from about 100 mL/min to 14 mL/min in the subendocardial Purkinje system 2 hours after occlusion (Karagueuzian et al. 1980). The flow is so reduced that injection of high concentrations of KCl into the coronary circulation does not depolarize the viable subendocardial fibers (Dangman et al. 1977; 1979). Yet despite this very low level of coronary blood flow, both muscle and Purkinje fibers survive during the first 6 hours after occlusion, a time period that is usually more than enough to kill myocardial cells deprived of their blood supply. It is possible that retrograde blood flow from the cavity into the subendocardial layers contributes to muscle and Purkinje survival. One might predict that if such retrograde perfusion of the subendocardium did occur, that it would increase after coronary occlusion when the pressure gradient from the left ventricle to the coronary vasculature is increased (increased left ventricular diastolic pressure and decreased coronary perfusion pressure). Moir (1969) found that there was only a small amount of luminal blood entering the subendocardium normally through arterioluminal connections and this amount did not increase significantly after coronary occlusion. Nevertheless, even if there is only a small amount of blood, some contribution to subendocardial cell survival may still occur.

It is also possible that subendocardial cardiac cells survive coronary occlusion because there is diffusion of oxygen and nutrients into the myocardium which is not dependent on retrograde blood flow. The amount of tissue that may survive from simple diffusion alone has been predicted from *in vitro* studies. For isolated quiescent preparations of cardiac muscle placed in a tissue bath and superfused with oxygenated Tyrode's solution (95% O_2 = pO_2 of 500–800 mm Hg), the rate of diffusion of oxygen and small molecules like glucose into the preparation becomes critical when a cylindrical preparation is more than about 600 μm in diameter (Cranefield and Greenspan 1960). An ischemic central core forms when the diameter is larger than this amount. In a plane sheet of tissue which is more analogous to the endocardial border zone, this critical distance is even less, because for a thickness of the sheet equal to the diameter of the cylinder, the surface area per unit volume across the sheet is half of that of a unit volume along the cylinder. Thus, in experiments on isolated sheet-like preparations over which oxygenated Tyrode's solution was flowing, the layer of cells that remained morphologically normal after prolonged periods of superfusion was not thicker than 150 μm, which would be about 7–10 cell layers (Janse et al. 1978). To determine how much of the subendocardium might remain viable because of diffusion in an experimental situation designed to mimic the events occurring after a coronary occlusion, Wilensky et al. (1986) perfused isolated preparations of rabbit interventricular septa with Tyrode's through the coronary vasculature while immersing the preparations in a tissue chamber and superfusing the surface of the tissue with a solution of the same composition. The superfusate took the place of the cavity blood. Transmembrane potentials could be recorded from the endocardial surface while coronary perfusion was interrupted. Superfusion was maintained, mimicking what we think occurs *in situ* during a coronary occlusion where the endocardial surface of the ventricles is still superfused with cavity blood. Moderately ischemic changes in action potentials under these conditions (reduction of membrane potential to between -78 and -68 mV) occurred at depths of 150–650 μm beneath the endocardial surface. At greater depths severe ischemia occurred causing the reduction of membrane potentials to values more positive than -60 mV and the cells became inexcitable. The phosphocreatine levels in the cells fell off to about 40% of normal by a depth of 600 μm from the surface, but even this amount shows that there is still a considerable amount of oxygen available at this depth. A depth of 600 μm corresponds to about 30 to 40 layers of ventricular muscle cells, which remain viable because of diffusion in the isolated preparations. However, *in situ* after a coronary occlusion, usually only 1–5 cell layers are viable and these layers are comprised only of Purkinje fibers and not muscle. The thickness of the surviving border zone is 50 to 300 μm. Why doesn't diffusion maintain a thicker endocardial border zone *in situ* as it does *in vitro*? Some possible answers to this question are: (1) *In vivo*, the muscle fibers may be expending more energy than *in vitro* since they are still contracting and pumping blood. Thus, they require more oxygen to remain alive. (2) The pO_2 that is the main driving force for diffusion is lower in blood (50 to 80 mm Hg) than in Tyrode's oxygenated with 95% O_2 (500–800 mm Hg). In any case, even if there is not an exact agreement between the results of experiments on isolated tissues and what happens in infarcts, these experimental studies do provide convincing evidence that diffusion plays an important role in maintaining the viability of subendocardial fibers. The ability of cells of the specialized conducting system to withstand hypoxia, probably because Purkinje fibers utilize less oxygen than do ventricular muscle (Bagdonas et al. 1961), might further enhance their ability to survive. The higher oxygen requirements of muscle cells and their greater distance from the cavity may cause them to die eventually, although cavitary blood may sustain their viability for hours.

Diffusion of oxygen and nutrients from the ventricular cavity to the surviving Purkinje cells is not sufficient to maintain normal electrophysiological properties, although it is adequate to keep them alive. The diffusion only keeps the muscle fibers alive for a limited period of time. During this time the muscle is also electrophysiologically abnormal. The transient abnormal electrophysiology prior to death of the muscle and the longer-lasting electrophysiological abnormalities in the Purkinje fibers are likely to be caused by ischemic alterations in cellular metabolism.

Mechanisms for the Development of Abnormal Electrical Activity in the Endocardial Border Zone

Alterations in Lipid Metabolism

Alterations in metabolism of Purkinje fibers in the endocardial border zone of canine infarcts are indicated by a progressive increase in intracellular lipid deposits in the cytoplasm that parallels the progressive changes in transmembrane potentials during the first 24 hours after coronary occlusion (Fenoglio et al. 1979). In Figure 3.41 (panel A) an electron micrograph of a Purkinje fiber in the first subendocardial layer of a noninfarcted left ventricle illustrates how the normal fine structure appears. There are the characteristic sparse, disordered bundles of myofilaments (F) and extensive areas of cytoplasm containing rich deposits of glycogen (G). There are no lipid droplets, which can be seen to be present in abundance in the electron micrograph of a subendocardial Purkinje fiber in a 1-day-old infarct (labeled L in panel B). Similarly, lipid droplets have been described in the Purkinje fibers of the endocardial border zone of human infarcts within the first week after acute coronary artery occlusion (Fenoglio et al. 1976). Lipid droplets also accumulate in any surviving ventricular muscle. The lipid deposits in the canine infarcts disappear during the next 7 weeks as the transmembrane potentials return to normal (Friedman et al. 1975). Figure 3.42, panels A and B, shows the relatively normal ultrastructural appearance of subendocardial Purkinje fibers in a 10-day-old (A) and a 7-week-old (B) infarct after the lipid disappeared. Abnormal metabolism in the Purkinje fibers leading to the accumulation of lipid may be a major cause of the delayed arrhythmias. The relationship between lipid accumulation and the prolongation of the action potential duration is further suggested by the ultrastructural studies on the cells in the endocardial border zone of reperfused infarcts. These Purkinje fibers do not have increased lipid deposits; apparently the two hours of occlusion is not sufficient to cause the lasting metabolic changes that lead to lipid formation (Karagueuzian et al. 1980). Concomitantly, action potential duration is only slightly prolonged 1 day after occlusion and reperfusion and does not prolong further between 1 and 3 days as occurs in Purkinje fibers in infarcts caused by permanent occlusion. Changes in other parameters of the Purkinje fiber action potentials such as the reduction in maximum diastolic potential and action potential amplitude are also less marked. Lipid droplets do accumulate in the surviving muscle cells in the endocardial border zone of reperfused infarcts, which have prolonged action potential duration (Karagueuzian et al. 1980).

The accumulation of the lipid droplets is a result of the effects of ischemia on the cellular metabolism and may be related to a number of the electrophysiological abnormalities that develop with the same time course. Lipid (free fatty acids and neutral fat) accumulates in hypoxic myocardium within 1 hour and can be found in ischemic ventricular muscle around the peripheral zones of

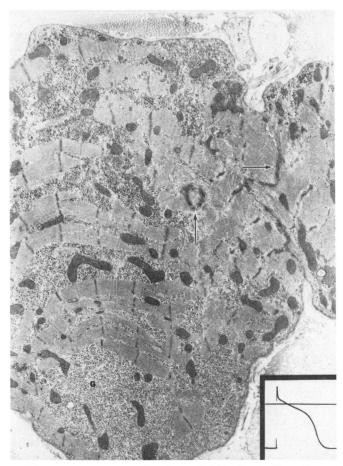

Figure 3.41: A: Ultrastructure of a subendocardial Purkinje fiber (first subendocardial cell layer) from the noninfarcted region at the tip of the anterior papillary muscle of an infarcted canine heart 7 weeks after coronary artery occlusion. The transmembrane action potential recorded in this region is shown in the bottom right corner. By electron microscopy, this subendocardial Purkinje fiber is entirely normal in appearance. G = glycogen; black and white arrows = intercalated disks. (Reproduced from Friedman et al. (1975) with permission.)

developing infarcts within 3 hours (Katz and Messineo 1981). The endocardial border zone is part of this peripheral zone. The lipid is derived from several sources. One source is the increase in plasma free fatty acids that accompany a myocardial infarction (Kurien and Oliver 1970). This elevation is a consequence of an increase in sympathetic discharge and an increase in circulating plasma catecholamines. The catecholamines activate a glyceride lipase that increases hydrolysis of triglycerides in the fat depots, releasing the free fatty acids (Katz and Messineo 1981). Because there is an elevation of plasma free fatty acids there is an increase in their uptake by the myocardial cells, which

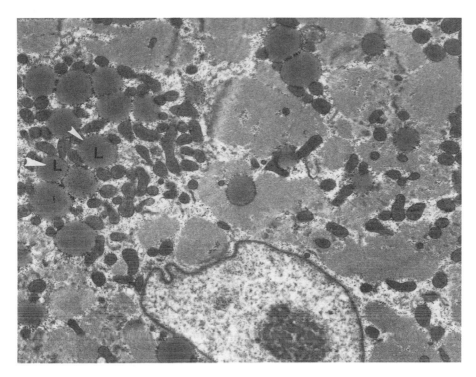

Figure 3.41: B: Ultrastructure of a subendocardial Purkinje fiber in the second cell layer of the subendocardial border zone of a 24-hour-old canine infarct. There are a large number of lipid droplets (L and white arrows) in the cytoplasm.

normally use them as a primary source of high-energy phosphates. Some of the increased intracellular lipid may also come from endogenous sources. Lipid synthesis in cardiac cells occurs when there is a lack of molecular oxygen for electron transport as occurs during hypoxia and ischemia. β-Oxidation of fatty acids, which is the primary pathway for generation of the high-energy phosphates is inhibited because of the lack of ATP coming from the citric acid cycle. Lurie et al. (1987) have found that there was a 30% reduction in ATP, ADP, and AMP in the surviving subendocardial Purkinje fibers and a 45% fall in the phosphate potential. They also measured a 25% decline in phosphocreatine and an increase in inorganic phosphate. Although these data show a profound change in Purkinje fiber metabolism, the changes are much less than those that occur in infarcting muscle (Reimer et al. 1977). Thus, long-chain fatty acids are not degraded but accumulate in the cell as long-chain fatty acyl derivatives. Some of these fatty acids may be stored as triglycerides that we assume is the composition of the lipid droplets identified in the electron micrographs (Figure 3.41B). There is also inhibition of tissue triglyceride lipase in ischemic cells, which prevents the breakdown of the triglycerides and favors the deposition of the fat droplets.

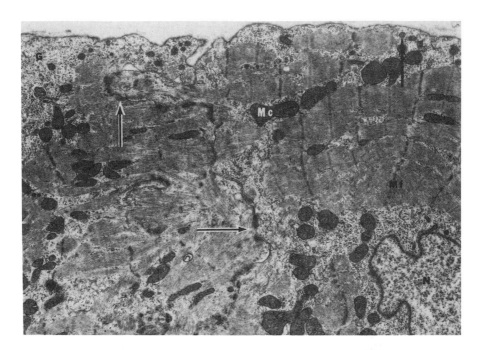

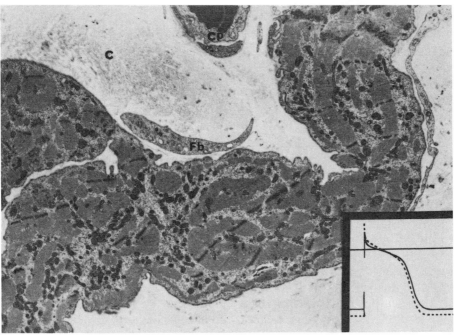

Figure 3.42: A: Ultrastructure of a surviving subendocardial Purkinje fiber in the endocardial border zone of a 10-day-old canine infarct. At 10 days, large numbers of lipid droplets are no longer present. B: Ultrastructure of a surviving subendocardial Purkinje fiber in the endocardial border zone of a 7-week-old canine infarct. The fiber is encircled by collagen (C), but no lipid is present. A fibroblast (Fb) and a capillary (C$_p$) can be seen. At the lower right, the action potential recorded from this region (solid trace) is superimposed on the action potential recorded from a noninfarcted heart and is not different. (Reproduced from Friedman et al. (1975) with permission.)

Intracellular accumulation of free fatty acids and lipids may lead to changes in the structure and function of membrane systems in the cardiac cell, which have profound effects on the ionic currents that flow during the generation of an action potential. Although we do not yet know the relationship between abnormal lipid metabolism and accumulation in the cells of the endocardial border zone to the abnormal membrane potentials and the genesis of arrhythmias, there are several possibilities that can be considered. Many of the lipid substances that accumulate in ischemic myocardial cells are soluble amphiphiles. At low concentrations they exist in solution as monomers, which can be inserted into the hydrophobic portion of the lipid membrane that forms the sarcolemma (Katz and Messineo 1981). This insertion is predicted to change the physical properties of the sarcolemma. Such changes in properties have been demonstrated in experiments using artificial membranes that are made from lipid bilayers and proteins, the same as the natural sarcolemma (Guyton 1986). At high concentrations, incorporation of the amphiphiles into the membranes can cause their physical disruption (known as a detergent effect) (Katz and Messineo 1981). Thus we can speculate that as the ischemic wave front moves into the endocardial region, the initial accumulation of low concentrations of amphiphiles in the membranes of the ventricular muscle cells may contribute to the development of abnormal electrophysiological properties because the function of membrane channels is altered, but as ischemia worsens higher concentrations lead to membrane disruption and contribute to cell death. In the Purkinje system the concentrations of the amphiphiles in the sarcolemma never reach the concentrations that cause membrane disruption, but only alter the properties of the sarcolemma.

The effects of amphiphiles on the electrical properties of membranes of excitable cells have been investigated in a number of experimental preparations. The results of some of these studies can be used to predict what they might do to the electrical activity of the cardiac fibers in the endocardial border zone. These compounds have a so-called "membrane stabilizing effect" which has been used to explain the mechanism of action of some of the lipid, soluble anesthetics that they resemble. They may exert this effect through the alterations in the lipid bilayer of the membrane, which in turn affects the mobility and conformation of the membrane proteins that form the ion channels. Katz and Messineo (1981) describe three possible ways that membrane function may be influenced: (1) The membrane volume may be expanded causing conformational changes in ion channel proteins; (2) Calcium may be displaced from negatively charged binding sites. Calcium binding has important influences on channel function; and (3) The phospholipid environment around the hydrophobic region of the membrane protein can influence the activity of the proteins. As a result, membrane permeability to ions that flow through the channels may be changed. In particular, a decrease in sodium conductance has been associated with such membrane stabilizing effects. There is a decrease in the inward sodium current in the cells of the endocardial border zone as indicated by the reduced rate of depolarization of phase 0 and the decreased action potential amplitude.

In addition to the physical alterations in membrane properties, fatty acids may also have biochemical effects on enzymes and metabolic pathways that may lead to changes in electrical properties of cardiac cells. Unsaturated fatty acids have been reported to inhibit adenyl cyclase activity (Lamers and Hülsmann 1977). Adenyl cyclase is involved in the phosphorylation of L-type calcium channels through which the slow inward calcium current flows during the action potential plateau. The marked changes in the time course for repolarization in the cells of the endocardial border zone suggest possible alterations in the functioning of these channels. Free fatty acids and long-chain acyl carnitines also inhibit Na^+-K^+ ATPase and thereby diminish the function of the rheogenic pump (Lamers and Hülsmann 1977). A decrease in the Na/K pump current would be expected to cause a reduction in resting membrane potential, prolongation of the action potential and enhanced diastolic depolarization (Gadsby and Cranefield 1979a; 1979b). Acute exposure of cardiac fibers to high levels of fatty acids in a superfusate has some effects that do occur in the fibers of the endocardial border zone such as prolongation of the action potential duration (Aomine et al. 1989). However, *in situ* it takes many hours for the electrophysiological changes in the endocardial border zone to be fully expressed and, therefore, we should not expect that acute exposure to elevated lipids *in vitro* would mimic the events occurring *in vivo*. Prolonged superfusion of sheep or dog Purkinje fibers with solutions containing elevated free fatty acids does cause a significant prolongation in the action potential duration (Karagueuzian et al. 1982). Products of lipid metabolism also influence the function of the sarcoplasmic reticulum. Palmityl carnitine inhibits the calcium pump of the sarcoplasmic reticulum and high oleic acid concentrations increase its calcium permeability. Abnormal sarcoplasmic reticulum function may be linked to the occurrence of the delayed afterdepolarizations in the subendocardial Purkinje fibers in infarcts.

The accumulation of lipid droplets in muscle fibers in an ischemic area is usually the precursor to eventual cell death, perhaps partly due to the detergent effects of the lipids described above. However, in the Purkinje fibers the lipid deposits eventually disappear as normal cellular electrophysiological properties return. We assume that the eventual disappearance of lipid droplets and return of normal transmembrane potentials indicates a restoration of normal metabolism in these cells. Most likely, this return of function does not represent adaptation of Purkinje fibers to ischemic conditions, but results from restoration of capillary flow to the surviving endocardial cells (Dangman et al. 1979). Whereas at around 6 hours after coronary occlusion it appears that there is very little if any flow through capillaries to the subendocardial Purkinje fibers and therefore they must be nourished entirely by blood in the ventricular cavity, at 24 hours some return of capillary blood flow can already be demonstrated. After several days the capillary blood flow to the Purkinje fibers is restored (Dangman et al. 1979). The restoration of coronary flow to this ischemic region may be through collateral vessels and intercoronary anastomoses which gradually open after the coronary occlusion. The time course for the increase in blood flow to the Purkinje fibers in the infarcts is the same as the increase in collateral blood flow to epicardial and peripheral regions of infarcts (Pasyk et al. 1971; Cox et al. 1975; Bishop et al. 1976; Rivas et al. 1976; Schaper and Pasyk 1976).

Ionic Mechanisms Causing Abnormal Purkinje Fiber Electrophysiology

The abnormalities in the transmembrane potentials of the Purkinje fibers in the endocardial border zone that cause arrhythmias result from the effects of prolonged ischemia on cell metabolism (described above) and membrane function. A consequence of these alterations is abnormalities in transmembrane ion distributions and membrane currents. In this section we discuss what is known about these specific alterations.

Depolarization of the Membrane Potential   The maximum diastolic or resting potential of cardiac cells is to a large extent determined by the potassium equilibrium potential, which can be calculated from the Nernst equation based on the intracellular and extracellular free potassium ion concentrations or activities. Normal intracellular potassium ion activity (a_K) in free running canine and sheep Purkinje fiber strands, determined with K^+ sensitive microelectrodes, is 110–130 mmol/L (Miura et al. 1977; Sheu et al. 1980), which translates into a free K^+ concentration of 149–176 mmol/L using an activity coefficient of 0.74. Canine subendocardial Purkinje cells have a mean intracellular K^+ activity of 112 mmol/L (Dresdner et al. 1987). Based on these values, the calculated potassium equilibrium potential (E_K) is −97 to −101 mV at 37°C. For normal canine subendocardial Purkinje cells stimulated at a cycle length of 800 msec, the maximum diastolic potential averages around −85 mV when the extracellular K^+ concentration is 4 mmol/L. Thus the membrane potential is more than 10 mV positive to E_K. This characteristic is generally true of most cardiac cells at a normal extracellular K^+ of around 4 mmol/L; membrane potential is positive to E_K because the sarcolemma has significant permeability to other ions in addition to potassium. Of particular importance is an inward leakage of sodium ions that has a depolarizing influence (Baumgarten and Fozzard 1986).

In addition to the important role of the relative concentrations and permeabilities to the different ions in determining the membrane potential, the Na/K pump plays an important role. The intracellular Na^+ activity (a_{Na}^i) of cardiac cells is at least tenfold lower than the extracellular Na^+ activity because this pump continuously transports Na^+ out of the cell. Normal intracellular Na^+ activity in Purkinje fibers paced at cycle lengths between 500 and 1000 msec is between 7.6 and 9.8 mmol/L but increases at more rapid rates. The membrane Na/K pump is electrogenic because the coupling ratio between Na^+ and K^+ is 3:2, generating an outward Na^+ current across the cell membrane. This may contribute between 3 and 10 mV to the membrane potential (Eisner

1986), and also accelerates the time course of repolarization (Gadsby and Cranefield 1982).

A primary alteration in the transmembrane potential of Purkinje fibers in the endocardial border zone, which is caused by prolonged exposure to ischemia is a depolarization of the resting potential, which is progressive during the first 24 hours. The decrease in membrane potential may have many secondary consequences such as leading to a decrease in the depolarizing inward Na^+ current during the action potential upstroke (because of voltage-dependent inactivation of the Na^+ channels), and increasing the automatic firing of these cells. The mechanism for the decrease in resting potential has been investigated with double-barrel ion-selective microelectrodes in isolated, superfused preparations of infarcted canine left ventricle. With this technique the transmembrane potential is recorded with one barrel and ion activity with the other, thus enabling the two to be related for the same cell (Dresdner et al. 1987). During the first hour of superfusion of subendocardial Purkinje fibers in 24-hour-old infarcts, when maximum diastolic potential was in the range of -50 mV (about 35 mV less than normal), intracellular K^+ activity was found to be 62 mmol/L (Dresdner et al. 1987). The intracellular potassium activity (aK_i) is plotted in panel A of Figure 3.43 (24 hours, solid circle) and compared to normal. Thus, there is a substantial loss of K^+ (approximately 50 mmol/L). Because of this loss, the K^+ equilibrium potential is decreased to about 82 mV (calculated with the Nernst equation using K_o = 4 mmol/L and K_i = 62 mmol/L). The measured reduction in the membrane potential, however, is more than the reduction in the K^+ equilibrium potential that accounts for only about one half of the reduction in the maximum diastolic potential. This is shown in panel B of Figure 3.43 where the maximum diastolic potential (MDP) of Purkinje fibers in 24-hour-old infarcts (solid circle, 24 hours) is plotted versus the potassium equilibrium potential (E_K). The point on the graph falls far below the straight line that describes a relationship between MDP and E_K that has a slope of 1. Therefore, membrane conductance changes must also occur to account for part of the depolarization.

The decrease in the intracellular K^+ may itself lead to a change in the membrane conductance that contributes to the depolarization, by virtue of its effects on the inwardly rectifying K^+ channels (Cohen et al. 1989). In Purkinje fibers, the membrane current, I_{K1}, which sets the resting potential near the membrane equilibrium potential for K^+ is an inwardly rectifying current. The inwardly rectifying channels activate when membrane potential moves in the negative direction and deactivate when the membrane potential moves in the positive direction. The intracellular K^+ concentration, $[K^+]_i$ (as well as the extracellular K^+ $[K^+]_o$) affects the kinetics of activation, the voltage dependence of steady state activation, and the kinetics and voltage dependence of deactivation of the inward rectifier. When $[K^+]_i$ of isolated Purkinje fiber myocytes was reduced from 145 to 25 mmol/L by intracellular dialysis, it decreased the rate of activation of I_{K1} at a given voltage by severalfold, reversed the voltage dependence of recovery from deactivation so that the deactivation rate decreased with depolarization, and caused a positive shift in the midpoint

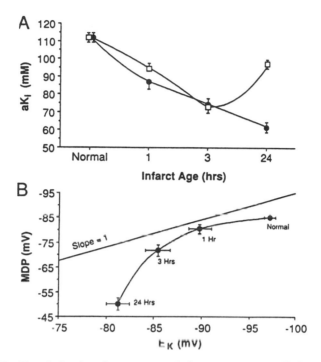

Figure 3.43: In Panel A, the time course of change in intracellular K^+ activity in Purkinje fibers in the endocardial border zone of canine infarcts is shown. Intracellular K^+ activity (a_{Ki}) is plotted on the ordinate and infarct age is on the abscissa. The measurements indicated by the filled symbols were made soon after the infarct was isolated and superfusion was begun in the tissue chamber. The measurements indicated by the unfilled symbols were obtained after several hours of superfusion. In Panel B the maximum diastolic potential (MDP) of Purkinje fibers in the endocardial border zone of infarcts of different ages is plotted on the ordinate as the solid circles versus E_K in millivolts on the abscissa. The straight line indicates a theoretical relationship between the two with a slope of 1. (Reproduced from Kline et al. (1992) with permission).

of the activation curve of I_{K1}, which was several fold smaller than the associated shift of reversal potential (Cohen et al. 1989). From these results it is predicted that the reduction of intracellular K^+ in the Purkinje fibers of the endocardial border zone to around 50 mmol/L should slow both activation and deactivation of the inward rectifier K^+ current with little shift of the activation curve on the voltage axis. When intracellular K^+ declines, E_K and thus the resting potential becomes more positive. At these more positive potentials the conductance due to I_{K1}, and hence the membrane conductance should be significantly reduced.

The membrane potential of the depolarized Purkinje fibers in 24-hour-old infarcts hyperpolarizes during tissue bath superfusion for 6 hours. E_K also increases simultaneously because of an increase in intracellular K^+ activity. The intracellular K^+ activity after prolonged superfusion is shown by the un filled square at 24 hours in Figure 3.43A (compare with solid circle at 24 hours

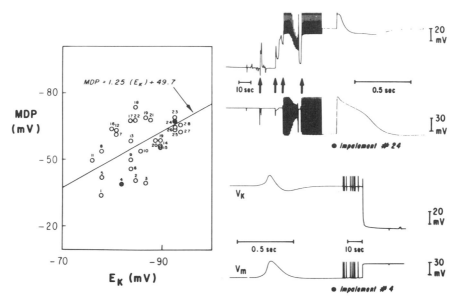

Figure 3.44: The graph on the left displays data points from double-barrel potassium microelectrode impalements in subendocardial Purkinje fibers from a canine infarct. Points are numbered in the order in which they were obtained during the experiment. During superfusion, both the maximum diastolic potential (MDP) and E_K became more negative. Records from impalements numbers 4 and 24 are shown at right (see solid points on left side plot). For each record the bottom trace, V_m, is the recording from the reference barrel and the top trace, V_K, is the differential output from the electrode (synonymous with K^+ activity). Upward arrows on these records indicated electrode advancement into the cell. Note that cell number 4 has a low maximum diastolic potential and depressed action potential waveform and that cell number 24 has a more polarized maximum diastolic potential and partially recovered action potential waveform. The straight line is the linear regression (r = 0.72, p < 0.001). (Reproduced from Dresdner et al. (1987) with permission.)

to see the magnitude of change). Therefore, the loss of K^+, which is a consequence of the prolonged ischemia can be reversed by exposure to an environment that is not ischemic. The results of an experiment showing this are also displayed in Figure 3.44. For each cell impalement with the double-barrel microelectrode, the maximum diastolic potential (MDP) and potassium equilibrium potential (E_K) are plotted and numbered in the order in which the recording was obtained during the experiment. The figure shows that with time during superfusion, both the MDP and E_K values become more negative. On the right-hand side of the figure are representative recordings from a depressed cell obtained within the first hour of tissue bath superfusion (impalement #4) and from a more recovered cell obtained several hours later (impalement #24). Therefore, there is uptake of K^+ with time. This may result from increased activity of the Na/K pump during superfusion of the isolated tissue (see below). As the cells take up K^+ and hyperpolarize, the difference between the MDP and E_K diminishes, indicating a change in the membrane conductance. This may be a result of the hyperpolarization itself, changes in the properties of the membrane channels, or the direct effects of increasing the intracellular K^+ concentration. After prolonged tissue bath superfusion (> 6 hours) intracellular K^+ activity is restored to normal although membrane potential is still depolarized by 5 to 10 mV (Dresdner et al. 1987). The persistent depolarization reflects persistent altered membrane conductance. An increase in membrane resistance has been measured in the Purkinje fibers in 24-hour-old infarcts, which is indicative of a decrease in resting membrane conductance (Argentieri et al. 1990), as might be caused by a decrease in K^+ conductance. In experiments on disaggregated, single Purkinje cells from 24-hour-old infarcts more than 2 hours after removal from the heart, a similar depolarization in the presence of an unaltered intracellular K^+ activity has also been found by Boyden et al. (1989a). The input resistance measured in the single cells was increased suggesting a decrease in membrane conductance causing the depolarization (rather than an increase in conductance, possibly to Na^+). The results can be explained by a decrease in potassium permeability. Therefore, a decrease in I_{K1} may persist even after the cells regain their intracellular K^+ (Boyden et al. 1989a). These experimental results also confirm that there are alterations in membrane properties that persist outside of the environment of the infarcted heart.

The loss of intracellular K^+, which is so severe in the surviving Purkinje fibers 1 day after coronary occlusion, actually begins early after the onset of ischemia. We have described this K^+ loss in ventricular muscle and how it contributes to the occurrence of the early ischemic arrhythmias in Chapter 11. During the early arrhythmias, the depolarization of the membrane potential of the muscle is mostly a result of an increase in the extracellular K^+ and not a reduction in the intracellular K^+. The amount of K^+ lost from the cells is only a small fraction of the intracellular K^+ concentration or activity, yet because of the restricted extracellular spaces it can cause a marked elevation of extracellular K^+. A simultaneous loss of K^+ from subendocardial Purkinje fibers has not been measured in the early minutes of ischemia and it is not known whether the depolarization that occurs in the Purkinje system during acute ischemia is related to K^+ loss from the Purkinje cells or from diffusion of K^+ from adjacent ischemic, ventricular muscle cells. Eventually ischemic cells that remain viable over prolonged periods of time but continue to lose K^+ do have a significant reduction in the intracellular K^+, which affects the resting potential. One hour after coronary occlusion, intracellular K^+ activity of the subendocardial Purkinje fibers, measured *in vitro* with ion-sensitive microelectrodes was 87 mmol/L shortly after superfusion was begun in the experiments of Kline et al. (1992). This value is plotted on the graph in Figure 3.43A (solid circle at 1 hour). The reduction in intracellular K^+ accounts for almost the entire depolarization of the membrane potential at this time (which decreases to -80 mV) since the K^+ equilibrium potential is reduced by the same amount (see Figure 3.43B, solid circle at 1 hour). The loss of K^+ continues during the subsequent hours after coronary occlusion and it is reduced to around 74 mmol/L by 3 hours after the occlusion (Figure 3.43A) (Kline et al. 1992). Up to this time the reduction of the K^+ equilibrium potential explains the decrease in the maximum diastolic potential. For times later than 3 hours, additional changes in the membrane conductance have begun to occur. This is indicated in Figure 3.43B by the solid circle showing the relationship between MDP and E_K at 24 hours. At this time the reduction of E_K is no longer sufficient to explain the large depolarization of the membrane potential.

How is the K^+ lost from the Purkinje cells in the endocardial border zone after coronary occlusion? It is possible that the same increase in K^+ channel conductance and passive K^+ efflux that has been proposed for ventricular muscle occurs (see Chapter II). What is clear is that K^+ lost from the Purkinje cells during the early hours of ischemia cannot all be pumped back into the cells because of a depression in the activity of the Na/K exchange pump. This depression is evident by 3 hours after the coronary occlusion (Dresdner et al. 1988). In the depolarized Purkinje fibers at 24 hours, intracellular Na^+ activity is elevated by about 6 mmol/L, to a level of 15 mmol/L (Dresdner et al. 1987). This suggests an inhibition of the pump at that time but may not be an accurate indication of the magnitude of this inhibition. Because the Purkinje cells begin to depolarize shortly after the onset of ischemia and continue to depolarize further with time the electrical gradient that drives Na^+ into the intracellular space continues to decrease during the first 24 hours after occlusion. Therefore, even in the presence of a depressed pump, the intracellular Na^+ does not go to very high values. Boyden and Dresdner (1990) have studied Na/K pump function in enzymatically dispersed single Purkinje cells from the subendocardial border zone of 24-hour old infarcts and found no abnormalities in its ability to extrude Na^+ from the cell or to generate current. However, the cells that were studied may not have had low membrane potentials and a significant elevation of intracellular Na^+. It is these very depressed cells found in the endocardial border zone that are expected to have abnormal pump activity and not those cells of the border zone with more normal membrane potentials. It is also possible that the Na/H exchange pump contributes to the elevated Na^+. This exchanger transports Na^+ into cells in exchange for extruded H^+ (Lazdunski et al. 1985).

The mechanism for K^+ loss from the subendocardial Purkinje cells that leads to depolarization still needs to be explained, as does the mechanism for maintenance of intracellular electroneutrality since positively charged Na^+ does not replace the lost K^+ ions (Dresdner et al. 1987). It was described in our discussion on the electrophysiological effects of acute ischemia how pH changes caused by alterations of metabolism may contribute to the electrophysiological changes in the ventricular muscle. Intracellular acidification, which is a consequence of ischemia in ventricular muscle may be coupled to the loss of K^+ from the cells and, in addition, an acid environment has a direct depolarizing effect through the actions of protons on the sarcolemma from both the intracellular and extracellular surfaces (Lauer et al. 1984). However, a decrease in intracellular pH caused by ischemic-induced changes in metabolism has not been found in the subendocardial Purkinje fibers within 1 hour after coronary occlusion (Kline et al. 1992).

The intracellular measurements of pH had to be made in fibers in the isolated superfused preparations with the earliest measurements recorded after about 20 minutes in the tissue chamber. The possibility exists, therefore, that some ischemic changes in pH reverted back towards normal in the Tyrode's superfusate, since intracellular pH is quite sensitive to extracellular pH that was normal in the superfusate. Intracellular measurements at 3 and 24 hours after coronary occlusion showed that the intracellular pH of subendocardial Purkinje fibers in infarcts was no different from normal Purkinje fibers when superfused with a 12 mmol/L bicarbonate Tyrode's that had a pH of 7.2 (Dresdner et al. 1989; Kline et al. 1992). At 24 hours, the Purkinje fiber intracellular pH was slightly alkaline compared to normal in a 24 mmol/L bicarbonate Tyrode's that had a pH of 7.4.

The surface pH of the Purkinje cells in infarcts (the pH just outside the sarcolemma) was also similar to the normal Purkinje cells implying that the steady state rate of production of acid equivalents was the same as in normal. The surface pH layer arises from the accumulation of weak acids and/or dissolved CO_2 produced by cellular metabolism (de Hemptinne 1980; de Hemptinne and Huguenin 1984; Vanheel and de Hemptinne 1985). Increased glycolysis due to ischemia or hypoxia should acidify the surface pH layer as it acidifies intracellular pH. Since these measurements *in vitro* were not made immediately after the tissue was removed from the heart, there is still the possibility that an acidic pH present *in situ* may have reverted to normal during the period in the oxygenated Tyrode's solution before the measurements were made.

Thus, acidification may still be the mechanism by which K^+ is lost from the cells without a comparable gain in Na^+, but it is not the mechanism for the maintenance of the lowered intracellular K^+ once it is lost. Cellular K^+ loss may occur from the Purkinje fibers in the endocardial border zone during acute ischemia and may be accompanied by intracellular acidification but the acidification then subsides by 24 hours due to unknown metabolic adjustments leaving the intracellular K^+ still reduced. This is consistent with observations that 75% of the total intracellular K^+ reduction has already occurred by 3 hours after the occlusion (Kline et al. 1992). The Purkinje cells in the infarcts may not remain acidic since they are separated from normal oxygenated cavity blood only by a thin endothelial sheath and are at most 1 to 3 cell layers from the endocardial surface. Or the effects of ischemia may occur gradually as indicated by the gradual build-up in the intracellular lipid droplets and this gradual effect is not associated with persistent cellular acidification.

We can then hypothesize how membrane depolarization and the reduction in intracellular K^+ can be sustained once cellular acidification has subsided. This mechanism may be related to our discussion on the effects of low intracellular K^+ on membrane conductance. After the acute phase of net cellular K^+ loss, the resulting low intracellular K^+ may be sustained as the result of the altered membrane conductance coupled with the suppression of the Na/K pump (Dresdner et al. 1987; Kline et al. 1992).

Prolongation of the Action Potential Duration   The ionic mechanism for the prolongation of the Purkinje fiber action potential duration that occurs after coronary occlusion is unknown. In our discussion on lipid metabolism, we have mentioned the possibility that depression of the Na/K pump by free fatty acids would be expected to cause prolongation because of a decrease in outward pump current. However, Boyden and Dresdner (1990) did not find a decrease in pump current in well-polarized, single Purkinje cells from the subendocardial border zone even though these cells have a prolonged action potential duration (Boyden et al. 1989a). Another possible cause for the prolongation that has been considered is the uncoupling of the surviving Purkinje cells from the underlying dying ventricular muscle. If uncoupling occurs, the repolarizing influence of electrotonic current flow from ventricular muscle with shorter action potential durations should be lost, leading to prolongation of Purkinje fiber action potential duration. However, Purkinje fiber action potential duration in the subendocardial border zone eventually returns to normal after several weeks (Friedman et al. 1975), after collateral blood flow returns to this region (Dangman et al. 1979), even though the Purkinje cells remain uncoupled from the muscle cells. Also, enzymatically dispersed Purkinje myocytes from the endocardial border zone have a longer action potential duration than myocytes from normal subendocardium (Boyden et al. 1989a). Therefore, although uncoupling may contribute to the initial appearance of a prolonged action potential duration, other more important factors must be responsible, such as alterations in membrane channels causing repolarization. Elucidation of these alterations awaits the result of voltage-clamp studies on inward and outward currents during repolarization, in the enzymatically dispersed single Purkinje cells. An indication that the action potential prolongation is not a result of a significant increase in Na^+ window current (Attwell et al. 1979) is the small effect that lidocaine (Allen et al. 1978) and tetrodotoxin (Bril et al. 1989) have on the prolonged action potential duration, whereas both compounds significantly shorten normal Purkinje fiber action potentials by blocking this Na^+ current (Colatsky 1982; Coraboeuf et al. 1976). Alternatively the membrane channels affected by lidocaine and TTX may be altered so that they are no longer sensitive to these agents.

Reduction in Action Potential Upstroke and Enhanced Impulse Initiation
The causes of the reduction in action potential upstroke have not been elucidated. It may simply result from depolarization of the membrane potential. Alternatively, it may result from effects of prolonged ischemia on the function of the fast Na^+ channels.

Likewise, the cause of automaticity is uncertain. It also may result because of depolarization of the membrane potential since abnormal automaticity does occur in normal Purkinje fibers when they are depolarized. Another possibility that is worth testing is that an increase in intracellular calcium leads to spontaneous firing in much the same way described for atrial muscle by Escande et al. (1987) (see Chapter I). We suspect that intracellular calcium in the Purkinje fibers of the subendocardial border zone 24 hours after occlusion is elevated. Part of this elevation may be a consequence of the depolarized membrane potential since it has been shown that depolarization of sheep Purkinje cells (Sheu and Fozzard 1982) and rat ventricular cells (Sheu et al. 1987) elevates free intracellular calcium. In addition, depolarization of the membrane potential may alter net calcium fluxes by the Na/Ca exchanger, decreasing outward calcium transport and adding to intracellular stores (Mullins 1981; Sheu and Fozzard 1982; DiFrancesco and Noble 1985). Since the concentration of ATP also falls during prolonged ischemia, calcium ATPase activity may also decrease, resulting in a decrease of extrusion of calcium from the cell by the sarcolemmal calcium pump (Sheu and Blaustein 1986). The increased intracellular calcium may also be the cause of delayed afterdepolarizations and triggered activity when it occurs (Gough and El-Sherif 1989). In fact, the mechanisms causing abnormal automaticity and delayed afterdepolarization may be related as we discussed in Chapter I. The level of membrane potential may determine which mechanism occurs; at more depolarized levels the elevated intracellular calcium may not be oscillatory, leading to sustained activity.

Electrophysiological Properties of Surviving Myocardial Fibers in the Epicardial Border Zone

We mentioned that there is some evidence that 24 hours after coronary occlusion, some ventricular ectopic impulses might arise in epicardial muscle over the infarct (the epicardial border zone). At 24 hours, epicardial border zone muscle cells studied *in vitro* in isolated superfused tissue preparations have low resting potentials (-60 to -80 mV) (Ursell et al. 1985; Dangman et al. 1988), which is at least partly a result of a significant decrease in intracellular K^+ (Hanna et al. 1987). Spontaneous diastolic depolarization causing abnormal impulse initiation has been recorded in these cells, most often after exposure to catecholamines (Dangman et al. 1988). Cells with very low membrane potentials (less than -65 mV) did not require the presence of catecholamines to initiate impulses spontaneously. Delayed afterdepolarizations and triggered activity were also caused by catecholamines in those cells with membrane potentials more negative than -70 mV (Dangman et al. 1988). These findings in the isolated preparations may explain how ventricular impulses of epicardial origin can occur during accelerated idioventricular rhythms.

The epicardial border zone has a much more important role as being the site of probable origin of the rapid ventricular tachycardias that lead to sudden death between 12 and 18 hours after the coronary occlusion. We described how these tachycardias are often initiated by several closely coupled premature impulses. The tachycardias are accompanied by continuous electrical activity in the epicardial border zone that indicates the occurrence of reentrant excitation in this region (Scherlag et al. 1989). Reentrant tachycardias arising in the epicardial border zone can also be initiated by a short burst of electrical stimuli applied to the ventricles (El-Sherif et al. 1982; Scherlag et al. 1983). The reentrant circuits have been mapped and characterized (El-Sherif et al. 1982) and are very similar to those which have been studied 1 week or more after occlusion in healing infarcts. These characteristics are described in the next chapter along with the characteristics of reentrant circuits in the older infarcts.

Chapter IV

Later Phases of Ventricular Arrhythmias: Late Hospital and Chronic Ventricular Arrhythmias

The effects of a period of ischemia caused by obstruction of a coronary artery on the electrophysiology of cardiac cells may occur quickly, causing the acute or prehospital arrhythmias that we discussed in Chapter II. The effects of ischemia may also progress over a number of hours, leading to the spontaneous delayed arrhythmias that generally occur within the first 1–2 days after coronary occlusion, as described in Chapter III. It has also been documented that arrhythmias may continue to occur after these early periods in patients who have an infarction (Bigger et al. 1977). We will discuss both the clinical and experimental evidence that shows that these later phases of arrhythmias have still different underlying electrophysiology than the earlier phases and detail what is known about their mechanisms. The later phases of clinical arrhythmias can be subdivided into "late hospital" arrhythmias, which are arrhythmias documented just prior to hospital discharge, and posthospital arrhythmias—also referred to as chronic arrhythmias—which occur after the patient is discharged from the hospital. Experimental animal models have been developed to study the electrophysiology of each of these periods.

Some Clinical Characteristics of Late Hospital and Chronic Ventricular Arrhythmias

Late Hospital Arrhythmias

Although the time of discharge from the hospital for patients treated for infarction has changed over the years, the time period for the classification of late hospital arrhythmias may be considered to be about 1 to 3 weeks after admission for an acute myocardial infarction. During this period, changes that occur in the electrophysiological properties of the myocardial cells surviving in and around the infarcted region as the infarct starts to heal may result in the occurrence of these arrhythmias. The documentation of late hospital

357

arrhythmias occurred after it became easier to record continuous electrocardi-ograms for long periods of time (6–72-hour Holter recordings) since some of the late arrhythmias appear only infrequently and can only be detected during long periods of continuous monitoring (Bigger et al. 1986a). Bigger et al. (1977; 1986a; 1986b) have summarized the data in the literature describing the fre-quency of occurrence of ventricular arrhythmias in the late hospital period. Although the incidence of arrhythmias decreases between the acute phase and 5 days after hospital admission, it increases again during the subsequent late hospital period so that about 20% of patients have more than ten ventricular premature depolarizations (VPDs) per hour, 43% have multiform VPDs, and 10% have ventricular tachycardia (Bigger et al. 1981; 1986a). Most tachycar-dias (3 or more consecutive ventricular beats at rates greater than 100 per minute) begin with ventricular premature beats that occur after the T wave (late coupled) and terminate spontaneously (Bigger et al. 1981). Late hospital ventricular tachycardia often occurs in those patients with the most severe infarction as indicated by high serum enzyme levels, and depressed left ventric-ular function (Schulze et al. 1977).

There is not always a relationship between the occurrence of tachycardia in the late hospital period and the severity of the early acute arrhythmias in the coronary care unit; patients with the most severe acute arrhythmias are not always the patients that have tachycardias in the late hospital period (Moss et al. 1971; Vismara et al. 1975). For those patients that have severe acute arrhythmias as well as late arrhythmias, we could find no published clinical data to document whether the electrocardiographic characteristics of the late arrhythmias are the same or different from the acute arrhythmias, e.g., rate, QRS morphology, patterns of onset, and termination. A comparison of the two periods might indicate whether the site of origin and mechanism of the arrhyth-mias remain the same or change. As we will discuss, we believe that both mechanism and site of origin change with time.

Subsequent mortality during the first year after discharge from the hospi-tal has been related to the incidence and type of the late hospital arrhythmias. There is a significant increase in subsequent mortality in patients with large numbers of late hospital VPDs (10–30 VPDs per hour) (Bigger et al. 1986a) or ventricular tachycardia (Ruberman et al. 1977; Bigger et al. 1981; 1984; Kleiger et al. 1981). Figure 4.1, from the studies of Bigger and his group (1986b), shows the relationship between survival and time after infarction for four groups of patients who had 24-hour continuous ECG recording taken approximately 11 days after myocardial infarction. The curve labeled 0 is sur-vival of those patients with no detected VPDs; curve 1 is survival of those patients with single VPDs; curve 2 is survival of those patients with paired VPDs; and curve 3 is survival of those patients with runs of VPDs or ventricular tachycardia. Clearly, survival is reduced as the incidence and severity of ar-rhythmias increases. Ventricular tachycardia is a significant risk factor for cardiac death independent of depressed left ventricular function (Moss et al. 1979; Bigger et al. 1984; Mukharji et al. 1984). However, the lack of arrhyth-mias in the late hospital period does not preclude the later development of

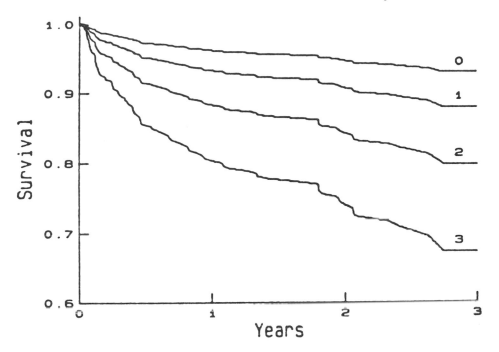

Figure 4.1: Relationship between 2-year mortality (survival) and repetitive ventricular premature depolarizations (VPDs) detected in 820 24-hour continuous ECG recordings made 11 ± 3 days after myocardial infarction. The percentages of patients in the categories are as follows: 0 = no VPDs at all (14%); 1 = only single VPDs (58%); 2 = paired VPDs (17%); 3 = runs of VPDs 11%. (Reproduced from Bigger et al. (1986b) with permission.)

potentially lethal arrhythmias. Some patients who do not have late hospital arrhythmias go on to develop ventricular arrhythmias during the posthospital period and these arrhythmias may also be fatal. Many of the patients who later develop ventricular tachycardia have large myocardial scars or aneurysms, which form as the infarct heals and, which may become a source of the tachycardias.

Exercise stress testing has been used in an attempt to identify some of the patients who do not show spontaneously occurring ventricular arrhythmias during the late hospital period, but may be at risk for subsequent arrhythmic death (Théroux et al. 1979). The theoretical consideration behind this procedure is that an ischemic electrophysiological milieu that is capable of causing lethal arrhythmias may be provoked to do so by the sympathetic nervous system, whereas sympathetic influences on the heart do not usually cause ventricular arrhythmias in the absence of an ischemic substrate. The provocation of arrhythmias by the sympathetics may occur spontaneously in some patients with ischemic heart disease during the course of their natural activities. The exercise test is a way of provoking the interaction between the sympathetics and the ischemic myocardium under controlled conditions. When exercise provokes the occurrence of both ST segment abnormalities and ventricular arrhythmias in people who have not had a myocardial infarct, then there is likely to be extensive underlying ischemic heart disease (Helfant et al. 1974; Weld et al. 1981). Exercise testing of patients in the late hospital phase of myocardial infarction can provoke arrhythmias when none are present or increase the severity of arrhythmias (Ericsson et al. 1973). The data indicate that patients with arrhythmias provoked by the testing are at an increased risk for subsequent cardiac death with a greater risk in those patients with more than ten VPDs per hour, paired VPDs, or ventricular tachycardia (Granath et al. 1977; Weld et al. 1981).

Chronic Ventricular Arrhythmias

After discharge from the hospital, ventricular arrhythmias that are documented in the late hospital period may persist with similar characteristics (Kotler et al. 1973; Moss et al. 1976; Van Durme and Pannier 1976; Kleiger et al. 1981), may persist but change their characteristics (Oliver et al. 1975; Ripley et al. 1975; Moss et al. 1976), or may disappear. Arrhythmias may also begin to occur in some of the patients who had no documented late hospital arrhythmias (Marchlinski 1988). Changes in the characteristics of arrhythmias, or disappearance or appearance of arrhythmias are all possible because of the continued evolution of the infarct structure and electrophysiology during infarct healing. Although it is not yet possible to directly relate the occurrence of chronic arrhythmias to particular features of the infarct from the clinical studies, we will point out later how the results of experimental laboratory studies suggest special structural and electrophysiological characteristics of the infarct that favor arrhythmogenesis. These characteristics may not develop until later in the healing process (after several weeks), or if they are present early during healing, they may subsequently disappear. Sometimes the occurrence of chronic arrhythmias can be related to the extent of the coronary disease (Lown et al. 1975).

From the data available from various epidemiological studies, it seems that approximately 60% of patients who have had a myocardial infarction have some kind of documented ventricular arrhythmias after hospital discharge, with sustained ventricular tachycardia present in about 3% (Kotler et al. 1973; Wellens et al. 1983) and nonsustained ventricular tachycardia present in 10% to 20% (for review see Willems 1990). Ventricular arrhythmias can also be induced by exercise testing in some of those patients who do not have spontaneously occurring arrhythmias (Califf et al. 1983). As with the late hospital arrhythmias, it has been shown that there is a relationship between the occurrence and severity of arrhythmias and the occurrence of sudden death both in the first year after discharge and later (Kotler et al. 1973; Bigger et al. 1977; Cobb et al. 1980; Myerburg et al. 1980; Ruskin et al. 1980). The risk is greater when premature ventricular depolarizations are frequent or complex (multiform QRS morphologies) (Ruberman et al. 1977; Moss et al. 1979; Bigger et al.

1982). According to some observations, frequent ventricular premature depolarizations may trigger ventricular fibrillation. The highest mortality is associated with the presence of ventricular tachycardia (Bigger et al. 1982). The prognosis of patients developing sustained tachycardia is poor: despite intensive antiarrhythmic therapy, including surgery, overall 1-year mortality is in the order of 20% (Wellens et al. 1983; Willems et al. 1990). Sustained ventricular tachycardia may either directly cause a marked decrease in blood pressure and hemodynamic collapse or may eventually degenerate into ventricular fibrillation with the same hemodynamic results. Many of these patients are characterized by the presence of multivessel coronary artery disease, extensive anteroseptal myocardial infarction, right bundle branch block, the presence of a left ventricular aneurysm, and severe left ventricular dysfunction (Lie et al. 1978; Marchlinski et al. 1983).

Some Characteristics of Late Hospital and Chronic Ventricular Arrhythmias from Clinical Electrophysiological Studies: An Overview

Limited information that is helpful in determining the mechanisms causing the late hospital and chronic arrhythmias has been obtained from the analysis of the electrocardiograms during the spontaneous occurrence of these arrhythmias. The major contribution of the electrocardiographic studies has been to show that these arrhythmias occur and are related to subsequent sudden death. The information that is essential for determining these mechanisms comes from clinical electrophysiological studies. There is much more information from clinical studies on electrophysiological mechanisms causing the late hospital and chronic ventricular arrhythmias than there is on the acute and subacute arrhythmias. The results of a large number of clinical electrophysiological studies, beginning with the initial investigation by Wellens and his collaborators in 1972, have provided data showing that reentrant excitation is the principal causative mechanism. The techniques that have been used to elucidate the pathophysiology causing the arrhythmias and to locate the reentrant circuits in these clinical studies include: (1) programmed electrical stimulation; (2) extracellular electrical recordings, e.g., electrogram characteristics, activation maps, signal averaging; and (3) ablation of arrhythmogenic regions with surgery or with catheter techniques. These clinical studies have been done either during cardiac catheterization or open heart surgery when the heart can be electrically stimulated and local extracellular electrical activity recorded. Each of these approaches has provided pieces of the puzzle that has been put together to arrive at the conclusion that the primary arrhythmogenic mechanism is reentry. For the most part, reentry has not been directly demonstrated in the clinical studies by the methods one would choose to use under ideal conditions in the experimental laboratory so that Mines' criteria for proving reentry could be fulfilled, e.g., the movement of the excitation wave around the circuit has not usually been followed and then the circuit severed to terminate the arrhythmia. However, the responses of the cardiac rhythm to electrical stimulation, as well as the characteristics of local electrical activity provide a convincing argument for a reentrant mechanism. This is further supported by the results of more detailed laboratory experiments on similar kinds of arrhythmias in experimental animals.

Since there has been the opportunity for so much clinical investigation of the electrophysiology of these later phases of ischemic arrhythmias (unlike the earlier phases), information on mechanisms from laboratory experiments has not been dominant as was the case for the acute and subacute arrhythmias discussed in Chapters II and III. Instead, the experimental laboratory studies have been closely intertwined with the clinical studies, and the synthesis of the two provides an overall picture of electrophysiological mechanisms. Since there is such a close relationship between the clinical and the experimental data, we find it difficult to discuss each aspect separately as we did in the previous chapters on the earlier arrhythmia phases. In this chapter, we discuss both the experimental laboratory data and the results of the clinical studies together in an attempt to synthesize an overall view of the arrhythmia mechanisms. We have tried to be careful to clearly point out which information is from human studies and which is from laboratory studies to avoid confusion.

Induction of Ventricular Arrhythmias by Programmed Electrical Stimulation

Sustained Ventricular Tachycardia

Sustained monomorphic tachycardia (tachycardia with a single, uniform QRS complex lasting for more than 30 seconds or requiring termination because of hemodynamic compromise) can be initiated by programmed electrical stimulation in more than 90% of patients who have documented spontaneously occurring episodes of this arrhythmia either in the late hospital or chronic phases after myocardial infarction. The induced tachycardias are often the same as the spontaneously occurring tachycardias, as indicated by the same QRS morphology and rate. The initiation of tachycardia by electrical stimulation is very important evidence supporting a reentrant mechanism and excluding an automatic mechanism. According to Josephson et al. (1984) sustained ventricular tachycardia can be induced by premature electrical stimuli delivered during sinus rhythm in 15% to 25% of patients with spontaneously occurring sustained ventricular tachycardia. During basic ventricular pacing and stimulation from the right ventricle, a single premature stimulus can induce tachycardia in about 20% to 30% of patients; two successive premature stimuli can induce sustained tachycardia in an additional 55% of patients; and three successive premature stimuli are necessary to induce tachycardia in still an additional 20% of patients (Brugada et al. 1984; Buxton et al. 1984a; Mann et al. 1985; Kudenchuk et al. 1986). In patients in whom tachycardias cannot be induced, the infusion of isoproterenol may sometimes enable successful induction (Reddy and Gettes 1979; Freedman et al. 1984). The premature stimuli must be appropriately timed to occur at a certain critical location in the basic cycle length, usually near the descending limb of the T wave of the previous impulse. This characteristic is illustrated in Figure 4.2, which shows the initiation of ventricular tachycardia by a single premature stimulus. We need only be concerned with the ECG recordings now, which are the top two traces in each panel. The first two ECG complexes from left to right are a result of the basic pacing stimuli and are followed by a premature stimulus at the arrow. The coupling interval of the premature stimulus is shorter in panel B than in panel A, and still shorter in panel C. Whereas in panels A and B the prematurely stimulated depolarizations are followed by the resumption of sinus rhythm, in panel C a sustained monomorphic ventricular tachycardia follows the prematurely stimulated QRS complex. Tachycardias may be initiated over a range of premature coupling intervals similar to the initiation of supraventricular tachycardia that we discussed in Chapter I. Figure 4.3 shows an example of a tachycardia induced by two successive premature stimuli (S_2 and S_3) during basic drive of the ventricle at a constant cycle length (S_1-S_1). The top panel shows that when the stimuli were delivered to the right ventricular apex no tachycardia was induced. In the bottom panel, two premature stimuli delivered at the exact same coupling intervals to the left ventricle induced tachycardia. When one to two premature stimuli delivered to the right ventricle fail to induce tachyarrhythmias, the same stimulus pattern delivered to the left ventricle may succeed in some patients not induced from the right side (Robertson et al. 1981; Morady et al. 1984a). In a small percentage of patients with spontaneously occurring sustained tachycardia, premature stimulation may not induce the arrhythmia, but it can be induced by rapid pacing of the ventricles (Josephson et al. 1985). A tachycardia induced in this way is shown in Figure 4.4; the first five QRS complexes in the top two traces are stimulated at a cycle length of 300 msec, followed by a tachycardia with a slightly longer cycle length. In most patients it is easier to induce tachycardia with premature stimuli than with rapid pacing or even not possible to induce tachycardia with rapid pacing when it can be induced by premature stimulation. This characteristic is reasonable evidence that the tachycardias are not caused by triggered activity dependent on delayed afterdepolarizations, which are expected to be more easily initiated by rapid stimulation.

In addition to the induction of sustained monomorphic ventricular tachycardia with the same QRS morphology as the spontaneously occurring tachycardia, sustained monomorphic tachycardias with other morphologies can sometimes be induced (Buxton et al. 1984a). The induction of sustained tachycardias with QRS morphologies other than the spontaneously occurring one is still considered to be a result of the ischemic disease.

Sustained monomorphic ventricular tachycardia has also been induced by programmed stimulation in more than 50% of patients without documented spontaneously occurring sustained tachycardia, who have been revived from an

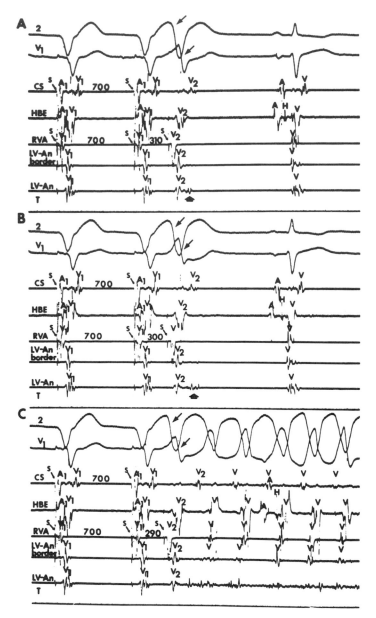

Figure 4.2: Initiation of ventricular tachycardia (VT) in a patient with myocardial infarct by stimulated ventricular premature depolarizations. Each panel is organized from top to bottom as follows: ECG leads 2 and V_1 and electrograms from the coronary sinus (CS), His bundle region (HBE), right ventricular apex (RVA), the border of a left ventricular aneurysm (LV-An), and within the LV-An. In panels A to C, progressively premature ventricular stimuli (arrows and V_2) were delivered during a ventricular paced cycle length of 700 msec (V_1-V_1). An increasing degree of fragmentation and delay can be seen in the LV-An as the premature coupling interval was decreased (broad arrow). At a premature coupling interval of 290 msec, continuous fractionated activity developed and VT ensued (panel C). (Reproduced from Josephson and Seides (1979) with permission.)

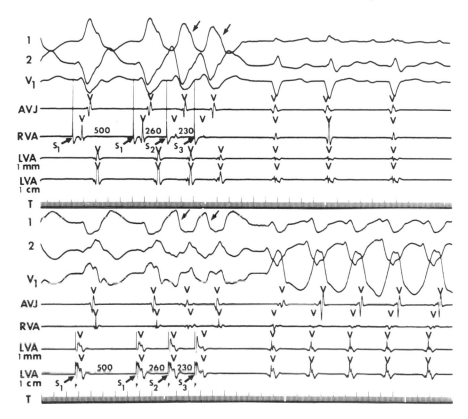

Figure 4.3: Initiation of ventricular tachycardia in a patient with a myocardial infarct by two premature stimuli. In both panels, surface leads I, II, and V_1 are shown along with electrogram recordings from the atrioventricular junction (AVJ), right ventricular apex (RVA), and left ventricular apex (LVA). In the top panel, two ventricular extrastimuli (arrows and S_2, S_3) delivered from the right ventricular apex failed to initiate a tachycardia. In the bottom panel, two ventricular premature stimuli (arrows and S_2, S_3) delivered at the exact same coupling intervals to the left ventricle initiated ventricular tachycardia. (T = time lines). (Reproduced from Robertson et al. (1981) with permission.)

episode of cardiac arrest attributed to ventricular fibrillation. In these patients, triple premature stimuli have been required to induce tachycardia more frequently than in patients with documented sustained ventricular tachycardia that is hemodynamically tolerated and induction by single extrastimuli is rare. The triple extrastimuli are also more effective when applied to the left ventricle than to the right ventricle (Buxton et al. 1984a). The rate of the induced tachycardias is usually very fast and they may eventually cause fibrillation.

Until now, this discussion has been concerned with the induction of sustained monomorphic tachycardia by programmed electrical stimulation in patients with documented spontaneously occurring ventricular tachycardia or sudden death. Sustained monomorphic ventricular tachycardia may also be

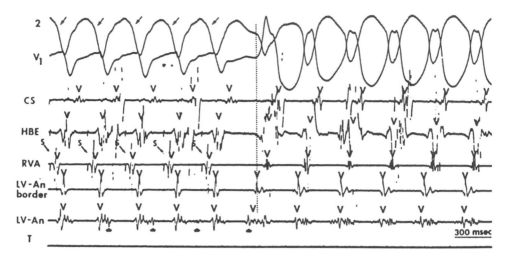

Figure 4.4: Ventricular tachycardia (VT) induced by ventricular pacing in a patient with a myocardial infarct. The figure is organized as in Figure 4.2. Ventricular pacing from the right ventricle (arrows and S) produced gradual fragmentation and delay in the LV-An electrogram (broad arrows), that resulted in VT when pacing was discontinued. During ventricular pacing, the electrogram in the LV-An occurred late in the QRS complex but appeared prior to the first beat of the tachycardia; thus, reentry may have occurred in the area recorded by the LV-An electrogram. (Reproduced from Josephson et al. (1978c) with permission.)

induced during the late hospital phase of myocardial infarction in some patients who do not have spontaneous occurrence of this arrhythmia (Hamer et al. 1982; Marchlinski et al. 1983; Richards et al. 1983; Breithardt et al. 1985; Denniss et al. 1985; Roy et al. 1985; 1986; Waspe et al. 1985b; Brugada et al. 1986). Sustained monomorphic ventricular tachycardia is also occasionally induced in patients with a healed myocardial infarct and a left ventricular aneurysm when the occurrence of spontaneous episodes of tachycardia has not been documented (Buxton et al. 1984a). The ability to initiate sustained ventricular tachycardia in these patients indicates that the heart contains an electrophysiological substrate that is capable of causing the arrhythmia. This substrate is the reentrant circuit that we will discuss in detail in a later section. It is commonly believed (and supported by evidence) that sustained monomorphic tachycardias cannot be induced in hearts without either ischemic or structural disease, or evidence of spontaneously occurring tachycardia (Brugada et al. 1984; Buxton et al. 1984a; 1984b; Morady et al. 1984b). Although spontaneously occurring tachycardias may not have been documented at the time tachycardias are induced by stimulation, the presence of a potential reentrant circuit may eventually result in the spontaneous occurrence of the arrhythmia.

Polymorphic ventricular tachycardia, characterized by a changing QRS morphology, can also be induced in patients with ischemic heart disease and a prior myocardial infarction. In this setting, the tachycardia is not usually associated with a prolonged QT interval as it is in other clinical situations (for example, torsade de pointes). Polymorphic tachycardia may be induced in patients with documented spontaneous episodes of the arrhythmias or in survivors of cardiac arrest (Josephson et al. 1980; Ruskin et al. 1980; Buxton et al. 1984a; Stevenson et al. 1986). In the latter cases, the induced tachycardia often degenerates into ventricular fibrillation. Induction usually requires two or three premature stimuli delivered during regular ventricular pacing. Although polymorphic tachycardia may sometimes be a nonspecific arrhythmia induced by aggressive stimulation protocols (Brugada et al. 1983; 1984; Brugada and Wellens 1984b), its occurrence in the presence of a prior myocardial infarction and either documentation of the spontaneous occurrence of the arrhythmia or a history of prior syncope or cardiac arrest is evidence for it being caused by ischemia (Josephson 1992).

Although it was initially thought that the induction of ventricular tachycardia by stimulated premature impulses was simply mimicking the way in which tachycardias were naturally induced by spontaneously occurring premature impulses, this does not always seem to be the case. In many instances, spontaneous onset of tachycardia follows late coupled premature ventricular depolarizations, often with the same ECG morphology as the depolarizations during the tachycardia (Berger et al. 1988). The relationship between the mechanism for spontaneous and induced onset of tachycardia is not yet understood.

Nonsustained Ventricular Tachycardia

Nonsustained ventricular tachycardia (tachycardia lasting at least three beats and terminating spontaneously within approximately 30 seconds or less), may occur during the late hospital or chronic phases of infarction. It may be asymptomatic or may be associated with palpitations. The tachycardias might lead to fibrillation and sudden death, although proof awaits the results of ongoing clinical trials. Nonsustained tachycardias can be induced in these patients by programmed stimulation, which along with other characteristics, is evidence that they are caused by reentry. In general, the characteristics of initiation are similar to sustained tachycardias. Single, double, or triple premature stimuli might be needed for induction with the incidence of induction increasing with the number of stimuli. The stimuli must be properly timed in the cardiac cycle. The tachycardias can either be polymorphic or monomorphic (Buxton et al. 1984b). Figure 4.5 shows an example of both a spontaneously occurring polymorphic nonsustained tachycardia (top panel) and a similar nonsustained tachycardia that was induced in the same patient by programmed stimulation (bottom panel). Two extrastimuli applied to the right ventricle during basic pacing induced the tachycardia.

There is probably some mechanistic relationship between nonsustained and sustained ventricular tachycardia. Nonsustained ventricular tachycardia can also be induced in patients with sustained ventricular tachycardia (Vandepol et al. 1980; Livelli et al. 1982). It might occur at premature stimulus coup-

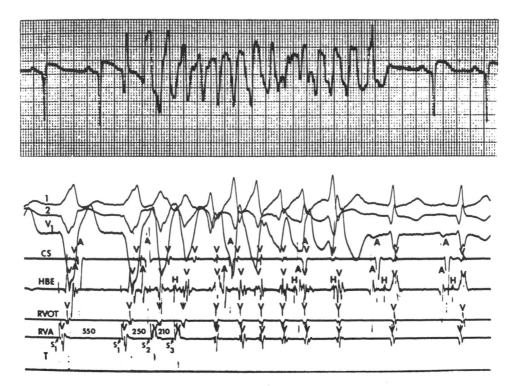

Figure 4.5: The electrocardiogram at the top shows a spontaneous episode of polymorphic nonsustained ventricular tachycardia initiated in a patient with a myocardial infarct by a late coupled ventricular premature depolarization. Underneath it is shown induction of polymorphic nonsustained ventricular tachycardia in the same patient by two right ventricular extrastimuli delivered while pacing at a cycle length of 550 msec. Surface electrocardiographic leads 1, 2, and V_1 are shown in addition to intracardiac recordings from the coronary sinus (CS), His bundle electrogram (HBE), right ventricular outflow tract (RVOT), and right ventricular apex (RVA). S denotes stimulus artifact with S_1 being the basic drive stimuli and S_2 and S_3 being the premature stimuli. A denotes atrial electrograms. V denotes ventricular electrograms. (Reproduced from Buxton et al. (1984b) with permission.)

ling intervals that are slightly longer than those necessary to induce the sustained tachycardia. In some patients with spontaneously occurring nonsustained ventricular tachycardia, sustained ventricular tachycardia can be induced by programmed stimulation even though sustained tachycardia does not occur spontaneously. The substrate for sustained tachycardia is therefore present. In patients with good left ventricular function, the available evidence shows a low risk of sudden death (Gomes et al. 1984; Veltri et al. 1985; Zheutlin et al. 1986; Buxton et al. 1987), but in patients with an ejection fraction < 40%, the induction of sustained tachycardia by programmed stimulation is associated with a significant risk of subsequent sudden death if effective antiarrhythmic therapy is not instituted (Buxton et al. 1987; Klein and Machell 1989; Wilber et al. 1990). These patients, therefore, are likely to have a spontaneous episode of the tachycardia that may precipitate fibrillation. Since nonsustained tachycardia can also be induced in some hearts without ischemic disease (Brugada et al. 1983; Morady et al. 1984b), it may not always be caused by ischemia and is sometimes considered to be a nonclinical arrhythmia. This is particularly true when it is induced by three or four premature stimuli (Morady et al. 1984a; Kudenchuk et al. 1986). When induced by a "nonaggressive" stimulation protocol (1–2 premature stimuli) in patients with ischemic heart disease and documented sustained or nonsustained tachycardia, it is most likely a result of the ischemic disease (Brugada and Wellens, 1984a).

Ventricular Fibrillation

Ventricular fibrillation can be induced in survivors of out-of-hospital cardiac arrest believed to have resulted from a spontaneous episode of fibrillation (Ruskin et al. 1980). Often an aggressive stimulation protocol using three premature stimuli is required to initiate the arrhythmia (Buxton et al. 1984a). Inducible ventricular fibrillation does not appear to be a very specific response, since fibrillation can also be induced by an aggressive stimulation protocol in patients without ischemic or structural heart disease, although it is not a common response (5 of 52 patients in the study of Brugada et al. 1984; 1 of 52 patients in the study of Morady et al. 1984b).

Ventricular Premature Depolarizations

Most of the clinical electrophysiological data do not address the cause of ventricular premature depolarizations, but rather are focused on ventricular tachycardia. Gomes et al. (1984) found that reentrant ventricular tachyarrhythmias could be induced by programmed stimulation in 27% of their patient study group with high-grade (Lown scoring system [Lown and Wolf 1971]) ventricular premature beats (also see Zheutlin et al. 1986). In this group, circuits most likely existed in which reentry could occur. The same circuits that caused tachycardia might also cause the ventricular premature depolarizations although this has not been proven. Many of these patients subsequently went on to develop spontaneous episodes of tachyarrhythmias. Other patients with high-grade ventricular premature beats did not have inducible arrhythmias nor did they develop spontaneous episodes of tachyarrhythmias.

Termination of Ventricular Arrhythmias by Programmed Stimulation

Once initiated, sustained ventricular tachycardias can also be terminated by electrical stimulation of the ventricles (Josephson et al. 1978b), which is additional evidence that the arrhythmias are reentrant. Termination of non-sustained tachycardia by stimulation cannot be demonstrated because of the transient nature of the arrhythmias and therefore, cannot provide evidence that these arrhythmias are caused by reentry. One means of terminating sustained tachycardia is with appropriately timed premature stimuli (Wellens 1971; Wellens et al. 1972; 1974; 1976; Josephson et al. 1978b; 1978d). The number of premature stimuli needed to terminate a tachycardia is dependent on the rate of the tachycardia. Tachycardias with rates slower than about 175 per minute can be terminated by single stimulated premature impulses (Josephson et al. 1978d; 1985; 1987). An example of termination of ventricular tachycardia by a single stimulated premature impulse is shown in Figure 4.6. The QRS complexes during tachycardia are labeled "T" and the prematurely stimulated QRS complex is labeled "S". Sinus rhythm resumed following this stimulated impulse. It usually takes two or more premature impulses stimulated in succession to terminate tachycardias with more rapid rates (Wellens et al. 1976; Josephson et al. 1978b; 1978d; Josephson et al. 1985) and rapid tachycardias may sometimes not be terminated by premature stimulation at all. It may require overdrive stimulation which, in general, is more effective in terminating most reentrant tachycardias (Fisher et al. 1978; Almendral et al. 1986a; 1986b). When a tachycardia can be terminated by a premature stimulus, the critical location where the premature depolarization must occur in the tachycardia cycle is quite variable from patient to patient. However this location is usually less than 50% of the cycle length. The critical location may in fact be a zone of coupling intervals. The site of stimulation also has an

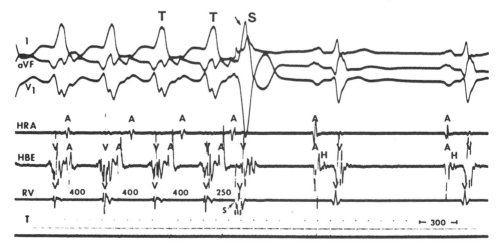

Figure 4.6: Termination of ventricular tachycardia (VT) by a single prematurely stimulated impulse (S) in a patient with a myocardial infarct. The figure is organized from top to bottom as follows: ECG leads 1, aVF, and V₁, and electrograms from the high right atrium (HRA), His bundle region (HBE), and right ventricle (RV). VT was terminated by a single VPD (S, arrow) delivered at a coupling interval of 250 msec. (Reproduced from Josephson and Seides (1979) with permission.)

important influence on the ability of premature impulses to terminate tachycardias (Rosenthal et al. 1986). For example, Josephson et al. (1985) showed results of a study in which single premature stimuli delivered to the right ventricular outflow tract terminated tachycardia while stimuli delivered to the right ventricular apex failed to terminate the arrhythmia.

As indicated above, overdrive stimulation (a train of stimuli applied to the ventricles at a rate faster than the tachycardia rate) is very effective in terminating sustained ventricular tachycardia. An appropriate rate and duration of stimulation is necessary for successful termination of the arrhythmias.

Summary

The preceding discussion is just a brief overview of some of the electrophysiological characteristics of the late hospital and posthospital ventricular arrhythmias to provide the background for our discussion of the animal models developed to investigate the arrhythmia mechanisms. These characteristics of initiation and termination by stimulation of the ventricles have been considered to be evidence, albeit indirect, that the underlying mechanism causing tachycardia is reentry. This conclusion is based on many of the experimental studies discussed in Chapter 1 showing that premature stimuli may set up the necessary conditions of unidirectional conduction block and slow conduction that are prerequisites for most kinds of reentry (Wit et al. 1976; Hoffman and Rosen 1981; Janse 1986a) and that during continuous reentry, a stimulated impulse that enters a reentrant circuit can render the circuit refractory to the circulating wave front, causing it to block (Mines 1913, 1914). Later in this chapter we will discuss in more detail how the responses to electrical stimulation can be used as evidence for a reentrant mechanism and show direct electrical measurements during tachycardias in hearts with infarcts that strongly suggest that this supposition is correct. However, the reader should also keep in mind that arrhythmias caused by delayed afterdepolarization-dependent triggered activity are expected to have some similar characteristics (see Chapter I). Initiation and termination of tachycardias by electrical stimulation alone does not prove that the arrhythmias are caused by reentry.

Animal Models of Late Hospital and Chronic Ventricular Arrhythmias

Goals of Experimental Studies

The results of the clinical studies summarized in the previous section indicate that many of the arrhythmias associated with the later phases of infarction require an appropriate trigger for initiation, which is sometimes a premature depolarization. Later, we will discuss the evidence that the arrhythmias arise from reentrant circuits in the infarcted region—the electrophysiological substrate. Therefore, both a trigger and an appropriate substrate may be necessary for occurrence of tachyarrhythmias. The premature ventricular depolarizations (trigger) may occur spontaneously or they may be provided by the stimulated impulses during programmed stimulation protocols. Arrhythmias however, do not occur in all patients with ischemic heart disease or healed myocardial infarcts even when the "trigger" is supplied from an external stimulus (Vandepol et al. 1980). What is special about certain infarcts that provide the appropriate electrophysiological substrate that enables arrhythmias to occur? This question has provided the impetus for the experimental studies that have had the goal of producing laboratory models of these arrhythmias. It has been the aim of the experimental electrophysiologist to develop animal models that have arrhythmias with characteristics similar to those that occur in humans, so that the models could be used to help elucidate the mechanisms causing the clinical arrhythmias with the additional techniques available in the experimental laboratory (Spear et al. 1982). In the development of these animal models, attempts have been made to fulfill a number of criteria that would make the models a realistic representation of the clinical events. These criteria include the following:

(1) The arrhythmias should occur in hearts with a healing or healed myocardial infarct since this is the pathophysiological setting of the clinical arrhythmias. In the clinical late hospital phase of myocardial infarction, the healing process in the damaged region of the heart is well underway and continues into the posthospital phase. The healing process may not be complete for more than 1 year.

(2) Ventricular premature depolarizations, tachycardia, and fibrillation should occur spontaneously and sometimes cause sudden death, as they do in humans.

(3) Ventricular arrhythmias should be initiated by the "triggers" that have been shown or suggested to initiate them in humans, including spontaneous or stimulated premature ventricular depolarizations and stress or other factors that may lead to an increase in sympathetic discharge. Unfortunately all the initiating events in humans are not known and therefore, cannot be built into the experimental models.

(4) The characteristics of the tachyarrhythmias should be similar to the clinical arrhythmias. Characteristics include appearance on the electrocardiogram and the response of the arrhythmias to programmed stimulation protocols.

(5) Reproducibility of arrhythmias over a long period of time, as has been shown to occur in some humans, is suggestive of a stable electrophysiological substrate and is necessary for evaluation of new and experimental antiarrhythmic drugs (Lynch and Lucchesi 1987).

There are a number of laboratory models using experimental animals that have been developed in an attempt to achieve the goals listed above. Although they have all fallen short in one respect or another, each has provided important information that has improved our understanding of the physiology of arrhythmias in healing and healed infarcts. All of the models have in common the fact that they involve an experimental occlusion of one or more coronary arteries. The exact method of occlusion, site of occlusion, and duration of occlusion differ among the models as they did for the acute ischemic models discussed in Chapter II. These different procedures of occlusion, in general, all result in infarcts, but the anatomical characteristics of the infarcts among models are different with particular reference to infarct size and location, the amount of surviving myocardial fibers in the infarcted region, and the location of these surviving fibers. These anatomical features are important in determining whether or not arrhythmias occur and the characteristics of arrhythmias that do occur (Gardner et al. 1984). Arrhythmias may not occur without the presence of surviving myocardial fibers in the infarcted region that act as the arrhythmogenic source (Euler et al. 1981; Wetstein et al. 1985b). The spatial arrangement of the surviving fibers may be important to provide reentrant circuits. The size of the circuits may influence the arrhythmia characteristics, for example, determine whether tachyarrhythmias are nonsustained or sustained or whether ventricular fibrillation occurs. All of these possibilities will be discussed in more detail and examples shown when the results of the experimental studies are described.

The size of the infarct and location of surviving myocardium might also influence whether autonomic nervous system dysfunction contributes to arrhythmogenesis. Since efferent sympathetic fibers travel in the subepicardium of the left ventricle, transmural infarcts that extend to the epicardial surface may damage them and produce heterogeneous sympathetic denervation of normal myocardium apical to the infarct (Barber et al. 1983; Zipes 1990). Afferent denervation of the autonomics might also occur (Barber et al. 1985; Stanton et al. 1989). Heterogeneous sympathetic influences on refractoriness as a result of chronic infarction may be arrhythmogenic (Gaide et al. 1983; Kozlovskis et al. 1986; Herre et al. 1988). Infarcts that do not extend to the epicardial surface should leave sympathetic efferents and normal function intact.

Our discussion will concentrate on the experimental studies utilizing canine models of infarction. These are the models with which we have had the most experience, and therefore, can contribute a discussion of the results of our own experiments. Important contributions to our understanding of the mechanisms of arrhythmias associated with healing and healed infarcts have also come from experimental studies on a feline model in the laboratory of Myerburg and Bassett (Myerburg et al. 1977; 1982a; 1982b; 1982c) and we will also utilize their data in an attempt to provide an overall view of mechanisms causing these arrhythmias. Other animal models of healing and healed infarcts have not been used extensively for electrophysiological studies.

Characteristics of Arrhythmias in Animal Models of Healing and Healed Infarction

In general, spontaneously occurring arrhythmias have not been studied to a large extent in the canine models of healing and healed infarction that have been used most frequently for the investigation of the mechanisms causing arrhythmias. There are some exceptions that will be discussed later. Spontaneously occurring arrhythmias have been studied in the feline model in which ventricular premature depolarizations and nonsustained tachycardia often occur. In most of the experiments on canine models, programmed stimulation protocols have been utilized to induce arrhythmias. The stimulation protocols are patterned after the clinical ones described previously. Single or multiple premature stimuli with durations of 5 msec or less and strengths usually less than four times diastolic threshold are applied to the ventricles at progressively decreasing coupling intervals with the previous beat, either during sinus rhythm or during stimulation of the ventricles at a regular rate. Short rapid trains of stimuli (burst pacing) are also effective for inducing arrhythmias (Kaplinsky et al. 1972). Programmed stimulation studies have been done both in conscious and anesthetized animals. Therefore, a consideration of the effects of anesthesia on the induction and characteristics of the arrhythmias is important. We will discuss these effects later. Once again, we point out that it is also necessary to keep in mind the effects of these same stimulation protocols on normal hearts (see Chapter I) as an aid for determining which arrhythmias induced by stimulation are a specific product of the ischemia and infarction.

Although the specific methods used to cause infarction differ in different studies (see below), the characteristics of the arrhythmias induced by stimulation in the different canine models are remarkably similar (El-Sherif et al. 1977a; 1977b; Karagueuzian et al. 1979; 1986a; Garan et al. 1980; 1985; 1987; Garan and Ruskin 1984; Michelson et al. 1980; 1981a; 1981b; 1981c; 1981d; Davis et al. 1982; Gang et al. 1982; Cobbe et al. 1983; Echt et al. 1983; Bardy et al. 1984; Wetstein et al. 1984; Ogawa et al. 1986; Duff et al. 1988; Hunt and Ross 1989). They are also similar to the arrhythmias that occur in humans. Ventricular arrhythmias can be induced by single premature stimuli in these models during sinus rhythm or stimulation of the ventricles at a regular cycle length. Induction of the arrhythmias usually happens when the premature stimuli occur somewhere near the descending limb of the T wave, although arrhythmias also can be induced by premature stimuli occurring at longer coupling intervals. In Figure 4.7, induction of ventricular arrhythmias during programmed stimulation of a canine heart with a healing infarct caused by coronary occlusion and subsequent reperfusion of the infarcted region is shown. This animal model is described in more detail later. The occurrence of a single nonstimulated ventricular depolarization following the stimulated premature ventricular depolarization delivered at a coupling interval of 205 msec, in panel A (arrow) defines the outer boundary of the "repetitive response" zone. As the coupling interval of the premature stimulus was decreased (to 195 msec in panel B), the number of nonstimulated impulses that it induced increased, resulting in nonsustained tachycardia. Nonsustained tachycardias may have either a multiform QRS morphology and an irregular cycle length or a uniform QRS morphology and regular cycle length. They terminate spontaneously within approximately 30 seconds. At shorter premature stimulus coupling intervals sustained tachycardia may occur. This is shown in panel C where the

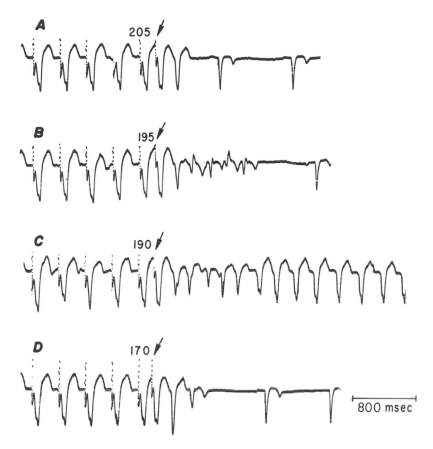

Figure 4.7: Initiation of ventricular tachycardia in a dog on the third day after occlusion of the left anterior descending coronary artery for 2 hours followed by reperfusion. The ECG is shown in each panel. Panels A-D show records in which the ventricles are driven at a cycle length of 350 msec, and a single stimulated premature impulse (arrows) is stimulated. In panel A, the coupling interval of the induced premature impulse is 205 msec; this is followed by a nondriven impulse. Sinus rhythm resumes after a pause of 390 msec. In panel B, the coupling interval of the stimulated premature impulse is 195 msec; this is followed by five nondriven impulses. After a pause of 720 msec sinus rhythm reoccurs. In panel C, the coupling interval of the stimulated premature impulse is 190 msec and a long period of tachycardia follows. The cycle length of the initial eight beats varies between 175–260 msec. Thereafter, the QRS during tachycardia is uniform and there is a stable cycle length (275 msec). The tachycardia lasted for 10 minutes. In panel D, a single stimulated premature impulse, induced at a coupling interval of 170 msec, is followed by two nondriven impulses. Sinus rhythm occurs after a pause of 760 msec. (Reproduced from Karagueuzian et al. (1979) with permission.)

premature stimulus was applied with a coupling interval of 190 msec. Sustained ventricular tachycardias have been defined differently by different investigators and include stable tachycardias lasting longer than 30 seconds that do not lead to hemodynamic collapse as well as tachycardias requiring termination by an intervention such as overdrive stimulation or countershock because of severe hemodynamic impairment. They may begin with several multiform QRS complexes with an irregular cycle length, but then often become monomorphic with very regular cycle lengths as shown in Figure 4.7C. The cycle lengths of the tachycardias usually range from 140–250 msec, significantly shorter than most human sustained tachycardias. A possible explanation for the faster tachycardia rates is the smaller heart size and therefore smaller infarcts and reentrant circuits than in humans. On occasion the QRS morphology may change during the tachycardia. In some experiments, tachycardias with different QRS morphologies can be induced in the same heart. Sustained tachycardias may also degenerate into fibrillation, particularly when the tachycardia cycle length is very short. Ventricular fibrillation may also be initiated by a single premature stimulus without a prior period of sustained tachycardia. The inner boundary of the repetitive response zone occurs when shorter coupled premature stimuli no longer induce sustained or nonsustained tachycardia or the premature stimulus coupling interval reaches the effective refractory period of the ventricles. This is shown in Figure 4.7D, where a premature impulse with a coupling interval of 170 msec induced only several repetitive responses. Often, if arrhythmias are not induced by single premature stimuli, a more aggressive protocol involving a second and possibly a third premature stimulus may induce arrhythmias similar to those shown in Figure 4.7. Up to seven premature stimuli delivered in succession have been used (Hunt and Ross 1989). The arrhythmias that are induced by either single or multiple premature stimuli are caused by the ischemia and the presence of the infarct since, as we have discussed, they do not usually occur in noninfarcted hearts. In addition to premature stimuli, rapid stimulation can also initiate arrhythmias, such as nonsustained and sustained ventricular tachycardia or ventricular fibrillation. There may be a critical number of stimuli and a critical cycle length in a burst needed to start a nonsustained or sustained tachycardia. An example of the induction of sustained ventricular tachycardia by a burst of stimuli is shown in Figure 4.8; a train of eight stimuli at a cycle length of 180 msec was successful in initiating tachycardia. This protocol does not initiate sustained tachycardias in normal hearts. Ventricular fibrillation may also be initiated by burst pacing in the infarcted heart. It is difficult to ascribe ventricular fibrillation induced by burst pacing to ischemia since very rapid bursts of stimuli can also fibrillate normal hearts (Moore and Spear 1975).

In the canine models, the site in the ventricles where the stimuli are applied is sometimes an important determinant of whether arrhythmias are induced, as we pointed out for the clinical studies. When the myocardial infarct is located in the left ventricle, stimulation of right ventricular sites at a distance from the infarct, for example the free wall, is often not as effective as stimulation close to the infarct, for example in the right ventricular apex for

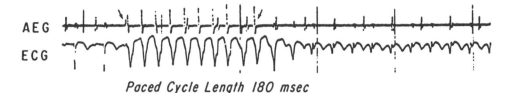

AEG

ECG

Paced Cycle Length 180 msec

Figure 4.8: Induction of ventricular tachycardia by rapid pacing of the ventricles in a canine heart 5 days after complete occlusion of the left anterior descending coronary artery for 2 hours followed by reperfusion. An atrial electrogram (AEG) and the electrocardiogram (ECG) are shown. The first two QRS complexes are of sinus origin, followed by a period of pacing (between the two arrows) at a 180-msec cycle length. After pacing, a rapid sustained tachycardia occurred. (Reproduced from Davis et al. (1982) with permission.)

an anteroseptal infarct (Hunt and Ross 1990). Stimuli applied in the left ventricle at the border of infarcted and noninfarcted myocardium are often most effective. Even at these locations, arrhythmias may be induced by stimuli applied at some sites and not at others. In general, considering the different stimulation protocols and sites of stimulation, stimuli applied to the left ventricle (particularly) at the infarct borders are more effective than stimuli applied to the right ventricle, multiple premature stimuli are more effective than single premature stimuli, and bursts of stimuli may be the most effective method for inducing tachycardia (Duff et al. 1988; Michelson et al. 1981d). Many of these characteristics are similar to the experience with programmed stimulation in the clinical studies.

Tachycardias that do not terminate spontaneously can often be terminated by single or multiple ventricular stimuli occurring at an appropriate time in the cardiac cycle. Termination of sustained ventricular tachycardia by single and double premature stimuli in the canine model of a reperfused infarct is shown in Figure 4.9. The single premature impulse (top panel) delivered at a coupling interval of 175 msec (arrow) did not terminate tachycardia, but it did when initiated with a coupling interval of 144 msec (arrow). The double premature stimuli (bottom panel) at coupling intervals of 200 msec (arrows) did not terminate tachycardia, but did when initiated with coupling intervals of 160 and 200 msec (arrows). Bursts of stimuli (overdrive stimulation) are also effective in stopping tachycardias.

Infarct Models

Now that we have described the kinds of arrhythmias that occur in the canine models of healing and healed infarcts, we will describe the different models. A number of different methods for causing myocardial ischemia and infarction have been used to produce experimental models in which arrhyth-

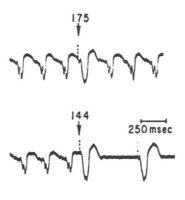

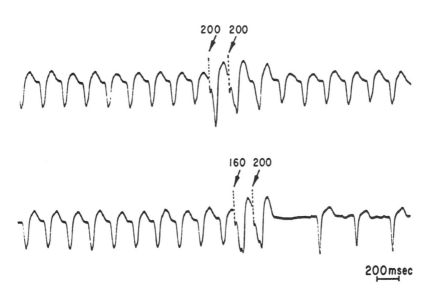

Figure 4.9: Effects of ventricular stimulation on induced ventricular tachycardia. The ECG records from a dog 4 days after coronary artery occlusion and reperfusion are in the top panel. The application of a single stimulated premature impulse (arrow) at a coupling interval of 175 msec is followed by continuation of tachycardia, whereas the application of a premature stimulus at a coupling interval of 144 msec terminates the tachycardia. There is a pause of 360 msec after the premature stimulus that terminated tachycardia, and then a driven ventricular depolarization occurs. The bottom panel shows the effects in another dog of two successive premature stimuli on tachycardia that could not be terminated by a single stimulus. The upper ECG trace in the panel shows that the application of the two closely coupled stimuli (200 msec) does not interrupt the tachycardia. When the coupling interval of the first premature impulse was made shorter (160 msec) without changing the coupling interval of the second stimulus (lower trace), tachycardia was abruptly terminated. (Reproduced from Karagueuzian et al. (1979) with permission.)

mias can be initiated by ventricular stimulation. The different methods cause infarcts with different anatomical features and this has an important influence on arrhythmogenicity. The models are in many ways similar to those used to study acute ischemia, except that the electrophysiological measurements are made days to weeks after the coronary occlusion.

We should add an explanatory note here on the terminology that we will use for discussing the animal models. Since it is inappropriate to use the term "late hospital" for the laboratory experiments, we have equated late hospital in patients with the healing phase in the experimental models. During this period, which begins within several days after coronary occlusion, there is a continuing remodeling of the ischemic and infarcted region caused by the healing response to the injury. This response includes phagocytosis of the dead myocardial fibers and the deposition of connective tissue for scar formation. Healing continues in the canine heart for a number of weeks before the gross structure of the infarct is relatively stable. Experimental studies on the healing phase of infarction are generally within the first several weeks after the coronary occlusion. After this time we refer to the laboratory models as being either healed or chronic. This definition may not be entirely accurate since there is some evidence that structural changes may continue to occur for as long as several years (Duff et al. 1988; Hanich et al. 1988a) after occlusion in the canine heart, but the nature of these changes is uncertain.

Permanent Coronary Artery Occlusion

The technique of permanently occluding a major coronary artery (as opposed to transiently occluding it followed by reperfusion) has been widely used for investigating the effects of acute and subacute ischemia on cardiac rhythm in the dog as well as in other laboratory animals as we have already discussed in Chapters II and III. Permanent coronary occlusion also causes arrhythmias during the healing and healed phases of infarction. Permanent occlusion is usually accomplished by ligating the artery with a suture under anesthesia with the chest open and then repairing the chest wound. Careful postoperative care is then necessary to maintain the dogs while the infarcts develop. Infarcts with different anatomical characteristics produced by permanent coronary occlusion at different sites have been studied in the canine heart. Occlusion of the left anterior descending coronary artery near its origin (usually just distal to the first septal branch so that atrioventricular conduction is maintained, and proximal to the first main diagonal branch so that the infarct is large) is a widely used technique. The occlusion can be done with either a two-stage Harris procedure that was described in Chapter III (Harris 1950) where the artery is first narrowed and then later completely occluded, or a single-stage technique in which the artery is occluded all at once. Both procedures produce a similar anteroseptal infarct. Survival after the acute ischemic arrhythmias, which occur immediately after occlusion, is probably better with the two-stage technique. The size of the infarct that results after left anterior descending artery occlusion is variable, and depends on the anatomy and distribution of the coronary and collateral circulation (Uemura et al. 1989). In mongrel dogs, this can be quite different among animals. Infarcts may be large and transmural and occupy up to 40% of the left ventricle (El-Sherif et al. 1977a; 1977b; Karagueuzian et al. 1979; Wit et al. 1982a; Kramer et al. 1985). Several layers (2–5) of Purkinje fibers survive on the endocardial surface of the infarct (the Purkinje fibers responsible for automatic arrhythmias 1–2 days after coronary occlusion, which were discussed in Chapter III). A variable number of layers of muscle cells (1–40) also survive on the epicardial surface because of persisting collateral blood flow (Wit et al. 1981a; Mehra et al. 1983; Kramer et al. 1985; Ursell et al. 1985). The epicardial muscle plays an important role as the site of origin of arrhythmias during the healing phase and its anatomical and electrophysiological characteristics will be described later. Nontransmural infarcts may also result from this technique and involve only the subendocardial muscle or inner two thirds of the ventricular wall (Karagueuzian et al. 1979). Nontransmural infarcts probably occur when there is extensive collateral circulation. Nonsustained and sustained ventricular tachycardias, induced by programmed stimulation, are more frequently associated with large transmural infarcts than with the nontransmural infarcts (Harrison et al. 1980; Scherlag et al. 1985; Denniss et al. 1989). Therefore, to insure the occurrence of a large infarct, a second ligation of the left anterior descending coronary artery, 2–3 cm distal to the proximal ligation has been done, and the diagonal branches between the two points have also been occluded (Hunt and Ross 1989; 1990). The additional ligations may decrease collateral blood flow to the ischemic region. Ventricular fibrillation induced by programmed stimulation occurs in hearts with both large and small infarcts (Denniss et al. 1989). However, below a minimum infarct size that has not yet been quantified, no arrhythmias related to infarction can be induced. Also, the thinner the layer of surviving epicardial muscle in hearts with transmural infarcts, the more likely the occurrence of arrhythmias (Scherlag et al. 1985). The relationship between the thickness of this surviving layer and occurrence of arrhythmias may be explained by the effect of thickness on conduction properties in this region where arrhythmias originate, which will be described later. Occlusion of the right coronary artery in the dog, resulting in right ventricular infarction may also result in arrhythmias that can be induced by programmed stimulation during the healing phase of infarction (Karagueuzian et al. 1986a). Similar studies are not usually done with main left circumflex artery occlusion because of the high mortality rate that results from the resulting extensive left ventricular infarction.

Ventricular arrhythmias (nonsustained and sustained tachycardias or fibrillation) can be induced by stimulation of the ventricles using the stimulation protocols described previously, during the healing and healed phases of infarction following permanent left anterior descending coronary artery occlusion (El-Sherif et al. 1977a; 1977b; Hope et al. 1977; 1978; Karagueuzian et al. 1979; Denniss et al. 1989; Hunt and Ross 1989). The period of arrhythmia inducibility includes the first 2 days after occlusion, the same time when the delayed spontaneous arrhythmias occur (El-Sherif et al. 1982; Scherlag et al. 1983). When only single premature impulses are stimulated from the right ventricle (Karagueuzian et al. 1979), the zone of premature coupling intervals for arrhythmia induction decreases during the first week after occlusion until no arrhythmias are induced after 5–8 days. Figure 4.10 shows the range of coupling intervals of premature stimuli applied to the right ventricle, which induced nonsustained and sustained tachycardia over a 3-day period, in the same group of animals. By day 4, there was a marked decrease in the ability of the single premature impulse to induce tachycardia. This period of arrhythmia induction might be considered to be analogous to the late hospital period in patients. When multiple premature stimuli applied to the right or left ventricle are used, there may still be a decrease in inducibility of arrhythmias after 1 week in some hearts with eventual disappearance of arrhythmias (Hunt and Ross 1990), similar to some observations in humans (Denniss et al. 1985; Bhandari et al. 1987). In

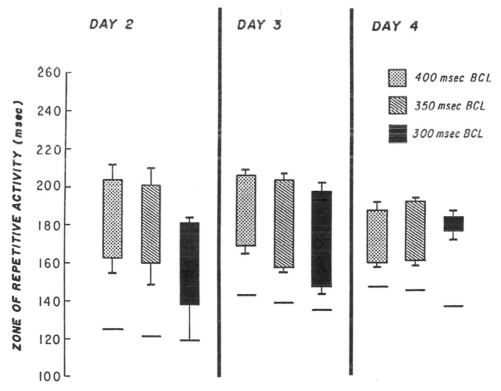

Figure 4.10: The range of coupling intervals of single premature impulses applied to the right ventricle that induced nonsustained and sustained ventricular tachycardia (zone of repetitive activity) in dogs with permanent occlusion of the left anterior descending coronary artery is shown by the bar graphs. This range of coupling intervals was determined at three different basic drive cycle lengths and on three different days after occlusion. (Reproduced from Karagueuzian et al. (1979) with permission.)

others however, reproducible ventricular arrhythmias may be induced for as long as 4 months (Denniss et al. 1989; Hunt and Ross 1990), corresponding to the chronic infarction arrhythmias in humans. The level of autonomic nerve activity also influences the occurrence of arrhythmias. An increase in sympathetic activity has been shown to facilitate the induction of ventricular tachycardia in 3-week-old transmural infarcts (Herre et al. 1988).

Ventricular stimulation to initiate arrhythmias after permanent left anterior descending coronary artery occlusion has been done in both anesthetized dogs with the chest open and the heart exposed (El-Sherif et al. 1977a; 1977b) and in unanesthetized dogs in which the coronary artery was previously occluded surgically (Karagueuzian et al. 1979; Hunt and Ross 1989). Under the former experimental conditions, anesthesia is expected to have some influence, either arrhythmogenic or antiarrhythmic (Dawson et al. 1980). Hunt and Ross (1988) found that both halothane and pentobarbital anesthesia prevented induction of tachycardia in 40% to 50% of dogs that were inducible prior to anesthesia. Halothane also slowed the rate of tachycardia, while pentobarbital increased the incidence of ventricular fibrillation. The combination of fentanyl-droperidol plus nitrous oxide did not suppress the induction of tachycardia in this study (Hunt and Ross 1988). The attenuation of baroreceptor reflexes under some types of anesthesia such as pentobarbital might influence the kinds of arrhythmias induced, since an uncompensated fall in blood pressure during tachycardia may decrease coronary perfusion. This in turn might superimpose an acute ischemic insult on top of the more chronic substrate for arrhythmias formed by the healing infarct. In addition, a decline in blood pressure during rapid tachycardia, which is most often seen during anesthesia, is expected to cause reflex sympathetic discharge, which may influence the arrhythmias. With these effects in mind it is expected that the characteristics and/or inducibility of arrhythmias would be different in anesthetized dogs compared to unanesthetized dogs. Cooling of the epicardial surface of the heart when the chest is open also may influence arrhythmia induction.

It is difficult to determine from an analysis of the literature the exact incidence of the different kinds of arrhythmias (nonsustained and sustained tachycardia and ventricular fibrillation) that can be induced in hearts with infarcts caused by left anterior descending coronary artery occlusion. This analysis is complicated by the use of anesthesia in some studies and not in others and by the variability in inducibility with time. Our estimate is that nonsustained tachycardia is initiated in 50% to 60% of dogs, and sustained tachycardia in about 20%. We are uncertain about the frequency of induction of fibrillation that can occur immediately after premature stimulation or following a period of tachycardia. In the remaining dogs, no arrhythmias are induced even though an infarct is present (Karagueuzian et al. 1979; Kramer et al. 1985; Scherlag et al. 1985). Arrhythmia induction can be increased by the infusion of isoproterenol during programmed stimulation (Hunt and Ross 1990), an effect similar to the one described in patients (Reddy and Gettes 1979; Freedman et al. 1984). The incidence of the different arrhythmias probably reflects the random occurrence of infarcts of different sizes and with different anatomical characteristics.

Spontaneously occurring ventricular arrhythmias with the same characteristics as the induced arrhythmias have rarely been reported for this model. However, Denniss et al. (1989) observed spontaneously occurring ventricular tachycardia 3–9 days after infarction and we have also seen it on occasion during this time period. Hunt and Ross (1989) found that in many of the dogs with healed infarcts in whom tachycardia could be induced, similar arrhythmias also occurred spontaneously in the first 2 months after infarction. The failure to consistently document spontaneously occurring tachycardia may be a result of inadequate ECG monitoring of dogs during the normal daily routine outside the laboratory. As we mentioned in our discussion of the clinical arrhythmias, late hospital arrhythmias were first appreciated when patients were continuously monitored with the Holter technique and Holter monitoring has rarely been used to study dogs with healing infarcts.

A modification of the canine infarct model caused by permanent occlusion of the left anterior descending coronary artery involves administration of methylprednisolone prior to the ligation. This procedure significantly increases the incidence of inducible sustained tachycardias (Guse et al. 1979; Gessman et al. 1981; Brachmann et al. 1983a; Cobbe et al. 1983; Cardinal et al. 1984; Cobbe et al. 1985; Scherlag et al. 1985), to as high as 75% of experiments (Scherlag et al. 1985). The electrocardiographic characteristics of the arrhythmias are similar to arrhythmias induced without methylprednisolone, except that the rate of tachycardia may be more rapid. Following pretreatment with methylprednisolone, Cobbe et al. (1985) found that arrhythmias were induced only during the first week after coronary occlusion and not thereafter. The same variability in induction of arrhythmias over a longer period of time that occurs without methylprednisolone might still be expected. The reason why sustained ventricular tachycardia is more easily inducible after methylprednisolone is not entirely clear. It may be related to its effects on the size and morphology of the infarct (Scherlag et al. 1985). Methylprednisolone pretreatment can cause expansion of infarcts (Roberts et al. 1976; Vogel et al. 1977) and hearts with larger transmural infarcts are more susceptible to inducible ventricular tachycardia. Not only the size of the infarct, but also the distribution of surviving myocardium is an important factor for the inducibility of tachycardia. The survival of a narrow rim of muscle fibers on the epicardial surface of the infarct is crucial for arrhythmogenesis in this animal model, while arrhythmias may not occur if there is no surviving rim or if the rim is too thick (discussed later). Methylprednisolone pretreatment may for some unknown reason increase the likelihood of survival of the narrow rim of muscle (Scherlag et al. 1985).

The survival of the epicardial rim of muscle and the origination of many of the arrhythmias in this muscle in the canine model of infarction caused by permanent left anterior descending coronary artery occlusion with or without methylprednisolone is a very important favorable property for the study of arrhythmia mechanisms. The epicardial origin of arrhythmias has permitted detailed activation maps to be constructed of reentrant circuits without the necessity of determining transmural or endocardial activation patterns. Detailed measurements have also been made of the cellular electrophysiological properties at the site of arrhythmia origin. Data derived from this model form much of the basis for our description of the mechanisms causing ventricular arrhythmias in healing infarcts later in this chapter.

The reasons why arrhythmias are usually no longer inducible after a week in many of the experiments on dogs with infarcts caused by left anterior descending coronary artery occlusion have not been determined. One possibility that has been considered is the lack of real aneurysm formation during infarct healing as sometimes occurs in humans. Patients with chronic ventricular tachycardia often have ventricular aneurysms, which may be involved in the arrhythmogenesis. Klein et al. (1979) fed dogs a protein-deficient diet after causing infarction by ligation of one or more diagonal or obtuse marginal arteries to promote the occurrence of aneurysms. The effects of stimulating the hearts was studied 1–10 months after coronary ligation. Nonsustained and sustained ventricular tachycardias were induced in 45% of the dogs and in 63% of the dogs in which tachycardia could be induced, they lasted for greater than 50 beats. It is uncertain from the description of the results in this paper whether the induction of tachycardias was reproducible. Tachycardias were also not initiated on a number of different days to determine if they maintained stable characteristics. The usefulness of this animal model is therefore questionable.

In another experimental canine model developed by Garan and Ruskin, the site of the permanent occlusion (done by ligation) of the left anterior descending coronary artery is distal to the first diagonal branch, resulting in a smaller area of ischemia than when the left anterior descending coronary artery is occluded near its origin as described above. In addition, the epicardial branches from the circumflex and posterior descending coronary artery to the left ventricular apical area are occluded in this model by ligating each of the individual branches (Garan et al. 1980; 1981; Garan and Ruskin 1984; Garan et al. 1985; 1987). This method produces an infarct that has some different morphological characteristics from the infarct caused by the more proximal occlusion of the left anterior descending coronary artery alone. The infarct involves mostly the anteroapical left ventricle (5% to 25% of the left ventricle) and the interventricular septum is usually spared (Garan et al. 1980). Successful arrhythmia induction requires that the infarct be transmural (Garan et al. 1985). There is probably less surviving epicardial muscle compared to infarcts caused by left anterior coronary artery occlusion alone as a consequence of ligation of the epicardial branches from the circumflex, since these branches may be an important source of collateral blood flow. However, a detailed histologic study of the subepicardial region has not been reported. There is some surviving intramural muscle, subendocardial muscle and Purkinje fibers. This difference in infarct anatomy may cause a difference in the site of origin of some of the arrhythmias; arrhythmias may originate in the intramural or subendocardial muscle in this model in addition to the subepicardial muscle (discussed in more detail later). The electrocardiographic characteristics of the arrhythmias remain the same as for the other models of infarcts caused by permanent occlusion. Although no spontaneously occurring tachycardias have been reported, programmed electrical stimulation in the unanesthetized dogs during the first week after coronary occlusion showed that sustained ventricular tachycardias could be induced in 45% to 50% of experiments (Garan et al. 1985) and similar tachycardias could be induced for at least a month thereafter (Garan et al. 1981; Garan and Ruskin 1984; Garan et al. 1985). Nonsustained polymorphic ventricular tachycardia could be induced in 25% to 35% of experiments (Garan et al. 1981). The higher incidence of arrhythmia induction over a longer period of time compared to left anterior descending coronary artery occlusion alone seems to make this a better model of truly chronic ventricular tachycardia. However, the endocardial (and sometimes intramural) origin of the arrhythmias makes it more difficult to study arrhythmia mechanisms.

In addition to the canine, the cat has been used to study the effects on cardiac rhythm of healing and healed infarction caused by permanent coronary artery occlusion. Myerburg et al. (1977; 1982a; 1982b) have developed a model in which two or three distal branches of the left ventrolateral artery (equivalent to the left anterior descending coronary artery in the dog) are ligated causing either transmural infarction of the anteroapical left ventricle, or nontransmural infarction involving more than 50% of the wall thickness. Subendocardial muscle and Purkinje fibers survive in the infarct scar as they do in human infarcts. In this model, spontaneous premature ventricular depolarizations and ventricular tachycardia occur during a 1-week to 6-month period, (Myerburg et al. 1977). Several examples of electrocardiograms recorded at different times after coronary occlusion are shown in Figure 4.11. Programmed premature stimulation of the ventricles of feline hearts with 2-week-old infarcts caused by proximal occlusion of the left ventral artery resulted in induction of ventricular tachyarrhythmias (ventricular tachycardia and fibrillation) in one reported study (Wetstein et al. 1985a) although sustained ventricular tachycardia occurred only occasionally. This infarct model has contributed a great deal of important information about cellular electrophysiological changes in surviving cardiac fibers in infarcts that we will show later.

Coronary Artery Occlusion and Reperfusion

Ventricular tachyarrhythmias can be induced in canine hearts with healing or healed infarcts caused by temporary occlusion of the left anterior descending coronary artery for 90 to 120 minutes and subsequent release of the occlusion resulting in reperfusion of the ischemic region (Karagueuzian et al. 1979; Michelson et al. 1980; Gang et al. 1982). The occlusion can be accomplished by surgical ligation of the artery with the chest open and then later releasing the ligation before closing the chest wound (Karagueuzian et al. 1979). It has also been done with the chest closed by inserting a balloon catheter through an artery into the aortic root and coronary ostium, inflating the balloon for a period of time and then removing the catheter (Gang et al. 1982).

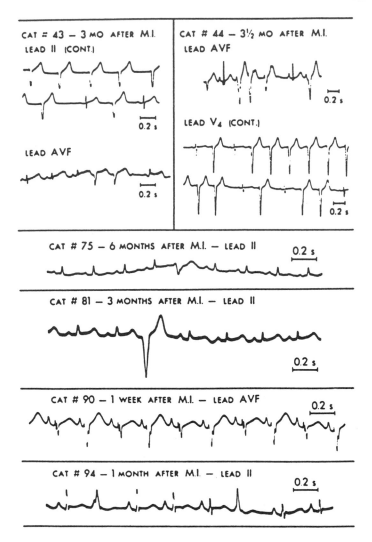

Figure 4.11: Representative ECG rhythm strips demonstrating spontaneous ventricular ectopic activity in cats with myocardial infarction. The abnormalities include ventricular tachycardia (cats 43 and 44, 3 to 3 1/2 months after coronary occlusion), single premature ventricular beats (cats 75 and 81, 6 and 3 months after coronary occlusion), bigeminy (cat 90, 1 week after coronary occlusion), and frequent unifocal premature ventricular beats (cat 94, 1 month after coronary occlusion). (Reproduced from Myerburg et al. (1977) with permission.)

The electrocardiographic characteristics of the arrhythmias remain the same as in the permanent occlusion models. Occlusion of a coronary artery by a thrombus and subsequent dissolution of the thrombus causing reperfusion may occur spontaneously in patients or after thrombolytic therapy, providing the clinical counterpart to this animal model. Sustained ventricular tachycardia can sometimes be induced by programmed stimulation in patients who received streptokinase for reopening occluded arteries (Kersschot et al. 1986).

The temporary occlusion and reperfusion produces an infarct with different anatomical features than those caused by permanent occlusion and the different anatomy may influence the site of origin of the arrhythmias. When a coronary artery is occluded the myocardial cells in the region of the ventricle supplied by that artery do not die immediately and simultaneously. Cell death continues for at least several hours and as we indicated in Chapter III, the wave front of necrosis progresses from the most vulnerable region near the subendocardium (Lowe et al. 1983) towards both the epicardial surface (Reimer et al. 1977) and the endocardial surface (Fenoglio et al. 1979). If blood flow is restored prior to complete death of all the cells, salvage of some of the ischemic cells (prevention of cell death) may be accomplished (Maroko et al. 1972; Mathur et al. 1975). Reperfusion usually must be instituted within a 2–3 hour period for "effective" reflow to the ischemic region and myocardial salvage (Constantini et al. 1975). If occlusion is maintained for a longer time period, ischemic damage to the myocardial cells may be irreversible or fragile ischemic capillary walls may break during the reperfusion. If the capillaries break, the restored blood flow never reaches its intended target, the myocardial cells. Hemorrhagic areas caused by capillary fragility are often found even when reperfusion occurs after less than 3 hours (Bresnahan et al. 1974). As a result of myocardial cell salvage, the reperfused infarct is not homogeneously necrotic as may often occur after a permanent occlusion (Karagueuzian et al. 1979, Michelson et al. 1980; 1981a; 1981c; Wetstein et al. 1982; 1985b; Duff et al. 1988). At 2–4 days after occlusion and reperfusion, viable myocardium with normal histologic characteristics may be found interspersed among necrotic myocardium giving it a mottled appearance. These regions of viable myocardium either appear to be completely surrounded by ischemic or necrotic myocardium or are continuous with viable myocardium bordering the infarct. In older healed infarcts, the viable cells are trapped in the proliferating connective tissue. It has been proposed that surviving intramural fibers form reentrant pathways that lead to arrhythmias (Karaguezian et al. 1979; Michelson et al. 1980). The lateral margins of the reperfused infarcts are irregular. The endocardial and epicardial border zones often appear thicker than after left anterior descending coronary artery occlusion with more muscle cells surviving on each surface. Reperfused infarcts may also occasionally extend to the epicardial surface. If adequate reperfusion does not occur after the occlusion is released, because of the "no reflow" phenomenon, the anatomy of the infarct may not be much different than after permanent occlusion. This may have occurred in some of the studies in which intramural cell survival was not prominent (Kramer et al. 1985; Scherlag et al. 1985; Duff et al. 1988). Successful reflow is indicated by the appearance of ectopic ventricular premature depolarizations within several minutes after release of the coronary occlusion, which gradually increase in number over the next several hours (Mathur et al. 1975; Karagueuzian et al. 1979). We have discussed these arrhythmias in Chapter III.

When the left anterior descending coronary artery is occluded above the first diagonal branch (Karagueuzian et al. 1979; Wetstein et al. 1985b; Duff et al. 1988), or at its origin (Gang et al. 1982; 1984), and then reperfused after 2 hours, large infarcts involving up to 30% of the left ventricle may still occur despite the increased surviving myocardium within the infarcted region. The borders of the reperfused infarct may be extended and encompass more of the left ventricle than after permanent occlusion. The incidence of all ventricular tachycardias, inducible by programmed stimulation, during the first week is usually greater than 50% of experiments, and the incidence of sustained ventricular tachycardia has been reported to range from 39% to 61% of experiments (higher than after permanent occlusion) (Karagueuzian et al. 1979; Davis et al. 1982; Gang et al. 1982; Jackman and Zipes 1982; Cardinal et al. 1988). Sustained tachycardias occur most frequently in hearts with large infarcts (Karagueuzian et al. 1979; Gang et al. 1983; Wilber et al. 1985; Duff et al. 1988). Arrhythmia inducibility has been studied in the same dogs over a number of days. Karagueuzian et al. (1979), using single right ventricular premature stimuli, found inducibility of sustained tachycardias to be greatest 3–4 days after occlusion and the incidence decreased thereafter. Figure 4.12, which is from their study, shows the effects of infarct age on the repetitive response zone for a group of dogs with infarcts caused by temporary left anterior descending coronary artery occlusion and inducible sustained ventricular tachycardia. The bars indicate the range of coupling intervals of single premature impulses which induced repetitive responses at each of three basic drive cycle lengths. Within each bar, the white area is the range of coupling intervals of premature impulses which induced sustained ventricular tachycardia. Both the repetitive response zone and the zone of coupling intervals at which sustained tachycardia could be induced decreased significantly from day 3 to day 4, and then to day 5. After day 5, sustained tachycardia could not be initiated although in some dogs repetitive responses could be initiated for several more days. The failure to find inducible tachycardias after 5 days in this study may be a consequence of the nonaggressive programmed stimulation protocol that was used, i.e., single premature stimuli applied to the base of the right ventricle, rather than multiple left ventricular premature stimuli. Duff et al. (1988) were able to induce tachycardias on 5 different study days over a 24-day period and Hanich et al. (1988a) induced tachycardias after 4–6 years. In the experiments of Duff et al. (1988), as time progressed it was necessary to use multiple right or left ventricular stimuli to induce arrhythmias, whereas at 4 days single right ventricular stimuli were effective. The results of these studies lead to the conclusion that during infarct healing, electrophysiological changes occur that may cause a decreased propensity for induction of arrhythmias. This finding is similar to the results of Bhandari et al. (1987) in humans.

In the reperfusion model developed by Michelson et al. (1981a; 1981b), occlusion by surgical ligation of the left anterior descending coronary artery is done distal to one or all of the diagonal branches, and as a consequence, the ischemic region is confined to the left ventricular apex. Although the same kind of mottled infarct characterized by survival of intramural myocardial cells results as with a more proximal occlusion, the total area covered by this infarct

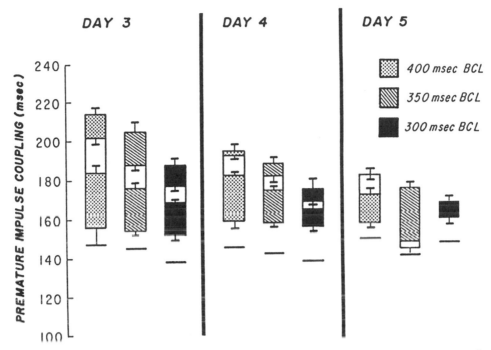

Figure 4.12: Vertical bars indicate the range of coupling intervals of premature impulses that induced repetitive responses in dogs with occlusion of a coronary artery for 2 hours followed by reperfusion, at each of three basic drive cycle lengths: 400 msec (stippled bar), 350 msec (striped bar), and 300 msec (solid bar). Within each bar, the white area is the range of coupling intervals of premature impulses that induced sustained ventricular tachycardia. Repetitive response zones and tachycardia zones are shown for days 3, 4, and 5 after reperfusion. The thick horizontal line below each bar is the effective refractory period of the ventricular muscle under the stimulating electrode at each of the basic cycle lengths. (Reproduced from Karagueuzian et al. (1979) with permission.)

is much smaller, usually 5% to 25% of the left ventricle. Sustained ventricular tachycardia could be induced in 38% of the experiments of Michelson et al. (1981a; 1981b), comparable to the results of the studies utilizing a proximal left anterior descending coronary artery ligation. Fibrillation occurred more frequently than tachycardia. Fibrillation was also more easily induced in hearts with smaller infarcts than with larger ones (Michelson et al. 1981a; 1981b). Tachyarrhythmias could also be initiated by multiple premature stimuli or burst pacing for several months after coronary occlusion, but since each dog was studied at only one time and not on a number of different days, it is not known whether tachycardias can consistently be induced over this prolonged time period (Hanich et al. 1988a). These results appear to be contradictory to the results of the studies using a more proximal occlusion of the left anterior descending coronary artery followed by reperfusion in which tachyarrhythmias could not be induced in hearts with small infarcts. However, one possible explanation for the differences may be the different locations of the small infarcts. After a proximal occlusion and reperfusion, small infarcts usually result from the salvage of too much myocardium, perhaps related to extensive collateral flow persisting during the occlusion period. The infarcts are usually small and subendocardial. Reperfusion after the more distal occlusion still results in a transmural but small infarct with cell survival in the infarcted region. To the extent that reentrant pathways are a result of intramural cell survival, in a transmural infarct the propensity for tachyarrhythmias may be maintained.

Another method, using coronary occlusion and reperfusion to cause arrhythmias in healing infarcts, has been described by Lucchesi and his colleagues (Gibson and Lucchesi 1980; Patterson et al. 1980; 1981a; 1981b). Prior to complete occlusion by surgical ligation, a critical stenosis is placed around the left anterior descending coronary artery and maintained there so the maximum hyperemic response that follows release of the complete occlusion is reduced by at least 60%. The stenosis is not severe enough to impair resting coronary flow. Presumably, the decreased hyperemia reduces the amount of capillary damage during reperfusion and thereby reduces hemorrhage into the infarct. The infarcts that resulted were around 20% of the left ventricular mass but no additional histologic data has been published to enable comparison with the studies on other occlusion-reperfusion models. We assume that the reperfusion results in the survival of intramural muscle. Ventricular arrhythmias have been induced in greater than 90% of experiments 3–7 days after reperfusion (nonsustained ventricular tachycardia: 41%; ventricular fibrillation: 15% to 30%; and sustained ventricular tachycardia: 40%). The incidence of sustained ventricular tachycardia is similar to that reported for other models of occlusion and reperfusion.

Healed Infarcts and Acute Ischemia

We described in Chapter II that several experimental models of ventricular arrhythmias involve the imposition of an acute ischemic stimulus on a heart with a healing or healed infarct (Patterson et al. 1982; Kabell et al. 1984; Wilber et al. 1985). These models attempt to replicate a situation that is sometimes thought to cause sudden death in humans.

Further Contributions of Programmed Stimulation Studies to Elucidation of Pathophysiological Mechanisms

Evidence for Reentry from Programmed Stimulation Studies

We have indicated that arrhythmias occurring in hearts with healing and healed infarcts are, to a large extent, the result of reentrant excitation. The earliest evidence suggesting that this mechanism is important in these stages of infarction in both humans and the experimental models comes from the programmed stimulation studies. Initially, simply the ability to initiate and terminate the arrhythmias with electrical stimuli in both the clinical and experimental studies was considered sufficient proof of reentry. Many of the initial studies were done in the early and mid-1970s, prior to the availability of data suggesting a possible role of delayed afterdepolarization-dependent triggered activity as an arrhythmogenic mechanism. Later, additional characteristics of the arrhythmias in infarcted hearts, also derived from the stimulation studies, were useful as further evidence for a reentrant mechanism and to help distinguish reentry from triggered activity, since triggered activity can also be started and stopped by stimulation. To distinguish reentry from triggered activity, we must utilize what we know about the properties of both mechanisms from the experimental studies discussed in Chapter I. Many of these distinguishing features of infarction-related arrhythmias have been pointed out by Josephson et al. (Josephson et al. 1978a; 1978c; 1984; 1985; Josephson 1992).

Characteristics of Initiation

One of the most prominent characteristics of late hospital (healing infarct) and chronic (healed infarct) ventricular tachycardias is that they can be initiated by programmed stimulation. This characteristic alone is indicative of either triggered activity caused by delayed afterdepolarizations or reentrant excitation being the cause of the arrhythmia. It eliminates both automaticity (normal and abnormal) and triggered activity caused by early afterdepolarizations, which cannot be initiated by stimulation. As described in Chapter I, programmed stimulation may establish slow conduction and transient conduction block for the initiation of reentry or may increase delayed afterdepolarization amplitude for the initiation of triggered activity. But to distinguish reentry from triggered activity caused by delayed afterdepolarizations, one must look at additional features of initiation. One such feature is a comparison of the effect of premature stimulation versus rapid pacing. Triggered activity caused by delayed afterdepolarizations in the various experimental models that have been studied is induced more easily by rapid pacing than by single or multiple premature impulses (Wit and Rosen 1986). It often takes a number of short cycle lengths in succession to increase the amplitude of the delayed afterdepolarizations sufficiently to reach threshold. It is rare that triggered activity can be induced by 1–3 premature stimuli, but not by rapid pacing. On the other hand, in only a small percentage of the patients studied by the Josephson laboratory has sustained ventricular tachycardia been initiated by rapid pacing (Josephson et al. 1985), but it has often been initiated by 1–3 premature stimuli. Nonsustained tachycardias are also more easily initiated by premature stimuli than rapid pacing in patients. Why premature stimulation induces reentry and rapid pacing does not could be explained if conduction properties are not rate-sensitive enough to result in the prerequisite slow conduction and conduction block at the rapid rates of stimulation tested. Block of a premature impulse might occur more easily, because at an appropriately short cycle length of prematurity, the impulse might conduct into tissue with a long refractory period, the duration of which is a property of the longer basic drive cycle length. In the canine models, tachycardia is also not easily induced by rapid pacing over a range of cycle lengths from 180–250 msec but is readily induced by premature stimuli. It is however, more easily induced by bursts of up to seven premature stimuli in a row than by two or three premature stimuli.

When triggered activity caused by delayed afterdepolarizations can be induced by premature impulses, it is easier to do so at a fast basic pacing rate than at a slow one because at the faster rate the amplitude of the delayed afterdepolarizations is usually larger, and therefore, threshold for firing is more easily reached. However, it is sometimes easier to induce tachycardia in hearts with healing or healed infarcts in both clinical and experimental studies, with premature stimuli delivered during slower basic pacing rates than at fast ones. Josephson et al. (1985) described an example of a case to make this point, in which sustained ventricular tachycardia was more easily induced by a single premature stimulus delivered during a long basic cycle length than triple premature stimuli during a shorter basic cycle length. This would not be expected of triggered activity. In some of our experimental studies on the canine heart with a healing infarct, it has also been possible to induce tachycardia by premature stimuli delivered during a long basic drive cycle, but not during a short one. At the longer basic cycle length, the action potential duration and refractory period of cardiac fibers in the reentrant circuit may be longer or more heterogeneous, establishing the conditions for slow conduction and block of the premature impulse and the initiation of reentry. Ventricular tachycardia (clinical and experimental) is sometimes more easily initiated by premature stimuli delivered during fast basic pacing rates than slow ones (Morady et al. 1984a; Summitt et al. 1990). If it is still assumed that tachycardia is caused by reentry, then it must be assumed that in some hearts the faster pacing rate establishes conditions that are more favorable for slow conduction and block of the premature impulses. There may be a rate-dependent increase in the refractory period, for example, caused by an increase in postrepolarization refractoriness. This might seem to contradict what we said about a possible reason for the failure of rapid pacing alone to induce tachycardia, but it is conceivable that the increase in refractoriness might only be sufficient to influence the propagation of premature impulses and not the basic impulses. Therefore, the variable effect of basic pacing rate (cycle length) on inducibility of tachyarrhythmias with premature stimuli indicates that the electrophysiological properties of the arrhythmogenic area vary in different hearts. The evidence favors reentry in those hearts where it is easier to induce arrhythmias at a long basic cycle length.

In about one third of patients in whom single stimulated premature impulses can induce sustained tachycardia, an inverse relationship exists between the coupling intervals of the premature impulses with the last basic drive impulse (the S_1-S_2 interval), and the coupling intervals of the premature impulses and the first beat of tachycardia (the S_2-T_1 interval) (Wellens et al. 1976; Josephson et al. 1978b; 1984). Stated another way, over the range of premature coupling intervals at which tachycardia is induced, as the interval between the premature impulse and the last basic drive impulse decreases, the interval between that premature impulse and the first beat of tachycardia increases. An example of this relationship from a study by Wellens et al. (1976) is shown in Figure 4.13. The top two traces in each panel are leads I and III of the ECG, the middle two traces are a right atrial (RA) and His bundle electrogram, and the bottom two traces are leads V_1, and V_6 of the ECG. The inverse relationship can be seen by concentrating on lead V_6 (bottom trace). The basic drive cycle length was 550 msec and a premature depolarization was stimulated at a coupling interval of 290 msec in the top panel. The first impulse of tachycardia occurred at a coupling interval of 420 msec to the stimulated premature impulse and then the sustained tachycardia eventually assumed a cycle length of 350 msec. In the bottom panel, the premature depolarization was stimulated at a shorter coupling interval of 230 msec. The first impulse of tachycardia

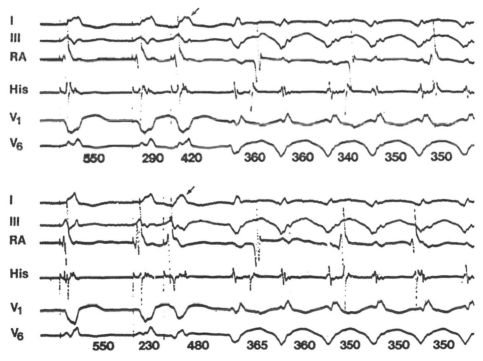

Figure 4.13: Prolongation of the interval between the initiating ventricular premature beat (arrows) and the first beat of tachycardia when the prematurity of the initiating beat is decreased in a patient with a myocardial infarct. The interval from the premature beat to the first beat of tachycardia measures 420 msec after a premature beat interval of 290 msec (upper part of figure), and 480 msec when the premature beat interval is 230 msec (lower part of figure). (Reproduced from Wellens et al. (1976) with permission.)

occurred at a longer coupling interval of 480 msec to the stimulated premature impulse. This inverse relationship is also sometimes apparent in the animal models, but we do not have data indicating the exact frequency of its occurrence. This feature of an inverse relationship is predicted to be a characteristic of reentry and not triggered activity. As we have described in Chapter I, in some studies the coupling intervals of delayed afterdepolarizations to the preceding action potentials are not altered by the degree of prematurity (Johnson and Rosen 1987) while occasionally the rate of rise of the delayed afterdepolarizations may increase after shorter coupled premature impulses, causing the afterdepolarizations to reach their peak sooner. Therefore, there may be no change in the interval from the premature impulse to the first impulse of triggered tachycardia (S_2-T_1) over a range of premature coupling intervals (Johnson and Rosen 1987) or there may be a direct relationship between the premature coupling intervals (S_1-S_2) and interval from the premature impulse to the first impulse of triggered tachycardia (S_2-T_1). On the other hand, the inverse relationship is an expected characteristic of reentry. As the prematurity of the stimulated impulse increases (the coupling interval decreases), the impulse is expected to conduct more slowly through the reentrant circuit because it encounters more refractory tissue. The more slowly the impulse conducts through the reentrant circuit, the longer it takes to reemerge from the circuit to cause the first impulse of tachycardia; thus the coupling interval between the premature impulse and the first impulse of tachycardia lengthens. The slow conduction of the premature impulses was easily demonstrated in the studies on paroxysmal supraventricular tachycardia in which the slowly conducting part of the reentrant circuit is in the AV node and conduction through this part of the circuit could be estimated by the A-H interval on the His bundle electrogram (Bigger and Goldreyer 1970). However, measurements of conduction in the slowly conducting part of the circuit causing ventricular tachycardia are more difficult to make and rely on local electrogram recordings from the vicinity of the reentrant circuit in the infarct. Such recordings are not always available. In about two thirds of the clinical cases of sustained ventricular tachycardia, there is no inverse relationship between premature impulse coupling interval and the first cycle length of the tachycardia. In these cases there is usually no change in the cycle length between the premature impulse and the first impulse of tachycardia as the premature coupling decreases. A direct relationship is rarely seen. There are a number of theoretical reasons why the inverse relationship might not be seen in some cases of ventricular tachycardia even when reentry is still the mechanism. For example, there may be intervening regions of slow conduction between the site of stimulation and the reentrant circuit or between the circuit and the rest of the ventricles. Slowing of conduction of the premature impulse before entering or after leaving the circuit may distort the expected relationship. Also, when the reentrant circuit is functional, it may change its size or shape after very early premature impulses. A change in the length of the reentrant pathway would then alter the interval between premature and first tachycardia impulse in an unexpected way.

The characteristics of initiation by rapid pacing of tachycardias caused by triggered activity and by reentry are also expected to be different. During rapid pacing, afterdepolarizations have a faster rate of rise and attain threshold more quickly than at slow rates of pacing. Therefore, the interval between the first impulse of triggered tachycardia and the last stimulated impulse should be directly related to the rate of stimulation (shorter at faster rates). This is not a characteristic of reentry and has not been shown to occur when ventricular tachycardia can be initiated by rapid pacing in hearts with healing or healed infarcts. The rate of ventricular tachycardia in the setting of infarction is also not dependent on the pacing rate that induces it, a feature that is expected of tachycardia caused by delayed afterdepolarizations that result from digitalis (see Chapter I).

The initiation of nonsustained and sustained ventricular tachycardia by programmed stimulation is often dependent on the site of stimulation in both clinical and experimental studies. Stimulation from some right ventricular sites is more effective than from others. Left ventricular stimulation may be more effective than right ventricular stimulation, particularly when only one or two premature stimuli are applied. We would not expect triggered activity caused by delayed afterdepolarizations to be dependent on the site of stimulation, whereas there are plausible explanations to explain possible influences of the site of stimulation on the initiation of reentry. In order for a premature impulse to induce triggered tachycardia, it need only reach the triggerable fibers at the required coupling interval. One might propose that areas of conduction block between the site of stimulation and the triggerable focus could prevent triggering from some stimulation sites and not others (Josephson et al. 1984). However, in order to postulate that failure to induce a tachycardia arising in the left ventricle by stimulation of the right ventricle but not the left ventricle is the result of conduction block between the site of stimulation and a triggerable focus, the area of conduction block needs to be enormous and such large areas of block have not been demonstrated. In fact, during failure to induce tachycardia from a particular stimulation site, local electrogram recordings from the site of the proposed arrhythmia origin have shown that the premature impulse reached that site. On the other hand, induction of reentry can be influenced by the stimulation site in experimental studies because the site of stimulation influences the ability of the stimulated impulse to enter the circuit and block.

Experimental evidence derived from studies on isolated cardiac preparations with delayed afterdepolarizations shows that a period of inactivity after a period of triggered activity facilitates another induction of triggered activity. Repeated inductions of ventricular tachycardia in both the clinical and experimental studies does not require intervening periods of inactivity or slow sinus rhythm as may be necessary for repeated inductions of triggered activity.

Characteristics of Termination, Resetting, and Entrainment

The effects of stimulation can only be studied on sustained, hemodynamically stable tachycardia. In many (but not all) investigations of sustained ventricular tachycardias in both experimental animal models and in humans, it has been found that the tachycardias can be reproducibly terminated by one or several premature stimuli delivered during a critical time in the tachycardia cycle length. This is a property expected of a reentrant mechanism, but not impulse initiation caused by automaticity. Triggered activity caused by delayed afterdepolarizations might also be terminated by premature impulses and triggered activity caused by early afterdepolarizations might rarely be terminated. Since delayed afterdepolarization-dependent triggered activity can be terminated by premature impulses (Wit and Rosen 1986) (Chapter I) additional characteristics of the termination are necessary to make a stronger case for reentry. In our experience with studies on experimental models of triggered activity not caused by digitalis intoxication, it has been very difficult to terminate triggered rhythms with single or multiple premature stimuli, although occasionally this can be accomplished (Wit and Cranefield 1976). This is also the experience of the Rosen laboratory with experiments on both digitalis and nondigitalis models of triggered activity (Johnson and Rosen 1987). Therefore, termination of an arrhythmia by one or two premature impulses seems to be reasonable evidence for reentry.

Termination of a reentrant tachycardia by an impulse arising outside the reentrant circuit (at a site of stimulation) is dependent on several factors: (1) the ability of the impulse to reach the reentrant circuit; (2) the ability of that impulse to enter into the reentrant circuit when it is able to reach it; (3) the ability of the impulse to enter the circuit at an appropriate time relative to the location of the reentrant wave front in order to extinguish that reentrant wave front. In the case of tachycardias caused by myocardial infarction, the reentrant circuit is usually in the left ventricle. During stimulation from right ventricular sites, the premature impulse often has a long distance to travel to reach the circuit. (An exception is those tachycardias with a left bundle branch block pattern. The exit route from the circuit may be in the intraventricular septum. Some right ventricular stimulation sites may be close to the circuit in this situation (Rosenthal et al. 1986; Stamato et al. 1987)). Premature impulses initiated at a short coupling interval to the previous QRS are sometimes not able to reach the reentrant circuit on time to terminate the tachycardia when the intervening tissue has a long refractory period, causing conduction of the premature impulses to block before reaching the circuit (Wellens et al. 1971). This problem may sometimes be overcome by stimulating multiple premature impulses to "peel back" the refractory period (Almendral et al. 1986a; Stamato et al. 1987). The first of two premature impulses may conduct part of the way to the circuit and block, but the refractory period following it is short because of the prematurity. A second premature impulse may succeed in reaching the circuit because of the shortening of the refractory period. Electrogram recordings in clinical studies have shown the failure of right ventricular single premature stimuli to reach the left ventricle while the second of two premature stimuli succeeded (Josephson et al. 1978b). Therefore, several premature impulses in succession may be necessary to stop a tachycardia.

When there is a long distance between the site of stimulation and the circuit, reentrant impulses have more of a chance of leaving the circuit and depolarizing large areas surrounding the circuit before the premature impulse arrives. The premature impulse might then be prevented from reaching the circuit because it collides with the tachycardia impulse. The last of a series of multiple premature impulses, however, might succeed in reaching the circuit. If a single premature impulse collides with the excitation wave emanating from the circuit, at a distance from the circuit, a second closely coupled premature impulse may be able to advance further towards the circuit and even reach the circuit. The refractory period of the first stimulated premature impulse is short because of the preceding short cycle length. This enables the second premature impulse to propagate to the circuit prior to the exit from the circuit of the next reentrant impulse.

It is usually easier to terminate tachycardias with premature stimuli from left ventricular sites since they are often near the reentrant circuits as long as the circuit has an excitable gap. Rapid tachycardias are more difficult to terminate with single prematurely stimulated impulses than slow tachycardias, even if the site of stimulation is close to the circuit (Stamato et al. 1987). Often, a rapid tachycardia cannot be terminated by a single premature impulse. One possible explanation is that at the more rapid rate of tachycardia, impulses leaving the circuit prevent single premature impulses from reaching it by rendering the tissue around the circuit refractory. In addition, the excitable gap of rapid tachycardias may have a shorter duration than the gap of tachycardias with longer cycle lengths because the rapid rate is the result of either a smaller circuit or more rapid propagation in the circuit; both tend to decrease the size of the excitable gap. Rapid tachycardias can be terminated by several premature impulses in succession. However, sometimes neither a slow nor a rapid tachycardia can be terminated by one or several prematurely stimulated impulses and overdrive stimulation is required to stop the tachycardia (Josephson et al. 1978b).

Premature impulses terminate tachycardia only when their coupling is decreased to a critical interval that enables the stimulated impulse to block in the antegrade pathway of the reentrant circuit while colliding with the reentrant impulse in the retrograde pathway. The longer coupled premature impulses may still affect the reentrant circuit and tachycardia without terminating it. Effects on the reentrant circuit are manifested by transient alterations in the tachycardia cycle length following the premature impulse. The effects of premature impulses on subsequent tachycardia cycles are of interest because they also help distinguish reentry from other arrhythmogenic mechanisms as well as provide information about the properties of the reentrant circuit (Almendral et al. 1986a; Rosenthal et al. 1986; 1988; Stamato et al. 1987) (See Chapter I). Since these studies have been done without mapping the propagation of the reentrant impulse in the circuit, it must be kept in mind that many of the conclusions that have been drawn are inferred rather than proven.

The responses of sustained ventricular tachycardia to premature impulses have been determined in patients with healed myocardial infarction (Almendral et al. 1986b; Rosenthal et al. 1986; Stamato et al. 1987). Unfortunately, comparable data have not been reported for experimental models. In all patients studied there was a range of long premature coupling intervals during which resetting of the tachycardias did not occur, e.g., the tachycardia impulse following the premature impulse came exactly on time (it was compensatory), indicating that the circuit was not affected. Capture of the ventricles without affecting the tachycardia also implies small or localized circuits and is evidence that the bundle branches are usually not part of the circuit (Josephson et al. 1978d). Resetting of 50% to 60% of the tachycardias studied occurred following a single premature impulse, although the range of premature coupling intervals at which resetting occurred in each patient was quite variable. When resetting occurred, the QRS following the premature impulse came earlier than expected and was less than compensatory. Some tachycardias that could not be reset by single premature impulses could be reset by two premature impulses delivered in succession (Almendral et al. 1986a; Stamato et al. 1987). The first of the two premature impulses did not reach the reentrant circuit and was followed by a fully compensatory pause at all coupling intervals. Addition of the second premature impulse resulted in the resetting. The increased incidence of resetting with multiple premature impulses over single premature impulses is similar to the increased incidence of termination with multiple premature impulses and is probably a result of the same mechanism (Almendral et al. 1986a). The first of the premature impulses "peels" back the refractory period and reverses the direction of spread of the activation wave from the circuit, enabling the second of the premature impulses to reach the circuit. In tachycardias that can be reset by single premature impulses, the zone of resetting can be extended by adding a second premature impulse (preceding it). The preceding impulse need not perturb the circuit itself, but it "peels" back the refractory period of the intervening tissue, allowing earlier coupled impulses following it to reach the circuit (Stamato et al. 1987).

The occurrence of resetting is also dependent on the site of stimulation. In the study of Rosenthal et al. (1986), some tachycardias could be reset by stimuli applied to the right ventricular apex and not the outflow tract and vice versa. As we have discussed previously, the site of stimulation may influence the ability of the premature impulse to reach the circuit.

The pattern of the resetting response of tachycardias to premature impulses varies, but is often different from that expected of impulse initiation caused by automaticity or triggered activity. The first cycle length of some tachycardias following the premature impulse (either a single premature or the second of two prematures) is the same as before the premature impulse and remains constant as the prematurity of the stimulus is decreased. This pattern has been called a "flat response pattern" by Josephson's group and is illustrated in the top panel of Figure 4.14 (Almendral et al. 1986a; Stamato et al. 1987). During a reentrant tachycardia, the cycle length following the premature impulse is likely to reflect propagation time of that impulse through the reentrant circuit. Therefore, it is proposed that when there is a "flat response pattern", the circuits have a wide, fully excitable gap since there is no evidence for slowing of conduction of the premature impulse in the circuit. Over the wide range of

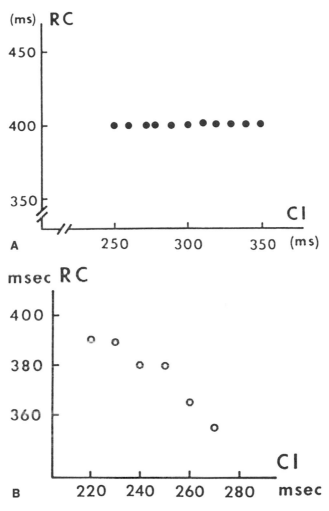

Figure 4.14: Response patterns of ventricular tachycardia to premature stimulation, as determined in clinical electrophysiology studies. The return cycle length (RC) following the premature stimulus is on the ordinate and the premature impulse coupling interval (CI) to the preceding tachycardia QRS is on the abscissa. The flat response shown in the top panel occurs when the return cycle does not change over a range of premature coupling intervals. The increasing response shown in the bottom panel occurs when the return cycle increases over the range of premature coupling intervals. (Reproduced from Almendral et al. (1986b) with permission.)

coupling intervals (more than 100 msec in Figure 4.14, top panel), the premature impulses were not able to enter the circuit early enough to encroach on relatively refractory tissue in the circuit. It must also be assumed that the entrance and exit routes of the premature impulses into and out of the circuit remain constant. A fixed exit route is suggested by a constant morphology of the QRS complex following the prematurely stimulated one that is the same as the tachycardia QRS morphology. A change in the entrance site would be expected to cause a change in the conduction time around the circuit and therefore, a change in the return cycle (Almendral et al. 1986a). The duration of the fully excitable gap in these patients is at least as long as the range of coupling intervals over which the flat return response was obtained. However, the excitable gap may exceed the resetting interval since the refractoriness between the stimulus site and the reentrant circuit may limit the prematurity with which the stimulated impulse arrives at the circuit (Almendral et al. 1986b). Because of the extensive fully excitable gap, the mechanism causing reentry is probably not the leading circle mechanism in a functional pathway since the leading circle mechanism is not expected to have a fully excitable gap. A fully excitable gap is usually thought to be associated with an anatomical circuit, but it can also occur in functional, anisotropic circuits. A "flat response pattern" is not, in and of itself, characteristic of only reentry. As we described in Chapter I, it may also occur during automatic or triggered activity. It therefore cannot be used alone to prove that reentry is the arrhythmogenic mechanism.

In other patients, the cycle following the premature impulse increases as the premature coupling interval decreases as shown by the increasing response patterns in the bottom panel of Figure 4.14. This pattern suggests that there is slowing of conduction in the reentrant circuit, which is dependent on prematurity (Almendral et al. 1986a; Stamato et al. 1987). Although circuits having this response pattern have an excitable gap allowing the stimulated impulse to enter the circuit, the slowing of conduction indicates that the gap is not fully excitable and that the premature impulse conducts in increasingly relatively refractory tissue in the circuit, as it enters the circuit earlier and earlier. This can also occur in either anatomical circuits or functional circuits caused by anisotropic reentry. An increasing response pattern over a wide range of premature coupling intervals (60 msec in Figure 4.14, bottom panel) is not characteristic of arrhythmogenic mechanisms other than reentry. The rate of increase of the return cycle after more prematurely stimulated impulses, as shown by the slope of the line, has been found to be an indicator of the "ease" with which tachycardia can be terminated by premature impulses. The slope of the resetting curves of tachycardias that can be terminated by premature impulses is steeper than the slope of resetting curves of tachycardias that cannot be terminated (Gottlieb et al. 1990). The slope is thus a predictor of the potential for conduction block of the premature impulse in the circuit.

Another response pattern that has been found to occur in these patients is that the cycle length following the premature impulse is flat at long premature coupling intervals and then increases as the coupling intervals are decreased further (a mixed curve). This response pattern is expected to be characteristic of a circuit with a small fully excitable gap enabling a narrow range of long coupled premature impulses to propagate in fully excitable tissue in the circuit, but short coupled premature impulses propagate in relatively refractory tissue (Almendral et al. 1986b). The mixed response curves are also not characteristic of arrhythmogenic mechanisms other than reentry. The tachycardias with the increasing return cycles or the mixed flat and increasing return cycles usually demonstrated resetting over 10% of the tachycardia cycle length (Almendral et al. 1986a). This would not be expected of the leading circle mechanism where any partially excitable gap would be expected to have a very narrow duration. The size of the excitable gap might have an important effect on the efficacy of antiarrhythmic drugs. Thus, a class III antiarrhythmic agent, which prolongs the refractory period, may be expected to be more effective the smaller the excitable gap.

The return cycle after the premature impulse as measured on the ECG has been less than the tachycardia cycle in a significant number of tachycardias (Almendral et al. 1986a; Rosenthal et al. 1988). It has been proposed that this would occur if the stimulated impulse penetrates the tachycardia circuit at a site different than the exit site and then reaches the exit site before completing a full revolution in the reentrant pathway (Almendral et al. 1986a). If there was only one common entrance and exit point into and out of the circuit, the return cycle would need to be at least the same as the tachycardia cycle length because the stimulated impulse would have to traverse the entire circuit.

As mentioned above, the resetting patterns described for sustained ventricular tachycardia are different from those that occur during automaticity or triggered activity caused by delayed afterdepolarizations. Although, with those mechanisms of impulse initiation, the cycle length following the premature impulse is also less than compensatory, it is not expected to show a progressive increase as is characteristic of many of the ventricular tachycardias caused by infarction. However, despite the increase in the return cycle following early premature impulses in the studies on ventricular tachycardias, the responses were usually less than compensatory, unlike the results of studies on atrioventricular nodal reentrant tachycardia (Bigger and Goldreyer 1970). Conduction of premature impulses in the atrioventricular node appears to be slowed to a much greater extent than in the reentrant circuits of the ventricles.

Sustained ventricular tachycardia in hearts with healing or healed infarcts (in patients or the experimental animal models) can also be terminated by overdriving the ventricles (stimulating at a rate faster than the tachycardia rate) (Escher and Furman 1970; Bennett and Pentecost 1971; Fisher et al. 1978). The success rate in terminating tachycardia with this procedure is greater than for premature stimulation. In early attempts to utilize overdrive as clinical therapy, it was recognized that a critical rate of overdrive is necessary to terminate tachycardia and that rates slower than the critical rate are not effective. The period of overdrive must also last for a critical duration. As a research tool, the effects of overdrive on tachycardia have also provided important information about the arrhythmogenic mechanism. Termination of an arrhythmia by overdrive is suggestive of a reentrant mechanism and eliminates the possibility of an automatic mechanism. Triggered activity caused by delayed afterdepolarizations (and sometimes early afterdepolarizations) is terminated as well, so some additional features of the effects of overdrive are needed to distinguish triggered activity from reentry. In some experimental models of delayed afterdepolarization-dependent triggered activity, once overdrive is stopped the rate gradually slows for 10 to 20 beats prior to cessation of the tachycardia (Wit and Rosen 1986). This characteristic is not expected of reentry, which should most often terminate immediately after overdrive stimulation is stopped; there might occasionally be several additional impulses before termination. Sustained monomorphic ventricular tachycardia associated with infarction often does terminate immediately after a period of overdrive stimulation. Overdrive stimulation that does not terminate ventricular tachycardia associated with infarction may entrain it, a characteristic of reentrant excitation (MacLean et al. 1981; Anderson et al. 1984; Waldo et al. 1984; Almendral et al. 1985; Mann et al. 1985; Okumura et al. 1985; 1987; 1988; Kay et al. 1988). Entrainment is not expected to occur during overdrive of triggered activity.

The phenomenon of entrainment has been shown to occur in studies on sustained ventricular tachycardia in patients with old myocardial infarcts and/ or ventricular aneurysms (MacLean et al. 1981; Anderson et al. 1984; Waldo et al. 1984; Almendral et al. 1985; 1988; Mann et al. 1985; Okumura et al. 1987; Kay et al. 1988). Reports of entrainment of tachycardias during the late hospital phase of infarct healing have not yet been published. The concept of transient entrainment as developed by Waldo and his colleagues was discussed in Chapter I. Transient entrainment is defined as an increase in the rate of the tachycardia during overdrive pacing to the pacing rate, with resumption of the same tachycardia after termination of pacing. According to this definition, the ECG morphology during entrainment should resemble the ECG of the tachycardia. By indirect methods involving analysis of the electrocardiogram and locally recorded electrograms in the clinical studies it can be argued that during entrainment of a reentrant tachycardia, each of the overdrive (stimulated) impulses enters the reentrant circuit, travels through it to the normal exit route from the circuit (which may be different from the entrance route), and activates the ventricle from this exit route. At a critical rate of overdrive, a stimulated impulse causes conduction block in the circuit and terminates the tachycardia (Waldo et al. 1984). Mapping studies on reentrant circuits in experimental models of ventricular tachycardia in hearts with healing infarcts have, for the most part, confirmed interpretation of the clinical results (El-Sherif et al. 1987; Waldecker et al. 1993). The "increase in the rate of the tachycardia" distinguishes a reentrant mechanism from simple overdrive of an arrhythmogenic mechanism such as a pacemaker where the ECG morphology assumes the characteristic of the pacing site.

Figure 4.15 shows an example of entrainment of a ventricular tachycardia from a clinical study (Anderson et al. 1984). In panel A, five leads of the ECG recorded from a patient with a healed myocardial infarction are shown during a sustained ventricular tachycardia induced by programmed electrical stimulation. The QRS has a right bundle branch block morphology and a cycle length of 410 msec. Panel B shows the ECGs and electrograms during overdrive pacing of the tachycardia at a cycle length of 380 msec by stimuli applied to the right ventricle. The ventricular rate has increased to the pacing rate and the morphology of the QRS complexes on the ECG has assumed a right bundle branch block pattern with a rightward axis. The ECG has changed slightly

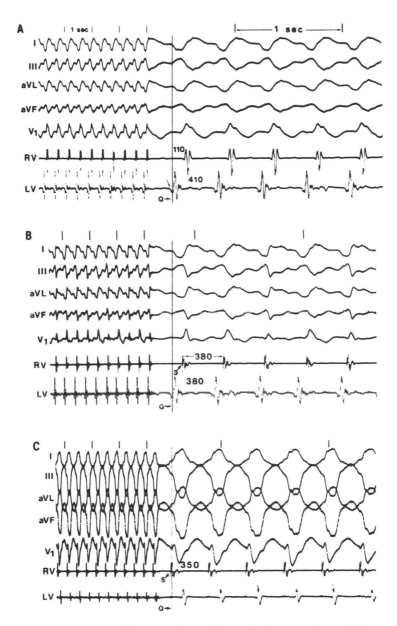

Figure 4.15: Entrainment of ventricular tachycardia in a patient with a myocardial infarct. In each panel, five electrocardiographic leads and electrograms recorded from the right (RV) and left (LV) ventricles are shown. Panel A shows the ECGs and electrograms during sustained tachycardia at a cycle length of 410 msec. Panel B shows the ECGs and electrograms during overdrive pacing from the right ventricle at a cycle length of 380 msec that entrains the tachycardia. Panel C shows the ECGs and electrograms during pacing from the right ventricle at a cycle length of 350 msec in the absence of tachycardia. (Reproduced from Anderson et al. (1984) with permission.)

from that of the unperturbed tachycardia that was shown in A, but still resembles the ECG of the tachycardia. Thus, the rate of the tachycardia has been increased to the pacing rate. The ECG during overdrive does not show the ECG characteristics of stimulation from the overdrive pacing site in the right ventricle. The characteristics of the ECG during right ventricular pacing at a cycle length of 350 msec in the absence of tachycardia is shown in panel C. The morphology of the QRS complex is a left bundle branch block pattern. The QRS during entrainment is a fusion QRS resulting from combined activation of the ventricles by stimulated impulses that entered the reentrant circuit and then left the circuit from its normal exit route as well as excitation waves coming directly from the pacing site without passing through the circuit (see Chapter I). Although ECG fusion during overdrive was one of the original criteria for entrainment it is only likely to occur when activation of the ventricles from the stimulus site (in the absence of tachycardia) produces a markedly different QRS than the tachycardia QRS (Waldo et al. 1984; Almendral et al. 1985; Mann et al. 1985). Entrainment of a reentrant tachycardia without ECG fusion can also occur and can be identified from electrogram recordings in the vicinity of the circuit (Okumura et al. 1987; Almendral et al. 1988).

Another characteristic of entrainment of ventricular tachycardia is that termination of overdrive is followed by resumption of tachycardia with the same QRS morphology as prior to overdrive. This feature is shown in panel A of Figure 4.16, which shows ECG recordings from another patient (Mann et al. 1985). The ECG morphology of a tachycardia with a cycle length of 310 msec is apparent at the left (first two complexes). Overdrive from the right ventricular apex began at the "S" (arrow), at a cycle length of 280 msec. During pacing, the QRS configuration was similar to that of the ventricular tachycardia. On termination of overdrive at the right (arrow), tachycardia continued at its initial cycle length, with an unchanged QRS morphology. After entrainment, the cycle length from the last fused complex during overdrive to the first QRS, which is not fused is usually shorter than the spontaneous tachycardia cycle length and sometimes equal to the overdrive cycle length. The first QRS which is identical to the tachycardia QRS is a nonfused QRS that is still an entrained impulse resulting from the last paced beat emerging from the reentrant circuit (see Chapter I). The cycle length between the last fused QRS and the first QRS that is not fused is dependent on the conduction time of the last stimulated impulse in the reentrant circuit and the time it takes for this impulse to begin activating the rest of the ventricles after leaving the circuit (Almendral et al. 1985; Mann et al. 1985).

Another feature of entrainment is that when a tachycardia is overdriven at a critically rapid rate, fusion no longer occurs and the tachycardia is terminated after overdrive is stopped. Figure 4.16 demonstrates this characteristic (Mann et al. 1985). In panel B the ECG recorded during a tachycardia with a cycle length of 320 msec is shown at the left. Pacing was initiated at the right ventricular apex at a cycle length of 280 msec (arrow) and accelerated the ventricular rate to this cycle length. During pacing, the configuration of the QRS complexes is similar to the configuration during tachycardia. Without stopping the pac-

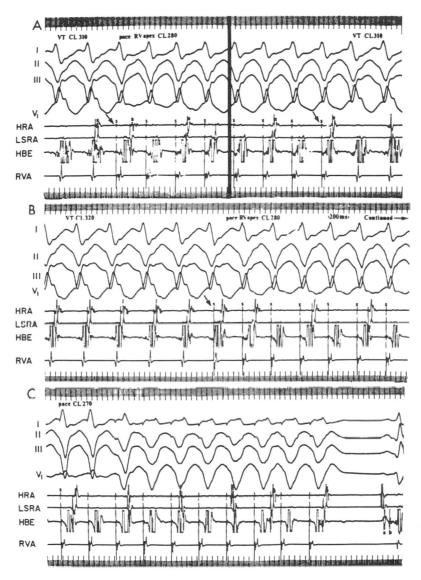

Figure 4.16: Entrainment and termination of ventricular tachycardia in a patient with a myocardial infarct. In each panel are shown four electrocardiographic leads and electrograms recorded from the high right atrium (HRA), low septal right atrium (LSRA), His bundle (HBE), and right ventricular apex (RVA). In panel A, the first two complexes at the left are those of the tachycardia with a cycle length of 310 msec. Overdrive pacing from the right ventricular apex at a cycle length of 280 msec began at the left arrow (on HRA trace) and stopped at the right arrow. Panel B shows another episode of tachycardia at a cycle length of 320 msec. Overdrive pacing from the right ventricular apex, at a cycle length of 280 msec, began at the arrow on the HRA trace. The recordings in panel C show the effects of decreasing the pacing cycle length to 270 msec. (Reproduced from Mann et al. (1985) with permission.)

ing, the pacing cycle length was decreased to 270 msec (panel C) causing a sudden change in the QRS to a left bundle branch block morphology. This is the morphology that occurred when the ventricles were paced from the right ventricular apex in the absence of tachycardia. When overdrive was stopped (at the right) tachycardia did not resume. The interpretation is that the tachycardia terminates because conduction block of a stimulated impulse occurs simultaneously in the antegrade and retrograde direction of the reentrant circuit (see Chapter I).

Failure of termination of tachycardia to occur (Fisher et al. 1978) may indicate a small, protected circuit (Josephson 1978d) into which the stimulated impulse cannot penetrate. At rapid rates of overdrive stimulation, changes may also occur in the circuits to cause acceleration of the rhythm rather than termination or to cause a new tachycardia with a different QRS complex (Fisher et al. 1978). Later, we will return to an additional discussion of entrainment since, besides being used as an indicator of reentry, it has also provided information about the electrophysiological properties of reentrant circuits causing ventricular tachycardia.

Development of the Pathophysiological Substrate for Reentry as Determined from Programmed Stimulation Studies

From the studies on induction of tachyarrhythmias by programmed stimulation in patients who have had a myocardial infarction, we can formulate a picture of when the reentrant circuits develop that lead to the late hospital and chronic ventricular tachycardias. These reentrant circuits are, in all likelihood, not the same circuits that cause the acute ischemic arrhythmias. The time of occurrence of these later arrhythmias, after the acute phase of early arrhythmias subsides, is dependent both on the formation of the appropriate anatomical substrate for the reentrant circuits and the development of special electrophysiological properties in the surviving cardiac muscle forming this substrate. After an acute myocardial infarction, the reentrant circuits develop in and around the infarcted region during the healing process. Some myocardial fibers survive in the healing infarct and the reentrant circuits form in the surviving fibers. We will provide more information on the specific anatomical features of these circuits later.

Sustained and nonsustained tachycardias have been induced in about 10% of patients studied by programmed stimulation, as early as 5 days after infarction (Kuck et al. 1986) and in an increasing number of patients (20% to 50%) by 3 weeks after infarction (Breithardt et al. 1985; Roy et al. 1985; Waspe et al. 1985b; Kuck et al. 1986). Many of these patients in whom tachycardia could be induced by programmed stimulation did not show spontaneously occurring tachyarrhythmias (Richards et al. 1983; Breithardt et al. 1985; Denniss et al. 1985; Roy et al. 1985; 1986;). In those patients, it can be assumed that the anatomical and electrophysiological substrate for reentry has developed at this stage of infarct healing, but that there is no spontaneously occurring "triggering" event to initiate the arrhythmias. Other patients have both spontaneous and inducible tachycardias at this time, and therefore, have both the pathophysiological substrate (the reentrant circuit) and the spontaneous trigger (Hamer et al. 1982; Waspe et al. 1985a). What this trigger is, is uncertain. It might sometimes be appropriately timed, spontaneously occurring premature impulses that the programmed stimulation protocols mimic. However, this is not always the case and may not even be the usual trigger (Berger et al. 1988). Other factors that are candidates for the spontaneously occurring trigger include an increase in sympathetic discharge or a transient period of acute ischemia.

Why some patients develop the appropriate substrate (both anatomical and electrophysiological) for the occurrence of late hospital ventricular tachyarrhythmias and others do not is an important, but as yet unanswered question. Left ventricular function in some patients with inducible tachycardia but no spontaneously occurring tachycardia may be depressed (Richards et al. 1983; Denniss et al. 1985) and some of these patients may have more spontaneously occurring ventricular premature depolarizations than patients without inducible arrhythmias (Marchlinski et al. 1983). However, these distinguishing features do not always characterize the patients with inducible tachycardia in the late hospital period (Breithardt et al. 1985; Roy et al. 1985; 1986; Kuck et al. 1986). In several studies, it has been shown that the patients who have inducible late hospital sustained tachycardia in the absence of spontaneously occurring tachycardia cannot be distinguished from those who do not have inducible or spontaneously occurring tachycardia either by virtue of the occurrence of spontaneous ventricular tachycardia or fibrillation during the first 48 hours after the acute myocardial infarction (Denniss et al. 1985), infarct size (assessed by enzymes), or by severity of coronary disease assessed by angiographic studies (Marchlinski et al. 1983; Breithardt et al. 1985; Roy et al. 1985; 1986; Waspe et al. 1985b; Kuck et al. 1986). Thus, the development of the ability to sustain reentry at this time of infarct healing is not necessarily related to the amount of ischemic damage. However, patients with both spontaneously occurring sustained tachycardia and inducible sustained tachycardia in the late hospital period are more likely to have larger infarcts and depressed left ventricular function than patients without spontaneously occurring arrhythmias. Therefore, it seems that the larger the infarct, the more likely there will be spontaneously occurring triggering events. However, larger infarcts are not necessary for the appropriate anatomical substrate for reentry to be present.

Pathological studies on the healing of human infarcts show that changes in infarct anatomy associated with infarct healing may continue for as long as several years until the final scar is formed. One would expect that the healing process would therefore change the anatomy or electrophysiological properties of reentrant circuits with time and change the arrhythmias that the circuits cause. However, despite these continuing changes expected in the pathological anatomy, reentrant circuits that develop during the first 3 weeks can persist with fairly stable electrophysiological properties for many months in some patients (Roy et al. 1986). In most of these patients, the QRS morphology of tachycardia remained the same, but in some it did change. In other patients, there is evidence for changes in the circuits after the late hospital period, caused by infarct healing. These changes may either be anatomical or electrophysiological. Often the cycle length of tachycardia induced in-hospital is shorter than the cycle length of tachycardia that is induced later (Hamer et al. 1982; Marchlinski et al. 1983; Kuck et al. 1986; Roy et al. 1986). These changes in the arrhythmias suggest that some changes may be occurring in either the anatomy or the electrophysiology of the circuit with time. However, other factors may cause changes in arrhythmia characteristics such as differences in autonomic tone or plasma electrolytes between the time of the first and subsequent electrophysiological studies.

There are other patients whose responses to programmed stimulation suggest time-dependent changes in the anatomical or electrophysiological substrate for reentry. In those patients who have inducible tachycardias in-hospital, but not after hospital discharge, the anatomical changes that occur during the healing of the infarcted region may obliterate the reentrant circuit that is formed during early healing. Changes in electrophysiological properties during healing may also make it impossible for reentrant excitation to occur (Marchlinski et al. 1983). In other patients, the development of the reentrant circuit or the electrophysiological properties that cause reentry may occur late during the time course of infarct healing. These are patients who do not have inducible tachycardia in the hospital, but do have inducible tachycardia months or years later when spontaneously occurring tachycardia develops. The reentrant circuit may then remain stable for years. In patients who develop spontaneously occurring sustained ventricular tachycardia in the setting of a ventricular aneurysm, the same tachycardia (QRS morphology, rate) often remains inducible and reoccurs over long periods of time (Schoenfeld et al. 1984) indicating that the circuit anatomy and electrophysiology remain stable. Patients who do not have inducible sustained tachycardia in the hospital may also die suddenly during the subsequent follow-up period (Roy et al. 1985) indicating that reentrant circuits or appropriate electrophysiology may develop later during the infarct healing period.

Finally, in addition to changes in the reentrant circuit, there may be changes in the arrhythmia "trigger" as the infarct heals. Some of the patients who have inducible sustained tachycardia, but no spontaneous ones during the late hospital period may go on to develop spontaneously occurring tachycardia and/or sudden death months later (Richards et al. 1983; Borgreffe et al. 1985; Breithardt et al. 1985; Denniss et al. 1985, Roy et al. 1985; 1986; Waspe et al. 1985b). Although, in some of the patients who die suddenly after discharge from the hospital, there may be new episodes of acute ischemia that are responsible for the arrhythmias, a large number of deaths during the first year after acute myocardial infarction are unexpected and are not associated with clinical or postmortem evidence of fresh myocardial ischemia or infarction (Denniss et al. 1985). It appears that the reentrant substrate that was present during the healing phase of infarction as shown by the inducibility of arrhythmias by programmed stimulation remained, and a spontaneous trigger—the nature of which has not yet been elucidated—developed.

The animal models of arrhythmias in hearts with healing or healed infarcts mimic some of these time-dependent changes in arrhythmogenesis that occur in patients. Sustained ventricular tachycardia can be induced during the first week after coronary occlusion, often without evidence of spontaneously occurring tachycardia. Thus, the substrate for reentry is present without the trigger. In some hearts, inducibility of tachycardia decreases with time until it can no longer be induced after 1–2 weeks. This kind of response resembles those patients who have inducible arrhythmias during the late hospital period, but not later. Studies on canine models have also shown that tachycardias may be induced for months or years in some hearts, similar to some of the patients described above. Therefore, further study of these animal models might answer many of the questions concerning time-dependent changes in the arrhythmogenic substrate, both anatomical and electrophysiological, that have been raised by the results of the clinical electrophysiological studies.

Location of Reentrant Circuits Causing Ventricular Tachyarrhythmias

Where is the site of origin of the ventricular tachyarrhythmias in hearts with healing and healed infarcts? To answer this question we rely to a large extent on the results of electrophysiological mapping studies that have located "early activity" during tachycardia. The location of reentrant circuits has also been inferred from the location of sites where extracellular electrograms have been recorded with characteristics that are equated with reentrant excitation; that is, sites where electrograms show continuous activity are often considered to be sites of reentry even in the absence of mapping data. Here, we would like to again stress an important principle that was also discussed with relation to the subacute arrhythmias in Chapter III: the site of arrhythmia origin is dependent on the location of surviving myocardial cells in and around the infarcted region. It is necessary to have these surviving cells in order to have arrhythmias. These cells may have electrophysiological properties that are favorable for the occurrence of reentry as a result of being exposed to the trauma of the ischemic environment for a long period of time; the geometrical arrangement of the cells that survive may be favorable for the formation of reentrant circuits, or some combination of the two. The location of the surviving cells in the infarct region is influenced by the particular coronary artery that is occluded, by the location of the occlusion along the length of the coronary artery (proximal or distal), by the presence and location of collateral blood supply, and by the duration of the occlusion (permanent versus temporary with reperfusion). The results of the experimental studies have emphasized this concept, since in those studies it has been possible to vary the location and duration of the coronary occlusion and show how these variables influence the location of the surviving myocardial cells and origin of the arrhythmias.

Anatomical Characteristics of Healing and Healed Infarcts: Relationship to Arrhythmia Origin

Before discussing the electrophysiological data that show where the arrhythmias originate, we will discuss some of the anatomical characteristics of the healing and healed infarcts in both the experimental models and in humans. The purpose is to describe where the surviving myocardial cells are located. This information will later be correlated with the site of origin shown by the electrophysiological studies.

Experimental Infarcts

We will first describe the experimental infarcts before the human infarcts because of the more detailed information that is available about the anatomical characteristics of the sites of arrhythmia origin. After the experimental studies showed the relationship between arrhythmia origin and infarct anatomy, studies on human infarcts indicated that the relationship applies to clinical arrhythmias as well. Some of what we say here has been mentioned previously, but we will now provide more details.

In the experimental models in which the effects of prolonged ischemia and infarction have been studied, it has been shown that myocardial fibers may survive on either or both the epicardial and endocardial surfaces of healing and healed infarcts, even when the coronary artery is occluded near its origin and the infarct is transmural (Lazzara et al. 1973; Friedman et al. 1975; Myerburg et al. 1977; Karagueuzian et al. 1979; 1980; Mehra et al. 1983; Wetstein et al. 1984; Kramer et al. 1985; Ursell et al. 1985; Wetstein et al. 1985b). These regions of surviving myocardial cells are called the epicardial and endocardial border zones (Wit et al. 1981a). Muscle fibers may also survive in intramural regions of the infarct, particularly if there is reperfusion of the ischemic region before intramural cell death is complete (Karagueuzian et al. 1979; Michelson et al. 1980; 1981c). Both epicardial and endocardial border zones, as well as the intramural fibers are important sites of arrhythmogenesis. Similar patterns of cell survival also occur in human infarcts. There is also the possibility that myocardial cells surviving along lateral aspects of infarcts may have abnormal electrophysiological properties that may cause arrhythmias. The presence of such a lateral border zone in acutely ischemic regions is controversial (see Chapter II), but there is some evidence for its existence in healed infarcts (Denniss et al 1989).

Epicardial Border Zone　　The epicardial border zone is an important site of arrhythmia origin in healing canine infarcts. Muscle fibers on the epicardial surface of transmural anteroseptal canine infarcts caused by permanent occlusion of the left anterior descending coronary artery near its origin survive because they still receive blood flow from epicardial branches of the circumflex artery or from collaterals of the left anterior descending coronary artery that anastomose with the patent circumflex. A redistribution of coronary blood flow from necrotic endocardial layers to surviving epicardial ones may also maintain their viability (Hirzel et al. 1976). Therefore, if the circumflex branches are occluded along with the left anterior descending coronary artery, epicardial muscle may not survive. Since occlusion of the main circumflex artery has not been extensively used for arrhythmia studies in canine hearts with healing and healed infarcts, we do not know if there would be similar epicardial muscle survival after occlusion of this artery. Muscle fibers on the epicardial surface of reperfused infarcts, that is, infarcts caused by a 2- to 3-hour occlusion of the left anterior descending coronary artery followed by reperfusion, also survive because the wave front of ischemic cell death (see Chapter III) does not reach them for more than several hours after occlusion (Reimer et al. 1977; Reimer and Jennings 1979) and therefore, they are still viable when blood flow is reestablished.

The microscopic anatomy of the border zone of surviving epicardial muscle in canine infarcts has important influences on the electrophysiological properties of this region that cause arrhythmias. Two aspects of the anatomy influence properties of impulse conduction: thickness of the surviving rim of muscle and orientation of the muscle bundles that form the rim. In infarcts resulting from permanent occlusion and occlusion and reperfusion, the border zone of surviving epicardial muscle cells on the anterior surface of the left ventricle has a thickness of from one to several hundred cells. The number of surviving cell layers is fewest towards the center and increases towards the margin with normal myocardium (Karagueuzian et al. 1977; Wit et al. 1982a; Mehra et al. 1983; Ursell et al. 1985). This pattern is shown in Figure 4.17 in which the number of muscle cell layers that survived on the epicardial surface of the anterior left ventricle of a healing, transmural canine infarct caused by permanent left anterior descending coronary artery occlusion is plotted. The top of the oval area that represents the epicardial border zone is the base of the left ventricle, the margin to the left is adjacent to the left anterior descending coronary artery, and the margin towards the right is on the lateral left ventricle. Each pattern of shading indicates the number of surviving epicardial cell layers that was counted from histologic sections, according to the key at the bottom of the Figure. In this infarct, there was an extensive center region where only 2 to 10 cell layers survived forming a narrow sheet, which increased in thickness to more than 100 cell layers towards the margins with noninfarcted myocardium. At the right is a photomicrograph of the infarcted region near the center of the oval with the epicardial surface at the top. The surviving epicardial muscle cells beneath this surface are delineated by the thin arrows. There are 10–15 surviving cell layers at this site. The thick arrows towards

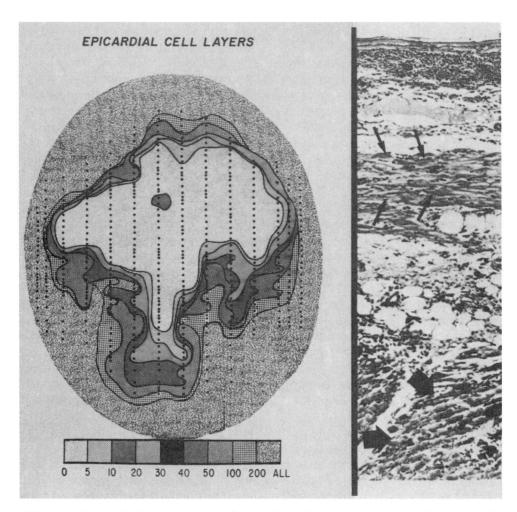

Figure 4.17: At the left is a map of the number of surviving muscle cell layers in the epicardial border zone of a healing canine infarct. The oval represents a large region of the epicardial surface of the anterolateral left ventricle. Each pattern of shading indicates the number of surviving epicardial cell layers (thickness) according to the key at the bottom of the figure. Thus, there is an extensive central region where only 2–10 cell layers survived, whereas toward the margins, the surviving cells constitute a layer greater than 100 cells thick. At the right is a photomicrograph of the infarcted region. At the top is the epicardial surface. The surviving epicardial muscle cells beneath the surface are delineated by the thin arrows. The thick arrows toward the bottom of the photomicrograph show infarcted muscle. (Reproduced from Wit et al. (1982a) with permission.)

the bottom of the photomicrograph show infarcted muscle. There is some variability in this pattern of cell survival among hearts, even when the site of occlusion is exactly the same. In occasional hearts, the infarct may extend all the way to the epicardial surface at some sites, forming a "hole" that interrupts the continuity of the epicardial rim of muscle. This inexcitable area may sometimes form the center of a reentrant circuit (Saltman 1990; 1993). In some hearts, the entire surviving epicardial rim may be much thicker, several hundred cell layers or more. In reperfused infarcts the epicardial border zone may sometimes be thicker than after a permanent occlusion (Karagueuzian et al. 1977; Wit et al. 1982b). Thickness after reperfusion is dependent on how much myocardium is salvaged by the return of coronary blood flow. If reflow is not complete, the surviving epicardial border zone may not be much different than after permanent occlusion. Very narrow or thin epicardial border zones have properties that favor the occurrence of reentry more than the thick ones as we describe later.

The surviving epicardial muscle fibers are arranged parallel to one another during the healing phase (first 2 weeks) after infarction. The long axis of the muscle fiber bundles is perpendicular to the left anterior descending coronary artery and extends from the coronary artery towards the lateral left ventricle and apex, the same orientation as epicardial muscle fibers in the noninfarcted anterior left ventricle (Roberts et al. 1979). The muscle fibers may be either tightly packed together, as they are in the normal subepicardium, or they may be separated by edema, which is commonly seen in a healing infarct. Examples of both kinds of arrangement are shown in Figure 4.18. In the top panel, the muscle fibers are widely separated by edema, while in the bottom panel they are closely packed together. The parallel orientation forms an anisotropic structure that has important influences on conduction properties that may cause reentry in this region.

The ultrastructure characteristics of the surviving subepicardial muscle cells in canine infarcts caused by permanent left anterior descending coronary artery occlusion have been studied during the first week. These characteristics show that, despite the normal histologic appearance, the cells have been affected by the prolonged ischemia (Ursell et al. 1985). Electron micrographs of the epicardial muscle cells in 1- and 5-day-old infarcts in Figure 4.19 show numerous nonmembrane-bound lipid droplets (labeled "L") within the sarcoplasm of most cells while other ultrastructural features are normal. The presence of lipid may indicate that ischemia has altered cellular metabolism (see Chapter III), which in turn might be related to some of the changes in transmembrane action potentials during the healing phase, which we discuss later. While it appears that in permanent occlusion infarcts all the epicardial cells have been influenced by ischemia, since lipid droplets can be found in almost all cells examined, it is uncertain whether this is the situation in reperfused infarcts. Spear et al. (1983a) have suggested that there might be intermingling of normal and abnormal muscle fibers.

As the infarct continues to heal, there are further changes in the structure of the epicardial border zone as determined by the studies on the canine models.

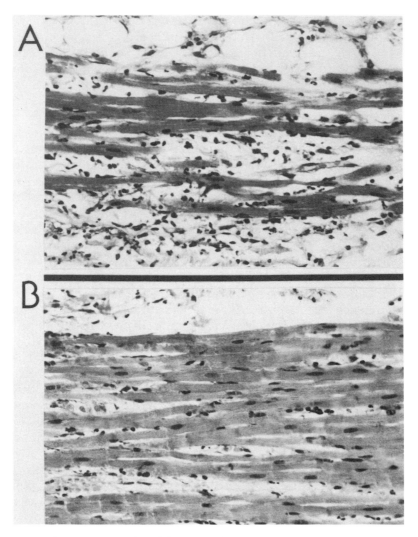

Figure 4.18: Photomicrographs of the parallel surviving muscle fibers in the epicardial border zone of a healing canine infarct. In some regions (A) muscle fibers are widely separated, while in others (B) they are packed more closely together. However, in both cases the fibers are oriented parallel to each other. (Reproduced from Dillon et al. (1988) with permission.)

Surviving epicardial muscle fibers in a 2-week-old infarct are shown in panels A and B of Figure 4.20. In panel A, the thin rim of the epicardial border zone consists of several layers of ventricular muscle cells between the epicardium and the granulation tissue of the healing infarct (arrows). These surviving cells are now separated by increased fibrous tissue, especially adjacent to the infarct below. The parallel orientation of the fibers, however, is generally maintained at this time. At high magnification (panel B), the myocardial cells appear to be intact with distinct cross-striations (Ursell et al. 1985). After 2 weeks, these surviving muscle cells display a range of ultrastructural appearances ranging from normal to highly abnormal. Figure 4.21 shows that the myocardial cells have an intact sarcolemma, but a moderate to marked loss of contractile elements and T tubules. The myofibrils that remain are in disarray. These changes may be a consequence of the reduced contractile activity. A few scattered lipid droplets remain in some cells, but no cells contain the extensive amount of lipid that is present during the first week after coronary occlusion. Thus, there may be recovery of more normal metabolism. There may be a relationship between the changing ultrastructural abnormalities and the changing abnormalities in the transmembrane potentials during this time period (see below).

Epicardial muscle also survives on the surface of healed permanent occlusion and reperfused infarcts more than 2 weeks after coronary artery occlusion (Gardner et al. 1984; 1985; Ursell et al. 1985; Duff et al. 1988; Hanich et al. 1988a). Further changes in the structure of the epicardial border zone evolve as the infarct continues to heal. Panels C and D of Figure 4.20 show that the muscle cells become trapped in the dense scar tissue formed from the infarct below and the pericarditis above. The organization of these muscle fibers in regions where they are present in relatively large numbers (20–30 cell layers) is similar to the 2-week-old infarcts; parallel-oriented fibers are separated by increased connective tissue (Ursell et al. 1985). In regions with fewer cell layers, myocardial fibers become markedly separated from each other along their length to such an extent that side-to-side connections between bundles are not always apparent (Gardner et al. 1984, 1985; Ursell et al. 1985). The individual cells and their orientation are also deformed by the growth of fibrous tissue. As is apparent in Figure 4.20C and D, the fibers are no longer parallel to one another, but rather are oriented in many different directions. The surviving subepicardial cells in healed infarcts have a range of ultrastructural appearances. Some have normal shapes and intracellular components. Others have markedly distorted shapes because the interstitium is expanded by abundant collagen that separates and isolates individual cells and portions of cells. An electron micrograph of muscle fibers in the surviving epicardial border zone over a 2-month-old infarct is shown in Figure 4.22 to illustrate this point. Despite their abnormal shape, intracellular structure, including contractile elements, is normal and lipid droplets are not present in abnormal amounts (Ursell et al. 1985). Further changes in anatomy may also occur during subsequent years relating to contraction of the size of the infarct, hypertrophy of myocardial cells, or aneurysm formation (Jugdutt and Amy 1986). There are no detailed anatomical studies on the epicardial border zone at these times in canine hearts, although Hanich et al. (1988a) have described more surviving muscle in reperfused infarcts at 4 years than at 2–24 weeks. This may be the result of contraction of the infarct scar in canine hearts (Choong et al. 1989).

The changes in the morphology of the epicardial border zone of canine infarcts that occur as the infarcts heal are representative of changes that occur in other infarct regions where myocardial cells survive, and show the changes

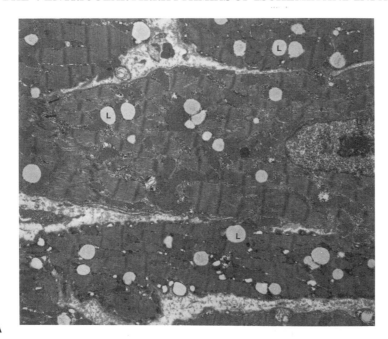

A

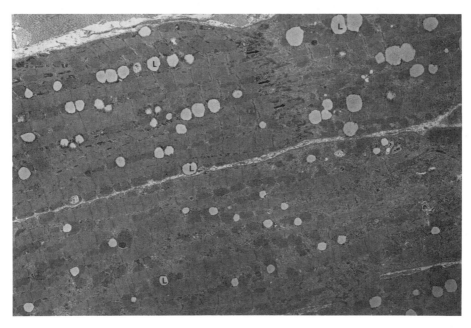

B

Figure 4.19: A: Ultrastructure of muscle fibers in the surviving epicardial rim of 1-day-old canine myocardial infarct. The only ultrastructural abnormality at this time is the presence of intrasarcoplasmic lipid droplets (L). The contractile elements, mito-chondria, and intercalated discs (arrows) appear normal. B: Ultrastructure of muscle fibers in the surviving epicardial rim of a 5-day-old canine myocardial infarct. As at 1 day, the only ultrastructural abnormality is the presence of intrasarcoplasmic lipid droplets (L).

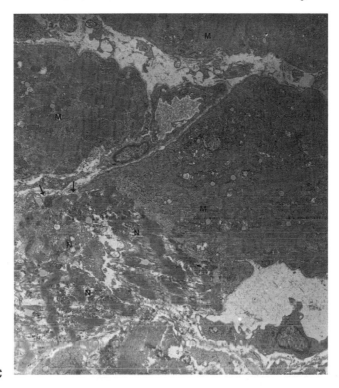

C

Figure 4.19: C: Ultrastructure at the interface between surviving muscle in the epicardial border zone and underlying necrotic muscle in a 5-day-old canine infarct. The cells at the top and right (M) are viable and have intact sarcolemmae and normal intracellular structure. The cells at the bottom (N) are necrotic and demonstrate ultrastructural features of irreversible cell injury. (Unpublished photographs of Philip C. Ursell.)

in the anatomical substrate of tachyarrhythmias that occur during infarct healing. One of the most important changes in morphology is the change in orientation of myocardial fibers from parallel bundles to complete disarray in some regions. As we will discuss in detail later, where there is parallel orientation of the muscle fibers, the epicardial border zone has the conduction properties of either a uniform or nonuniform anisotropic structure which may be important for reentry. Where the parallel orientation is lost, these conduction properties change drastically with no predictable directional differences, but the structure may still contribute to slow conduction that causes reentry. Therefore, the changes in the anatomical substrate during healing influence electrophysiological properties, which in turn may influence properties of the reentrant circuits and tachycardia.

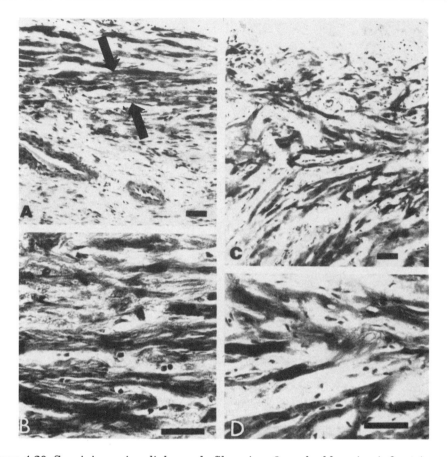

Figure 4.20: Surviving epicardial muscle fibers in a 2-week-old canine infarct (panels A and B) and in a 2-month-old canine infarct (panels C and D). In panel A, the thin surviving rim at 15 days (arrows) consists of several layers of ventricular muscle cells between the epicardium and the granulation tissue of the healing infarct. These surviving cells are separated by fibrous tissue, especially adjacent to the infarct. The parallel orientation of the fibers, however, is generally retained. At high magnification (panel B), these myocardial cells appear to be intact with distinct cross striations. In panel C, the disorganization of the surviving myocardial cells in the thin rim at 2 months is evident. The cells are widely separated and disoriented because of the ingrowth of fibrous tissue from the adjacent infarct. At high magnification (panel D), the myocardial cells have distinct cross-striations and central nuclei. The bars represent 50 μm. (Reproduced from Ursell et al. (1985) with permission.)

Endocardial Border Zone   Myocardial fibers survive on the endocardial surface of even extensive transmural infarcts. Some of the characteristics of this endocardial border zone have already been discussed in Chapter III in relation to the occurrence of the subacute arrhythmias that are mostly the result of automaticity. We will reiterate some points that are important for the reentrant arrhythmias that are the focus of discussion in this chapter. The survival of Purkinje fibers on the endocardial surface of transmural experimental ca-

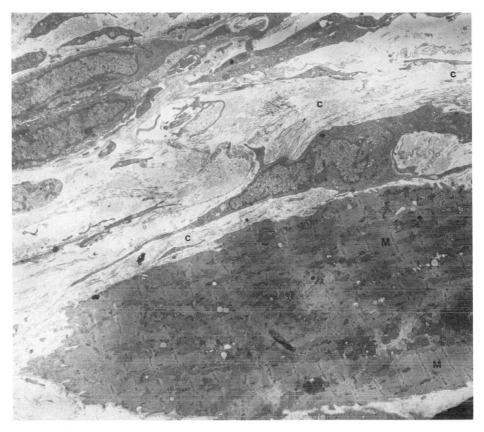

Figure 4.21: Ultrastructure of muscle fibers in surviving epicardial rim over a 2-week-old canine infarct. The most striking ultrastructural abnormalities of the myocardial cells at this time are the loss of some contractile elements (M) and replacement by large collections of monoparticulate glycogen and mitochondria. The sarcolemmae are intact, indicating cell viability. There are no longer large numbers of lipid droplets. (Unpublished photograph of Philip C. Ursell.)

nine infarcts caused by occlusion of the left anterior descending coronary artery can be attributed to a large extent to diffusion of oxygen and nutrients from the blood in the ventricular cavity but there are also other contributing factors that are discussed in Chapter III. Subendocardial ventricular muscle rarely survives in canine infarcts after permanent occlusion near the origin of the left anterior descending coronary artery, but may survive if the infarcts are reperfused after a period of occlusion lasting several hours, or if the occlusion is below one or more of the diagonal branches. Reperfusion restores coronary blood flow before the wave front of necrosis reaches the subendocardial muscle. More distal occlusions may spare some branches of the left anterior descending coronary artery that supply the subendocardial muscle. The details of the microscopic anatomy of this region during the healing phase of infarction are

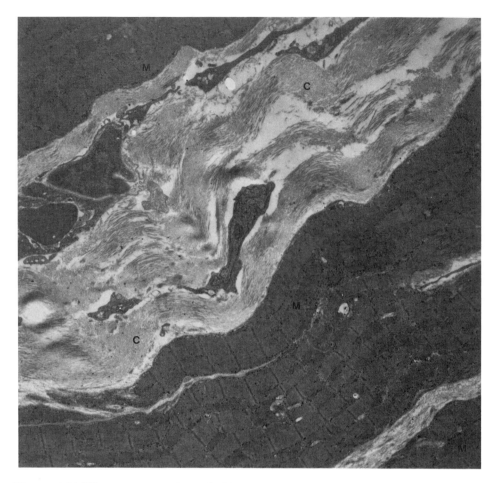

Figure 4.22: Ultrastructure of muscle fibers in surviving epicardial rim over a 2-month-old infarct. At this time, abundant collagen (C) in the interstitium separates the cells. The intracellular components—contractile elements, mitochondria, and glycogen—are intact and normal. (Unpublished photograph of Philip C. Ursell.)

discussed in Chapter III. The main structural feature of the surviving cells 1–3 days after occlusion, which we equated with the abnormal electrophysiology that causes the subacute automatic arrhythmias, was the accumulation of lipid droplets in the cytoplasm of the Purkinje cells. By 1 to 2 months, the ultrastructure of Purkinje cells that form the endocardial border zone is normal, as are the transmembrane potentials of these cells (Friedman et al. 1975). However, other structural changes that occur in this region during healing are similar to the changes in the epicardial border zone. After proximal occlusion, subendocardial fibrosis resulting from the healing process separates the bundles of Purkinje cells. When there is surviving subendocardial muscle, subendocardial fibrosis has similar effects on geometrical arrangement and intercellular connections as in the epicardial border zone, separating the muscle fibers and sometimes distorting their orientation. The fibrosis does not significantly affect conduction in the Purkinje system, which is normal during the later stages of healing, but it may influence conduction at Purkinje muscle junctions or in the subendocardial muscle where connections among cells may be disrupted by fibrosis (Kienzle et al. 1987), as we describe in detail later. Whether only Purkinje fibers survive on the endocardial surface or whether both Purkinje fibers and muscle survive may be important for arrhythmogenesis in the healing and healed phases. When only Purkinje fibers survive, their activation is normal and rapid and may not lead to arrhythmias. However, when subendocardial muscle also survives, conduction in the muscle may be abnormal as it is in the muscle of the epicardial border zone because of the structural changes, causing arrhythmias.

Arrhythmias in healing and healed infarcts have also been studied in a feline model of infarction caused by distal ligation of the left ventral artery in the cat (Bassett et al. 1977; Myerburg et al. 1977). Multiple layers of surviving subendocardial cells become trapped in the endocardial scar of the healed, transmural infarct forming an endocardial border zone where arrhythmias may originate. Some of the surviving cells are Purkinje fibers and other cells are ventricular muscle. The fibrous tissue from the healing infarct encroaches between the surviving cells in a similar way as we described for the epicardial and endocardial border zones of canine infarcts. Thus, myocardial fibers may be pulled apart and their orientation changed, and it is possible, although not explicitly shown by these studies, that intercellular connections are diminished and conduction properties altered.

Lateral Border Zone and Intramural Cell Survival   Viable muscle bundles may protrude into the infarct from its lateral edge and interdigitate with scar tissue in canine infarcts caused by either permanent occlusion of the left anterior descending coronary artery or by occlusion and reperfusion and may be an important factor in arrhythmogenesis (Karagueuzian et al. 1979; Michelson et al. 1980; 1981c; Denniss et al. 1989). The muscle bundles may extend as far as the center of the infarcted wall and appear as surviving intramural muscle. In the experimental healing and healed canine infarcts caused by permanent occlusion of the left anterior descending coronary artery near its origin, there is usually very little myocardial cell survival in intramural regions of the infarcts because extensive lateral bundle penetration is absent, and therefore, arrhythmias cannot originate at intramural sites. Arrhythmogenesis is dependent on the survival of the epicardial rim of muscle. More distal occlusions may leave some of the intramural branches from the left anterior descending coronary artery unobstructed resulting in intramural cell survival from penetrating lateral bundles (Denniss et al. 1989) just as it also results in subendocardial muscle survival. Reperfusion, if accomplished prior to irreversible intramural myocardial cell death, may salvage ischemic intramural cells. The lateral margins of the reperfused infarcts are very irregular (Karageuezian et al. 1979; Kramer et al. 1985) and peninsulas of surviving myocardial cells from the lateral margins penetrate well into the infarcted region. The surviving muscle in a transmural infarct caused by occlusion and reperfusion was shown in Figure 3.18 in Chapter III. Within the infarct, these myocardial cells are surrounded by the necrotic myocardium (Karageuezian et al. 1979; Michelson et al. 1980). Some viable intramural muscle cells may also form islands that are disconnected from the bordering noninfarcted myocardium (Karageuezian et al. 1979; Michelson et al. 1980). During the early healing stages (2–4 days) the surviving intramural cells can be distinguished from necrotic cells by the continued presence of centrally located nuclei and well demarcated cross striations as can be seen in panel C of Figure 3.18 (in Chapter III). These characteristics are maintained at later stages of healing during connective tissue proliferation (Karageuezian et al. 1979; Michelson et al. 1980). The connective tissue separates and distorts the orientation of the myocardial fiber bundles, which is expected to have the same effects on conduction as in the epicardial border zone; conduction may be slowed because of disruption of connections between cells. These effects of connective tissue separation on conduction properties are discussed in a later section. Surviving intramural muscle fiber bundles may form complex conduction pathways and reentrant circuits.

Human Infarcts

The information derived from the experimental studies indicates that there can be survival of myocardial fibers in subepicardial, subendocardial, and intramural regions of healing and healed infarcts depending on the location and duration of the coronary occlusion. These regions have abnormalities in electrophysiological properties that cause arrhythmias, which are discussed later. It was the establishment of the relationship between myocardial cell survival and arrhythmogenesis in these experimental models that prompted a search for similar cell survival in humans with ventricular arrhythmias. Although large infarcts have been equated with the occurrence of ventricular tachyarrhythmias in humans (Roberts et al. 1975), arrhythmias do not occur in all patients with large infarcts (Bolick et al. 1986). The survival of myocardial fibers in some, but not all large infarcts, or the location or organization of the surviving fibers might explain why arrhythmias occur in some of these hearts and not in others.

Epicardial Border Zone   There is sometimes an epicardial border zone in healing and healed human infarcts that plays a role in arrhythmogenesis. Figure 4.23 shows schematic diagrams of the morphology of healing and healed myocardial infarcts from a group of patients, some with ventricular tachycardia and some without (from the study of Bolick et al. 1986). Panel A represents hearts with no tachycardia, panel B represents hearts with healing infarcts

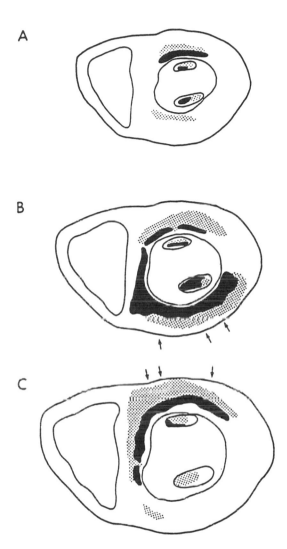

Figure 4.23: Illustration of cross-sectional slices from the infarcted hearts of patients with no ventricular tachycardia (A), subacute ventricular tachycardia (B), and chronic ventricular tachycardia (C). The subacute group (B) had predominantly large solid myocardial infarcts with a ribbon of spared subendocardium. Surviving muscle also occurred on the epicardial surface of the infarcts (arrow). The chronic ventricular tachycardia group (C) had predominantly large patchy myocardial infarcts with irregular spared subendocardium and some surviving epicardial muscle (arrows). The group without tachycardia (A) had smaller hearts and smaller more randomly distributed patchy myocardial infarcts. Black represents solid myocardial infarct, and stippling represents patchy myocardial infarct. Slices are seen from the basal aspect. (Reproduced from Bolick et al. (1986) with permission.)

(approximately 1 week) with tachycardia, and panel C represents hearts with healed infarcts with tachycardia. Patients with sustained ventricular tachycardia (panels B and C) often had a large area of solid, homogeneous infarct (black region) that usually included the septum and extended around much of the circumference of the ventricular cavity, from the anterior to the lateral wall. The solid infarct was transmural in that it extended from the subendocardium into the subepicardium and was larger in the healing than in the healed group. On the subepicardial surface over solid infarct, there was patchy infarct (stippled regions) and surviving subepicardial muscle (unshaded regions indicated by arrows) similar to the epicardial border zone in the canine infarction models. Older infarcts were composed of larger areas of patchy infarct and thinner epicardial border zones. The differences in some of these structural features may be related to different properties of reentrant circuits in healing versus healed infarcts as we inferred when we described the characteristics of the arrhythmias. Surviving subepicardial muscle cells can be found even in ventricular aneurysms. Surviving muscle in the epicardial border zone of two patients of Littmann et al. (1991) who had subepicardial reentrant circuits causing tachycardia is shown in Figure 4.24. The photomicrographs show strands

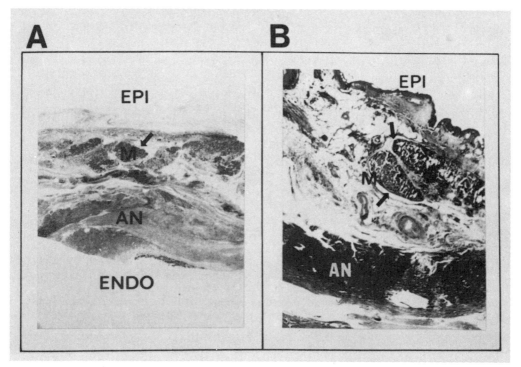

Figure 4.24: Histologic sections from two patients with left ventricular aneurysm and ventricular tachycardia related to subepicardial reentry. Both panels show strands of myocardial fibers (M and arrows) embedded in subepicardial fat and connective tissue. The epicardial surface (EPI) is at the top. (Reproduced from Littmann et al. (1991) with permission.)

of surviving myocardial fibers (M) at the border of a left ventricular aneurysm and normal myocardium. The myocardial fibers are embedded in subepicardial fat and connective tissue. There are no additional detailed microanatomy studies of the organization of the subepicardial muscle fibers nor of the changes that occur in these muscle fibers during the healing process. We suppose that there are similarities to the anatomy in canine hearts since the healing process in dogs and humans has many similar features. However, in healed human anteroseptal infarcts, particularly with aneurysms, the subepicardial muscle does not always form a continuous rim, but is sometimes discontinuous. This difference between some human and canine infarcts may explain some of the differences in the sites of arrhythmia origin between the experimental models and the human infarcts. As we show in the next section, many human tachycardias arise in the endocardial border zone, while canine tachycardias often arise in the epicardial border zone. If there is no continuous rim of subepicardial muscle in some human infarcts, there may be no possibility for reentrant circuits to form. Reentry then may occur in other regions where more muscle survives such as intramurally or in the subendocardium.

Endocardial Border Zone   As we have already discussed in Chapter III, a narrow "ribbon" consisting of both Purkinje fibers and ventricular muscle survives between the endocardial surface of the solid infarct and the ventricular cavity, the endocardial border zone of human infarcts (Fenoglio et al. 1983: Bolick et al. 1986). The surviving ribbon is shown in the diagrams in Figure 4.23. The surviving cells are then trapped in the scar as necrotic myocardial cells are replaced by fibrous tissue. Figure 4.25 shows some histologic pictures of muscle cells in the endocardial border zone from an endocardial resection that abolished chronic, sustained ventricular tachycardia in a patient with a 1-year-old infarct. Many of the surviving cells have a normal appearance (centrally located nuclei and cross-striations) (Fenoglio et al. 1983) although hydropic and vacuolar changes are also evident in some cells (Bolick et al. 1986). The myocardial fiber bundles and the cells within the bundles are widely separated by the fibrous tissue in some areas (panel B) where they are no longer oriented parallel to each other. In other areas, where they are packed more closely together (panel A) the fiber bundles maintain a parallel arrangement. These features are similar to the arrangement of muscle fibers in the healed epicardial and endocardial border zones of canine and feline hearts, and may provide the basis for similar electrophysiological properties that cause arrhythmias, i.e., slow, inhomogeneous propagation. However, Purkinje fibers are also present in the endocardial border zone and not the epicardial border zone, and influence activation so that some conduction properties of the two border zones may be different. These Purkinje fibers in healed infarcts look very similar to the canine Purkinje fibers in healed infarcts: their ultrastructure is essentially normal (Fenoglio et al. 1983). Subendocardial scarring and trapping of myocardial fibers in a subendocardial scar may also extend into areas around the periphery of infarcts, outside the region of transmural infarction, because coro-

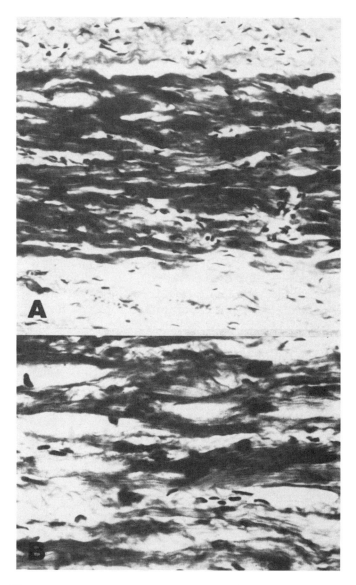

Figure 4.25: Histology of the subendocardial border zone in a patient with a healed transmural myocardial infarction and ventricular tachycardia. In tightly packed bundles (A) the myocardial cells are closely apposed. In this bundle the myocardial cells are well preserved and filled with myofibrils. In loosely packed bundles (B) the myocardial cells are separated by abundant interstitial connective tissue. In this bundle many of the myocardial cells are vacuolated. (Reproduced from Fenoglio et al. (1983) with permission.)

nary flow to this surrounding subendocardium may also be reduced (Geer et al. 1980). The trapped subendocardial muscle and Purkinje fibers in these peripheral regions are separated from the intramural muscle by the extensive subendocardial scar. Arrhythmias may arise in these peripheral regions since subendocardial resection of scarred areas around infarcts may stop tachycardia (Josephson et al. 1979). In patients with aneurysms and chronic, sustained ventricular tachycardia, survival of both subepicardial and subendocardial myocardial fibers occurs both within the aneurysm and in the infarcted regions bordering the aneurysms. Both regions may be involved in arrhythmogenesis, since aneurysmectomy alone does not abolish tachycardia in many cases (Thind et al. 1971). A surviving endocardial border zone can also be found in infarcted hearts without ventricular tachycardia so its presence alone is not the distinguishing factor between arrhythmic and nonarrhythmic hearts. The area of spared subendocardium was found to be larger in patients with ventricular tachycardia than in those without by Bolick et al. (1986) because it extended around more of the circumference of the left ventricular cavity. Whether this is the reason why arrhythmias occur is uncertain at this time.

In some hearts, bundles of myocardial fibers extend from the endocardial border zone deeper into the subendocardium and also into midmyocardial regions of the solid infarct, forming subendocardial or intramural conducting pathways (De Bakker et al. 1990). Similarly, muscle bundles may also extend from the lateral borders of the infarcted region, penetrating the solid infarct. Tracts of subendocardial and intramural muscle bundles may sometimes form reentrant circuits.

In summary, the pathological anatomy of human hearts with a healing or healed infarct has many similarities to the animal models. There are surviving myocardial cells in the infarcted region that form an epicardial and endocardial border zone. An irregular lateral border zone may also exist, projecting bundles of viable cells into the infarct. Since arrhythmias arise in viable cells in infarcted regions, all these sites are possible candidates for the arrhythmogenic substrate. Differences in the infarct anatomy among hearts should influence the site of arrhythmia origin.

Origin of Ventricular Tachyarrhythmias

Early in this century, in experiments to locate the origin of the heart beat during normal sinus rhythm, investigators such as Lewis and his collaborators (1910) and Eyster and Meek (1921) studied the atrial activation sequence. The origin of the heart beat was assigned to a region where the earliest extracellular electrical activity was recorded (see Chapter II). In this region of the pacemaker, the unipolar extracellular wave form was entirely negative (primary negativity) since the wave front propagates away from the recording site in all directions in a region of impulse origin. Similar characteristics are expected at an ectopic pacemaker site causing a tachycardia: earliest electrical activity and a negative unipolar extracellular waveform. In locating the site of origin of tachycardia impulses that result from a reentrant rhythm rather than a pacemaker, the concepts of earliest electrical activity and primary negativity as indicators of the site of arrhythmia origin require some modification. First, tissue anisotropy due to differences in fiber orientation may give rise to negative initial deflections at sites where an activation front is passing beneath the electrode; propagation in the direction perpendicular to the long fiber axis generates QS complexes even at sites that are not at the origin of the impulse (Corbin and Scher 1977). Secondly, in a reentrant circuit, the propagating excitation wave continuously conducts throughout the cardiac cycle in the circuitous pathway. Thus, electrical activity at this "site of origin" is continuous and may occur both early and late with respect to activation of the rest of the heart. The wave form of unipolar electrograms recorded at the origin in a reentrant circuit would not also be expected to show primary negativity since at any site in the circuit excitation would be leaving that site at one point in time giving rise to a negative wave form, while approaching that site at another point in time giving rise to a positive wave form. Electrograms therefore should have composite waveforms consisting of positive and negative components. In a small reentrant circuit, the electrical activity recorded at any one site might also seem to persist throughout the entire cardiac cycle if the recording electrode also senses some of the electrical activity in the rest of the circuit surrounding it.

When a reentrant circuit is the origin of a ventricular arrhythmia, the reentrant impulse must exit the circuit in order to activate the rest of the ventricles. There may be only one exit route from the circuit during a monomorphic ventricular tachycardia, but sometimes a number of different exit routes during polymorphic tachycardias. Different monomorphic tachycardias in the same heart may also utilize different exit routes from the same circuit. The conducting pathway that is activated by the excitation wave leaving the circuit is expected to be activated the earliest with respect to the rest of the ventricles (discounting activation in the reentrant circuit). A small unipolar electrode placed here would not be expected to record primary negativity since the wave front is approaching this site from the circuit and leaving this site as it moves out to the rest of the heart. However, since the tissue mass comprising the reentrant circuit is often small compared to the large mass of noninfarcted myocardium, initial negativity can be recorded at the site of "earliest" activation (the exit route from the circuit) at the border of an infarct (De Bakker et al. 1987).

Some additional explanation is required here to distinguish between very early activation and very late activation during ventricular tachycardias, both of which might occur some time during the diastolic interval at the site of origin if activity is being recorded from the reentrant circuit. Early activation of a recording site has been arbitrarily defined in many clinical electrophysiological studies as being confined to the last half of the diastolic interval before the onset of the following QRS complex while late activation occurs in the first half of the diastolic interval after the preceding QRS complex. Both kinds of activity are called diastolic potentials. However, it is quite possible that some sites that are considered to be activated late by this definition might actually be the early site for the following QRS complex. A diastolic potential may also reflect activity from a "dead-end pathway" that is not actually part of the reentrant circuit (and be "late" with respect to the preceding beat and not causally related to the next one). One way to distinguish whether a diastolic potential is part of the circuit or not is to introduce premature beats during the tachycardia. If the tachycardia is reset and the time interval between diastolic potential and the postextrasystolic beat of the tachycardia is unchanged, the diastolic potential is most likely caused by activity in the reentrant circuit (Josephson and Wit 1984). If the tachycardia is terminated and the diastolic potential disappears, that also is evidence for a causal relationship between diastolic potential and reentrant circuit (Josephson and Wit 1984). If despite termination of the tachycardia the diastolic potential is still present following the premature beat, it probably is due to activity in a "dead-end pathway" (Hauer et al. 1986). Exact distinctions between early and late activity can also be made when many electrograms are simultaneously recorded continuously from the initiation of tachycardia and throughout the period of the sustained arrhythmia. There are only a few clinical mapping studies in which this has been done, although it has been done in a number of studies on experimental models.

Origin of Ventricular Arrhythmias in Experimental Animal Models and Ventricular Activation Patterns

Permanent Occlusion of the Left Anterior Descending Coronary Artery in the Canine Heart   Although ventricular premature depolarizations are a common arrhythmia during the healing and healed phases of myocardial infarction in humans, they do not occur consistently enough in the canine infarction models to allow their origin and mechanism to be elucidated. For similar reasons, spontaneously occurring tachyarrhythmias have not been studied in the canine models. Studies on origin and mechanism have been confined to tachycardias induced by programmed stimulation mostly during the healing phase of infarction (first week after occlusion). Many of the nonsustained and sustained ventricular tachycardias that are induced in the canine model of myocardial infarction caused by permanent occlusion of the left anterior descending coronary artery above the first diagonal branch during infarct healing arise in the rim of muscle that survives on the epicardial surface of the infarct, the epicardial border zone. The origin of the tachycardias is the same whether or not methylprednisolone is used to increase the incidence of tachycardia (Cardinal et al. 1984). This region was initially suggested to be the site of arrhythmia origin by El-Sherif et al. (1977a; 1977b) in the absence of mapping data, because they recorded continuous electrical activity here with a large composite electrode during tachycardia but not in the absence of arrhythmias. During initiation of tachycardia, either by ventricular pacing or premature stimulation, the continuous activity appeared with the stimulated impulse that started the arrhythmia (El-Sherif et al. 1977a; 1977b; Hope et al. 1977; El-Sherif 1978). The continuous activity is illustrated in Figure 4.26. Lead II (L-2) and aVR electrocardiograms are shown in the top two traces and the composite electrogram recordings from the epicardial border zone (IZeg) and noninfarcted left ventricle (NZeg) in the bottom two traces. Premature stimuli were applied to the His bundle during sinus rhythm. At the left, a premature impulse (PI) with a coupling interval of 205 msec did not induce an arrhythmia, while to the right, a premature impulse with a coupling interval of 190 msec induced ventricular tachycardia. This premature impulse was accompanied by fractionation of the IZeg "into a continuous series of multiple asynchronous spikes that extended in the diastolic interval up to the onset of the reentrant arrhythmia" (El-Sherif et al. 1977a). During the tachycardia fractionation of the IZeg persisted, although in this record it does not extend throughout diastole. The NZeg did not fractionate. Continuous activity in the composite electrogram from the epicardial border zone was interpreted to indicate that this was a site of reentry and thus the site of arrhythmia origin.

Activation maps of the entire ventricles confirm the conclusions resulting from composite electrogram studies, that arrhythmias induced by electrical stimulation of the canine heart with an infarct caused by left anterior descending coronary artery occlusion, originate in the surviving epicardial muscle

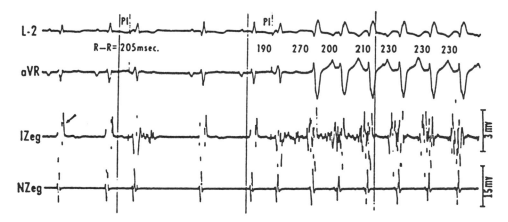

Figure 4.26: Continuous electrical activity in a composite electrogram recording during initiation of ventricular tachycardia. Recordings were obtained from the epicardial border zone of a canine heart approximately 1 week after occlusion of the left anterior descending coronary artery. The top two traces are electrocardiogram leads 2 and aVR, the next two traces are composite electrograms recorded from the epicardial border zone (IZeg) and the epicardial surface of adjacent noninfarcted myocardium (NZeg). Premature stimuli (PI) were delivered to the His bundle during sinus rhythm. A premature stimulus with a coupling interval of 190 msec induced tachycardia. During induction the IZeg shows continuous electrical activity. (Reproduced from El-Sherif et al. (1977b) with permission.)

(Wit et al. 1982a; 1982b; Kramer et al. 1985). Maps have been derived from experiments in which simultaneous electrogram recordings have been obtained from 60–250 sites with multiple electrode arrays. During sinus rhythm most of ventricular activation may be normal except that activation of epicardial muscle over the infarct takes longer than normal. In hearts with inducible ventricular tachycardia there may be regions of delayed activation or delayed potentials in the epicardial muscle over the infarct (Pagé et al. 1988). These regions are often located near the site of origin of ventricular tachycardia but they are not always a crucial part of the reentrant circuit (Assadi et al. 1990). During ventricular tachycardia, earliest activation of noninfarcted ventricular muscle occurs prior to the onset of the QRS, on the epicardial surface of the left ventricle at the border of the infarcted region with surrounding normal myocardium, either at its left anterior descending coronary artery or lateral margin (Wit et al. 1982a; 1982b; Kramer et al. 1985). This represents the exit route from the epicardial border zone. This activation pattern is shown in the maps of the epicardial surface in Figures 4.27A and 4.27B and 4.28A and 4.28B, derived from recordings obtained with a sock electrode array containing 196 recording contacts, during the initiation of a nonsustained tachycardia with a monomorphic QRS complex. Four views of the ventricles are shown for each ventricular depolarization: the anterior (Ant), the left lateral (Left), the posterior (Post) and the right lateral (Right). The infarcted region of the anterior and lateral left ventricular free wall is indicated by the oval-shaped area. During the basic drive (Figure 4.27A), earliest activation occurred at the base of the right ventricle near the stimulating electrode, 0–10 msec after the beginning of the QRS complex (anterior view), and activation spread away from the stimulating electrode on the anterior surface towards the apex, towards the left lateral ventricular wall and towards the right lateral ventricular wall. The margin of the infarct adjacent to the left anterior descending coronary artery and the margin towards the base of the heart were excited after 30–50 msec, whereas the apical and left lateral margins of the infarct were activated after 70 msec. Activation times and isochrones are not shown for epicardial muscle in the infarct zone because many of the unipolar recordings obtained from this region were difficult to interpret: local activity was masked by a large extrinsic deflection. However, at a few recording sites activation could be seen to occur after 40 to 90 msec. The posterior surface of the heart was activated last, after 90–110 msec. The ventricles were activated in a similar way by the stimulated premature impulse (Figure 4.27B) that initiated the tachycardia, but activation during the premature impulse took a longer time than during the basic drive impulse. Shortly after the ventricles were activated by the premature impulse the first tachycardia impulse occurred. Earliest activation of the non-infarcted epicardial surface of the ventricles occurred at the margin of the infarct adjacent to the left anterior descending coronary artery and the region of early activation included the anterior right ventricle adjacent to this artery as shown in the maps of the anterior and right lateral views in Figure 4.28A (Tach-1). From the region of early activation, excitation occurred in a direction towards both the base and the apex of the ventricles. The epicardium adjacent

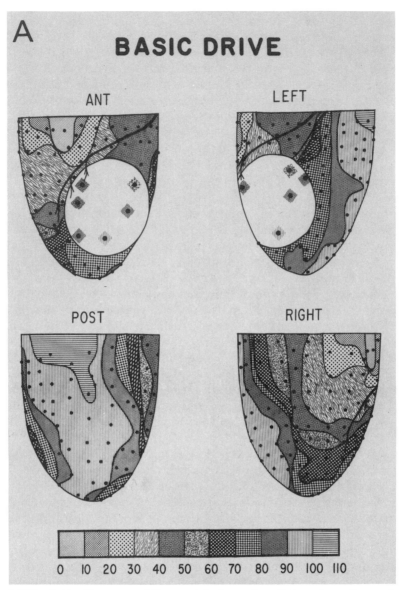

Figure 4.27A: Activation map of the ventricular epicardial surface of a canine heart with a 1-week-old infarct caused by permanent occlusion of the left anterior descending coronary artery during initiation of ventricular tachycardia. This figure shows activation during the last of a series of basic drive impulses. In each panel, four views of the ventricles are shown: anterior (ANT), left lateral (LEFT), posterior (POST), and right lateral (RIGHT). The location of the left anterior descending coronary artery is shown on the anterior, left, and right lateral projections, and the infarcted region of the antero-lateral left ventricle is indicated by the white oval area on the anterior and left lateral projections. Activation times from 0 to 150 msec are indicated by the shaded areas according to the keys below the panels. The dots on the maps indicate the locations of the recording sites where activation times were measured. (Reproduced from Wit et al. (1982a) with permission.)

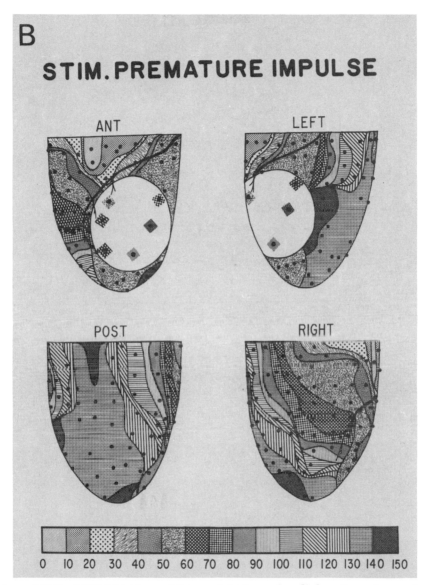

Figure 4.27B: Activation map of the ventricular epicardial surface of a canine heart with a 1-week-old infarct caused by permanent occlusion of the left anterior descending coronary artery during initiation of ventricular tachycardia. This figure shows activation during a stimulated premature impulse that induced a nonsustained tachycardia. In each panel four views of the ventricles are shown: anterior (ANT), left lateral (LEFT), posterior (POST), and right lateral (RIGHT). The location of the left anterior descending coronary artery is shown on the anterior, left, and right lateral projections, and the infarcted region of the anterolateral left ventricle is indicated by the white oval area on the anterior and left lateral projections. Activation times from 0 to 150 msec are indicated by the shaded areas according to the keys below the panels. The dots on the maps indicate the locations of the recording sites where activation times were measured. (Reproduced from Wit et al. (1982a) with permission.)

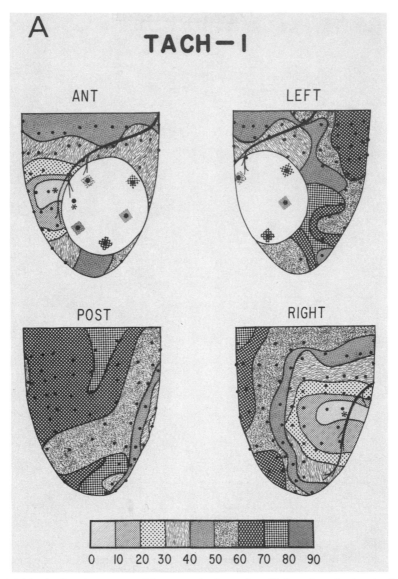

Figure 4.28A: Activation maps of the ventricular epicardial surface during tachycardia in the same heart shown in Figure 4.27. This figure shows activation during the first tachycardia impulse. The format of the figure is the same as in Figure 4.27. The asterisks on the anterior view indicate the sites of earliest epicardial excitation. (Reproduced from Wit et al. (1982a) with permission.)

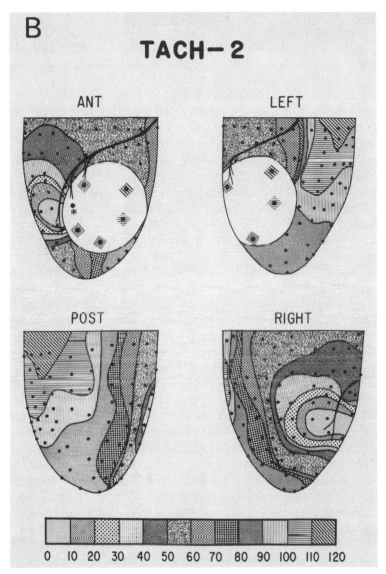

Figure 4.28B: Activation map of the ventricular epicardial surface during tachycardia in the same heart shown in Figure 4.27. This figure shows activation during the second tachycardia impulse. The format of the figure is the same as in Figure 4.27. The asterisks on the anterior view indicate the sites of earliest epicardial excitation. (Reproduced from Wit et al. (1982a) with permission.)

to the margin of the infarct towards the base of the heart was activated after 30 msec; the regions adjacent to the apical and the left lateral borders of the infarct were not activated until later. The posterior of the heart was activated between 60 and 90 msec. Activation of the ventricles during the second impulse of tachycardia (Figure 4.28B, Tach 2) was similar to activation during the first impulse of tachycardia; initial activation of the noninfarcted ventricle occurred near the anterior descending coronary artery although further towards the apex. It again appears that the impulse after emerging on the anterior surface spread along the margin of the infarcted region, both towards the base and the apex and reached the left lateral margin later. Similar sites of earliest activation and patterns of epicardial activation have been seen in maps obtained during sustained monomorphic ventricular tachycardia (Cardinal et al. 1984; Kramer et al. 1985).

From the site of earliest activation of noninfarcted subepicardial muscle, it can be inferred that the reentrant circuit is in the adjacent infarcted region. Since there is usually only surviving subepicardial muscle in this region, this muscle is a logical candidate for the source of the arrhythmia. When electrical activity is recorded from this subepicardial muscle during tachycardia, some sites are activated even earlier than the adjacent noninfarcted myocardium, while some sites are activated later. This is to be expected if these are different sites in the reentrant circuit. (Later, we will show detailed activation maps of these circuits in the epicardial border zone.) The earliest sites during tachycardia are often activated the latest during sinus rhythms; they are sites of delayed potentials (Denniss et al. 1989). Of course, epicardial maps alone can sometimes be misleading and do not eliminate a possible origin in the lateral or endocardial border zones. It is important to know how intramural and subendocardial regions are activated. These data have been obtained by inserting needle electrodes in and around the infarcted area so that transmural activity could be registered (Cardinal et al. 1984; Kramer et al. 1985). These studies indicate that earliest excitation during tachycardia usually occurs in the subepicardial layer and is followed later by subendocardial activation (Cardinal et al. 1984; Kramer et al. 1985). No intramural activity has usually been detected in the infarcted region caused by a proximal left anterior descending coronary artery occlusion because of the absence of viable muscle (Cardinal et al. 1984). Conformation of an epicardial site of origin is also provided by experiments in which cooling of a region of the epicardial border zone abolished tachycardia (El-Sherif et al. 1983a; Gessman et al. 1983).

The propagating impulse, often exiting myocardium adjacent to the left anterior descending coronary artery from the reentrant circuit in the epicardial border zone, conducts transmurally from subepicardium to subendocardium as soon as it encounters transmural myocardial pathways at the periphery of the infarct (Kramer et al. 1985). During monomorphic tachycardias, a consistent exit pathway is utilized, while during the initial polymorphic phase of tachycardia there are different exit sites into the subendocardium (Kramer et al. 1985). From the subendocardium, excitation can proceed through the Purkinje system to the noninfarcted regions of the left ventricle. Depolarization of a large part of the noninfarcted left ventricle can then occur in the direction from endocardium to epicardium. Impulse distribution in the Purkinje system might also lead to multiple areas of epicardial breakthrough (Smith et al. 1983). Some of these major features of ventricular activation are shown in Figure 4.29. A section through the epicardium and subendocardium is shown for three successive ventricular depolarizations: S_3 is the second of two premature stimuli that initiated tachycardia and T_1 and T_2 are the first two depolarizations of tachycardia (see ECG below). S_3 originated at the subendocardial base of the right ventricle (within isochrone 20) and propagated to the epicardium where reentry was initiated in the epicardial border zone as indicated by the arrows. The detailed pattern of reentry cannot be discerned because of the relatively low spatial resolution of the activation maps. However, the dashed arrow shows the impulse exiting from the circuit in the subepicardium at the lateral margin and the long arrow from the epicardium during S_3 to the subendocardium during T_1 shows it propagating to the subendocardium through the noninfarcted myocardium, arriving at the subendocardium at 240 msec (Panel T_1). While activating the subendocardium with a pattern shown by the arrows, activation also returned to the epicardial border zone where it arrived at

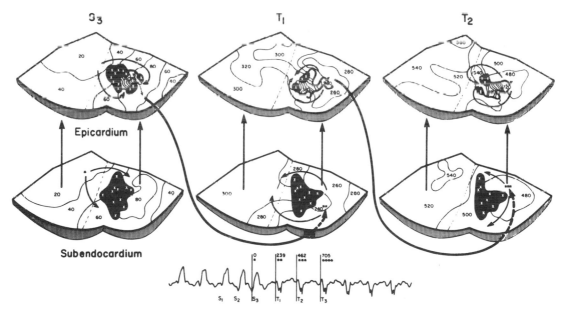

Figure 4.29: Activation patterns in the epicardium and subendocardium of a canine heart approximately 1 week after left anterior descending coronary occlusion. The electrocardiogram recorded during initiation of tachycardia is shown below: S_1 is the last of a series of basic drive impulses, S_2 and S_3 are two stimulated premature impulses, and T_1-T_3 are the first three impulses of the tachycardia. Above are shown the activation patterns of epicardium and subendocardium during S_3, T_1, and T_2. The arrows point out the pattern of impulse propagation. (Reproduced from Kramer et al. (1985) with permission.)

around 260 msec. Reentry again occurred in the epicardial muscle, shown by the black arrows. Exit from the circuit is at 480 msec, the wave front exiting from the circuit (dashed arrow) dipped down to the subendocardium (T_2) and then returned to the subepicardium as another reentry took place. In these activation maps, extensive regions of subendocardial block are indicated by the black areas in the subendocardial sections. We do not know why this block was found in this study of Kramer et al. (1985), since the subendocardial surface of transmural infarcts caused by permanent left anterior descending coronary artery occlusion is covered with surviving Purkinje cells that have relatively normal membrane potentials by 4–5 days after coronary occlusion. Examples of wave fronts emerging from the reentrant circuit almost simultaneously from the left anterior descending coronary artery margin of the epicardial border zone and the margin on the lateral left ventricle have also been reported (Kramer et al. 1985). Both wave fronts then rapidly activated towards the subendocardium. Activation of the ventricles was then a product of activation by these two wave fronts.

Right ventricular activation during tachycardia may sometimes result when the impulse from the reentrant circuit conducts retrograde from subendocardial ventricular muscle into the His bundle and then antegrade through the conducting system to the right ventricle (Cardinal et al. 1984). His bundle deflections, although occurring after the onset of the Q wave and initial excitation of the subendocardium, have sometimes been found to have a fixed coupling interval to the subsequent ventricular depolarization recorded on the His bundle electrogram, which represents right ventricular activity (Cardinal et al. 1984). Epicardial breakthrough on the right ventricle may occur in the same area as during sinus rhythm because of the activation through the right ventricular conducting system (Cardinal et al. 1984). When this occurs, activation of the right ventricle occurs in concentric isochrones that spread away from this area of breakthrough and collide near the septum with earlier impulses spreading from the left ventricle. Thus, the epicardial activation patterns can, to a large extent, represent activation dependent on distribution of the impulse by the subendocardial Purkinje system. Changes in QRS morphology during sustained tachycardia (switching from one monomorphic morphology to another) need not be accompanied by a change in the location of the reentrant circuit in the epicardial border zone, but rather can be caused by a change in the pattern of ventricular depolarization. One cause for this change in pattern has been shown to be an interruption in the participation of the conducting system in the transmission of excitation from the left to the right ventricle (Cardinal et al. 1984). This was indicated when suddenly, during tachycardia, His bundle deflections no longer regularly preceded right ventricular depolarization and right ventricular breakthrough no longer occurred in regions to which the conducting system distributed (Cardinal et al. 1984).

The exit route from the epicardial border zone to noninfarcted myocardium seems to occur mostly at either the left anterior descending coronary artery or the lateral-apical margins of the epicardial border zone (Kramer et al. 1985) although occasionally there is exit further toward the apex (Cardinal et al.

1984). This is not the consequence of well-defined anatomical pathways from the reentrant circuits since, as we will show later, the circuits are mostly functional and connected to the surrounding myocardium around their entire perimeter. Preferential exit routes may be a result of the orientation of the long axis of the myocardial fibers in the epicardial border zone. These fiber bundles are arranged with their long axis in the direction from the left anterior descending coronary artery towards the apex of the lateral left ventricle. Excitation occurs most rapidly along the long axis and very slowly transverse to the long axis (toward the base and the apex). Therefore, impulses circulating in reentrant pathways in the epicardial border zone may reach the normal myocardium most rapidly along the long axis of the bundles towards either the left anterior descending coronary artery or the apex of the lateral left ventricle, and begin to activate normal myocardium before the impulse exits the circuit from the apical or basal margins, routes that require conduction transverse to the long axis, which is very slow. We will illustrate this point more clearly when we show the maps of the reentrant circuits.

The origin of the tachycardias in the epicardial border zone of infarcts caused by permanent occlusion of the left anterior descending coronary artery above the first major diagonal branch is a consequence of the anatomy of the infarcted region in which a rim of surviving epicardial muscle lies on the surface of a transmural infarct. The subendocardial Purkinje network also survives in the infarcted region, but the available data indicate that it is rarely the site of reentrant circuits causing ventricular tachycardia in this experimental model. This may be because the conduction properties in the surviving Purkinje system are normal by this time. However, in the experiments of Garan et al. (1980; 1981) and Garan and Ruskin (1984) the permanent occlusion of the left anterior descending coronary artery was more distal, allowing myocardial perfusion through some of the diagonal branches and survival of some subendocardial and intramural muscle. In addition, they ligated many of the epicardial branches to the anterior ventricle wall. This may have resulted in infarction of the subepicardial muscle and either no epicardial border zone or a zone much diminished in size. As a result of the different infarct anatomy compared to the effects of proximal left anterior descending coronary artery occlusion, the origin of the ventricular tachycardias was sometimes either subendocardial or intramural. The surviving subendocardial or intramural muscle may have electrophysiological properties conducive to the occurrence of reentry while an anatomical substrate for reentry no longer exists on the epicardial surface. Mapping data showed that earliest activity sometimes occurred on the endocardial surface of the infarcted region during sustained ventricular tachycardia, and sites where electrograms with continuous activity were recorded were located close to the sites of earliest endocardial activity, suggesting arrhythmogenic impulse origin in these regions. Surgical ablation of regions where continuous electrical activity was recorded on the endocardial surface prevented induction of tachycardia (Garan et al. 1981; Garan and Ruskin 1984). However, epicardial reentrant circuits have also been described in this model (Garan et al. 1987). We suspect that this occurs when an epicardial border zone forms despite occlusion of epicardial branches, perhaps if ligation of some crucial branches is missed.

Coronary Reperfusion after a Period of Occlusion   One particular difference in the anatomy of those infarcts resulting from coronary occlusion and reperfusion and the anatomy of infarcts resulting from permanent coronary occlusion, particularly near the origin of the left anterior descending coronary artery, is the survival of salvaged intramural myocardium in the reperfused infarcted area that might represent protrusions from ragged lateral borders. These intramural fibers might provide conduction pathways that form reentrant circuits (Karagueuzian et al. 1979; Michelson et al. 1980). In addition, a thick epicardial border zone, which is not favorable for the occurrence of reentrant circuits because it lacks the appropriate conduction properties, often occurs after reperfusion (Wit et al. 1981a; Cardinal et al. 1984). Maps of ventricular activation during tachycardia still show that early activation of noninfarcted ventricle occurs on the epicardial surface adjacent to the infarct border (Wit et al. 1982a; Kramer et al. 1985), but there is also intramural electrical activity in the infarcted region, with low-amplitude rS complexes in unipolar electrograms (Cardinal et al. 1984). This local activity in an experiment described by Pagé et al. (1988), followed QS complexes during sinus rhythm and preceded them during ventricular tachycardia. Earliest activity occurred simultaneously at intramural and subepicardial sites during tachycardia with radial spread away from the epicardial area of early activity. In another experiment described by Cardinal et al. (1984), earliest excitation during monomorphic ventricular tachycardia occurred at intramural recording sites and preceded excitation of overlying epicardial sites by 20 msec. There was a radial pattern of excitation spread away from the epicardial breakthrough site on the left ventricle. One possible interpretation of these results is reentrant excitation in surviving intramural muscle bundles as the origin of tachycardia. On the other hand, Kramer et al. (1985) found activation patterns and the location of the site of origin of reentrant circuits in reperfused infarcts to be similar to the infarcts caused by permanent occlusion. They reported no evidence of intramural electrical activity or surviving intramural myocardium. Other studies have also shown reentrant circuits in the epicardial border zone of reperfused infarcts, particularly when this border zone is comprised of a thin rim of surviving muscle (Richards et al. 1984). The difference in the experimental results among laboratories is not completely understood. One possible reason that we have considered is variations in the adequacy of reperfusion. After a 2-hour period of occlusion there may not always be adequate reperfusion to salvage intramural muscle. Failure of reperfusion may result from the no-reflow phenomenon and from fragility of the capillaries caused by the period of ischemia, resulting in hemorrhage. Failure of reflow in some experiments would result in an infarct that is identical to an infarct caused by permanent occlusion. However, it is possible that even after adequate reperfusion, a thin epicardial border zone and minimal intramural muscle might sometimes occur.

Origin of Ventricular Tachycardia in Humans and Ventricular Activation
Patterns

Noninvasive methods such as analysis of the classic 12-lead electrocardiogram have not precisely localized the arrhythmogenic source during ventricular tachycardia (Josephson et al. 1981; Miller et al. 1988; Kuchar et al. 1989).
Body surface mapping, using a large number of thoracic leads, has the potential
for a much more precise localization of the earliest activated areas (Sippens-
Groenewegen 1990; SippensGroenewegen et al. 1990), but this technique has
not yet played a major role in clinical studies on activation of the heart in
patients with tachycardia. Rather, to locate the site of origin of ventricular
tachycardia in human hearts with healing or healed infarcts, activation has
been mapped by recording local electrograms both during catheterization and
cardiac surgery. From these maps the site of earliest activation has been determined and usually equated with the site of arrhythmia origin.

The use of catheters has permitted mapping of the endocardial surface of
the ventricles without the necessity for anesthesia, thoracotomy, or cardiopulmonary bypass, all of which are necessary for mapping excitation during surgery and which may sometimes interfere with the induction of the clinical
tachycardia by programmed stimulation. For catheter mapping, up to six multipolar electrode catheters have been inserted into the right and left ventricles
(Josephson et al. 1978b; Hauer 1987). Several of the catheters are left in a fixed
position to record reference electrograms, usually from at least one site in each
ventricle. One or more of the catheters are used as exploring electrodes and
are moved from site to site during a stable tachycardia. The position of the
catheter at each recording site can be verified by fluoroscopy. A special form of
mapping ("pace mapping") consists of stimulating the endocardium at different
sites when the heart is not in tachycardia, and identifying the site that produces
similar QRS complexes as those during spontaneous tachycardia. Its value is
sometimes limited in view of the variable results, and preference is given to a
direct mapping technique involving electrogram recordings (Josephson et al.
1982a). Catheter mapping can only be used for stable and uniform arrhythmias, not for polymorphic tachycardias or for transient events such as initia-
tions or terminations, since it depends on the recording of electrograms from
different sites during different beats. An example of the location and number
of recording sites that have been included in the activation maps in the studies
in Josephson's laboratory (1978b) is shown in Figure 4.30. This figure shows a
schematic view of the heart in serial sections, the inset shows the level of
transection of the heart from which each section comes. Recording sites 1–6
are in the right ventricle (RV) (1 = RV apex; 2 = RV midseptum; 3 = RV free
anterior wall; 4 = AV junction; 5 = RV inflow tract; 6 = RV outflow tract).
Sites 7–14 are in the left ventricle (LV) (7 = LV apex; 8 = LV low septum; 9
= LV midseptum 10 = LV anterior free wall; 11 = LV inferoposterior wall;
12 = LV high septum; 13 = LV lateral wall under the mitral valve; 14 =
posterobasal LV recorded from the coronary sinus). Additional sites might also

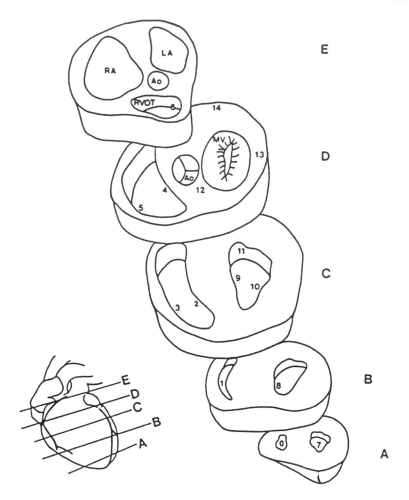

Figure 4.30: Schematic view of the heart in serial sections indicating recording sites for endocardial mapping with an electrode catheter. The inset at the lower left shows the level of transection for each section. The sites are (1) right ventricular (RV) apex; (2) RV midseptum; (3) RV free anterior wall; (4) A-V junction; (5) RV inflow tract; (6) RV outflow tract; (7) left ventricular (LV) apex; (8) LV low septum; (9) LV midseptum; (10) LV anterior free wall; (11) LV inferoposterior wall; (12) LV high septum (under aortic valve); (13) LV lateral wall (under mitral valve), and (14) posterobasilar LV (recorded from coronary sinus). Ao = aorta; MV = mitral valve; RVOT = right ventricular outflow tract; RA = right atrium; LA = left atrium. (Reproduced from Josephson et al. (1978b) with permission.)

be used to compose an activation map. One of the disadvantages of catheter mapping is the limited number of recording sites that can be obtained within a reasonable amount of time. As a result, activation maps have a relatively low spatial resolution. The site of origin, therefore, might not be pinpointed any better than a large area of 5–10 cm^2 (Josephson et al. 1978b) and the sequence of activation of the endocardial surface can only be described in general terms. Another disadvantage is the inability to map the epicardial surface of the heart, making it impossible to locate possible epicardial sites of arrhythmia origin and to determine the epicardial activation sequence. The morphology of the QRS has, therefore, been used as an indicator of epicardial activation sequence. Catheter mapping also might not detect some very low-amplitude signals arising in fibrous or scarred areas because of the relatively large interjyelectrode distance between poles of a bipolar catheter electrode and the limited amplification of the electrical signal that is usually used in the catheterization laboratory because it is sometimes difficult to keep electrical noise to the same low levels as in experimental laboratories. In some experimental studies in animals, it has been shown that cardiac fibers trapped in the scar of a healed infarct might generate extracellular signals less than 100 μV in amplitude (Gardner et al. 1985) and such signals might not be detected by the catheter mapping procedure.

Mapping during cardiac surgery usually provides higher resolution maps than catheter mapping. Mapping has been done with the roving probe technique (moving the electrode from site to site and recording electrograms during different beats of the tachycardia) including up to 75 epicardial sites and 55 endocardial sites (Horowitz et al. 1980; Mason et al. 1982). Mapping has also utilized simultaneous recordings from a number of sites ranging from 30–210 with multipolar electrode arrays (De Bakker et al. 1984; 1988; Downar et al. 1984; 1988; Kaltenbrunner et al. 1991). With the roving probe technique, epicardial maps have been obtained with the heart intact and the endocardial maps were then obtained by inserting the probe electrode through an incision in the aneurysm (Horowitz et al. 1980). Simultaneous recordings from the epicardial and endocardial surfaces have also been obtained, using up to 220 electrodes in patients on cardiopulmonary bypass (Harris et al. 1987; Downar et al. 1988; Kaltenbrunner et al. 1991). In Downar's laboratory (see Harris et al. 1987), a balloon covered with a mesh containing 2-mm unipolar electrodes at 1-cm intervals was inserted into the left ventricle through the mitral orifice via an atriotomy for endocardial mapping. The procedure did not necessitate a ventriculotomy, and therefore, there was no danger of cutting through the reentrant circuit. After the insertion, the balloon was expanded by filling it with dextrose solution. At the same time a nylon mesh sock containing 110 1.5-mm diameter electrodes was wrapped around the epicardium for the epicardial maps. A problem sometimes encountered with mapping during surgery is that tachycardia may not always be inducible under these conditions. Reasons for the failure to induce tachycardia are not always clear, but may include effects of the anesthesia, cooling of the heart on bypass, or incision through the arrhythmogenic site when a ventriculotomy is made for the insertion of an endocardial electrode (Horowitz et al. 1980; Downar et al. 1988).

Using these techniques for both catheter and surgical mapping, sustained monomorphic ventricular tachycardia induced by programmed stimulation has been mapped in patients with ischemic heart disease and usually healed infarcts with or without ventricular aneurysms. In most of the reported cases, acute infarction occurred more than several months prior to the mapping study.

No comparison has been made in the presentation of activation sequences between infarcts of different ages, for example between infarcts that are only several months old versus those that are several years old. Also, we are not aware of any mapping data from healing infarcts in the late hospital period, during which time ventricular tachycardia might also occur. At the present time it is apparently assumed that the age of the infarct does not influence the site of origin. However, the pathological anatomy of an infarct that can influence the location and properties of a reentrant circuit, may change significantly between the early weeks and the later months after infarction as we have already indicated, and this change might sometimes influence the origin of tachycardia.

The earliest site of activation (earliest activity during the second half of the diastolic interval) during monomorphic sustained ventricular tachycardia, found with both catheter and surgical mapping techniques, has often been located on the endocardial surface of the left ventricle in the surviving myocardial fibers of the endocardial border zone of the infarct (Wittig and Boineau 1975; Josephson et al. 1978b; Horowitz et al. 1980; Mason et al. 1982; Miller et al. 1985; Waspe et al. 1985b; Harris et al. 1987; De Bakker et al. 1988; Downar et al. 1988; Morady et al. 1988; Kaltenbrunner et al. 1991). Earliest endocardial activation does not necessarily mean that the entire reentrant circuit is located on the endocardial surface. Techniques for detecting intramural activity such as needle electrodes, have not been used routinely during the mapping studies and therefore, it has not been determined whether such activity exists, and if so, its relation to the endocardial activity that is recorded. The survival of deep subendocardial muscle fibers, and intramural fibers connected to the lateral infarct margins in some infarcted regions leaves open the possibility that parts of reentrant circuits are sometimes located in these regions (De Bakker et al. 1988). The early endocardial activity may sometimes only represent the exit route from the reentrant circuit to the rest of the ventricles. When endocardial activity is earliest, it occurs prior to the inscription of the QRS on the surface ECG, while earliest epicardial activation occurs after the onset of the QRS (Horowitz et al. 1980; Harris et al. 1987; Downar et al. 1988; Fitzgerald et al. 1988; Kaltenbrunner et al. 1991). Earliest right ventricular endocardial activation usually occurs after the earliest left ventricular endocardial activation, although it may sometimes occur simultaneously (Josephson et al. 1978b). Within the left ventricle the site of earliest activity can vary and this is likely to depend on the pathological anatomy of the infarct. In patients who have an aneurysm, the earliest endocardial site is usually near the margins of the aneurysm, either within the aneurysm or outside the aneurysm in the scarred tissue between aneurysm and noninfarcted myocardium (Josephson et al. 1978b; Horowitz et al. 1980; Waspe et al. 1985a). Figure 4.31 shows examples of catheter electrogram recordings used to located earliest activation in a patient with a left ventricular aneurysm during sustained monomorphic ventricular tachycardia (Josephson et al. 1978b). Electrocardiogram leads II and V_1 are shown in the top two traces followed by electrograms recorded from the high right atrium (HRA), coronary sinus (CS), atrioventricu-

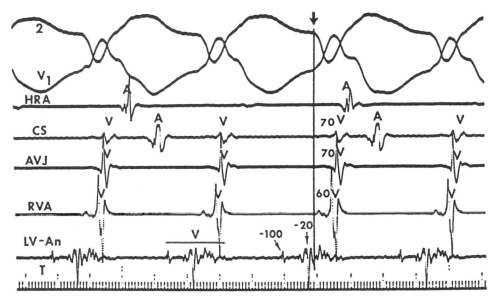

Figure 4.31: Some of the electrograms recorded from a patient with a left ventricular aneurysm during a catheter mapping study. The top two traces are electrocardiograms lead 2 and V_1, beneath which are electrograms recorded from the high right atrium (HRA), coronary sinus region (CS), atrioventricular junction (AVJ), right ventricle (RVA), and left ventricular aneurysm (LV-An). Note that electrical activity is present in the LV-An recording during systole and diastole with two sharp deflections occurring 100 and 20 msec prior to the onset of the QRS (arrows). (Reproduced from Josephson et al. (1978b) with permission.)

lar junction (AVJ), right ventricular apex (RVA), and the left ventricular aneurysm (LV-An). The electrogram recorded from the aneurysm (LV-An) has multiple components and a long duration, that is, it is fractionated. The first deflection in this recording occurs during diastole 100 msec prior to the onset of the QRS in lead II and prior to activity at all other recording sites (including the other left and right ventricular sites not shown in the figure), indicating that this region is "the site of origin". Fractionated electrograms like the one shown in Figure 4.31 are often recorded at the earliest site of activity (Morady et al. 1988). They can also be seen in the LV-An recordings in Figures 4.2 and 4.4. The multiple components represent the sum of electrical activity occurring in the muscle fibers within the recording field of the widely spaced bipoles. Some of the muscle bundles give rise to the earliest deflection but some are activated much later and give rise to the late LV-An deflections. These electrograms indicate slow and nonuniform activation of these regions, characteristics that are expected in areas where reentry is occurring. In fact, electrograms with this characteristic are not only located in reentrant circuits but may be located anywhere that there is slow and inhomogeneous activation. We will later discuss in more detail the electrophysiological basis for these fractionated electrograms. As mentioned above, the site of earliest activity may also be at a distance from the actual reentrant circuit. It sometimes occurs in more normal myocardium and when it does, it has relatively normal appearing rather than fractionated electrograms. In patients without aneurysms, earliest sites of activity on the endocardial surface are usually associated with scarred or dyskinetic areas. However, in both the aneurysms and scarred regions where sparse myocardial fibers may be trapped within a dense fibrous scar, the extracellular signal from the trapped fibers may be so small that it is not detected and therefore the real site of origin might sometimes be at some distance from the recorded one. The earliest site may also occur on the septum when it is involved in the infarction. In patients with a septal origin of tachycardia, the electrograms recorded from both the right and left side of the septum may occur nearly simultaneously, presumably because activity can spread very rapidly from the site of origin to both sides.

Sometimes the earliest site of activity may not be the site of origin of the tachycardia. Regions of the endocardial border zone at some distance from the reentrant circuit can be activated very slowly, so that activation occurs after the QRS during the diastolic interval. It may be fortuitous that this activity appears to occur in these regions prior to presystolic activity at the real site of origin. Sometimes activity at these sites can be shown to be unrelated to the generation of the tachycardia. For example, ventricular extrastimuli might not advance the occurrence of such electrograms while advancing the tachycardia QRS, or the diastolic activity might persist even after tachycardia terminates (Wit and Josephson 1985; Fitzgerald et al. 1988).

Several other observations provide additional evidence for the origin of ventricular tachycardias in the endocardial border zone. One is the characteristics of resetting and entrainment of the tachycardia that occurs when stimulating at some endocardial sites at which early presystolic, fractionated electrograms are recorded (Frank et al. 1987; Morady et al. 1988; Stevenson et al. 1988; 1989b). When single premature stimuli are applied during the diastolic interval, the tachycardia can be reset for the reasons described earlier. Stimulation at some of these sites results in a QRS complex that occurs earlier than the next expected QRS of the tachycardia and which has the same morphology as the tachycardia QRS. The advanced QRS complex follows the stimulus artifact with a long delay, up to several hundred msec. It has been proposed that these features result from the stimulation of a slowly conducting pathway in the reentrant circuit. The stimulated impulse conducts slowly out the exit route of the circuit to activate the ventricles in exactly the same way as the tachycardia impulse. This explains the morphology of the QRS being the same as that of the tachycardia and the long delay between stimulus and QRS (Frank et al. 1987; Morady et al. 1988; Stevenson et al. 1988; 1989b). The stimulated impulse cannot exit the circuit in any other way because of refractoriness in parts of the circuit recently excited by the reentrant wave front and because it collides with the oncoming reentrant wave front in the antidromic direction. Stimulation at the same location during sinus rhythm might give multiple QRS morphologies unlike the tachycardia QRS, because the slowly conducting pathway in the circuit, which is bounded by lines of block, is not established until tachycardia is initiated, if the circuit is functional (Frank et al. 1987). Stimulation at sites distant from the circuit can result in depolarization of large regions of the ventricles by the stimulated impulse spreading from the stimulation site and therefore alters the QRS morphology immediately after the stimulus. It is also possible that stimulation at a site within the circuit might alter the QRS if there is the potential for the stimulated impulse to exit the circuit through a pathway other than the one used by the tachycardia impulse (Stevenson et al. 1989b). Entrainment of the tachycardia can also be accomplished by stimulating sites on the endocardium which are in a slowly conducting region of the reentrant circuit. During overdrive stimulation at these sites, the rate of the tachycardia is increased to the pacing rate, there is a long delay between stimulus and QRS and the QRS complexes maintain the same morphology as the tachycardia. The reasons for these characteristics are the same as for the resetting responses described above; the stimulated impulses exit the circuit through the same route as the reentrant impulses causing tachycardia (Stevenson et al. 1987; Morady et al. 1988). There are no fusion QRS complexes when a tachycardia is entrained by stimulating at the site of origin because the stimulated impulses only activate the reentrant circuit and no part of the paced wave front directly activates other parts of the ventricles. On the other hand, when stimulating from sites that are not within the slowly conducting region of the reentrant circuit or not within the reentrant circuit, even at sites with presystolic or mid-diastolic activity, the stimulated QRS complex is altered and the delay between stimulus artifact and QRS is diminished (Stevenson et al. 1987; 1989b; Morady et al. 1988). These sites are not the true sites of origin of the tachycardia.

As we described in Chapter I, one of Mines' criteria for proving the occurrence of reentry is to cut through the circuit at one point to stop the circulating impulse. Although such a precise experiment has not been done at the site of origin of human tachycardia to determine if it is a site of reentry, destruction of relatively large subendocardial regions of early activation by surgical procedures has succeeded in abolishing tachycardia, providing further evidence for a subendocardial site of origin (Wittig and Boineau 1975; Josephson et al. 1979). Freezing the subendocardium (Gallagher et al. 1985; Pagé et al. 1989) or the application of high-energy shocks or laser photocoagulation through a catheter in contact with regions of early activity in the subendocardium have also succeeded in abolishing tachycardia or preventing its initiation (Morady et al. 1987; 1988; Fitzgerald et al. 1988; Stevenson et al. 1988). These effects also support the concept that some ventricular tachycardias originate in the endocardial border zone.

The site of arrhythmia origin may also be in the epicardial border zone. Presystolic or mid-diastolic earliest electrical activity has been recorded during tachycardia from the left ventricular epicardial surface of some patients with an inferior or posterior infarction with or without a discrete left ventricular aneurysm, near regions where delayed potentials were recorded during sinus rhythm (Mason et al. 1982; Svenson et al 1990; Littmann et al. 1991). The diastolic activity is over the infarct or at the border of the infarct and adjacent noninfarcted region. Epicardial activity may also occur throughout the diastolic interval as well as during systole and some of the epicardial electrograms may be fractionated (Svenson et al. 1990; Kaltenbrunner et al. 1991; Littmann et al. 1991). These are all characteristics similar to those of endocardial electrograms in those patients in which the site of origin is on the endocardial surface. An example of electrograms recorded from the epicardial surface of the left ventricle during tachycardia in a patient with an epicardial site of origin is shown in Figure 4.32. Panel A shows the epicardial activation map that we will describe later. The first eight traces from top to bottom in panels B, C, and D are electrograms recorded from the epicardial surface of the left ventricle and the bottom trace is the electrocardiogram (AVF). Panel B shows electrograms that occurred during diastole, and panels C and D show the electrograms that occurred during systole. Some of these electrograms are fractionated (for example recording G7). In the study of Kaltenbrunner et al. (1991),

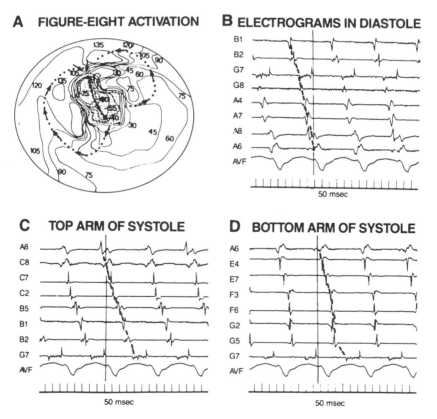

Figure 4.32: Activation map and electrograms recorded from epicardial surface of the left ventricle in a patient with a left ventricular site of origin of ventricular tachycardia. The map in A shows a figure-of-eight activation pattern. Panels B, C, and D show electrograms (first eight traces) and the electrocardiogram (AVF) in the bottom trace. (Reproduced from Littmann et al. (1991) with permission.)

simultaneous activation maps of the entire epicardial surface of both ventricles, and endocardial surface of the left ventricle showed that sites of early activation on the epicardial surface of the left ventricle (which occurred in diastole prior to the onset of the QRS), preceded earliest endocardial activation. The epicardial activation patterns of some of the patients with earliest epicardial activity has appeared to be in the form of reentrant circuits (Kaltenbrunner et al. 1991; Littmann et al. 1991), while in others the presystolic electrograms occurred in localized regions with subsequent spread from the region in a radial pattern (Harris et al. 1987; Littmann et al. 1991). We will discuss the reentrant patterns of excitation in detail later.

Further evidence for participation of the epicardial border zone as a site of tachycardia origin comes from demonstrations that tachycardias characterized by presystolic or diastolic epicardial activation can be terminated with epicardial cryoablation (Pagé et al. 1989; Kaltenbrunner et al. 1991) or by epicardial laser photocoagulation at these sites (Svenson et al. 1990; Littmann et al. 1991). Endocardial laser irradiation was not successful in terminating tachycardia in patients with electrophysiological evidence of an epicardial site of arrhythmia origin (Svenson et al. 1990). Also supporting an epicardial origin of tachycardia in these patients has been the ability to entrain the tachycardia by stimulating at the epicardial sites of presystolic activity (Littmann et al. 1991). Entrainment was characterized by the occurrence of QRS complexes during overdrive of the tachycardia that replicated the QRS complex of spontaneous tachycardia in all ECG leads, and a global epicardial activation pattern that was the same for the spontaneous and the entrained tachycardia. In addition, the stimulus artifact to the onset of the QRS during entrainment was the same as the interval between the local electrogram recorded at the stimulus site to the QRS complex during tachycardia (Littmann et al. 1991).

As with the tachycardias that are associated with earliest endocardial activation, earliest epicardial activation and termination by destruction of part of the epicardial border zone does not mean that the entire reentrant circuit is located in the epicardial border zone. Only a segment of the circuit may be located there and the remainder involves intramural pathways. Earliest epicardial activation might also sometimes occur when the entire circuit resides in the surviving intramural muscle fibers. This might be the case when earliest epicardial activation only slightly precedes earliest endocardial activation, because activation is spreading from an intramural site simultaneously towards the epicardium and endocardium. That intramural circuits may exist is also suggested when earliest epicardial and endocardial activation occur nearly simultaneously (Kaltenbrunner et al. 1991). Abolition of tachycardias arising in such reentrant circuits would seem to require extending ablation into intramural regions.

The sites of earliest activity of ventricular premature depolarizations, nonsustained ventricular tachycardia, and short periods of ventricular tachycardia that lead to fibrillation have not been located. These are transient events and therefore, determining activation sequences requires simultaneous electrogram recordings from large numbers of sites during the arrhythmias. This mapping technique is not yet widely utilized (as of 1992) for clinical studies. It is likely that these nonsustained arrhythmias also arise in the surviving myocardial fibers in the infarcted region, but the site of origin might sometimes be different from those for sustained, monomorphic ventricular tachycardia.

The site of earliest activation during sustained ventricular tachycardia is not related in a completely predictable way to the pattern of activation of the rest of the ventricles or to the morphology of the QRS on the ECG (Harris et al. 1987). When earliest activity occurs in a focal region (one region that may be as large as 10 cm^2) on the left ventricular endocardial surface, earliest epicardial activation is also usually in the left ventricle and may be focal with radial spread away from the site of breakthrough. An example of this activation pattern is shown in Figure 4.33, panels A and A' at the left (Harris et al. 1987). In Panel A, the epicardial surface is represented as a polar projection with the apex at the center. The locations of the right and left ventricular margins and the left anterior descending coronary artery are indicated on the diagram. In panel A', the endocardial surface of the left ventricle is also shown as a polar projection with the locations of the apex, left anterior descending coronary artery and septum indicated on the diagram. The earliest site of endocardial activation is at the 0 msec isochrone in panel A^1 near the apex while earliest epicardial breakthrough occurs 64 msec later in panel A, also near the apex. There is radial spread of excitation away from this earliest epicardial site. The endocardial activation pattern in this figure is in the form of a "figure-of-eight"; the possible significance of this pattern is discussed in the next section. When the earliest activation occurs on the endocardial surface of the free wall, epicardial breakthrough is also on the free wall (Horowitz et al. 1980) but otherwise, epicardial breakthrough may occur at a distance from the site of earliest activation. Breakthrough at a distance might result when the excitation wave must conduct to the subepicardium through long pathways that circumvent infarcted areas that lie between the surviving subendocardial muscle fibers and the subepicardium, the area of solid infarct described in the section on pathological anatomy. Therefore, epicardial activation maps are not always reliable for locating endocardial sites of arrhythmia origin. Two discrete sites of left ventricular epicardial breakthrough separated by some distance (4–7 cm), and also separated temporally by up to 50 msec have also been found to be associated with a focal site of early endocardial activation (Harris et al. 1987).

The earliest site of activity and global activation of the ventricles during sustained monomorphic ventricular tachycardia usually remains the same from beat to beat. However, sometimes the QRS morphology may change spontaneously from one form to another. In some instances, despite the change in QRS, the site of earliest activity remains the same (Josephson et al. 1978b; Horowitz et al. 1980; De Bakker 1985; Harris et al. 1987). The change in the QRS therefore, is likely to be a result of a change in the pattern of activation of the ventricles despite the same site of origin (presumably the same reentrant circuit). The interpretation of some of these results must be tempered by the recognition of the relatively low spatial resolution of many of the maps, and particularly the fact that the site of origin, even when described as focal, is

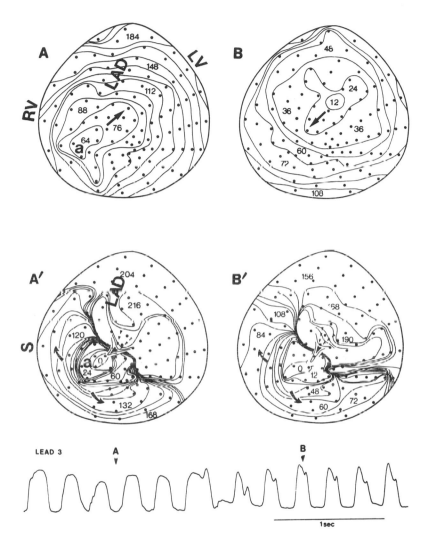

Figure 4.33: Activation of endocardial and epicardial surfaces of the left ventricle during ventricular tachycardia. The electrocardiogram is shown at the bottom. There was a spontaneous shift in the surface ECG configuration from a leftward to a rightward axis. Panels A and B show the epicardial activation maps (polar projection of the ventricles) during tachycardia with leftward axis (A) and rightward axis (B). The dots indicate sites at which electrograms were recorded and the numbers are activation times. Isochrones are drawn at 12-msec intervals. (A') and (B') are maps of the endocardial left ventricle (also polar projections) that show patterns of activation that occurred simultaneously with the epicardial maps above. Dots also show recording sites and isochrones are drawn at 12 msec intervals. RV = right ventricle; LV = left ventricle; LAD = left anterior descending coronary artery; S = septum; a = apex. (Reproduced from Harris et al. (1987) with permission.)

localized only to a relatively large area. The site of origin might therefore change within this area because of a change in the circuit or the exit route from the circuit, without being detected, and as a result subsequent ventricular activation is changed. Figure 4.33 is also an example of a change in QRS and epicardial activation during tachycardia that is not associated with an obvious change in "site of origin" (Harris et al. 1987). Panel A corresponds to the section of the ECG trace below that is labeled A and panel B to the section of the ECG trace labeled B. In A, epicardial breakthrough, indicated by the 64-msec isochrone, occurs at the apex with radial spread away from this region. In B, associated with the change in the ECG morphology is a shift in the site of epicardial breakthrough towards the base of the left ventricle (at 12 msec). Because of this shift, the epicardium of the left ventricle in B is activated differently than in A. The endocardial activation patterns associated with the two different epicardial patterns are shown in panels A′ and B′. There is a similar site of endocardial origin indicated by the 0-msec isochrone for both ECG morphologies. Therefore, after leaving the circuit, the route through which the wave front traveled to the epicardium must have changed, but the reason for this change is not apparent. In other studies a change in the ECG morphology during a sustained ventricular tachycardia has been associated with an obvious change in the site of earliest activity (Horowitz et al. 1980), which might also represent either a different exit route from the same circuit or a different circuit altogether. Why these changes might occur during a sustained tachycardia is a matter of speculation. One possible reason might be the development of conduction block in an exit route from the reentrant circuit caused by the rapid activity, forcing the impulse to take an alternative exit route.

Many of the patients with sustained monomorphic tachycardia also have more than one kind of tachycardia; that is, monomorphic sustained tachycardias induced at different times, with different rates and QRS morphologies. The site of origin may sometimes appear to be the same for the different tachycardias judging by similar sites of earliest activity (De Bakker 1985; Waspe et al. 1985a; Harris et al. 1987). This suggests the possibility of the same reentrant circuit with the same exit route from the circuit resulting in a different pattern of activation of the ventricles as was shown in Figure 4.33 for the change in QRS occurring during a tachycardia. However, again we must remember that the site of origin might sometimes change by up to several centimeters without being detected and such a shift might be associated with a change in the circuit or the exit route that would only be seen in high-resolution activation maps. Other patients have been shown to have widely separated sites of earliest endocardial activity associated with different tachycardias (greater than 4 cm between sites in the study of Waspe et al. 1985a) as well as different endocardial activation patterns (Harris et al. 1987). Although it is possible that the different tachycardias are associated with different circuits, it is also possible that despite the widely separated sites of origin there is only one rather large circuit that either has a subendocardial or intramural location, and that the site of exit from the circuit changes (Waspe et al. 1985a).

The QRS morphology during sustained ventricular tachycardia may have either a right or a left bundle branch block configuration. Traditionally, impulse origin in the left ventricle is expected to be associated with a QRS that has a right bundle branch block configuration because the right ventricle should be activated after the left. In patients with ventricular tachycardia with a right bundle branch block pattern, the site of origin is usually on the endocardial surface of the left ventricle as expected (left ventricular free wall or septum) (Josephson et al 1978b; Horowitz et al. 1980) and epicardial breakthrough on the left ventricle usually occurs along the epicardial margin of the aneurysm (Horowitz et al. 1980). Activation of the rest of the left ventricular epicardium results from the spread of excitation away from this region of breakthrough and left ventricular activation is usually completed before right ventricular activation (Horowitz et al. 1980). Traditionally, left bundle branch block is expected to be associated with right ventricular origin of a tachycardia because a right ventricular arrhythmogenic site should cause right ventricular activation before left. However, most instances of left bundle branch block in the patients with healing or healed infarcts have also been associated with earliest activity or site of origin in the left ventricle, usually on the septum (Horowitz et al. 1980) and it has been the right ventricle in only a few patients (Josephson et al. 1978b). The occurrence of left bundle branch block associated with left ventricular origin of the arrhythmias might occur if there is rapid activation across the septum to the right ventricle with slower activation of the diseased left ventricle (Josephson et al 1978b). Earliest right ventricular epicardial breakthrough in most of these patients often occurs along the interventricular groove before left ventricular epicardial breakthrough and right ventricular activation is completed before left ventricular activation (Horowitz et al. 1980). Left ventricular epicardial activation sometimes may extend beyond the limits of the QRS because of slow impulse conduction in diseased regions (Josephson et al. 1982b). Septal origin of tachycardia may also be associated with either a right or a left bundle branch block configuration and a QRS duration of less than 140 msec (less than the duration associated with other left ventricular sites of origin). Epicardial breakthrough occurs anteriorly or posteriorly, adjacent to the interventricular groove on either the right or the left ventricle (Horowitz et al. 1980).

Comparison of Origin of Ventricular Tachycardia in Humans and Experimental Animal Models

The electrophysiological studies indicate that many of the sustained tachycardias in humans with a healed myocardial infarct originate in the subendocardial region, particularly in hearts with anteroseptal infarcts and ventricular aneurysms. The endocardial border zone of these infarcts contains bundles of ventricular muscle as well as some Purkinje fibers. The muscle bundles provide a necessary substrate for the formation of reentrant circuits. Since they are separated by large amounts of connective tissue in the scar, they most likely have conduction properties characteristic of nonuniform anisotropy which causes the necessary slow conduction for reentry. We will discuss the conduction properties of this region later. Nonuniform anisotropic conduction is suggested by the fractionated electrograms. Hydropic intracellular changes in microanatomy of some muscle cells surviving in the endocardial border of human infarcts, as well as other changes in ultrastructure may mean that they are also chronically ischemic and have altered electrophysiological properties that may contribute to the occurrence of arrhythmias (Fenoglio et al. 1983; Bolick et al. 1986). Surviving Purkinje fibers may not be a crucial part of the reentrant circuits, because conduction in the Purkinje system may be normal. It seems that these kinds of infarcts do not have an epicardial border zone that is suitable for reentry. In regions of aneurysms, there may only be islands of surviving epicardial muscle fibers that do not form reentrant circuits. This is unlike the canine model of an anteroseptal infarct caused by permanent occlusion of the left anterior descending coronary artery near its origin, where tachycardias often arise in reentrant circuits formed in the subepicardial muscle. In this canine model, only Purkinje fibers form the endocardial border zone while muscle comprises the epicardial border zone. Conduction in the surviving Purkinje system does not seem to be abnormal in healing or healed infarcts (Kienzle et al. 1987) because Purkinje fibers are mostly recovered by this time from the ischemic insult that occurs soon after coronary occlusion (see Chapter III); there is no obvious electrophysiological cause for reentry in the endocardial border zone. Therefore, reentry occurs in the epicardial border zone where there is abnormal conduction in the surviving ventricular muscle because of the marked changes in the geometrical organization of the fibers resulting in nonuniform anisotropy as well as some changes in transmembrane potentials. It is only when ventricular muscle also survives in the endocardial border zone in experimental models as after a more distal left anterior descending coronary artery occlusion in the canine (Garan et al. 1980; 1981; 1987) or a ventral artery occlusion in the feline (Myerburg et al. 1977), that reentrant circuits may occur in the endocardial border zone. The bundles of surviving muscle cells in the endocardial border zone then are separated by increased amounts of fibrous tissue that may influence conduction properties in the same way as in the experimental epicardial border zone. Therefore, conduction properties of the endocardial border zone, when it is comprised of muscle bundles, may be analogous to those of the epicardial border zone in the canine hearts with a proximal left anterior descending coronary artery occlusion.

The epicardial border zone can be part of reentrant circuits in human hearts, particularly those with inferior infarcts. The epicardial border zone in these infarcts has structural similarities to the border zone in some canine infarcts where arrhythmias also originate in the epicardium. That is, there is a sufficient amount of muscle bundles with nonuniform anisotropic conduction properties to form reentrant circuits.

In both human and experimental infarcts, reentrant circuits and the site of arrhythmia origin may also be at intramural locations when there is survival of intramural muscle bundles projecting into the infarct from the lateral margins. Intramural muscle survival in infarcts may occur after more distal occlusions that do not deprive all intramural regions of their blood supply or after temporary occlusion followed by reperfusion. Reperfusion is induced in experimental studies by releasing the coronary ligation. Reperfusion of human infarcts can occur after spontaneous thrombolysis.

Why septal involvement in the infarct is frequently associated with the occurrence of sustained tachycardia in humans has not been explained (Bolick et al. 1986; Josephson 1992). The main difference between that septum and the anterior, lateral, or posterior left ventricular walls is the location of the specialized conducting system in the septum. This would seem to imply that the Purkinje system may play a role in the genesis of some ventricular tachycardias when the septum is involved.

Properties of Reentrant Circuits Causing Ventricular Tachyarrhythmias: Demonstration by Mapping Activation Sequences

The indirect evidence derived from electrical stimulation of the heart indicates that tachycardias associated with healing or healed infarcts are often caused by reentrant excitation. The site of origin of these arrhythmias, that is the location of the reentrant circuits, may vary and is determined, to a large extent by the pathological anatomy of the infarct. Activation patterns that have been obtained by a more detailed mapping of impulse propagation at these "sites of origin" further define the characteristics and properties of the reentrant circuits. More is known about the reentrant circuits from the experimental studies on the animal models than from human studies. However, integration of information obtained from both can explain many of the clinical electrophysiological characteristics of these arrhythmias.

Initiation of Tachyarrhythmias

One of the hallmark features of tachyarrhythmias in hearts with healing or healed infarcts is their initiation by programmed premature or overdrive stimulation of the ventricles. Spontaneous initiation of the arrhythmias may sometimes be triggered by premature beats, although the initiating impulse often has a long coupling interval (unlike the initiating stimulated impulse) (Berger et al. 1988). The initiation of tachyarrhythmias by stimulated impulses suggests that the reentrant circuit is either not present or not functioning until this initiating event occurs. If the circuit that causes the tachyarrhythmia is a functional circuit, it may not exist until a premature impulse causes it to form. If it is an anatomical circuit that always exists, it may still not cause reentrant arrhythmias until it is activated with a specific pattern that results from premature excitation. How do premature impulses initiate the reentrant excitation that causes the arrhythmias? This question is the basis for the first part of our discussion.

Mapping the excitation sequence of the impulse that initiates ventricular tachycardia shows how that impulse leads to reentry. This information must be obtained from simultaneous recordings at a large number of sites; that is a single beat must be accurately mapped. Sequential recordings from a number of sites during many beats, as can be done with a roving probe, is not sufficient. The canine model of proximal left anterior descending coronary artery occlusion has provided most of the data because the location of many of the reentrant circuits in the epicardial border zone allows for high-resolution mapping. The epicardial border zone can be treated as a two-dimensional structure because it is so thin and often lacks intramural connections, eliminating the need for three-dimensional mapping and enabling all the recording electrodes to be located on the epicardial surface of the heart. During sinus rhythm there is usually no evidence of activation of the epicardial border zone by transmurally conducting impulses because of this lack of intramural muscle bundles, but rather activation begins at the margins on the epicardial surface and proceeds towards the middle where the activation waves collide (Wit et al. 1982a; 1982b; Dillon et al. 1988). This pattern reflects the "two-dimensional structure". Time for total activation ranges from 40–80 msec but some regions may be activated considerably later. This is longer than the time for activation of the same region in normal ventricles where a large amount of epicardial muscle is activated nearly simultaneously by transmurally conducting activation waves from the subendocardium, hence, the longer duration of composite electrograms recorded in this region after occlusion of the left anterior descending coronary artery.

Activation maps of the epicardial border zone in the canine model have shown how premature stimuli can initiate arrhythmias. An example is shown in Figure 4.34. Activation times measured simultaneously at 196 sites within a 4 × 5 cm region went into the construction of these maps. The upper left panel shows that the basic drive stimuli, applied on the epicardial surface of the right ventricle adjacent to the left anterior descending coronary artery (at the pulse symbol) at a cycle length of 280 msec, initiated excitation wave fronts that spread over the epicardial border zone from this margin towards the opposite margin at the apex of the lateral free wall (arrows). The isochrones progress in sequence from 0 to 90 msec. There are no areas of block of the basic drive impulse in this map. Also, there is no evidence of a reentrant circuit in this region, judging by the activation pattern of the basic drive impulses. The prematurely stimulated impulses that initiate arrhythmias have very different activation patterns. Stimulated premature impulses that initiate tachycardias propagate into the epicardial border zone and block (El-Sherif et al. 1981; 1982; 1984; 1985; Wit et al. 1981a; 1982a; 1982b; Mehra et al. 1983; Cardinal et al. 1988; Dillon et al. 1988). The region of conduction block forms a line that extends for several centimeters, called the arc of conduction block by El-Sherif

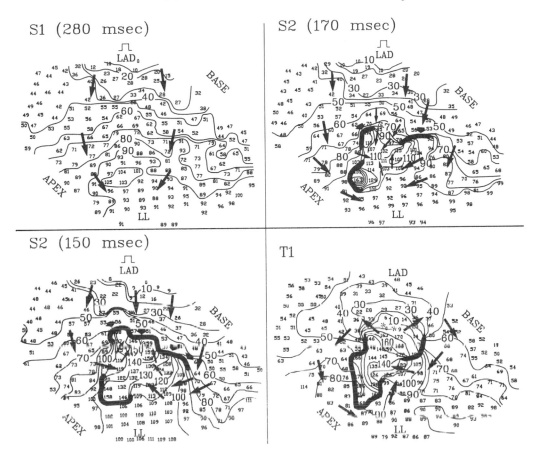

Figure 4.34: Activation maps of the epicardial border zone showing the initiation of reentrant ventricular tachycardia by a premature stimulus in a canine heart with a 4-day-old infarct. In each panel, the border of the electrode array adjacent to the left anterior descending coronary artery (LAD) is at the top, and the border of the electrode array on the lateral left ventricle (LL) is at the bottom. The base of the heart is to the right and the apex to the left. Activation times are plotted at each of the recording sites. The ventricles were driven at a regular cycle length (280 msec) by basic drive stimuli (S_1) applied through electrodes along the LAD margin of the epicardial border zone at the top of each map. The activation pattern of the epicardial border zone during the basic drive is shown in the top left panel (S_1, 280 msec). The arrows point out the direction of activation. The top right panel shows the activation pattern of a single premature impulse (S_2) elicited from the same stimulation site at the LAD margin at the coupling interval of 170 msec. This premature impulse did not initiate reentry, although there were local areas of conduction block indicated by the thick black lines (see text). The bottom left panel shows activation by another premature impulse elicited with a coupling interval of 150 msec. Conduction of this premature impulse blocked along the region indicated by the horizontal, thick black line (short thick arrow). Conduction around the line of block (large arrows) initiated reentry. The bottom right panel shows the reentrant excitation pattern of the first impulse of the tachycardia. Activation in this time window begins at the asterisk within the 10-msec isochrone, the point where the activation in the previous map and time window (lower left panel) ended. (Modified from Wit et al. (1990a) with permission.)

(1985). Conduction block of a premature impulse with a coupling interval of 150 msec to the last basic drive impulse that resulted in reentry is shown in the activation map in the lower left panel of Figure 4.34. Activation of the epicardial border zone by this premature impulse occurred from the left anterior descending coronary artery (LAD) margin, where it was initiated, to the 60-msec isochrone, about one third of the distance into the border zone before the block occurred. Conduction block is indicated by the thick black line. The line of conduction block sometimes occurs towards the margin of the border zone where there is a transition from the thick normal ventricular wall to the thin layer of surviving epicardial muscle (Mehra et al. 1983) although it also may occur well into the border zone as shown in the activation map of Figure 4.34. As the arc of block is approached, electrogram morphology changes as shown in Figure 4.35, which displays selected electrograms recorded along the pathway of propagation of the premature impulse. At the line of block, the wave form is monophasic which is characteristic of a wave form that has arrived at the end of its conduction pathway. Reentry occurs when stimulated wave fronts propagate around the extremities of the arc of conduction block and activate myocardium on the distal side of it after myocardium on the proximal side has recovered excitability. These wave fronts can then reexcite the myocardium on the proximal side. This pattern of activation is shown by the arrows in Figure 4.34 (lower left panel). The region on the distal side of the line of block was activated at between 150 and 160 msec by wave fronts propagating around both ends of the line of block. Activation on the distal side of the line of block occurred about 100 msec after block occurred at the proximal side (at 60 msec). This time lapse of 100 msec allowed the proximal side time to recover excitability. The map in the lower right panel of Figure 4.34 shows the wave front from the distal side of the line of block (beginning at the asterisk) propagating retrogradely across it to reexcite the proximal side (isochrones 10–30). The wave front returned to the left anterior descending coronary artery margin (40-msec isochrone) where it exited the border zone to excite the ventricles as the first tachycardia impulse (T_1). A functional reentrant circuit was therefore formed by the premature activation. Because of its transient nature, the arc of block acted as an area of unidirectional block that provided the return path for the reentrant impulse; conduction of the premature impulse blocked in the antegrade direction but not in the retrograde direction. During the initiation of reentry shown in Figure 4.34, there was electrical activity generated by the conducting premature impulse at one or another of the different recording sites in the reentrant circuit at all times, between the premature impulse and the first impulse of tachycardia. If a composite electrode had been located in this region, it would have shown continuous electrical activity similar to that described in Figure 4.26.

There is an interrelationship between the length of the arc of conduction block and the speed of activation around the arc of block that is an important determinant for the successful initiation of reentry (El-Sherif et al. 1981; 1984). If the length of the line of block is too short, activation of the distal side may occur too quickly, before the proximal side has recovered excitability. The prox-

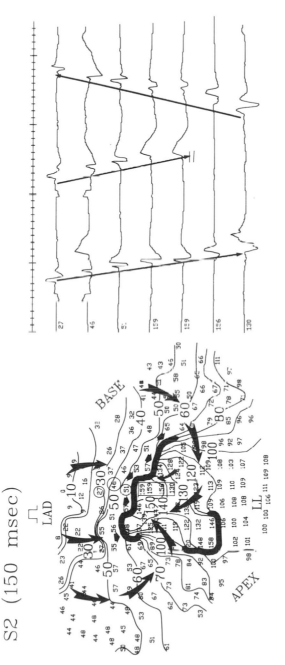

Figure 4.35: Electrograms recorded from the epicardial border zone during conduction block of a stimulated premature impulse that initiated ventricular tachycardia. The activation map at the left is the one previously shown in the lower left panel of Figure 4.34. The electrograms at the right were recorded at the sites on the map designated by the circles and the rectangle. The number at the left of each electrogram trace corresponds to the activation times on the map. The first group of electrograms (from top to bottom) resulted from the last basic drive stimulus, the second group resulted from the premature stimulus, and the third group resulted from the reentrant impulse. During propagation of the premature impulse, electrogram morphology changed from biphasic to monophasic at the site of block (electrograms 159). (Unpublished results of J. Coromilas and A.L. Wit.)

imal side of the region of block then cannot be reexcited and reentry cannot occur. The failure of a premature impulse to cause a sufficiently long arc of block and initiate reentry may occur if the coupling interval of the premature stimulus to the basic drive stimulus is too long. The arc of block lengthens as the premature coupling interval is decreased. In addition, conduction around the arc of block may be too rapid at long coupling intervals and slow as the premature coupling interval is decreased, facilitating the occurrence of reentry. These effects of prematurity explain why tachycardias are only initiated by appropriately timed stimulated premature impulses during programmed electrical stimulation. The top right panel in Figure 4.34 shows the activation pattern of a premature impulse, stimulated at a longer coupling interval of 170 msec that did not induce tachycardia (compared to the premature impulse with a coupling interval of 150 msec that did). Activation spread away from the left anterior descending coronary artery stimulation site and several small areas of conduction block developed as indicated by the thick black lines. The small areas of block were not confluent; activation moved towards the lateral margin between two of the small regions of block. The distal sides of the lines of block were activated with a delay of 20 to 50 msec beyond the activation time proximal to the lines of block, which was not sufficient to allow reentry to occur. It is likely that the muscle fibers proximal to the line of block did not have sufficient time to recover excitability, and therefore, excitation could not occur through this region in the retrograde direction to reactivate areas that were previously excited. Tachycardia might also not be initiated when the premature coupling interval is too short, rather than too long. The arc of block may then extend from one margin of the epicardial border zone to the opposite margin and there may be no way for the impulse to conduct around it, except in normal myocardium. Conduction in normal myocardium is too rapid for reentry to occur because it results in an insufficient delay of activation at the distal side of the block line.

Conduction of the premature impulses that initiate reentry in the epicardial border zone of canine infarcts may also block in the subendocardial layers of surviving muscle or Purkinje fibers although this block is probably not instrumental in causing tachycardia (Kramer et al. 1985). Even in the few examples in which activation maps indicate that the reentrant circuits in this canine model may involve intramural or subendocardial components (El-Sherif et al. 1985, Kramer et al. 1985), conduction block in the epicardial border zone as described above is the primary factor for initiation of reentry.

Two or three premature stimuli are often necessary to induce ventricular tachycardia. Sometimes the length of the arc of conduction block of single stimulated premature impulses at all possible coupling intervals may not be long enough or conduction around the arc of block may not be slow enough to permit the occurrence of reentry. However, a second or a second and third premature impulse may cause a sufficiently long arc of block or slow conduction or a combination of the two to initiate reentrant tachycardia (El-Sherif et al. 1984).

Another possible reason for the failure of a single premature impulse to induce tachycardia is that the premature impulse might not be able to reach the site of the potential reentrant circuit early enough for it to cause a line of block that would enable reentry to occur. If the stimulus site is at some distance from the potential circuit, early premature impulses might conduct in partially refractory muscle between the two points and arrival of the premature impulses at the circuit might be delayed. Conduction of even earlier premature impulses might block before reaching the site of reentry. Several premature impulses occurring in succession might then succeed in inducing reentry. A first premature impulse delivered at a coupling interval at which it can reach the circuit but not block, might enable a second premature impulse to arrive at the circuit early enough to cause an appropriate arc of block. The action potential duration of a premature impulse is shortened, and if the cells are well polarized, the refractory period of the premature impulses is shortened as well. Therefore, the first of a series of premature impulses is expected to shorten the refractory period of the tissue it traverses. The next premature impulse may then conduct through more fully recovered myocardium and succeed in reaching the circuit at an appropriate time to cause a sufficiently long arc of conduction block. The above discussion is speculative since we do not have activation maps from experimental or clinical studies to directly show this mechanism for tachycardia initiation.

Since the ability of premature impulses to reach the potential reentrant circuit early enough to cause the necessary unidirectional conduction block or slow conduction to initiate reentry is an important determinant of whether or not tachycardia is initiated, the site of stimulation may also have an important influence on the initiation of reentrant tachycardia. The clinical data indicate that tachycardia might sometimes be induced from one right ventricular stimulation site and not another. When premature stimuli delivered to the right ventricle fail to induce tachycardias, the same stimulus pattern delivered to the left ventricle may sometimes succeed (Robertson et al. 1981; Morady et al. 1984a). In the canine models, tachycardias are also sometimes more easily induced with left ventricular stimulation than with right. Left ventricular stimulation may be more effective than right ventricular stimulation because it is closer to the circuit and thus, there is less intervening tissue between the stimulus site and the circuit to influence conduction of premature impulses (Michelson et al. 1981d).

That tachycardia might be induced in some patients by one premature stimulus from the right ventricle and in others only by two or three or only by left ventricular stimulation may reflect on the electrophysiological properties of the circuit. These properties may be different in different hearts, depending on factors such as the stage of healing or the pathological anatomy. In some patients, the site of stimulation during the electrophysiological study may be farther from the circuit than in others, and therefore, more premature stimulated impulses may be necessary for the circuit to be reached or activated with sufficient prematurity to cause reentry. The results of some studies have shown no special characteristics to differentiate reentrant tachycardias that can be induced only by left ventricular stimulation from those that can be induced by one or two premature stimuli from the right ventricle (Robertson et al. 1981), suggesting that it is not different properties of the circuit itself that are responsible for these different characteristics of initiation. However, it has also been found that some tachycardias that require multiple premature stimuli for induction have faster rates than those induced by single premature stimuli (Buxton et al. 1984a). A faster rate may indicate that the reentrant circuit is smaller in patients that require multiple premature stimuli, or that impulse conduction in the circuit is faster. Therefore, two or three premature impulses may be needed to establish the slow conduction and block for initiation of reentry.

We described that the premature stimulation protocol used to initiate tachyarrhythmias is usually done at several different basic drive cycle lengths and that premature stimuli are sometimes able to initiate tachycardia at a long basic drive cycle but not at a short one or vice versa. It is likely that the basic drive cycle influences the characteristics of the line of block caused by the premature impulse. The basic drive cycle sets the refractory and conduction properties of the tissues in the reentrant circuit as well as between the site of stimulation and the circuit, both of which influence the ability of the premature impulse to induce tachycardia. The influence of the basic drive cycle length should be dependent on the characteristics of the transmembrane potentials in these regions. There are no experimental data to indicate how a long basic cycle length sometimes facilitates induction of tachycardia. The dispersion of refractoriness of normal ventricular muscle is not altered over the range of cycle lengths at which programmed stimulation studies are done (Janse 1971). It is possible that dispersion of refractoriness between normal muscle and muscle surviving in infarcts is influenced by the basic cycle length so that block is potentiated at long basic cycle lengths. This might occur if refractoriness of muscle surviving in the infarct prolonged more than normal muscle. A tachycardia might also be induced preferentially at a fast basic pacing rate over a slow rate. Although at more rapid basic drive rates, shorter coupled premature impulses can be initiated because of the shorter action potential duration and refractory period at the site of stimulation, this is not always the reason for the facilitation of tachycardia induction (Morady et al. 1989). In partially depolarized tissue, a rapid basic rate may slow conduction and prolong refractoriness, rather than shorten it much as it does in the atrioventricular node; that is, there may be an increase in postrepolarization recovery of excitability. Conduction of a premature impulse delivered during a more rapid basic pacing rate would then be slower than during a slow pacing rate. This might facilitate the occurrence of the appropriate amount of block or slow conduction to cause reentry. This, however, is speculative. Therefore, a number of factors might influence the effects of basic drive cycle length on induction of tachycardia by a premature impulse. The different effects of drive cycle length among hearts may reflect different electrophysiological properties of tissues in and around the reentrant circuits.

Rapid pacing at a constant cycle length without premature stimulation may also establish the necessary conditions that cause reentry, including a long arc of block and slow conduction around it. For rapid pacing to be effective, it requires a critical short cycle length and an appropriate number of stimulated impulses to establish the required conditions for reentry to occur (El-Sherif et al. 1984; Dillon et al. 1988). The initiation of tachycardia is also dependent on the cessation of the stimulation train at the appropriate time. Otherwise the reentering impulse may collide with the next stimulated impulse preventing occurrence of tachycardia (El-Sherif et al. 1984). Figure 4.36 shows the activation maps from a period of rapid stimulation that induced ventricular tachycardia. Activation of the epicardial border zone during the first two stimulated impulses occurred uniformly. Panel A shows the map of one of these stimulated beats; broad wave fronts moved from the site of stimulation, S, at the lateral margin (LL) to the left anterior descending coronary artery margin (LAD), from isochrones 10–60, as shown by the arrows. Activation by subsequent stimulated impulses slowed and a line of block then formed with a vertical orientation by the fifth stimulated impulse. The activation map of this stimulated impulse is shown in panel B; the vertical line of block is shown by the thick black line and unfilled arrows. Activation in this map occurred around the line of block in the direction indicated by the black arrows. The line of block then extended during each subsequent stimulated impulse until it was in the shape of a horseshoe with vertical and horizontal components by the eighth stimulated impulse, shown in panel C. Activation occurred around the line at both of its extremities towards the left anterior descending coronary artery (LAD) margin and moved back towards the lateral margin (LL) (isochrones 90–140). The activation wave reached the distal side of the vertical component of the block line at 150–160 msec. This wave front, returning towards the LL margin collided with the subsequent stimulated impulse and so could not start tachycardia; this pattern of activation continued for several more stimulated impulses. The activation map showing the collision is in panel D. The dotted area (10-msec isochrone) is the returning impulse resulting from the previous stimulus. This wave front collided with the antegradely conducting impulse evoked at site S. After the last stimulated impulse the returning wave front continued towards the LL margin (panel E, isochrones 10–50) and the reentrant circuit was established.

In some hearts with healing or healed infarcts, the conditions that cause conduction block and slow conduction necessary for reentry cannot be established by appropriately timed prematurely stimulated impulses or by rapid pacing. Drugs that influence conduction and refractoriness may sometimes assist in establishing the necessary conditions for reentry. In fact, this may be one mechanism by which some antiarrhythmic drugs are proarrhythmic (Velebit et al. 1982; Levine et al. 1989; Stanton et al. 1989). An example is the effect of flecainide. Both clinical and experimental studies have shown that flecainide can facilitate induction of ventricular tachycardia by programmed stimulation (Poser et al. 1985; Sakai et al. 1989b; Coromilas et al. 1993). The mechanism, as shown by mapping impulse propagation in the epicardial border zone of healing canine infarcts, may be the slowing of conduction around the arc of block to the critical degree necessary for successful reentry. Activation maps showing these effects are displayed in Figure 4.37. The electrocardiogram

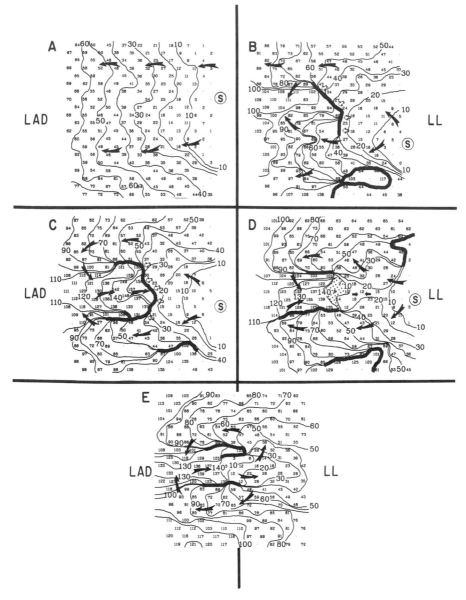

Figure 4.36: Activation maps of the epicardial border zone in a canine heart with a 4-day-old infarct during initiation of sustained ventricular tachycardia by rapid pacing. The margin of the epicardial border zone adjacent to the left anterior descending coronary artery (LAD) is at the left in each panel and the lateral-apical margin (LL) is at the right. Each number on the maps indicates an activation time. Panel A shows activation of the second stimulated impulse arising at (S), initiated at the lateral left ventricular margin (LL). Panel B shows the activation map of the fifth stimulated impulse, panel C of the eighth stimulated impulse, panel D of the tenth stimulated impulse, and panel E of the reentrant impulse after the last stimulated beat. (Reproduced from Dillon et al. (1988) with permission.)

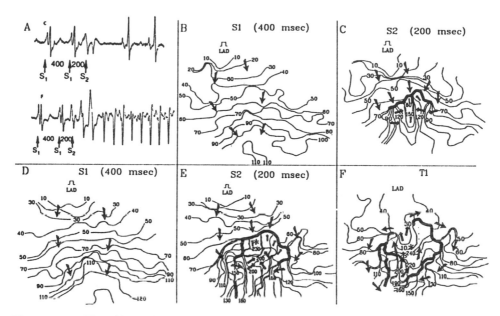

Figure 4.37: The effects of the antiarrhythmic drug flecainide on induction of ventricular tachycardia in an infarcted canine heart. In panel A, the top trace (c) shows the electrocardiogram prior to drug administration. The ventricles were stimulated at a basic cycle (S_1) of 400 msec and a premature stimulus (S_2) with a coupling interval of 200 msec, but tachycardia was not induced. In panel A, the bottom trace (f) shows that after flecainide administration, a premature impulse (S_2) with the same coupling interval induced ventricular tachycardia. The activation maps of the epicardial border zone of the control basic drive and premature impulse are shown in panels B and C, respectively. The activation maps of the epicardial border zone during the basic drive (S_1, 400 msec), premature impulse (S_2, 200 msec), and first impulse of tachycardia (T_1) after flecainide administration are shown in panels D, E, and F, respectively. The margin of the electrode array adjacent to the left anterior descending coronary artery (LAD) is at the top. The arrows indicate the sequence of activation. Isochrones are drawn at 10-msec intervals based on 196 activation times that are not shown. (Unpublished results of J. Coromilas and A.L. Wit.)

at the top of Figure 4.37A shows that the application of a premature stimulus (S_2) with a coupling interval of 200 msec did not induce tachycardia prior to administration of the drug. The activation maps in panels B and C show the reason why it did not. Panel B is the map for the basic drive impulse. It originated at the stimulus site near the left anterior descending coronary artery margin (LAD) and propagated across the epicardial border zone to the opposite side (isochrones 10 to 110). Panel C is the map for the premature impulse. It also originated at the left anterior descending coronary artery margin of the border zone, propagated to the 60–70-msec isochrone and blocked along the dark black line. Activation waves also propagated around the ends of this line of block (arrows), reaching the distal side after 160–170 msec. There was about a 100-msec time difference between activation on the proximal and distal side of the line of block. Reentry did not occur, probably because the epicardial muscle proximal to the block had not yet recovered excitability. The electrocardiogram in the lower trace in Figure 4.37A shows that after administration of flecainide, a prematurely stimulated impulse (S_2) with a coupling interval of 200 msec induced sustained ventricular tachycardia. The activation maps in panels D–F show how it did this. The activation map of the basic drive impulse, S_1, in panel D is similar to the one showing activation by the basic drive before flecainide except that activation takes 10–20 msec longer. The prematurely stimulated impulse, S_2 in panel E, after flecainide blocked as before (dark black line at the 60 msec isochrone). Conduction around the ends of the line of block was much slower so that the excitation wave did not reach the distal side until after 230 msec. This was sufficient time for recovery of excitability to occur and the wave front moved through the region where block was located, towards the left anterior descending coronary artery margin. This movement is shown in panel F (T_1), beginning at isochrone 10 (asterisk) and progressing to isochrone 40. The black arrows point out the reentrant circuit that was formed, excitation moving along the margins of the border zone to both the right and left (isochrones 50–150) and then returning towards the left anterior descending coronary artery margin to complete the first reentrant impulse of the tachycardia after 240 msec.

The discussion so far showing how tachyarrhythmias are initiated by stimulated impulses, has relied on activation maps obtained from a canine model. The differences between this model and clinical cases must always be kept in mind when applying data obtained from the model to clinical events. The canine model that was used is essentially a healing infarct rather than the healed infarct, often with an aneurysm from which much of the clinical electrophysiological data comes. There may be differences in the cellular electrophysiological properties between the two and there are differences in the anatomical substrate. Unfortunately very little mapping data exist from clinical studies showing activation patterns during the initiation of tachycardia because only a few clinical laboratories have the capability to map single beats. Downar and his coworkers (1988) have determined activation patterns during the initiation of ventricular tachycardia in patients with infarcts by mapping the epicardium and endocardium simultaneously with the sock and balloon electrode described earlier. An example of the initiation of a macroreentrant circuit in the endocardial border zone by several premature stimuli delivered in succession is shown in Figure 4.38. The endocardial surface of the left ventricle is depicted as a polar projection with the apex towards the center and the interventricular septum towards the left. The dots indicate the positions of the recording electrodes. No reentrant circuits were apparent prior to the application of the three premature impulses used to initiate the tachycardia (S2, S3, S4) shown in the electrocardiogram at the bottom of the figure. Panel S2 shows the activation pattern of the first stimulated premature impulse. Activity begins within the 0-msec isochrone around the site of stimulation and initially spreads radially away from it for 20–30 msec. After this time, activity does not appear again until 108 msec on the opposite side of the dark line formed by a number of

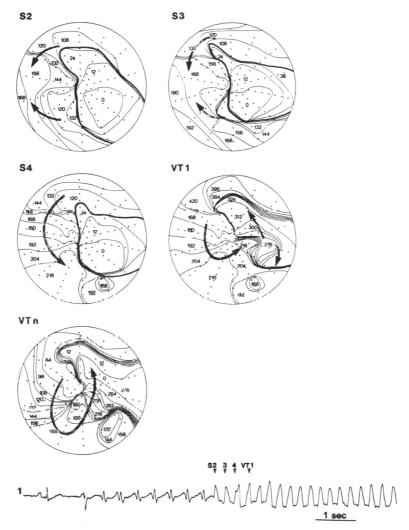

Figure 4.38: Activation maps of initiation of a rapid ventricular tachycardia by three premature stimuli in a human heart with a healed myocardial infarction. The endocardial surface of the ventricles is depicted as a polar projection in each panel. The dots indicate the positions of the recording electrodes, the numbers indicate activation times, and the arrows indicate patterns of activation. (Reproduced from Downar et al. (1988) with permission.)

isochrones closely bunched together. The investigators' interpretation was that activation became very slow in this region. The arrows show two wave fronts that cross this line. There is a time gap of 90–110 msec during which activity was not recorded, making it also possible that the activation wave took some other route, perhaps an intramural one before it reappeared at 108 msec above or 132 msec below. Activation during the S3 stimulated impulse (top right) has a similar pattern except for an increase in the activation time across the dark line. Activity proximal to the dark line is at 0–30 msec while it appears only after 108–132 msec distal to the line. Activation caused by the S4 stimulus initiated the reentry; block appears to extend along the lower part of the line while the excitation wave above still moves through the area of slow conduction from the 24-msec activation time to 120 msec. It then circles towards the lower region of functional block (arrow) and crosses it after about 220 msec to reactivate the stimulus site (at isochrone 0) as the first reentrant beat. The map labeled VT1 shows a time frame that overlaps the S4 map and shows the first reentrant impulse. It begins at the 168-msec isochrone, and shows the excitation wave reaching the line of initial block at 216 msec (this part of the activation sequence was also shown in map S4). After passing through the initial line of block, the wave front divides into two; the clockwise wave front appears to block (arrow pointing downward after 276 msec) while the one that moves counterclockwise towards the base (arrow pointing upward towards 324 msec) set up the large reentrant circuit. This excitation wave can be followed to the 420-msec isochrone in map VT1. Panel VTn shows the endocardial activation pattern during the sustained tachycardia. Activation begins at the 0-msec isochrone and the sequence of isochrones can be followed towards the left (septum) to the 96-msec isochrone, then downward around the apex (to the 192-msec isochrone) and upward to the region of initial activation (after the 276-msec isochrone). The arrow shows the pattern of activation. In this example, the cycle length of reentry is very short, 280 msec, indicating that the rhythm is probably ventricular flutter. Activity in the reentrant circuit shown in VTn occurred throughout the entire diastolic and systolic intervals. The region of the circuit activated at the beginning of the second half of the diastolic interval would be assigned as the site of earliest activity according to the conventions used for locating the site of arrhythmia origin that we described previously. At the same time, circulating activity was mapped on the epicardial surface. A gap of more then 100 msec occurred on the epicardium, during which activity could not be detected.

Despite the use of 112 electrodes to generate the activation maps shown in Figure 4.38, the spatial resolution of the maps is relatively low, leaving some of the interpretation uncertain, particularly in the region of very slow conduction and block. However, if the interpretation of the maps is correct, then conduction of the premature impulse that initiated the arrhythmia appeared to block in a localized critical region and it is this localized block that set up the reentrant circuit, very similar to the results of the experimental studies on the canine heart, which were described earlier.

The mechanism for the conduction block that results in the initiation of reentrant tachycardias by prematurely stimulated impulses, and the mechanism for the slow conduction around the line of block can be inferred from the results of studies on the permanent occlusion canine model. Block is dependent to a significant extent on dispersions of refractoriness of the surviving epicardial muscle fibers. Gough et al. (1985) determined the effective refractory period at a number of sites at which electrograms were recorded, which were used for constructing activation maps by applying premature stimuli through the electrodes. They found a graded increase in the effective refractory period progressing towards the center, from the margin of the epicardial border zone with normal myocardium. Refractory periods were also determined with this method on either side of the arc of conduction block that initiated reentry and it was found that block developed between adjacent sites of short and long refractoriness. Sites of long refractoriness were just distal to the arc of block. Therefore, it appears that the stimulated impulses block when they run into this region of increased effective refractory period. Slow conduction around the zone of conduction block may be attributed, at least partly, to propagation in regions with prolonged refractoriness which have partially recovered excitability (Gough et al. 1985; Restivo et al. 1990).

The anisotropic structure of the epicardial border zone in the canine model may also provide an additional mechanism for the block and slow conduction (Wit et al. 1987; Dillon et al. 1988; Wit 1989; Wit et al. 1990a). As we described in Chapter I, it has been shown in some studies on isolated tissues that the safety factor for conduction of premature impulses parallel to the long axis of muscle fiber orientation in nonuniformly anisotropic tissue is lower than transverse to the long axis, since current generated by the wave front must depolarize more membrane area for successful parallel propagation than transverse propagation (Spach et al. 1981; 1988; Spach and Dolber 1986; Spach 1987; Spach 1988). Therefore, conduction block of wave fronts moving in the parallel direction occurs more easily than in the transverse direction. Most of the arc of conduction block during initiation of tachycardia is usually oriented transverse to the long axis of the myocardial fibers that comprise the epicardial border zone, meaning that the blocked activation wave propagates in the same direction as the long axis of the myocardial fibers. This pattern is diagrammed in Figure 4.39. The left panel shows an activation map of a stimulated premature impulse in the epicardial border zone that initiated reentry; the pattern of conduction is shown by the arrows. The black arrow indicates that conduction of the premature impulse blocked in the epicardial border zone towards the left anterior descending coronary artery at 20 msec along the dark black line. The striped arrows show that wave fronts of the stimulated impulse also skirted around this area of block and reached the distal side of the line of block after 180 msec. These wave fronts then continued back into the normal ventricle along the left anterior descending coronary artery to cause the first reentrant beat. This pattern of activation is similar to the one shown in Figure 4.34. In the right panel, the direction of the long axis of the myocardial fibers is shown schematically. The arrows indicate the conduction pattern that was described for the left panel. The black arrow shows that the wave front that blocked was advancing parallel to the fiber orientation (hence, the line of block is oriented transverse to the long axis). Therefore, block might result from the effects of anisotropy in addition to the increase in refractory period at the region of block. Also shown in Figure 4.39 is that activation around the arc of block occurs first obliquely and then transversely to the long axis of the fibers. This direction of activation is then another cause of the slow conduction, in addition to propaga-

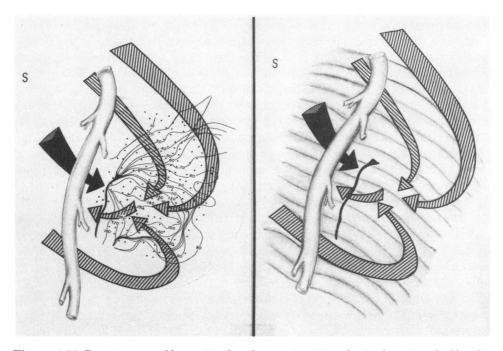

Figure 4.39: Reentry caused by a stimulated premature impulse in the epicardial border zone of a 5-day-old canine infarct after occlusion of the left anterior descending coronary artery (LAD). The stimulating electrodes were located toward the base of the anterior right ventricle at the "S". The left anterior descending coronary artery is shown schematically. The epicardial border zone is to the right of the artery. The pattern of impulse conduction is indicated by the arrows. The dots in the left panel indicate points where electrograms were recorded and activation times measured. The black arrow (left panel) indicates that conduction of the premature impulse was blocked along part of the infarct margin adjacent to the LAD at 20 msec along the dark black line. The striped arrows show that wave fronts of the stimulated impulse skirted this area of block and entered the epicardial border zone from the base at 10 msec and from the apex and left lateral margins at 80 msec. Activation then proceeded back toward the line of block and the margin along the LAD, which was reached after 180 msec. Conduction of the impulse then continued into the normal ventricle along the LAD to cause a reentrant beat. The relationship of the reentrant conduction pattern to the orientation of the myocardial fibers in the epicardial border zone is shown in the right panel. The long axis of the myocardial fibers is shown schematically to be perpendicular to the left anterior descending coronary artery. The arrows in the right panel indicate the conduction pattern that was shown in the left panel. (Reproduced from Gardner et al. (1984) with permission.)

tion in relatively refractory tissue, since transversely propagating wave fronts propagate slowly. If anisotropy plays a role in causing conduction block, it might influence the effects of stimulating at different sites to initiate tachycardia. Block would be predicted to occur more easily only when the stimulated wave front entered the region of the potential reentrant circuit in a direction parallel to the fiber bundle orientation and this orientation of the stimulated wave front might only occur from certain sites of stimulation and not others.

To summarize, limited clinical data and extensive experimental data show how stimulated impulses can initiate reentrant excitation in myocardial fibers surviving in infarcts. We already have mentioned that the experimental data come from studies on healing infarcts where the structure and electrophysiological properties are not exactly the same as in healed infarcts. Nevertheless, we suggest that the basic findings of conduction block and slow activation around the block shown in the experimental studies are likely to occur in human hearts. Both dispersions in effective refractory periods, and the anisotropic properties of the surviving muscle in the infarcts are likely to cause both block and slow conduction. The same mechanism might apply to initiation of tachyarrhythmias by spontaneously occurring premature impulses. However, these experimental results do not explain the mechanism for spontaneous onset of those clinical tachycardias that are not initiated by ventricular premature depolarizations. An area of transient unidirectional block similar to that caused by premature impulses must develop and a critical degree of slow conduction must occur, but the reason why is not readily apparent.

Reentrant Circuits Causing Ventricular Tachycardia

Activation Maps of Reentrant Circuits in Canine Models of Myocardial Infarction

The most detailed activation maps of reentrant circuits causing ventricular tachycardia have also been obtained from studies on canine models in which a large number of electrograms have been recorded simultaneously from the site of arrhythmia origin. We begin this section by discussing these data in detail because the data provide a framework for subsequently looking at maps of reentrant circuits in humans with infarcts. The clinical maps are by necessity usually less complete than the experimental ones, and their interpretation sometimes is not as clear. Seeing what has been done in the more ideal experimental studies provides a background that is helpful for a more critical evaluation of the clinical data. For our description of the experimental data we will again rely to a large extent on the canine model of infarction caused by ligation of the left anterior descending coronary artery in which the reentrant circuits are located for the most part in the epicardial border zone of surviving muscle fibers. This ideal location has enabled the detailed activation maps to be obtained. Reentrant circuits, however, cannot always be located, even in this model (Dillon et al. 1988). Many of these studies have been done during the healing phase of infarction. We will discuss later how these data might also apply to the healed phase in humans.

In our description of the initiation of tachycardia we showed how the conduction block of a stimulated impulse can lead to reentry. Following this first reentrant impulse a number of different events may occur. Tachycardia may be nonsustained or sustained, or ventricular fibrillation may result. The occurrence of each of these arrhythmias can be at least partly understood on the basis of the characteristics of the reentrant circuits. Excitation maps of the epicardial border zone in the canine infarct have shown that once the stimulated impulse that initiates reentry reexcites the region proximal to the arc of conduction block, the excitation wave may continue to propagate in a circuitous pattern to form a reentrant circuit. The location, size, and shape of this circuit is not usually the same as the circuit traversed by the initiating impulse (El-Sherif et al. 1981; 1982; Wit et al. 1982a; 1982b; Mehra et al. 1983; El-Sherif et al. 1984; 1985; Kramer et al 1985; Cardinal et al. 1988; Dillon et al. 1988). Initially, for the first few beats of the tachycardia, the location, size, and shape of the circuits may shift from beat to beat. When these shifts are also accompanied by some variations of the exit route from the circuit to the rest of the ventricles, the initial QRS morphologies of the tachycardia also change from beat to beat. Then if sustained monomorphic ventricular tachycardia has been initiated, the location and morphology of the circuit stabilizes and the pathway of conduction of the reentrant impulse repeats exactly for the subsequent beats of the tachycardia.

Figure 4.40 shows an activation map of a reentrant circuit in the epicardial border zone, obtained during one beat of a sustained and stable monomorphic ventricular tachycardia in a dog with a healing myocardial infarct. The border of the map at the top is adjacent to the left anterior descending coronary artery.

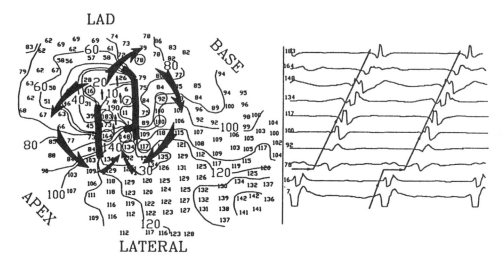

Figure 4.40: Activation map of a reentrant circuit in the epicardial border zone of a canine heart with a 4-day-old infarct. The margins of the electrode array are adjacent to the left anterior descending coronary artery (LAD), base, lateral left ventricle, and apex. Activation times at each of the recording sites are plotted for one impulse of tachycardia (small numbers). Isochrones are drawn at 10-msec intervals and labeled with large numbers. Arrows point out the direction of activation. At the right are selected electrograms recorded at sites in the reentrant circuit indicated by the circles on the activation map. The numbers at the left of the electrogram traces are the activation times on the map. (Unpublished results of J. Coromilas and A.L. Wit.)

The location of the base and apex of the anterior left ventricle is also indicated in the figure. In the time window that is shown, activation begins within the 10-msec isochrone (asterisk) and moves towards the left anterior descending coronary artery margin, where the wave front divides in two (black arrows). This time of activation is in diastole, 20 msec before the onset of the QRS. One wave front moves to the left on the map, which is the direction towards the apex of the left ventricle, the other moves towards the right, which is the direction towards the base. Activation by both wave fronts then moves towards the lateral left margin where the two wave fronts coalesce at around the 120-msec isochrone, and then progress back towards the left anterior descending coronary artery margin to the region where activation began. This sequence is illustrated by the black arrows. The reentrant circuit is completed after 183 msec, the cycle length of the tachycardia. The sequence of activation shown in this map repeated itself exactly for each beat of the tachycardia that lasted for several minutes.

The activation sequence shown in Figure 4.40 during reentry is around two long lines of conduction block (the two thick dark black lines in the figure) that are arranged parallel to each other. The lines are oriented parallel to the long axis of the myocardial fibers. The significance of this arrangement will be discussed later. This is not the same line of block that occurred during initiation of tachycardia by the premature impulse. In Figure 4.34, it can be seen how the line of block that occurs during initiation (panel S_2; 150 msec) changes to lines of block during tachycardia (panel T_1). The lines of block during tachycardia are located in a different region and are oriented at right angles to the line of block occurring during initiation. The lines of block in Figure 4.40 are formed from the interpolation of a large number of isochrones between adjacent electrodes at which there are very different activation times. For example, there is a 50–88-msec time difference between activation of the recording sites on either side of the right line of apparent block resulting in the interpolation of 5–9 isochrones that form the thick black line. By convention, the interpolation of a large number of isochrones has been interpreted as an indication of conduction block because such a large time difference between closely adjacent recording sites is often not compatible with conduction directly between these sites. As was described in Chapter I, a central zone of block is necessary for reentry to continue and if this zone is short-circuited, reentry will stop. This central zone may either be functional as in the leading circle model or it may be anatomical as in the Purkinje fiber bundle model. The parallel lines of block in Figure 4.40 form this central zone of block for the reentrant circuits. We will return to discuss the possible causes of the central region of block during sustained ventricular tachycardia later.

In Figure 4.40, there are actually two reentrant circuits causing the tachycardia. Each one is in the form of an oval that is characteristic of reentry in an anisotropic medium. One is rotating clockwise and the other counterclockwise around the long lines of apparent block and they share a common central pathway of conduction. This is the so-called "figure-of-eight pattern", named as such by El-Sherif (1985). Exit from the circuits to the rest of the ventricles is usually from one end of this common pathway (at the left anterior descending coronary artery or lateral-apical margins of the epicardial border zone) and therefore, there is only one excitation wave from the two circuits that is driving the ventricles. It would seem possible that excitation waves might also be able to emerge from the circuits simultaneously at other locations around their perimeter since the circuits may be in continuity with normal ventricle at the apex or base. If this occurred the ventricular rhythm would be chaotic. In all likelihood this does not usually happen because the spread of excitation from other sites around the perimeter of the circuits to normal ventricle is slow because it is transverse to the orientation of the myocardial fibers. Spread of excitation to normal myocardium from one end of the central common pathway, on the other hand, is rapid, because it is in a direction that is parallel to the myocardial fibers. Once in normal myocardium at the left anterior descending coronary artery or lateral-apical margin, the excitation wave quickly dips transmurally and enters the Purkinje system, which rapidly transports it to other regions of the ventricles, exciting them before excitation waves might slowly emerge from other margins of the circuit (Kramer et al. 1985).

The occurrence of such double circuits ("figure-of-eights") can have important influences on properties of the tachycardias. In particular, they affect the ability to terminate a tachycardia by interventions such as antiarrhythmic drugs, electrical stimulation, surgery, and cryoablation. To terminate tachycardia, such an intervention must cause either transient or complete block in the common central pathway, which would then interrupt both circuits. This has been done, for example, by cooling this region of the epicardial border zone with a cryoprobe until block occurred (Gessman et al. 1981; El-Sherif et al. 1983a; Garan et al. 1987). Cooling to cause block in another region, such as along the basal margin in Figure 4.40, only interrupts one circuit and the other might cause tachycardia to continue (El-Sherif et al. 1983a).

Sometimes, although it might seem that there is a figure-of-eight reentrant circuit from the activation pattern, in actuality only one circuit is completed and is responsible for causing the tachycardia. The second circuit is a "bystander" and is never completed. This can occur when one reentrant wave front arrives at the entrance to the common pathway slightly before the second reentrant wave front. For example, in Figure 4.40, if one wave front arrived at the lateral entrance of the common pathway at 120 msec, and the second arrived at 130–140 msec, the first wave front to have arrived would have completed the circuit while the second would have blocked. Although the second circuit is not actually completed, and is therefore not responsible for the tachycardia, its presence still has potential significance since interruption of the main circuit may lead to the second circuit taking over and controlling the rhythm of the heart. However, in order for this to occur, the central common pathway must remain intact and the primary circuit must be interrupted in a different region.

The reentrant circuits causing sustained tachycardia, illustrated in Figure 4.40, revolve around parallel lines of conduction block, oriented in the same direction as the long axis of the myocardial fiber bundles that form the epicardial border zone. The arrangement and orientation of these lines of block have implications for the mechanisms that are responsible for the block and the slow conduction that enables reentry to persist. Parallel lines of block oriented in the same direction as the long axis of the fibers are indicative of an anisotropic mechanism for reentry, a type of functional reentrant circuit. Why this is so will be discussed later. However, the lines of block are not always oriented parallel to the myocardial fiber bundles and the difference in orientation has some significance in relation to the mechanism causing block, also discussed later. An example of reentrant circuits with lines of block oriented in a different way, mapped in the epicardial border zone during tachycardia in a canine heart with an infarct, is shown in Figure 4.41. Activation in the time window shown in the figure begins at the 10-msec isochrone and moves in the directions shown

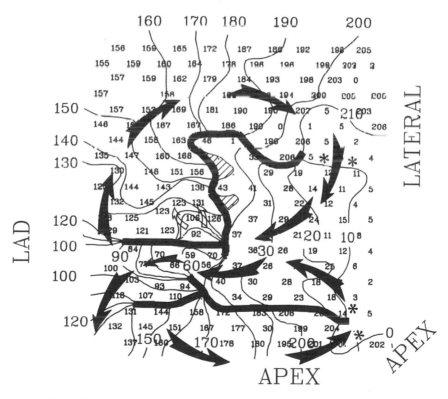

Figure 4.41: Activation map of a reentrant circuit of a single beat during sustained ventricular tachycardia in the epicardial border zone of a canine heart with a 4-day-old infarct. The location of the electrode margins is labeled. Activation times at each of the recording sites are plotted (small numbers). Isochrones are drawn at 10-msec intervals and labeled with large numbers. Arrows point out direction of activation. (Modified from Dillon et al. (1988) with permission.)

by the arrows. The sequence of isochrones shows that one wave front moved towards the LAD margin (isochrones 0 to 90), then towards the base (to the right), which it reaches after about 160 msec, and then towards the lateral margin to its point of origin after 190–200 msec. The other wave front (beginning at the 0 msec isochrone) moves towards the LAD margin, which it also reaches after 90 msec, then towards the apex and lateral margin and back to its point of origin after 200–210 msec. The two lines of block (thick black lines in the figure) that are formed are not straight lines and are not parallel to each other. The line of block above has a long segment extending in the direction from base towards apex that is perpendicular to the long axis of the myocardial fibers. It then makes a right-angle turn and extends towards the LAD margin of the epicardial border zone in a direction parallel to the long axis of the fibers. Because of this shape, the reentrant circuit around this line is nearly circular rather than elliptical. When lines of block are perpendicular to the long myocardial fiber axis, they may be functional but not caused by anisotropy, or they may be anatomical (discussed later). The second line of block near the apical margin, is oriented predominantly parallel to the long axis of the myocardial fibers and the circuit around it is elliptical.

Two simultaneous reentrant circuits or the figure-of-eight pattern do not always exist during the sustained tachycardias that have been mapped in the canine model of infarction. Figure 4.42 shows an example of a single reentrant circuit in the epicardial border zone that caused sustained tachycardia. Activation within the time frame that is shown begins within the 10-msec isochrone at the margin of the electrode array towards the lateral left ventricle (LL). The sequence of isochrones progresses from right to left along the base to the left anterior descending coronary artery margin (LAD) (arrows), which was activated after 90 msec. After reaching this margin, activation occurs back towards the LL margin (from left to right, isochrones 100 to 180). Electrograms were not recorded from a large part of the apical region because the infarct extended to the epicardial surface and there were few surviving epicardial muscle fibers, preventing the formation of a second reentrant circuit.

In the canine model of infarction caused by occlusion of the left anterior descending coronary artery towards its origin, the reentrant circuits are usually in the epicardial border zone as shown in Figures 4.40–4.42 and have rarely been found in the endocardial border zone (El-Sherif et al. 1982). Reentry may occur in the endocardial border zone after a more distal left anterior descending coronary artery occlusion in the canine model in which the epicardial branches of the circumflex are also ligated (Garan and Ruskin 1984; Garan et al. 1987). Although the anatomy has not been studied in detail, we suspect that survival of muscle fibers in the endocardial border zone after the more distal occlusion provides the appropriate electrophysiological substrate for reentry whereas subendocardial muscle does not survive after a more proximal occlusion. Reentry does not usually occur in the endocardial border zone when it is only formed by surviving Purkinje fibers as after the proximal occlusion. An example of a reentrant circuit that was located in the endocardial border zone during sustained ventricular tachycardia several weeks after the more distal

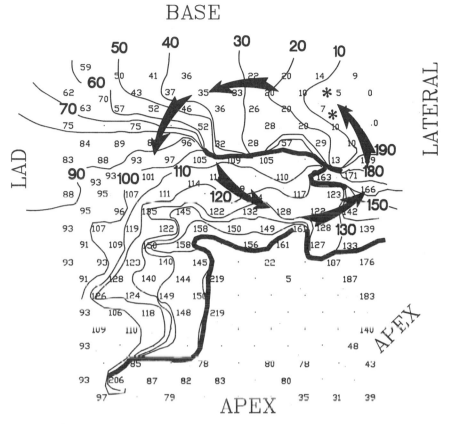

Figure 4.42: Activation map of a reentrant circuit during a single beat of sustained ventricular tachycardia in the epicardial border zone of a canine heart with a 4-day-old myocardial infarct. The location of the electrode margins is labeled. Activation times at each of the recording sites are plotted (small numbers). Isochrones are drawn at 10-msec intervals and labeled with large numbers. Arrows point out direction of activation. (Unpublished results of S.M. Dillon and A.L. Wit.)

left anterior descending coronary artery occlusion is shown in Figure 4.43. The maps are in the form of polar projections. Panel A is a map of endocardial activation, panel B is a map of epicardial activation. In panel A, activation by the endocardial wave front begins at time 0 (within the 10-msec isochrone), splits into two wave fronts, one moving to the right and the other to the left in the figure (arrows). These wave fronts form two reentrant circuits around two regions of block (outlined by dots) with a figure-of-eight configuration. Panel B shows the simultaneous activation of the epicardial border zone where there are two regions of epicardial breakthrough within two separate 10-msec isochrones. Activation spreads from these sites in a circuitous pattern as shown by the arrows, but a horseshoe-shaped arc of complete conduction block in the region of the dotted lines prevents epicardial circuits from being formed.

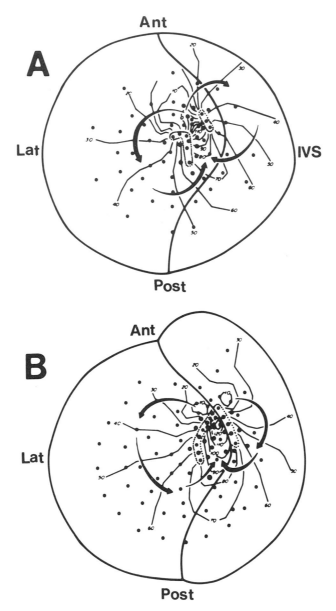

Figure 4.43: Endocardial (A) and epicardial (B) activation maps during one beat of a sustained ventricular tachycardia in a canine heart with a myocardial infarction. Each map is plotted on a polar projection of the ventricles. Ant: anterior surface of the left ventricle; IVS: interventricular septum; Lat: lateral margin; Post: posterior margin. The black dots show the location of the recording electrodes and the arrows point out the patterns of activation. Isochrones are labeled. (Reproduced from Garan et al. (1987) with permission.)

The lack of intramural muscle fiber survival often confines the reentrant circuits to the epicardial border zone in the canine infarct model of proximal left anterior descending coronary artery occlusion. Similar reentrant circuits in the epicardial border zone cause some of the ventricular tachycardias in the canine infarct models of a more distal left anterior descending coronary artery occlusion (Garan et al. 1987), or in the model of temporary left anterior descending coronary artery occlusion followed by reperfusion (Cardinal et al. 1984; Richards et al. 1984; Kramer et al. 1985). However, survival of intramural fiber bundles occasionally occurs after a proximal occlusion of the left anterior descending coronary artery because of the presence of some collaterals or anastomoses with the circumflex, or intramural muscle may survive after more distal occlusions or occlusion followed by reperfusion several hours later. When intramural muscle survival occurs, the opportunity for intramural reentrant pathways exists. Detailed mapping of the activation sequence in intramural reentrant pathways is a difficult problem. These circuits are three dimensional and therefore, a tremendously large number of electrodes are required to locate and map them with the same spatial resolution with which the circuits in the essentially two-dimensional epicardial border zone have been mapped. Therefore, the intramural maps that have been published, although suggestive of and consistent with intramural reentrant circuits, may not give a completely accurate representation of the circuits. An example of an activation pattern that has been interpreted to result from intramural reentry during sustained ventricular tachycardia in a dog several weeks after a more distal left anterior descending coronary artery occlusion is shown in Figure 4.44. On the epicardial surface in panel B there is a site of breakthrough within the 0-msec isochrone, where the impulse appears to arrive through transmural pathways. This wave front then circulates both clockwise and counterclockwise around a central region of functional block (within the area outlined by the dots) and the two wave fronts meet after 100 msec (indicated by the arrows). A similar pattern occurs on the endocardial surface shown in panel A, activation begins at the 0-msec isochrone and spreads in two directions shown by the arrows, around a region of block outlined by the dots, meeting after 110 msec. In both the endocardial and epicardial border zone maps, there is a gap of 30–60 msec, during the cycle of tachycardia during which no electrical activity was recorded. However, intramural recordings obtained beneath the epicardial region of central block from surviving myocardium that extended through the thickness of the transmural infarct showed electrical activity during the epicardial and endocardial gap period in a sequence from the sites adjacent to the endocardial and epicardial regions of convergence towards the sites adjacent to the endocardial and epicardial sites of breakthrough (Garan et al. 1987). That is, activation appeared to occur from the region activated at 110 msec in panel A, through an intramural pathway to the epicardial region activated at 0 msec in panel B, and from the region activated at 100 msec in panel B, back through an intramural pathway to the region activated at 0 msec in panel A. From these data, Garan et al. (1987) constructed models of intramural reentry, which are shown in the schematic diagram in Figure 4.45. These diagrams show that

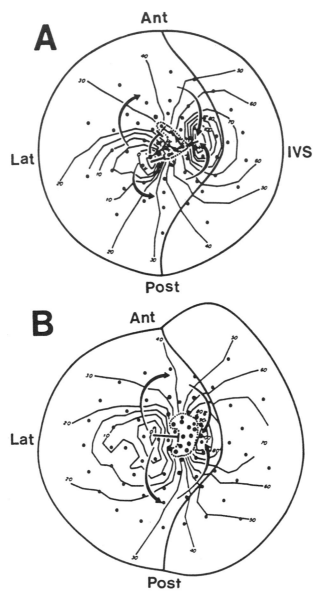

Figure 4.44: Endocardial (A) and epicardial (B) activation maps during one beat of a sustained ventricular tachycardia in canine heart with a myocardial infarct. Format is the same as for Figure 4.43. (Reproduced from Garan et al. (1987) with permission.)

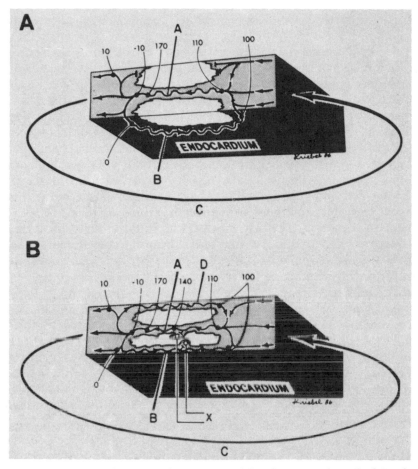

Figure 4.45: Schematic diagrams depicting models of reentry described in the text. Arrows and wavy lines represent slow conduction. Top panel shows endocardial conduction (B) at the periphery of the infarct as part of reentrant activity in series with an intramural pathway (A). Lower panel shows the same model with slow epicardial conduction (D) overlying the intramural pathway. The ventricular tachycardia cycle length is 180 msec. Zero time is arbitrarily chosen as the instant of earliest endocardial activation. A gap period, during which no epicardial electrograms were recorded, is from 110–170 msec in both diagrams when intramural activity occurs. "X" depicts an intramural bipolar electrode from which continuous electrical activity might be recorded during tachycardia. (Reproduced from Garan et al. (1987) with permission.)

epicardial and endocardial border zones may form only part of reentrant circuits that are completed through intramural pathways. In panel A of Figure 4.45, the infarct extends all the way to the epicardial and endocardial surface and there is no continuous epicardial or endocardial border zone. The arrows suggest a reentrant circuit involving part of the endocardial border zone and intramural pathways (follow the activation times from −10 to 0 to 100 to 110 to 170 to complete the circuit). In panel B, where there is both an endocardial and an epicardial border zone, an intramural component of the circuit still exits.

All of the patterns of reentrant excitation described above have been found during sustained monomorphic ventricular tachycardia. The repetition of an identical QRS complex for each tachycardia depolarization is a result of both an identical reentrant circuit for each beat as well as an identical exit route from the circuit. Whenever tachycardia occurs, the circuit assumes the same form, location, and conduction properties and the excitation wave exits the circuit in the same way. In some hearts (experimental animals and humans), there appears to be only one activation pattern that will result in sustained and stable tachycardia, that is, only one region within the infarct has the appropriate electrophysiological properties that will support reentry with only one possible exit route and therefore, the tachycardias are always the same. In other hearts, monomorphic tachycardias with different morphologies may occur. One cause may be different exit routes from the same circuit to activate the ventricles. For example, in the circuit described in Figure 4.40, the exit route was from the end of the central common pathway towards the left anterior descending coronary artery. However, if the exit switched to the end of the central common pathway facing the apex of the lateral left ventricle, as we have sometimes observed, the QRS morphology would change drastically because the ventricles are activated with a different pattern. A switch in the exit route might occur if conduction block developed between the central common pathway and normal myocardium at the left anterior descending coronary artery margin, for example as a result of the rapid rate. Reentrant circuits may also occur in different regions in the same heart, resulting in different ventricular activation patterns.

Activation maps of reentrant circuits causing nonsustained ventricular tachycardia have also been obtained in experimental studies on the canine models. Figure 4.46A shows an episode of nonsustained tachycardia induced by programmed stimulation in a canine heart with a healing myocardial infarct. Nonsustained tachycardias can be induced in the same hearts that have sus-

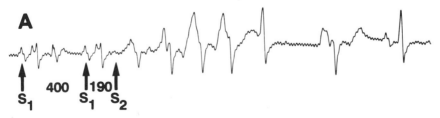

Figure 4.46A: The electrocardiogram recorded during an episode of nonsustained ventricular tachycardia induced by programmed stimulation in a canine heart with a 4-day-old infarct caused by permanent occlusion of the left anterior descending coronary artery. The basic drive cycle length (S_1-S_1) was 400 msec and the premature impulse coupling interval (S_1-S_2) was 190 msec. (Unpublished results of J. Coromilas and A.L. Wit.)

tained tachycardia or, as in Figure 4.46A, in hearts that do not have sustained tachycardia.

In Figure 4.46B, the activation maps of the epicardial border zone are shown for the nonsustained tachycardia in Figure 4.46A. Panel A is the activation map of the last basic drive that propagates from the margin adjacent to the left anterior descending coronary artery (LAD) toward the lateral left (LL) ventricle. Panel B is the premature impulse initiated at a coupling interval of 190 msec. It blocks at the dark horizontal black line (isochrones 60–80 msec), while propagating around the two ends of the line of block, to activate the distal side after 150 msec. Reentry then occurs as shown in panel C; the premature impulse passes through the original line of block in the retrograde direction (isochrones 10–40) and a figure-of-eight reentrant circuit is established (isochrones 40–180). The activation sequence that ends at the 190 msec isochrone in panel C is continued from the 10-msec isochrone (asterisks) in panel D. A second excursion around the reentrant circuit occurs (isochrones 10–160) before block at the dark horizontal line (isochrone 160). One more impulse of tachycardia then occurred. Activation in the epicardial border zone originates at the 30-msec isochrone in panel E and then blocks at the dark black horizontal line, terminating tachycardia. Panel F shows the activation of the epicardial

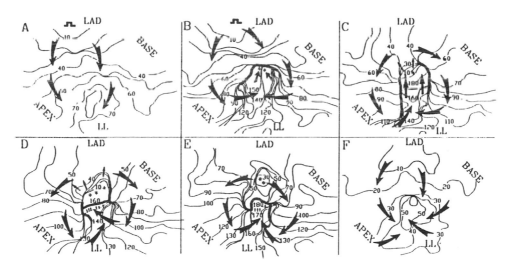

Figure 4.46B: Activation maps of the epicardial border zone during the nonsustained ventricular tachycardia shown in Figure 4.46A. The maps were constructed from activation times at 196 recording sites. Isochrones are drawn at 10-msec intervals and the arrows point out the activation patterns. The location of the margins of the electrode array on the epicardial border zone is labeled (LAD = left anterior descending coronary artery; LL = lateral left ventricle). Panel A is activation by the last basic drive impulse (S_1) originating at the LAD margin (pulse symbol). Panel B is activation by the premature impulse (S_2) at a coupling interval of 190 msec. Panels C-E are the activation patterns during three impulses of nonsustained tachycardia. Panel F is activation during a sinus beat that occurred immediately after the third tachycardia impulse. (Unpublished results of J. Coromilas and A.L. Wit.)

border zone by a subsequent sinus beat. Nonsustained tachycardias terminate spontaneously when conduction of the reentrant wave front blocks in the circuit. During a period of nonsustained tachycardia, the size, shape, location, and exit route of the circuit may be stable giving rise to a monomorphic nonsustained tachycardia, or the reentrant circuit causing each impulse of tachycardia may change as may the exit route from the circuit giving rise to polymorphic QRS complexes. When the circuit has a "figure-of-eight" shape, block of the reentrant wave front terminating the tachycardia usually occurs in the central common pathway (Figure 4.46B; panel D). Block may result if conduction velocity of the reentrant wave front is too rapid, causing the wave front to return to a region it has already excited before the region has recovered excitability. Nonsustained tachycardias induced in both experimental and clinical studies can sometimes be converted into sustained tachycardia if conduction in the circuit is slowed by the administration of an antiarrhythmic drug. As we discuss in more detail later, slow conduction enabling reentry to occur in the epicardial border zone of canine infarcts may be caused by propagation of the wave front transverse to the long axis of the myocardial fibers and the amount of slowing may be related to the effectiveness of the coupling of the muscle bundles in the transverse direction. Therefore, the amount of structural change in an infarct, resulting in separation of the muscle bundles may determine whether tachycardia is nonsustained or sustained.

Ventricular tachycardia in these canine models can lead to ventricular fibrillation, just as it does in clinical cases. There are at least two possible events associated with the transition from tachycardia to fibrillation. Very rapid tachycardias caused by either rapid conduction around a circuit or by reentry in a very small circuit can quickly cause fibrillation to begin in normal myocardium in the same way as fibrillation can be induced by stimulating a normal heart at very rapid rates. The beginning of fibrillation in normal myocardium is presumably the result of fragmentation of the rapid repetitive wave fronts leaving the circuit in the infarcted region, setting up additional reentrant circuits in the normal myocardium. This may be potentiated by a fall in blood pressure and a decreased coronary perfusion caused by the rapid rate that leads to ischemia in the noninfarcted regions. Fibrillation might also occur if a number of reentrant circuits form simultaneously in surviving myocardial fibers in an infarct, and impulses emanate from these circuits to normal myocardium causing it to fibrillate as well. This is a similar mechanism to the one that occurs during acute ischemia. The vulnerable property of normal myocardium is the final common pathway to fibrillation. The anatomical features and the electrophysiological properties of infarcts associated with fibrillation are most likely different than those associated with nonsustained or sustained tachycardia, but the differences have not yet been explicitly defined. It does seem that a larger area of slow conduction is necessary for the occurrence of sustained ventricular tachycardia while the small circuits that cause fibrillation can occur in smaller infarcts in which conduction may be more rapid.

We mentioned in our discussion of the clinical arrhythmias that there are very little data on the mechanisms causing ventricular premature depolarizations in the healing and healed phases of infarction. This is also true for premature depolarizations in the animal models. Spontaneously occurring premature depolarizations in the canine models can arise from reentry in the epicardial border zone since they are sometimes associated with continuous electrical activity in composite electrogram recordings from this region (El-Sherif et al. 1977a). They may sometimes be associated with a spontaneous increase in heart rate that presumably leads to the necessary slow conduction and block for reentry. However, ventricular premature depolarizations may also occur without any change in heart rate. The reason for their sudden appearance and disappearance is not known. They may not always be caused by the same mechanism causing tachycardias. The feline model of myocardial infarction (Myerburg et al. 1977) may offer the opportunity to investigate the mechanisms causing premature depolarizations because of their spontaneous occurrence in this model.

Activation Maps of Reentrant Circuits in Human Hearts

Although sites of earliest activity that have been found during mapping of ventricular activation during tachycardia in clinical studies have often been located in either the endocardial or in the epicardial border zone, indicating that these regions are likely exit routes from reentrant circuits, the location and size of the complete circuits have often not been apparent. Studies using more detailed intraoperative mapping techniques than those that have located "site of origin" have focused more on defining what the circuits look like. Catheter mapping does not have a high enough resolution to do this. The results of the intraoperative mapping studies suggest that the location, size, and shape of reentrant circuits varies in different patients. Some activation maps suggest a small circuit confined to a few square centimeters in the endocardial or epicardial border zone, some suggest a large circuit that might involve a large part of the left ventricle and that may extend into intramural regions. The different kinds of circuits probably reflect the variable pathological anatomy of human infarcts. The occurrence of different kinds of circuits may be responsible for the different properties of tachycardias, such as rate and responsiveness to drugs.

The site of earliest activity in maps of ventricular activation obtained during sustained monomorphic tachycardia often appears to be focal in the endocardial border zone with radial spread away from this site. No obvious reentrant circuit is evident (Josephson et al. 1980; Miller et al. 1985; Harris et al. 1987; De Bakker et al. 1988; Downar et al. 1988). Activation maps of the endocardial surface of the left ventricle with a healed infarct constructed from 64 simultaneously recorded endocardial electrograms showing this focal origin, is illustrated in Figure 4.47. The endocardial surface is depicted as though a cut were made along the left anterior descending coronary artery, from the base to the apex, and the walls then folded outward. Areas that appeared visually during the mapping procedure to be damaged (scarred) are shown by the

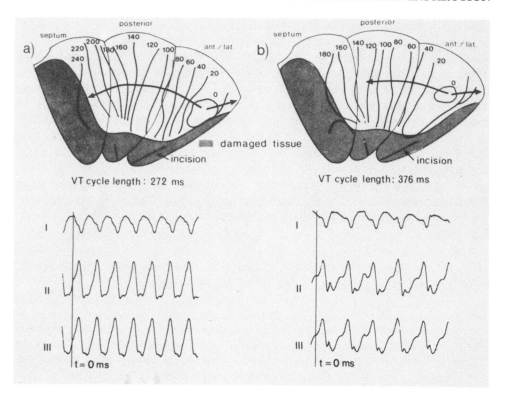

Figure 4.47: Endocardial activation maps of sustained ventricular tachycardias in a patient operated on for medically refractory tachycardia. The isochrone maps were constructed from endocardial electrograms that were recorded with a 64-point balloon electrode. The endocardial surface is depicted as though a cut were made along the left anterior descending artery, from base to apex, and the walls then folded outward. Isochrones are in milliseconds and are timed with respect to the onset of endocardial activation. Arrows indicate main spread of endocardial activation. Tracings below the maps are the surface leads I, II, and III. Areas that were visually abnormal to the surgeon are indicated as damaged tissue by the shading. Local activation in these areas was absent or obscured by remote activity in healthy tissue. The tachycardia in (a) arises from a small area in the anterior wall (0-msec isochrone). Spread of activation toward the septum is blocked. Activation toward the posterior wall arrives at the septum after 240 msec, which results in a gap of 30 msec between latest activation of one cycle and earliest activation of the following one. The tachycardia in (b), which has a morphology very similar to the one in (a), originates from the same area. The gap between earliest activity of one beat and latest activation of the preceding one was 196 msec in this case. (Reproduced from De Bakker et al. (1988) with permission.)

dark shading. Surface ECG leads I, II, and III are shown below. The arrows indicate the spread of activation. Earliest activity during the tachycardia in A is on the endocardial surface of the anterior wall, at the margin with damaged myocardium, at the 0-msec isochrone. Spread of activation on the anterior wall towards the septum was blocked (to the right in the map) presumably by the infarct that was located there. Activity also spreads towards the posterior wall in normal myocardium (to the left on the map) and arrives at the septum via this route after 240 msec. There was then a 30-msec gap in the time between this latest activation and the earliest activation of the next beat, which occurred at the same site (0-msec isochrone). Panel B shows endocardial activation during another episode of tachycardia with a similar QRS morphology and longer cycle length in the same patient. The site of earliest activation is also similar to the one shown in A, as is the pattern of excitation. However, the spread of activation towards the posterior wall and septum is completed after 180 msec, leaving a time gap of 196 msec prior to the onset of the next beat of tachycardia. In some patients two sites of origin have also been observed during a single beat of a tachycardia (De Bakker et al. 1988). When this occurred, the second site was found at some distance from the first, activity arising at this site was delayed compared to the first site, and it appeared from the activation maps that this site was not activated by impulses spreading from the first site (De Bakker et al. 1988).

There are several possible reasons for an apparent focal site of origin of tachycardia without an obvious reentrant circuit. Tachycardias caused by some kind of abnormal impulse initiation, triggered activity or automaticity for example, would be expected to have a focal origin but the other kinds of electrophysiological studies that we have already discussed strongly imply that this is not the usual arrhythmogenic mechanism. Since the "focal" origin may be up to 5–10 cm^2 in size because of the relatively low resolution in most of the clinical mapping studies (compared to experimental studies), it is also possible that an entire reentrant circuit is located within the "focus". For example, even though 64 simultaneous records were made to construct the map in Figure 4.47, the electrodes were 1.2 cm apart and therefore, a small circuit at the site of origin confined to an area several square centimeters within the focus would probably not have been detected. Such small reentrant circuits have been shown in experimental studies that utilized higher resolution activation maps (Richards et al. 1984). Fractionated electrograms recorded within the "focus" have sometimes extended throughout the cardiac cycle (Horowitz et al. 1980; Downar et al. 1988) suggesting the presence of a relatively small reentrant circuit at these sites. The extracellular electrical activity recorded on the endocardial surface may also have a very low amplitude (Downar et al. 1988; De Bakker et al. 1990), sometimes even on the order of 50 μV (De Bakker et al. 1988) as if arising from fibers embedded deep in the connective tissue scar that might form part of the circuit. A detailed analysis of electrical activity arising from muscle fibers within the scar cannot always be made because of the very low amplitude of the signals that are not always detected. Therefore, the focus might represent a narrow exit point from an intramural reentrant circuit.

Some reentrant circuits might also encompass a larger part of the left ventricle. On occasion, subendocardial electrograms have been recorded throughout the cardiac cycle around the perimeter of the aneurysm in a sequence compatible with that of a reentrant wave front progressing around the border of the aneurysm, much like a wave front conducting around a ring of tissue with an inexcitable hole at its center (Horowitz et al. 1980; Miller et al. 1985; Harris et al. 1987; De Bakker et al. 1988). This is a relatively rare occurrence. (In the experience of the Amsterdam group, it was found 5 times out of 400 ventricular tachycardias). Figure 4.48 shows an example of this kind of reentrant circuit. Four surface electrocardiographic leads recorded during tachycardia are shown at the top, and the map of the left ventricular endocardial activation sequence is at the bottom. The center "hole" in the map is the site of the aneurysm. Earliest activity is at −70 to −72 msec and continues around the aneurysm as indicated by the arrows, finishing one complete revolution after 330 msec, the cycle length of the tachycardia (Miller et al. 1985). In the map shown in Figure 4.47, the sequence of excitation is also compatible with a large circuit. One might postulate that after spread of excitation from the 0-msec isochrone to the septum in panel A, the wave front continued to spread from the posterior septum after 240 msec through deeper-lying, and therefore undetected, muscle bundles beneath the scar tissue (De Bakker et al. 1988) and eventually returned to the "site of origin", to reactivate it. The time for activation of the deeper pathway in this example needs to be 32 msec (the time of the gap during which no electrical activity was detected) in order for the wave front to arrive at the site of origin to begin the next tachycardia impulse.

There is evidence favoring the occurrence of deeper pathways of surviving muscle bundles at some distance beneath the endocardial surface, participating in large reentrant circuits when the site of origin appears to be on the endocardial surface. In the laboratory of one of us (MJJ), human hearts from patients with healed infarcts and a history of sustained ventricular tachycardia, were obtained at the time of cardiac transplantation and perfused by the Langendorff technique (De Bakker et al. 1988; 1990). Tachycardia could be induced in these isolated perfused hearts by programmed stimulation and the activation of the endocardium of the left ventricle carefully mapped with a balloon electrode. The activation map during one beat of a tachycardia is shown in Figure 4.49. Also shown are selected subendocardial electrograms recorded at the sites indicated on the figure. During this beat, the site of earliest activity was in a small endocardial area near the apex on the border of the septum and the posterior wall (the area encircled by the 0-msec isochrone). This was at the margin of the infarcted region that is shaded. Activation spread from this area to the left in the figure, towards the basal septum (from a to b) and continued to the anterior wall (from b to c to d to e). Spread of activation towards the posterior wall from the 0-msec isochrone (to the right) was prevented by the infarct that extended to the endocardial surface. Activation reached the lateral side of the infarcted zone via the anterior wall after 192 msec (near site e). This sequence of activity is seen in the electrograms a-e at the bottom. At the lateral side of the infarcted zone, subendocardial activation died out, as reflected in the slow positive deflection in the electrogram recorded at site e. The main component of the signals recorded at sites d and e are followed by small deflections (arrows in figure) that might have arisen from a tract of fibers deep beneath the endocardial surface. The sequence of the small deflections is such that it suggests that spread of activation continued via this tract of surviving muscle in the infarcted zone. In the signals recorded from sites f, g, and h, similar small

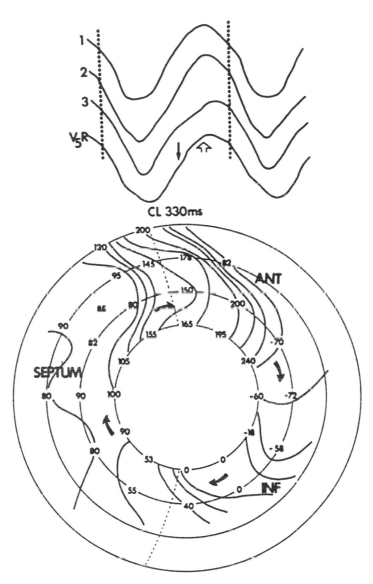

Figure 4.48: Reentrant excitation around an aneurysm in a patient with a healed infarct and sustained ventricular tachycardia. Four surface electrocardiographic leads are shown at the top. Below, the circular map represents a section through the ventricles around the aneurysm that forms the hole in the middle. Activation times are plotted and the arrows show the direction of wave front movement. Earliest activation is at − 70 msec and activation continues to 240 msec. INF is the inferior ventricular wall; ANT is the anterior wall. (Reproduced from Miller et al. (1985) with permission.)

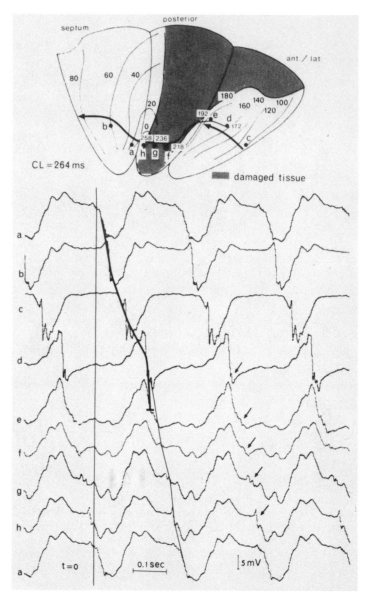

Figure 4.49: Endocardial activation pattern of one cycle of a sustained ventricular tachycardia induced in a Langendorff-perfused human heart with extensive infero-posterior infarction. Isochrones, which are constructed from endocardial electrograms recorded with the balloon electrode, are in milliseconds with respect to the time reference (t = 0) in the bottom panel. Thick arrows on the map indicate main spread of subendocardial activation; thin arrow indicates spread of activation via an isolated tract of surviving myocardial fibers in the infarcted zone. Numbers on the map are activation times. At the bottom, endocardial electrograms recorded at sites indicated in the top panel are shown. The thick line connects times of activation of subendocardial tissue at the sites a to e. At site d, the main deflection is followed by a second response of small amplitude (arrow). At sites e to h large signals mainly reflect remote activity, but in all signals small deflections are present (arrows). The timing of these small deflections is indicated by the thin line. (Reproduced from De Bakker et al. (1988) with permission.)

deflections were recorded (arrows on electrogram traces), suggesting that the path turned downward to site f, from where it advanced to the septum via g and h. Thereafter, the large muscle mass of the septum where activity originally began (0-msec isochrone) was reactivated from the small fiber tract, completing a large reentrant circuit around the circumferences of the ventricle. The presence of the connecting deep muscle tract in the scar was shown by histological studies of this region. Figure 4.50 illustrates that there was a continuous zone of viable myocardial cells that connected the myocardium of the lateral and septal wall. At the top left in the figure is a slice of the heart taken perpendicular to the long axis at the level of electrode b in Figure 4.49. The slice in the top right panel was taken about 1 cm beneath the one at the top left. Large bundles of myocardial fibers in the scar in both slices are pointed out by the arrows. The panels below are histological sections through the scar that show the surviving muscle bundle tracts. The cells in the tracts are arranged in a large bundle surrounded by connective tissue. Similar tracts of surviving muscle bundles were found embedded in the scar of the healed infarcts in other hearts as well, either in the subendocardium, subepicardium, or intramurally (De Bakker et al. 1990). These tracts connected viable tissue at either side of the infarct zone, possibly forming a return pathway for reentry. Impulse conduction in the tracts may be at normal velocity over long, circuitous or "zigzag" pathways formed by disruption of connections between bundles by the connective tissue of the scar. In some of the tracts, the myocardial fibers were arranged in a parallel fashion along the long axis of the tract, which favors rapid conduction. However, in other tracts myocardial fibers were oriented transverse to the direction of impulse propagation, accounting for slow activation through these regions (De Bakker et al. 1990). The surviving bundles assumed different geometries in different regions, which also might account for slow activation or unidirectional block. For example, block might be expected in regions where a thin bundle enters a larger one or at a branching site, but conduction in the other direction might succeed (De Bakker et al. 1990). The mechanisms for the effects of geometry on conduction properties were discussed in Chapter I. In other studies on *in situ* human hearts where extensive endocardial and epicardial mapping has been accomplished, gaps in activation of what appear to be possible reentrant circuits also suggest the possibility of intramural connections from which electrical activity could not be recorded (Harris et al. 1987).

Figure 4.51 shows selected drawings of another muscle bundle tract that probably formed part of the reentrant circuit in another Langendorff-perfused human heart. The time interval between latest and earliest endocardial activity during induced ventricular tachycardia was bridged by similar small amplitude deflections recorded from the infarct as those shown in Figure 4.49. In this heart, serial sections of 10 μm were made from the infarcted area where the small deflections were recorded. In drawing a, there is a peninsula of surviving myocardium (darkly shaded region) protruding from the posterior wall into the infarct. Drawing b, from a section 500 μm more towards the apex, shows that the peninsula has become an isolated island, which eventually merges with

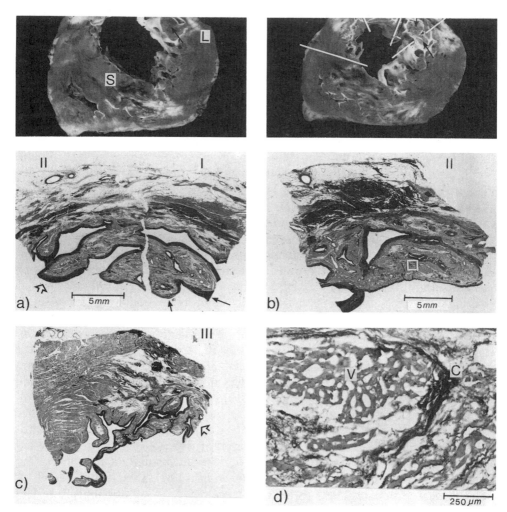

Figure 4.50: At the top, slices resected from the isolated human heart in Figure 4.49 are shown. The slice in the top left panel was taken perpendicular to the long axis of the heart at the level at which electrode terminal b in Figure 4.49 was located. The top right panel slice was taken about 1 cm beneath the other one. On the left a large bundle of viable myocardial fibers is present (arrow) that bifurcates in the panel on the right (arrows). Several other isolated bundles are present at this level in sectors II and III. Bundles are surrounded by fibrous tissue. S = septum; P = posterior wall; L = lateral wall. Bottom: panel (a) is a section taken 5.5 mm below the surface of the slice in the top right panel. The section shows that all bundles merge to one large coherent bundle. Arrows indicate the continuation of the bifurcated bundle. At this level, the joined bundle is isolated from remaining myocardial septal tissue by a thick endocardial layer (open arrow). (b) Photomicrograph taken 1.5 mm above (a) in sector II showing that the joined bundle merges with healthy offshoots of the septum in section III (open arrow in (c)). (d) Photomicrograph of the joined bundle (from the square in (b)) showing that it consists of areas with viable myocardial fibers (light areas as marked by V) and zones comprising connective tissue (dark areas as marked C). (Reproduced from De Bakker et al. (1988) with permission.)

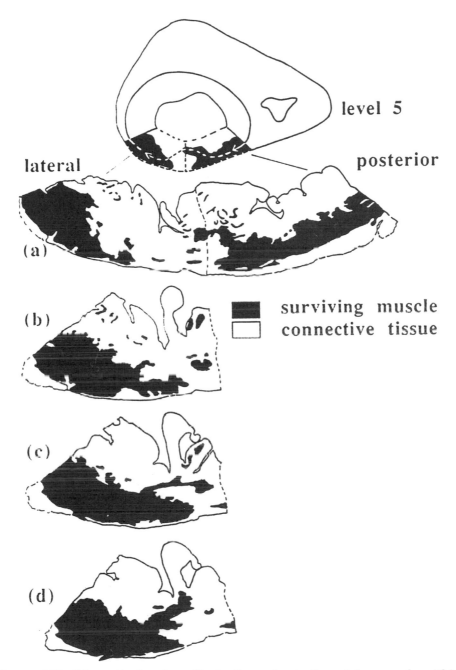

level 5

lateral

posterior

(a)

(b)

surviving muscle
connective tissue

(c)

(d)

Figure 4.51: Schematic drawings illustrating a tract of surviving muscle within a healed infarct in a human heart. At the top, a cross section through the left ventricle with the infarcted region outlined by the dashes is shown. Surviving muscle within the infarcted region is indicated by the dark area, connective tissue is not shaded. The arrows indicate a possible pathway of activation. (a), (b), (c), and (d) below are sections through the infarcted region showing the distribution of the surviving muscle tract (dark shaded) imbedded in connective tissue (white area). (Reproduced from De Bakker et al. (1990) with permission.)

the muscle fibers in the lateral wall in drawing c, (1,000 μm underneath a). To show that the tract was indeed continuous, all serial sections were examined and drawings were made of sections 100 μm apart throughout the lateral tissue block of Figure 4.51. A three-dimensional reconstruction of the tract of surviving tissue is shown in Figure 4.52. The schematic drawings of ten successive sections (a to k), each 100 μm apart, show that the tract (gray area) fuses with myocardium in the lateral wall (indicated in black) at level d. From here, the tract runs downward to level k, remains horizontal for about 6 mm and then ascends to merge with healthy tissue of the posterior wall at level a. Although the tract was continuous (as assessed by examining all intervening 10 μm sections), there were some narrow passages, especially in the ascending and descending parts. The smallest width of these bottlenecks, which possibly could be sites of unidirectional block permitting induction of reentry, was in the order of 250 μm.

In order for reentrant circuits like the one suggested in Figure 4.49 to occur, surviving muscle bundles must be present in the subendocardial scar tissue of the healed myocardial infarct. The surviving muscle in the endocardial border zone may also extend further intramurally. Intramural muscle bundles may also be projections from the lateral margin and provide conduction pathways through the scarred region. In Figure 4.49, myocardium outside the damaged region also formed part of the reentrant circuit, but it is possible that intramural bundles in the scar might sometimes form the complete circuit.

Clinical mapping studies have also provided data that suggest that the entire reentrant circuit may sometimes lie in the endocardial border zone near the endocardial surface. Downar and his coworkers (Harris et al. 1987; Downar et al. 1988) have described several patterns of subendocardial activation determined during simultaneous endocardial and epicardial mapping with the sock and balloon electrodes described earlier. One pattern is characterized by a large wave front of activation moving in a circular fashion or "vortex" forming a macroreentrant circuit in the endocardial border zone. An example of the initiation of this pattern was described in Figure 4.38 (Harris et al. 1987). Panel VTn shows the endocardial activation pattern during the sustained tachycardia. Activation begins at the 0-msec isochrone in the figure and the sequence of isochrones can be followed towards the left (septum) (0 to 84 msec), then downward around the apex (84 to 168 msec) and upward to the region of initial activation (168 to 276 msec). The arrow shows the pattern of activation. In this example, the cycle length of tachycardia is very short, 280 msec, indicating that the rhythm is probably ventricular flutter. During endocardial "vortex" reentry, circulating activity has been mapped on the epicardial surface moving in the same or opposite direction. However, large gaps of more then 100 msec occurred on the epicardium, during which activity could not be detected.

Excitation patterns in the endocardial border zone, resembling the "figure-of-eight" pattern, similar to those shown in the epicardial border zone of the canine heart, have also been described by Downar et al. (1988) in clinical mapping studies. Figure 4.53 shows an example of this pattern and its initiation by three premature stimuli. The maps are plotted on polar projections of the

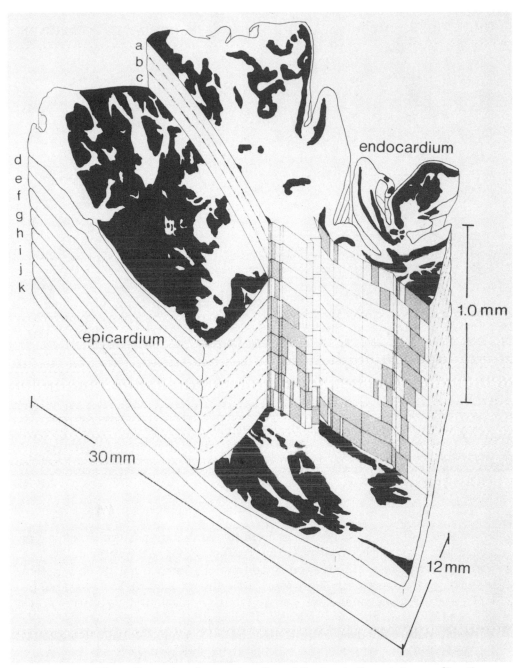

Figure 4.52: Three-dimensional reconstruction of the tract of surviving cardiac tissue traversing the infarct zone of the heart illustrated in Figure 4.51. Surviving tissue is indicated in black, and the surviving muscle of the tract is illustrated in gray. Eleven consecutive sections, 100 μm apart, and derived from the lateral tissue block in Figure 4.51 were used for the reconstruction. The left side of the tract is connected to the bulk of the surviving tissue of the lateral wall at level (d). The right side of the tract connects with surviving tissue of the posterior wall at level (a). By connecting the nonaffected lateral and posterior walls, the tract creates a possible return path for a reentrant circuit. The length of the tract is approximately 13 mm. (Reproduced from De Bakker et al. (1990) with permission.)

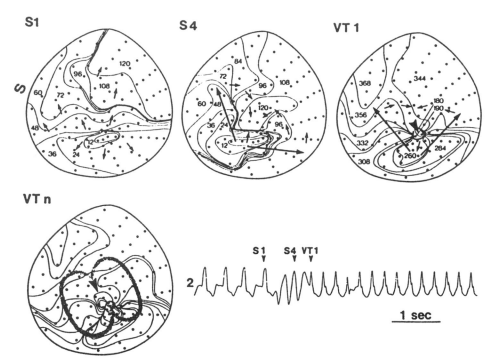

Figure 4.53: Figure-of-eight reentrant pattern in the subendocardial border zone of a healed human infarct. Initiation of the tachycardia by three premature impulses (S2, S3, S4) is shown in the lead 2 electrocardiogram at the bottom right. The panels show the endocardial activation sequence in response to S1 and S4 stimuli as well as the first (VT1) and subsequent beats (VTn) of the tachycardia. (Reproduced from Downar et al. (1988) with permission.)

left ventricle. Panel S_1 shows the endocardial activation pattern of the last of the train of basic drive impulses during stimulation at the left ventricular apex (isochrone at 12 msec). Activation spread radially away from the stimulation site towards the base of the heart as indicated by the arrows. There is a region of block or very slow conduction shown by the dark black line, separating areas activated at 60 and 108 msec. Panel S_4 shows the activation pattern of the fourth premature impulse that initiated the tachycardia. The spread of excitation away from the stimulus site was blocked along the dark black line. Wave fronts traveled around each end of this line of functional block. These two wave fronts joined on the opposite side of the line after 120 msec (arrows). Activation then continued retrogradely through the region of initial block and the region near the stimulation site was reactivated after 200 msec. This is indicated by the arrow in panel VT_1. This single return wave front then split in two, one of which traveled towards the lateral wall and then towards the base (to the right) and the other of which traveled towards the septum and towards the base (to the left). The two wave fronts then united again to return towards the apex establishing the figure-of-eight pattern (Panel Vtn) that persisted during the tachycardia.

The return pathway in the figure-of-eight map (Figure 4.53) was not associated with "unequivocal evidence of regenerative depolarization" according to Downar et al. (1988). "Instead there may be an apparent excitation gap of 80 to 120 msec over a distance of 1–2 cm". Details of the electrograms recorded in the region of the return pathway are shown in Figure 4.54. The 56-, 84-, 96-, and 108-msec isochrones are based on small potentials in the unipolar recordings (arrows pointing to the traces at the right). These small potentials are interpreted to indicate slow conduction along tracts of surviving fibers in the scar or "electrotonic potentials from decremental excitation". However, from the electrograms alone, it is difficult to be certain that activation occurred through this region to complete the reentrant circuit. Evidence that this region was important in the genesis of the tachycardia was obtained by applying the "Mines' test:" 100 J shocks delivered through these recording electrodes ablated this region and made it impossible to induce tachycardia (Downar et al. 1988).

Complete reentrant circuits have also been mapped in the epicardial border zone in patients with evidence of an epicardial site of origin of tachycardia.

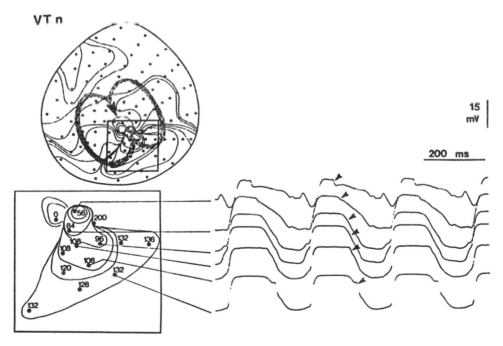

Figure 4.54: Activation of the return path in the figure-of-eight reentrant circuit shown in Figure 4.53. The figure-of-eight pattern is repeated above. The inset square shows activation times (in milliseconds) that followed latest activation of the previous cycle at the electrode marked 0. Local unipolar electrograms from the electrodes within the square are shown on the right. The lower four signals are partially clipped. (Reproduced from Downar et al. (1988) with permission.)

The figure-of-eight reentrant activation pattern has been documented (Kaltenbrunner et al. 1991; Littmann et al. 1991) as shown in panel A of Figure 4.32. We have already used this figure to point out that electrogram recordings have been obtained from the epicardium, throughout the diastolic period. Earliest activation on the map is at − 75 msec. From this point activation proceeds over a narrow path bracketed by arcs of block (from − 75 to − 40, dashed arrow), the narrow wave front then divides into two, one moving downward and the other upward on the map. The two separate wave fronts then return to the distal end of the narrow central pathway (isochrones 40 to 135) to complete the reentrant circuits. The shaded area on the map is the region where the electrograms were recorded throughout diastole (panel B). Panels C and D show the electrograms that were recorded during systole from each of the reentrant circuits that formed the figure-of-eight.

Other patterns of activation at epicardial sites of origin also resemble activation patterns at endocardial sites of origin (Littmann et al. 1991) including circular macroreentry in the shape of a vortex, reentry around the circumference of a left ventricular aneurysm, and focal sites of presystolic activity with activation spreading in a radial pattern away from the site. Epicardial laser photoablation at the common reentrant pathway in the figure-of-eight circuits terminated tachycardia, proving that this was indeed a part of the reentrant circuit (Littmann et al. 1991). However, laser ablation of the early presystolic region from which there was radial spread, did not terminate tachycardia, indicating this pattern represents an exit route from a reentrant circuit which probably has an intramural location (Littmann et al. 1991).

As yet, there are no clinical studies published that have been aimed at elucidating characteristics of reentrant circuits causing nonsustained ventricular tachycardias. The paucity of information is probably because most clinical electrophysiology laboratories do not have the instrumentation necessary for mapping single beats, a necessity for studying nonsustained events. In patients who have both nonsustained and sustained ventricular tachycardias, the same circuit might sometimes be responsible for both arrhythmias. Experimental studies on ventricular tachycardia show that this can occur. It is also conceivable that in these cases and in cases in which there is only documented nonsustained tachycardia, the circuits have different locations and properties than those causing sustained tachycardias. Also missing from the clinical studies are data on activation patterns of ventricular premature depolarizations and the transition of tachycardia to fibrillation.

At the time of this writing, the activation maps of clinical tachycardias that we discussed are the highest resolution maps that have been obtained from the *in situ* human heart and represent an outstanding contribution to the understanding of the mechanisms causing these arrhythmias. Nevertheless, the 1–3-cm spacing between the electrodes necessitates that many of the isochrones be drawn based on only one or two activation times and many isochrones are interpolated. This can be compared to the 1–3-mm spacing of electrodes in some of the experimental studies that results in a large number of data points forming the basis for each isochrone. Therefore, alternative pathways forming the reentrant circuits, not accurately depicted by the clinical maps, are sometimes possible. Nevertheless, the similarities of the activation patterns during some of the clinical tachycardias to activation patterns of experimental tachycardias are remarkable and lead us to conclude that the arrhythmogenic mechanism for both clinical and experimental arrhythmias is similar.

Termination of Tachycardias

We have discussed earlier that sustained monomorphic ventricular tachycardia in humans and in experimental animal models can be entrained and terminated by overdrive stimuli. The data obtained from electrocardiographic studies and from the recording of electrograms has been interpreted to indicate that the stimulated impulses enter the circuit during entrainment and activate it in a similar way as the reentrant impulse and that at a critical rate of stimulation, the stimulated wave front blocks in the circuit and causes the tachycardia to terminate. Studies in which excitation has been mapped in reentrant circuits in the canine heart with an infarct caused by a permanent occlusion of the left anterior descending coronary artery confirm many of the proposals made on the basis of the electrocardiographic studies (El-Sherif et al. 1987; Waldecker et al. 1993). Unfortunately, there are no clinical mapping studies of entrainment and termination of tachycardia by overdrive stimulation.

Figure 4.55 shows an electrocardiogram recorded from the canine model of permanent left anterior descending coronary artery occlusion during several periods of overdrive at different rates. In panel A, the tachycardia at the left has a cycle length of 150 msec. During overdrive at a cycle length of 140 msec the rate of the tachycardia is increased while there is only a small change in the morphology of the ECG complexes as is expected from fusion activation of the ventricles. When overdrive stimulation was terminated, the tachycardia continued with the same rate and morphology as prior to stimulation. In panel B, the QRS morphology markedly changes at a more rapid rate of stimulation (135 msec cycle length) to resemble the QRS morphology that occurred during stimulation from that site in the absence of tachycardia (panel C). When overdrive stimulation was stopped, the tachycardia did not continue (panel B). Figure 4.56 shows the activation maps of the reentrant circuit in the epicardial border zone during the period of entrainment. In panel A there is a map of the reentrant circuit prior to invasion by the first of the train of stimulated impulses. Activation begins at the asterisk and the sequence of activation is pointed out by the arrows. Activation during the first stimulated impulse that entered this region is shown in panel B. The stimulated wave front is indicated by the dashed isochrones (10 and 20 msec) at the lateral margin (LL) of the electrode array (pulse symbol) and the unfilled arrows while the reentrant wave fronts are indicated by isochrones formed by continuous lines and the black arrows. At the time the stimulated wave fronts entered this area (dashed isochrones

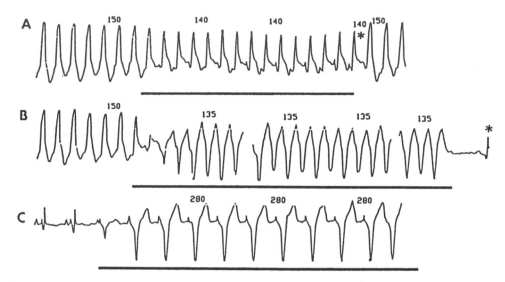

Figure 4.55: Electrocardiograms recorded from a canine heart with a 5-day-old myocardial infarction. The horizontal line below each trace indicates periods of overdrive stimulation from the lateral left ventricle. Panel A shows entrainment of the tachycardia by overdrive stimulation at a cycle length of 140 msec, 10 msec shorter than the tachycardia cycle length of 150 msec. Panel B shows termination of the tachycardia at an overdrive cycle length of 135 msec. The breaks in the trace indicate parts of the record that are not shown. Panel C shows the ECG morphology during stimulation from the same site as in A and B, but during sinus rhythm. (Unpublished results of B. Waldecker, J. Coromilas and A.L. Wit.)

10 and 20, unfilled arrows), the two reentrant wave fronts were moving along the apical and basal margins towards the lateral margin. Their position at this time is indicated by the asterisks. The reentrant wave fronts collided with the stimulated wave front near the entrance to the central common pathway, in the region indicated by the dashes. The merged wave front (reentrant and stimulated) entered the common pathway from the lateral side (isochrones 40–60), and subsequently activated the epicardial border zone with the same pattern as in panel A. Activation occurred around the left anterior descending coronary artery (LAD) ends of the lines of apparent block and returned toward the lateral margin (arrows) only to collide with the next stimulated wave front that is not shown in the figure. This pattern of collision between the wave fronts in the reentrant circuit and the next stimulated wave front continued throughout the period of overdrive. However, since the overdrive cycle length was shorter than the conduction time around the circuit, each stimulated wave front penetrated further into the central common pathway until the entire reentrant circuit was captured and reset. The activation map in panel C is from the last overdrive impulse and illustrates the pattern of activation during entrainment. The isochrones resulting from this overdrive stimulus are drawn with dashed lines, while those from the previously stimulated wave front in the circuit are drawn with continuous lines. When the new stimulated wave

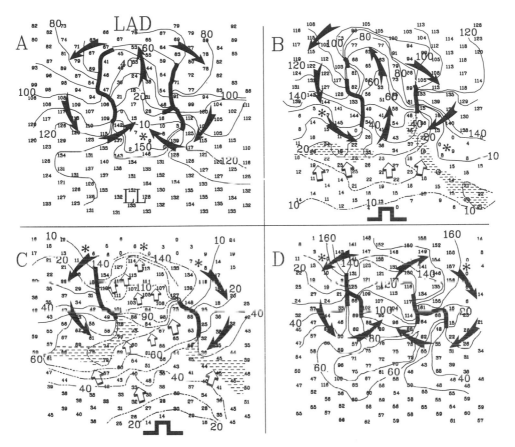

Figure 4.56: Activation maps from a reentrant circuit in the epicardial border zone of an infarcted canine heart showing overdrive pacing with entrainment. The small numbers are the activation times at each of the recording sites. Isochrones are drawn at 10-msec intervals and labeled with the larger numbers. The margins of the electrode array are labeled LAD = left anterior descending coronary artery; LL = lateral left ventricle. Panel A shows the activation map of the reentrant circuit during the sustained ventricular tachycardia shown in Figure 4.55. The black arrows indicate the sequence of activation. Activation during the first stimulated impulse from the lateral stimulation site (at the pulse symbol) is shown in panel B. The stimulated wave front is indicated by the dashed isochrones and unfilled arrows, the wave fronts from the reentrant impulse are indicated by the isochrones drawn with continuous lines and the black arrows. Regions of collision are shown by the horizontal dashes. The activation map during the last stimulated impulse is shown in panel C. The wave fronts resulting from the last stimulus are shown by the dashed isochrones and unfilled arrows. The wave fronts from the previous stimulated impulse are indicated by the continuous line isochrones and black arrows. The regions of collision are indicated by the dashed lines. Panel D shows activation during the first post-pacing cycle and the first impulse of tachycardia after pacing. (Reproduced from Waldecker et al. (1993) with permission.)

front entered the epicardial border zone (dashed 10-msec isochrone at the LL margin where the pulse symbol is located and unfilled arrows), the reentrant wave front resulting from the previous stimulus was at the LAD margin (continuous 10-msec isochrones and asterisks). The wave fronts in the circuit moved towards the stimulated wave fronts and they collided. The dashed lines show the approximate region of collision. Activation by the last stimulated impulse shown in Figure 4.56C continued through the central common pathway (the time window ends at the 140-msec isochrone, at which time the activation wave resulting from the last stimulated impulse is near the LAD margin). Figure 4.56D shows the continuation of this wave front beginning at the 10-msec isochrone (asterisks). The last stimulated wave front split into two, returned towards the LL margin along the base and apex, entered the common central pathway, and reentry continued resulting in the resumption of tachycardia with the same cycle length (see Figure 4.55A). The activation pattern during the first cycle following stimulation was nearly the same as the pattern before stimulation except that the lines of apparent block were slightly shorter. That the entire circuit was captured by the period of overdrive is also shown by the electrograms recorded from the circuit that is shown in Figure 4.57. The cycle length of the electrograms in the circuit was accelerated to that of the overdrive stimuli. The morphology of electrograms recorded in regions of the circuit that were activated in the same direction during overdrive as during tachycardia was unaltered (top four traces), while electrograms from regions activated retrogradely during overdrive have an altered morphology (bottom three traces).

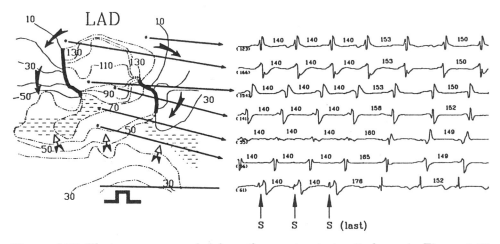

Figure 4.57: Electrograms recorded from the reentrant circuit shown in Figure 4.56 during overdrive stimulation and entrainment. At the left is the activation map previously shown in Figure 4.56C but without the individual activation times. At the right are electrograms recorded from sites in the circuit indicated by the long arrows. The cycle length at all the recording sites was decreased to the cycle length of the overdrive stimuli (140 msec) and returned to the cycle length of the tachycardia after the last stimulus. (Reproduced from Waldecker et al. (1993) with permission.)

Stimulation at a cycle length critically shorter than that necessary for entrainment usually terminates reentry by causing conduction block of the stimulated impulses in the central common pathway of the circuit. An example of this kind of termination is shown in Figure 4.58. This figure shows activation maps of a reentrant circuit in the canine epicardial border zone during overdrive from the lateral margin (LL), at a cycle length of 135 msec. The electrocardiogram during the period of stimulation that terminated tachycardia is shown in Figure 4.55B. During overdrive, the initial stimulated impulses entered the epicardial border zone from the lateral site (panel A) and moved towards the

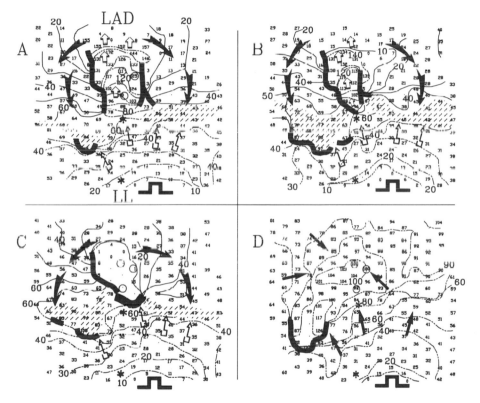

Figure 4.58: Activation maps of the epicardial border zone of an infarcted canine heart showing the mechanism for termination of reentrant ventricular tachycardia by overdrive stimulation. In each map, activation times are indicated by the small numbers, isochrones are drawn at 10-msec intervals and labeled with the larger numbers. Isochrones resulting from the current stimulated wave front are dashed and indicated by the unfilled arrows. Isochrones resulting from the previous stimulated wave front in the reentrant circuit are indicated by continuous lines and black arrows. Panel A shows the activation pattern during a stimulated impulse occurring early in the overdrive train. Panel B shows the activation pattern resulting from a subsequent stimulated impulse. Panel C shows the activation pattern resulting from the stimulated wave front that blocked in the circuit, causing termination of reentry. Panel D shows the activation pattern resulting from the next stimulated impulse. (Reproduced from Waldecker et al. (1993) with permission.)

left anterior descending coronary artery (LAD) margin in the central common pathway (dashed isochrones 10–120, unfilled arrows). Collision between the paced wave fronts moving towards the LAD and the reentrant wave fronts from the previous stimulus, moving towards the LL margin along the base and apex (continuous line isochrones and filled arrows) occurred in the regions indicated by the dashed lines. During subsequent stimulated impulses, the left line of block in the reentrant circuit shifted as shown in panel B. The entrance to the central common pathway was narrowed, but the stimulated impulse still followed the reentrant pathway as pointed out by the unfilled arrows. Collision with the previously stimulated impulse (continuous line isochrones and filled arrows) again occurred in the region of the dashed lines. The conduction of the following paced impulse (panel C), however, blocked at the dark black line and failed to activate the central common pathway. This stimulated wave front also collided with the returning wave fronts from the previous stimulus (continuous line isochrones and filled arrows) in the regions indicated by the dashes. Thereafter, the activation pattern of the epicardial border zone changed substantially as shown in the map in Figure 4.58D. Activation occurred around the peripheral margins of the epicardial border zone and proceeded towards the center where there was collision of the wave fronts. The lines of apparent block present during tachycardia and entrainment were no longer in existence. Tachycardia did not resume when pacing was discontinued.

Electrophysiological Mechanisms for Reentry

The next questions that we will consider are how and why reentry occurs during the healing and healed phases of infarction to cause ventricular arrhythmias. In Chapter I we discussed that reentry can have either an anatomical or functional basis, and that there is a variety of possible mechanisms for the necessary slow conduction and unidirectional conduction block. Are the reentrant circuits causing the tachyarrhythmias that we have discussed in the previous sections of this chapter anatomical or functional? What are the causes of the slow conduction and block? In an attempt to provide the answers to these questions, we rely on both experimental animal data and clinical data. In many instances only the former is available. When both kinds of data are available they are often complementary, although they sometimes disagree. First we will describe the cellular electrophysiological properties of regions in which the reentrant circuits have been located and then how these properties, as well as others, govern conduction and refractoriness in these regions. This will lead us into a discussion of the mechanisms causing reentry.

Cellular Electrophysiology

In our discussion of the acute ischemic arrhythmias in Chapter II, we pointed out that the transmembrane resting and action potentials of the muscle fibers in ischemic areas are severely depressed and that this is a primary cause of the reentrant ventricular arrhythmias. These data were obtained by micro-electrode recordings from *in situ* animal hearts and from isolated superfused tissue in an ischemic environment. In only one instance were microelectrode recordings obtained from an isolated, Langendorff-perfused human heart, showing similar changes during acute ischemia as in the animal studies (Janse and Kléber 1981). In addition, the characteristics of local extracellular record-ings in humans during acute ischemia, which reflect alterations in transmem-brane potentials, are in complete agreement with the experimental data. Like-wise, most of the information on characteristics of transmembrane potentials of myocardial cells in healing and healed infarcts comes from animal models, but these data do not come from the *in situ* heart. The characteristics of the transmembrane potentials of the cardiac cells that survive the acute ischemic insult and that are the cause of the subsequent arrhythmias have been deter-mined by microelectrode recordings from isolated tissue, superfused with a physiological solution (Lazzara et al. 1978b; El-Sherif and Lazzara 1979; Laz-zara and Scherlag 1980; Spear et al. 1983a; Ursell et al. 1985), as was the data for the subacute arrhythmic phase described in Chapter III. It is still necessary to obtain recordings *in vivo*, as has been done in the acute coronary occlusion experiments, to determine whether the results of *in vitro* studies are an accu-rate representation of the properties of these cells in the heart. The tendency of transmembrane potentials to change during superfusion in a tissue chamber, as we described for the subendocardial Purkinje fibers, again evokes the ques-tion as to whether some of the long-term effects of *in vivo* ischemia are reversed or altered in the normal, well-oxygenated Tyrode's solution usually used in these studies.

As was pointed out in Chapter II and at the beginning of this chapter, not all the cardiac cells subjected to the ischemic conditions of the acute phase die. Recovery of transmembrane potentials in some ischemic regions occurs as early as the first hour after coronary occlusion. Other cells probably begin to recover later, although the exact time is not known. The anatomical picture of surviv-ing cells in the ischemic and infarcted areas attests to this recovery. Recovery is attributed to an early increase in collateral blood flow, or in the case of infarcts that are reperfused, a return of coronary flow. In the experimental studies, reperfusion is controlled by the investigator. Spontaneous lysis of oc-cluding clots in humans is also expected to result in the return of coronary flow to acutely ischemic regions. As the surviving myocardial cells recover from the acute ischemia while the infarct heals, their transmembrane potentials undergo a progression of changes until a stable state is reached in the com-pletely healed infarct. The progression of changes in transmembrane potentials has been documented in the epicardial border zone of the canine model of com-plete occlusion of the left anterior descending coronary artery and the model of occlusion and subsequent reperfusion because the epicardial location of the surviving muscle enables the transmembrane potentials to be recorded (unlike surviving intramural cells). The action potential characteristics for both kinds of infarcts are similar (Spear et al. 1983a; Ursell et al. 1985). Furthermore, these recordings have been obtained from regions where the reentrant circuits causing tachycardia were located so the characteristics of the action potentials can eventually be related to the mechanism causing reentry.

The microelectrode studies have shown that the maximum diastolic potential and action potential amplitude of the surviving ventricular muscle cells in the epicardial border zone during the first week after permanent coronary occlusion or coronary occlusion and reperfusion are reduced. The amount of reduction is to some extent related to the thickness of the surviving epicardial rim of muscle, with greater reduction occurring in regions where fewer cells survive (Gardner et al. 1981). The amount of surviving cells may be a reflection of the regional severity of the ischemia, which also influences the membrane potentials. The bar graphs in Figure 4.59 show quantitative data for maximum diastolic potential (MDP), action potential amplitude (APA), and $\dot{V}_{max}$ of phase 0 for epicardial border zone muscle fibers at different times during healing after permanent occlusion. Maximum diastolic potential was in the range of

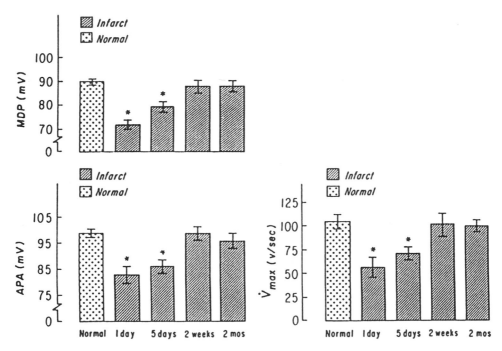

Figure 4.59: Changes in maximum diastolic potential (MDP), total action potential amplitude (APA), and the rate of phase 0 depolarization ($\dot{V}_{max}$) of surviving muscle fibers in the epicardial border zone of canine infarcts with increasing time after coronary occlusion. Column heights represent mean values for the first "layer" of muscle fibers beneath the epicardial surface in noninfarcted hearts (stippled columns) and in each group of infarcted hearts (striped columns) studied at the times after coronary occlusion indicated on the abscissa. Brackets indicate ± standard deviation. Asterisks denote values significantly different from controls (P < 0.01). (Reproduced from Ursell et al. (1985) with permission.)

-65 to -80 mV in preparations obtained from 5-day-old healing infarcts compared with -85 to -90 mV for normal epicardial ventricular muscle cells. Similar values have been reported for reperfused infarcts (Spear et al. 1983a). Severely depressed (depolarized) diastolic potentials of less than -70 mV were found in about 15% of cells in permanent occlusion infarcts by Ursell et al. (1985), but seem to be more prevalent in other studies, although no precise quantification of frequency of occurrence has been given (Lazzara et al. 1978b; El-Sherif and Lazzara 1979; Lazzara and Scherlag 1980). In infarcts caused by occlusion and reperfusion there may be a more heterogeneous population with a larger number of cells having very depolarized resting potentials (Spear et al. 1983a). Nevertheless, the degree of membrane potential depolarization at 5 days is less than during the height of the acute ischemic period. No data are available from muscle fibers surviving in human infarcts during this stage of healing. Along with the decrease in maximum diastolic potential, $\dot{V}_{max}$ of phase 0 is also decreased with average values of around 60 V/sec having been reported by 5 days after occlusion (Spear et al. 1983a; Ursell et al. 1985) compared to 100–120 V/sec for normal epicardial muscle (Figure 4.59). The rate of depolarization during phase 0 is higher than during acute ischemia and also represents a partial recovery from the acute ischemic period. Very slow rates of phase 0 depolarization, 10–15 V/sec, were found in the cells with the most severely depressed resting potentials. Interestingly, action potentials with low amplitudes and no overshoots were also found in cells with relatively normal resting potentials in cells from reperfused infarcts (Spear et al. 1983a). Another abnormality in these cells at 5 days that is shown in Figure 4.60 is that the action potentials have little plateau phase during repolarization and the action potential duration at the plateau is therefore decreased (action potential duration to 50% repolarization) (Spear et al. 1983a; Ursell et al. 1985; Boyden et al. 1988). This can be seen by comparing action potential C from a 5-day-old infarct to action potential A from a noninfarcted heart in Figure 4.60. This characteristic is similar to the reduction of the plateau during the acute ischemic period. Total action potential duration (to 90% repolarization in Figure 4.60) is also decreased as a consequence of the decrease in the plateau phase.

The maximum diastolic potential, action potential amplitude, and $\dot{V}_{max}$ of phase 0 return to normal by 2 weeks in both canine infarcts caused by permanent occlusion and by temporary occlusion. These data are also shown in the graphs in Figure 4.59. In contrast, the action potential duration is even shorter at 2 weeks than at 5 days and there is still little evidence of a plateau phase (in Figure 4.60, compare action potential D recorded at 2 weeks to action potential C recorded at 5 days) (Spear et al. 1983a; Ursell et al. 1985). Shortening of the action potential duration has also been suggested by shortening of the QT interval of local electrograms recorded *in vivo* near the margin of the epicardial border zone in reperfused infarcts although in some experiments QT intervals did not decrease (Duff et al. 1988).

After 2 weeks, the maximum diastolic potential, action potential amplitude, and $\dot{V}_{max}$ of phase 0 and action potential repolarization of the surviving muscle in the epicardial border zone, measured *in vitro*, is not significantly

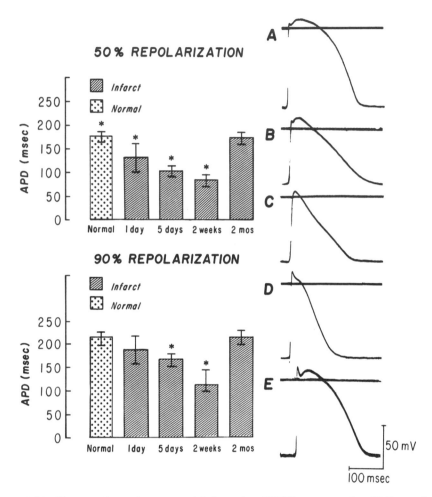

Figure 4.60: Changes in action potential duration (APD) measured to 50% repolarization (above left) and 90% repolarization (below left) of muscle fibers in the epicardial border zone of canine infarcts with increasing time after coronary artery ligation. Column heights represent mean values for the first layer of muscle fibers beneath the epicardial surface in normal noninfarcted left ventricles (stippled columns) and in each group of infarcted left ventricles (striped columns) studied at the times after coronary occlusion, indicated on the abscissa. Brackets indicate ± standard deviation. Asterisks denote values significantly different from control. At the right are shown representative epicardial muscle fiber transmembrane potential recordings; A is from a noninfarcted heart; B is from a 1-day-old infarct; C is from a 5-day-old infarct; D is from a 2-week-old infarct; and E is from a 2-month-old infarct. (Reproduced from Ursell et al. (1985) with permission.)

different from normal muscle fibers as shown in the bar graphs in Figures 4.59 and 4.60 (Gardner et al. 1984; 1985; Ursell et al. 1985). The action potential recorded from the epicardial border zone of a 2-month-old infarct in panel E of Figure 4.60 is nearly identical to the epicardial action potential from a noninfarcted heart in panel A.

The changes in membrane properties responsible for the changes in the epicardial muscle transmembrane potentials during the first several weeks of healing have not yet been elucidated in any detail. The alterations in membrane potentials may be related to ischemia induced changes in metabolism that cause the accumulation of lipid droplets that was described in Chapter III. These lipid droplets disappear by the time action potentials return to normal after several months (Ursell et al. 1985). Changes in metabolism can cause changes in membrane properties that influence current flow or ion pumps that maintain ion concentration gradients. The decrease in the resting potential during the healing phase is at least partially related to a decrease in the intracellular potassium concentration and potassium equilibrium potential as determined with potassium-sensitive microelectrodes in isolated superfused tissue preparations (Hanna et al. 1987). The potassium probably is lost mostly during the acute ischemic period and only gradually recovers during the subsequent weeks. The depressed upstroke of the action potentials appears to be dependent on Na^+ channel current rather than the slow inward calcium current since agents that block Na^+ channels such as TTX or lidocaine can abolish excitability while calcium channel blockers such as D600 do not (Lazzara et al. 1978b; Lazzara and Scherlag 1980). The reduced amplitude and absence of an overshoot in cells with nearly normal resting potentials in reperfused infarcts also suggest abnormalities in the Na^+ channels that prevent a normal inward Na^+ current from being generated. Some indirect evidence also suggests the possibility that the loss of the plateau phase of the action potential may be a result of a decrease in the slow inward (L-type calcium) current (Boyden et al. 1988). Precise determinations of the membrane current abnormalities await the results of voltage-clamp studies that cannot be done on the whole tissues because of the geometric complexities. Isolation of single myocytes by disaggregation of the whole tissues may provide a means by which membrane currents in these cells can be measured and the abnormalities that cause the changes in the action potentials can be determined (Lue and Boyden 1989).

In canine infarcts caused by permanent occlusion, Purkinje fibers survive on the endocardial surface of the infarcts and there is little if any ventricular muscle. The action potential characteristics of the Purkinje fibers have been studied 10 days after occlusion in isolated superfused infarct preparations, at which time the maximum diastolic potential, action potential amplitude, and $\dot{V}_{max}$ of phase 0 are only slightly less than normal (Friedman et al. 1975). The duration of the action potential plateau at this time is less than normal. None of these abnormalities in the action potentials have been identified as being a cause of arrhythmias. When there has been reperfusion of the occluded coronary artery, muscle survives on the endocardial surface of the infarct along with the Purkinje fibers. Transmembrane potentials of both cell types are normal during infarct healing (Karagueuzian et al. 1980).

The recovery of the transmembrane action potentials late in the healing phase of infarction and the persistence of this recovery in the healed phase has also been documented by microelectrode recordings obtained from the endocardial border zone of healed feline infarcts caused by distal ligation of the left ventral artery (Bassett et al. 1977; Myerburg et al. 1977). As described earlier, multiple layers of surviving endocardial cells become trapped in the endocardial scar of the healed, transmural infarct; some appear to be Purkinje fibers and others are ventricular muscle. The cellular electrophysiological characteristics of these surviving cardiac fibers have also been studied in Tyrode's superfused preparations *in vitro* at times ranging from 2 weeks to 6 months after occlusion (Myerburg et al. 1977; 1982a; 1982b; 1982c). Between 2 weeks and 3 months, many of the Purkinje fibers and ventricular muscle have normal resting membrane potentials and action potentials, although there are focal regions of cells that have partially depolarized membrane potentials. Between 3 and 6 months, cells with normal transmembrane potentials are also mixed with some abnormal cells, including depolarized ones with very short action potentials at the lateral border of the scar, and some cells with slow upstrokes that resemble slow responses. The nonuniformity in repolarization has been suggested to be an important factor in arrhythmogenesis (Wong et al. 1982). However, in general, most of the cells have been shown to have a normal resting potential and action potential upstroke. Cells overlying the central infarct have normal intracellular K^+ and Na^+ activities while abnormal cells at the margins have decreased intracellular K^+ and increased Na^+ activities, explaining the decreased resting potential (Kimura et al. 1986a).

Transmembrane potentials have also been recorded from myocardial cells trapped in regions of healed human infarcts that have been excised during arrhythmia surgery and studied *in vitro* with microelectrodes. Transmembrane resting and action potentials were found to be extremely heterogeneous. Normal appearing action potentials were recorded from some surviving Purkinje fibers and ventricular muscle cells with nearly normal resting potentials, while action potentials with slow upstrokes were recorded from other cells with depolarized resting potentials (Spear et al. 1979; De Bakker et al. 1988). Figure 4.61 shows an example of a transmembrane potential recorded from a surviving muscle fiber in the endocardial border zone of a healed human infarct. A picture of the resected subendocardial tissue from a patient who had ventricular tachycardia and from which the action potential was recorded is at the top. The (pulse) symbol on the picture is the site at which the isolated, Tyrode's superfused tissue was stimulated and the suture marks the site that was determined to be the origin of the tachycardia during the operation. The action potential shown below was recorded near the site of origin in the region marked by the asterisk. The maximum diastolic potential and amplitude of this action potential, and others recorded in the same region were nearly normal. An extracellular electrogram recorded at the site of the transmembrane potential recording, shown in the bottom trace, is characterized by fragmented activity,

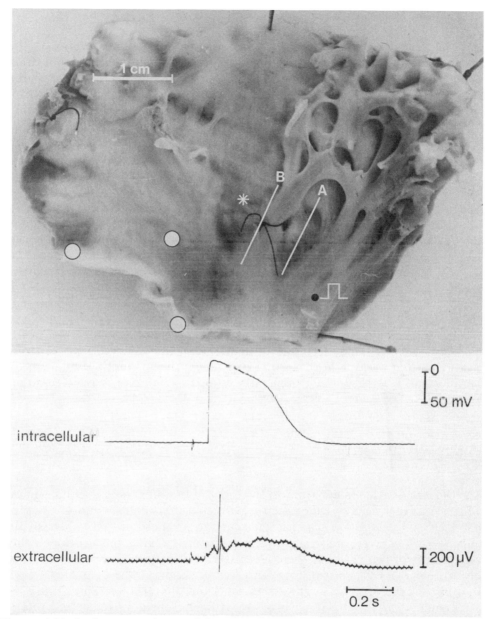

Figure 4.61: At the top, a picture of the resected endocardial tissue from the infarcted left ventricle of a patient who had ventricular tachycardia is shown. The specimen was placed in a tissue bath and superfused for electrophysiological investigations. Stimulation was performed at the site indicated by the pulse symbol at the bottom right. The suture in the middle of the resection (asterisk) marks the site that was determined to be the origin of the tachycardia by mapping during the operation. Black dots indicate the approximate sites at which presystolic activity was recorded during intraoperative mapping. At the bottom are the extra- and intracellular records from the site marked by the asterisk, which was close to the site of origin of the tachycardia. Action potentials were close to normal; extracellular recordings showed fragmentation. (Reproduced from De Bakker et al. (1988) with permission.)

indicating that even though action potentials were normal, activation of this region was slow and not uniform. Some cells with normal maximum diastolic potentials have been shown to have action potentials with fast upstrokes during activation from one direction and slow upstrokes during activation from another direction (De Bakker et al. 1988). Cells with normal resting potentials but very low amplitude action potentials also have been found (Spear et al. 1979). Action potential upstrokes sometimes have multiple components suggesting electrotonic interactions between closely adjacent sites.

To summarize our discussion on cellular electrophysiology, based on the data obtained from several experimental animal models as well as human infarcts, it appears that the transmembrane potentials of muscle fibers surviving in ischemic regions undergo a series of changes during healing of the infarct that eventually leads, for the most part, to the restoration of normal action potentials in the healed infarct. During both this period of healing and during the resultant healed phase, reentrant tachycardia can occur. Therefore, it seems that the cellular electrophysiological characteristics of the cardiac fibers supporting reentry may be different, depending on the time of occurrence of the arrhythmias relative to the acute event that causes the infarction. There is no one specific feature of the transmembrane potentials that can be tied to the occurrence of the arrhythmias. Furthermore, the occurrence of reentrant tachycardia in regions with normal transmembrane potentials might seem paradoxical. The conduction properties of healing infarcts provide some answers to the paradox.

Conduction Properties

Slow activation is apparent in the maps of the reentrant circuits causing ventricular tachycardia. Depression or reduction of the transmembrane resting potential and the action potential depolarization phase are probably not the only factors or even the most important factors causing the necessary slow conduction for rentry, as they are for the acute arrhythmias, since transmembrane potentials are not severely depressed in healing infarcts and are nearly normal in healed infarcts. The structure of the infarct, more specifically the arrangement of the surviving myocardial fibers, plays an important role in determining conduction properties. This structure is changing during infarct healing. As a result of the time-dependent changes in both transmembrane potentials and structure, conduction properties during different periods of the healing process are different.

First, we describe conduction properties during the healing phase (during the first several weeks after occlusion) when the surviving myocardial fibers are still organized in parallel bundles and the transmembrane resting potential and action potential upstroke may be somewhat reduced. Unfortunately, conduction measurements from human infarcts during the healing phase are not available, so we must rely on data obtained from experimental animal studies.

Conduction properties of the epicardial border zone of canine infarcts where the reentrant circuits are located have been characterized, both from *in vivo* and *in vitro* mapping studies during the first weeks after coronary occlusion and these data provide a good indication of conduction properties associated with reentry in healing infarcts. *In vitro* studies allow for very high resolution mapping with closely spaced extracellular electrodes and also permit the recording of transmembrane potentials with microelectrodes to determine the action potential characteristics associated with conduction abnormalities. A drawback of these kinds of studies is that data can only be obtained from a small part of the infarcted region since only a part of the infarct that participates in arrhythmogenesis can be fit into the tissue bath and still be well perfused. Therefore, inhomogeneities of properties in widely separated regions are not always apparent with this approach. On the other hand, *in vivo* mapping of impulse propagation may be done over the entire infarct, but microscale details at local sites may be missed because of the limited spatial resolution of an electrode array that must cover a larger region. However, by synthesizing results from both types of approaches an overall picture can be formulated.

Conduction in the epicardial border zone of healing canine infarcts is anisotropic, that is, it is influenced markedly by the direction of propagation relative to the orientation of the long axis of the myocardial fiber bundles which, as we mentioned above, are still arranged parallel to one another. This influence of myocardial fiber orientation is also likely to apply to other regions of healing infarcts in which there are surviving myocardial cells, such as endocardial border zone or intramural fiber bundles. Conduction properties in different infarcts at the same stage of healing may also be different from one another. In some infarcts stimulated wave fronts traveling parallel to the long axis of the muscle fiber bundles in the epicardial border zone may travel at normal conduction velocities of 50–60 cm/sec in regions where reentrant circuits are located during periods of tachycardia (Ursell et al. 1985; Cardinal et al. 1988; Saltman 1990; Saltman et al. 1993). Wave fronts traveling transverse to the long axis of the fibers have also been shown to propagate at normal average velocities of 20–30 cm/sec in some regions (Saltman 1990), but transverse conduction velocity may be as slow as 5 cm/sec in others (Ursell et al. 1985; Dillon et al. 1988). An activation map of the epicardial border zone illustrating the marked directional differences in conduction is shown in Figure 4.62. The map shows the excitation pattern of the epicardial border zone of a healing canine infarct following stimuli applied in the center where the pulse symbol is located. The mapped region is where a reentrant circuit was located during tachycardia. Activation of the border zone by the stimulated impulse spreads away from the stimulus site in all directions (arrows). The excitation wave fronts reached the left anterior descending coronary artery and lateral margins quickly (after 40–50 msec) but the basal and apical margins slowly (after 70–80 msec). The rapid excitation spread towards the left anterior descending coronary artery and lateral margins is in a direction that is parallel to the orientation of the long axis of the myocardial fiber bundles, while the slow spread of excitation towards the apex and base is transverse to this long axis. Conduction

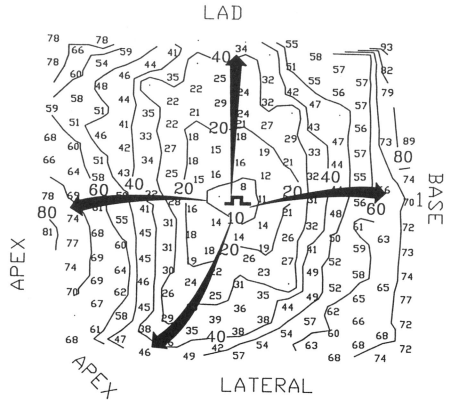

Figure 4.62: Activation pattern during stimulation of the epicardial border zone of a 4-day-old infarct in a canine heart. The margins of the epicardial electrode array adjacent to the left anterior descending coronary artery (LAD), base of the left ventricle, lateral left ventricle, and apex are labeled. The stimulus site is indicated by the pulse symbol at the center. Activation times at all recording sites are indicated by the small numbers. Isochrones are drawn at 10-msec intervals and labeled by the large numbers. Activation spread away from the stimulus site in all directions as indicated by the arrows. (Unpublished results of J. Coromilas, A.E. Saltman, S.M. Dillon, and A.L. Wit.)

velocities calculated in both the longitudinal and the transverse directions in this experiment are normal, approximately 60 cm/sec in the fast direction and 30 cm/sec in the slow direction.

Regions of the epicardial border zone that have normal conduction velocities during activation parallel to the long axis of myocardial fiber orientation most likely have normal or nearly normal transmembrane resting potentials and action potential upstrokes. Even at rapid rates of stimulation, conduction velocities in these regions slow only slightly, no more than in normal myocardium (Saltman 1990). Significant rate-dependent slowing of conduction would be expected if the transmembrane potentials were depressed. The same regions are activated slowly by wave fronts propagating transverse to the fiber long axis. The slow activation is a result of the anisotropic properties of the tissue.

Where there is very slow activation in the transverse direction such as those regions with conduction velocities of 5 cm/sec or less, the myocardial fiber bundles may be more widely separated by edema or connective tissue and some of the transverse connections may be disrupted. Slow conduction, primarily caused by anisotropic properties may contribute to reentrant excitation as we will discuss later.

Normal conduction velocities do not always occur in the epicardial border zone of healing canine infarcts. Conduction can be depressed in marked contrast to the conduction properties that are described above (Saltman et al. 1990). An activation map in Figure 4.63 of excitation during stimulation at the center of the border zone, at a rate that was only slightly faster than sinus rate, illustrates the occurrence of slow conduction and block. Activation moved away from the central stimulation site (pulse symbol) only towards the base without block as indicated by the arrows, reaching this margin after 80–100 msec. Activation towards the left anterior descending coronary artery margin progressed up to the 40-msec isochrone but there was block between the 40- and

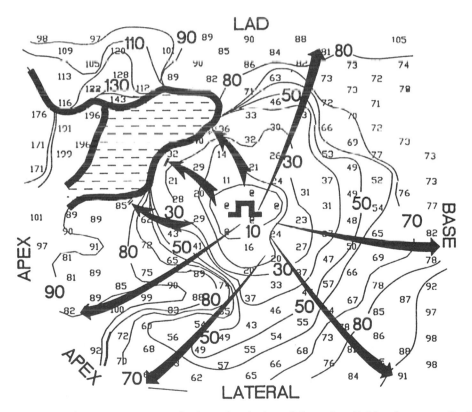

Figure 4.63: Activation pattern during stimulation of the epicardial border zone of a 5-day-old infarct in a canine heart. The format and labeling is the same as Figure 4.62. The region indicated by dashed lines is an area of conduction block. (Unpublished results of J. Coromilas, A.E. Saltman, S.M. Dillon, and A.L. Wit.)

80-msec isochrone. Activation did not reach the far left anterior descending coronary artery margin until after 90 msec. Activation spread towards the apical and apicoseptal margins of the border zone for only the first 30 msec following stimulation and then block occurred. For all experiments within the group showing these characteristics, the conduction velocity parallel to the long axis of the fibers (the fast direction) in regions where there was no block was around 30–35 cm/sec, which was half that found in epicardial border zones with normal conduction properties. Conduction in the transverse (slow) axis was around 10–15 cm/sec, also about half of normal (Saltman 1990). At increased pacing rates, areas of block present during sinus rhythm or slow stimulation increased in extent and new areas of block appeared in some regions exhibiting slow activation at the slower rates (Saltman 1990). These regions were also activated with delay during sinus rhythm and were the sites where late potentials were recorded.

The conduction properties of the epicardial border zone during healing in canine infarcts caused by coronary occlusion and subsequent reperfusion are somewhat different than those of the epicardial border zone of infarcts caused by permanent occlusion. Conduction velocity measured in experiments on isolated superfused preparations from infarcts up to 2 weeks old was depressed both parallel and transverse to myocardial fiber orientation in local regions (0.015–0.02 m/sec) and was normal in others (Spear et al. 1983a). There may be several mechanisms causing the localized regions of slow conduction. In some areas, slow conduction occurred where resting membrane potential and action potential amplitude were severely depressed. Within these areas the slow conduction was uniform and correlated with these membrane properties (Spear et al. 1985). In other regions, slowing of conduction may have resulted from changes in coupling between the myocardial cells because slowing of conduction was greater than predicted from the amount of depression of the transmembrane potentials (Spear et al. 1983a). Large increases in activation times occurred between closely adjacent sites where action potential upstrokes were preceded by prepotentials. This characteristic suggests transmission between poorly coupled cells. Space constants measured in these regions with suction electrodes were reduced to less than 0.5 mm (from normal values of about 1.0 mm) (Spear et al. 1983b). Changes in the properties of the gap junctions caused by ischemia or disruption of cell interconnections by fibrosis or edema may be responsible for the slow conduction. From these data it appears that conduction in the epicardial border zone of reperfused infarcts may be more irregular and have more regions of very slow activation than in infarcts caused by permanent occlusion. However, such a comparison is necessarily subjective and not quantitative and is complicated by the fact that there is also slow and irregular conduction in the epicardial border zone of some infarcts caused by permanent occlusion. When reperfusion salvages a thick rim of subepicardial muscle over the infarct rather than only a narrow zone of surviving muscle, activation of this region can be very rapid even during tachycardia and the reentrant circuits are probably located elsewhere (Wit et al. 1982a).

The description of conduction in healing infarcts indicates that conduction properties and the causes for slow conduction may be different in different hearts. In some hearts there may be nearly normal action potentials and slow conduction may result only from anisotropic properties of infarct anatomy, e.g., slow conduction transverse to the long axis of the myocardial fibers. In other hearts transmembrane potentials may be depressed, and along with anisotropy, cause slow conduction. The reason why transmembrane potentials are only sometimes depressed is not obvious. The implication of the variety of mechanisms for slow conduction is that reentrant circuits causing tachyarrhythmias may have different electrophysiological properties in different hearts. The different conduction properties may influence the rate and stability of the arrhythmia as well as explain a variable response to drugs. The different electrophysiological properties of the reentrant circuits are discussed in more detail later.

The conduction properties of healed infarcts are still different from those of healing infarcts. As we described earlier, surviving myocardial bundles in some regions of healed infarcts are no longer packed together in a parallel arrangement, but are widely separated by connective tissue and are in disarray. As a consequence, there are fewer connections among fiber bundles. Parallel orientation may be maintained in other regions. This change in anatomy from the healing to the healed stage is partly responsible for a change in conduction properties. Detailed measurements of activation patterns and transmembrane potentials in isolated superfused preparations of the epicardial border zone from healed canine infarcts in regions of myocardial fiber disarray have illustrated the conduction properties which are also expected to occur in other regions of healed infarcts with a similar anatomy (Gardner et al. 1985). Figure 4.64 compares activation of the epicardial border zone in a healed infarct (2 months, right panel) with activation in a healing infarct (5 days, left panel). The points at which action potentials were recorded to construct the activation maps are shown by the dots and the activation times are indicated. A distance scale is below each map. In the 2-month-old infarct, activation moving in the directions indicated by the arrows was very slow as is shown by the close bunching of the isochrones. In some regions, it required 10 msec for the activation wave to move a distance of 0.5 mm, a conduction velocity of 0.05 cm/sec. This velocity is much slower than in healing infarcts as exemplified in the left panel where conduction velocity in the direction of the arrows is 20–40 cm/sec; in the direction of the long axis of the muscle fibers. (The isochrones are much more widely spaced, reflecting the faster conduction velocity.) The very slow conduction velocity occurred in the healed infarct despite the normal transmembrane potentials recorded at most sites as exemplified by the record of the action potential above that was recorded at the site indicated by the circle on the map. The slow activation is dependent on the structural alterations that occur as the infarct heals rather than abnormalities in transmembrane potentials; the separation and disorganization of the muscle bundles in the epicardial border zone that occurs as it is invaded by fibrous tissue from the adjacent infarct disrupts intercellular connections, thereby slowing conduction (Gardner et al. 1985). In these regions there are no longer the well defined anisotropic

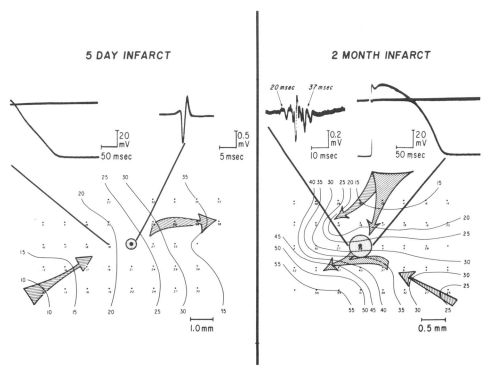

Figure 4.64: Activation maps of regions around bipolar electrodes in two different epicardial border zones, one from a 5-day-old infarct at the left, and one from a 2-month-old infarct at the right. The location and size of the electrodes is indicated by the stippled circles and the electrograms recorded in each experiment are shown above. The points at which action potentials were recorded are indicated by the dots and small numbers in each panel. Representative action potentials are also shown. The arrows and isochrones show the direction of activation. The stimulus sites are not included on the maps. The distance scale for each panel is shown below; note that the scale is two times larger for the 5-day-old infarct preparation than for the 2-month-old infarct preparation. (Reproduced from Gardner et al. (1985) with permission.)

properties seen in healing infarcts, that is, conduction is slow in all directions rather than just transverse to the long axis of parallel organized muscle bundles. In other regions of the epicardial border zone where the parallel arrangement of the muscle bundles is maintained, conduction properties and anisotropic properties are more similar to those of healing infarcts. These same structural features found in the epicardial border zone of canine infarcts, regions of sparse, poorly connected, myocardial fibers in disarray and regions of parallel oriented bundles of fibers, also occur in the epicardial and endocardial border zone of human infarcts. They are expected to affect conduction properties in the same way that they do in the experimental infarcts. The epicardial border zone is a model for conduction in surviving ventricular muscle in healed infarcts, no matter where that surviving muscle is located (epicardial, subendocardial, or intramural).

Some of the extracellular electrograms recorded in regions of slow activation in the isolated canine preparations of epicardial border zone in healed infarcts have a characteristic long duration and fractionated appearance (Gardner et al. 1985), which is illustrated at the top of the right panel in Figure 4.64. Similar electrograms have been recorded from healing and healed regions of infarction in all of the experimental animal models. The electrogram shown in Figure 4.64 was recorded with a bipolar electrode (1-mm distance between poles) at the site indicated by the shaded circle on the activation map. Activation of the small region around the electrode (several millimeters) was very slow and required almost 20 msec, causing the long duration of the electrogram compared to electrograms recorded from other regions that were activated more quickly. For example, the electrogram shown above the left panel was recorded from a region in the healing infarct that was activated in less than 5 msec. The duration of the electrogram is directly related to the time it takes the propagating wave front to pass beneath the recording electrode, being very long when activation is slow. It is influenced by the distance between the bipoles since, when they are farther apart, they sense electrical activity in more myocardium. In addition to the very slow activation causing electrograms with a long duration, it has been shown in these experimental healed infarcts that activation is not homogeneous and this property causes the fractionated nature of the electrogram (Gardner et al. 1985). The diagram in Figure 4.65 offers a simplistic explanation for the relationship of nonhomogeneous, slow activation to the occurrence of fractionated electrograms. It applies to other regions of healed infarcts as well. Three functional bundles of surviving muscle embedded in the infarct scar are shown. In panel A there are very few connections between the bundles because of their separation by the connective tissue. Interconnections occur at distant sites not shown in the figure. The larger circles represent the location of the bipolar electrodes and the arrows show the pattern of impulse propagation between bundles. This model assumes circuitous conduction in the vicinity of the bipolar electrode. Conduction velocity in each of the three functional bundles can be normal because of the normal transmembrane potentials in healed infarcts but total activation of the region is slow because of the circuitous pathway of propagation made necessary by the lack of interconnections. Isoelectric intervals in the fractionated electrogram at the right (between deflections a, b, and c) occur during the time the impulse is out of the recording field of the bipolar electrode; components of the fractionated electrogram (a, b, and c) occur when the impulse returns in one of the muscle bundles. The model in panel B shows a different possible mechanism for the fractionated electrogram. The arrows again show the propagation pattern in the vicinity of the bipolar recording site indicated by the large circles. This model assumes that there are long pauses as excitation passes across connections between adjacent muscle bundles. The pauses might occur if the resistance at intercellular contacts between myocardial fibers is high causing slow impulse transmission across high resistance junctions or barriers (Spach et al. 1981; Joyner et al. 1984a; 1984b). A high resistance might result from the effects of prolonged ischemia on the gap junctions or from a decrease in size or number of interca-

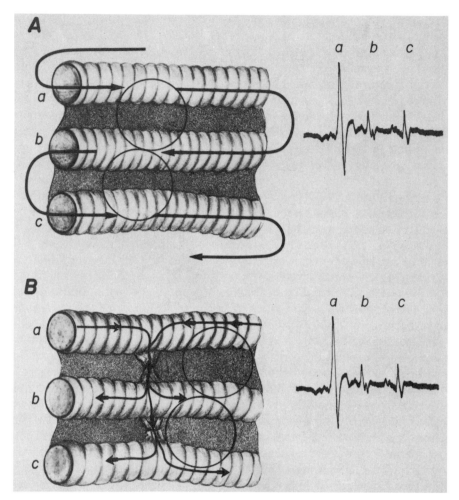

Figure 4.65: Two models that might explain the occurrence of fractionated electrograms. In A, three cardiac fibers or bundles are indicated by the cylindrical structures. These fibers are separated by connective tissue (shaded regions) and are not interconnected in the region shown by the diagram. However, interconnections do occur at a distant site. The large circles represent the location of a bipolar electrode and the dark arrows show impulse propagation. In B, the three cardiac fibers are connected in the field of the diagram and impulse propagation occurs in a relatively straight line through these connections as indicated by the arrows. If it is assumed that the resistance at the connections is high, there might be a delay in conduction from one fiber to another. The model does not explain the different amplitudes of the electrogram components that may result from different diameters of the bundles or different distances of each bundle from the recording electrodes. (Reproduced from Gardner et al. (1985) with permission.)

lated discs because of the increased amount of connective tissue associated with formation of the scar. Other possible causes for such exaggerated discontinuous conduction include abrupt changes in cell size or surface to volume ratios, marked differences in the number of cells connected across high-resistance barriers, and abrupt cell branching (Joyner et al. 1984a; 1984b). Discontinuities in conduction are often evident by prepotentials or notches on the action potential upstrokes in the healed infarcts in regions where fractionaed electrograms are recorded (Gardner et al. 1985). Therefore, each component of a fractionated electrogram indicates a functional muscle bundle that is activated out of synchrony with adjacent bundles because of their separation by connective tissue scar during infarct healing. The individual "spikes" of the fractionated electrograms may be rapid because of the fast upstrokes of the underlying action potentials. The amplitude of fractionated electrograms is also much lower than electrograms recorded from normal regions, because of the paucity of muscle fibers trapped in the large amount of scar tissue where they are recorded. Extracellular current flow in these regions is small. Low-amplitude electrograms that are not fractionated have also been recorded from other regions with few muscle bundles that are still activated in synchrony (Gardner et al. 1985). Low-amplitude electrograms that are not fractionated can also be recorded in regions where the transmembrane potentials are depressed, and thus, extracellular currents are small, but conduction may still be homogeneous.

Similarly, nonhomogeneous slow activation, normal appearing transmembrane potentials and fractionated electrograms have been recorded in isolated preparations of healed infarcts obtained from human hearts (De Bakker et al. 1988). Figure 4.66 shows data obtained from the heart of a patient studied in Amsterdam who underwent cardiac transplantation because of congestive heart failure as a result of extensive myocardial infarction. After removal, the heart was perfused through the aortic root in a Langendorff apparatus and monomorphic, nonsustained ventricular tachycardia was induced by programmed stimulation. The earliest activated area during tachycardia was on the endocardial surface of the left ventricle, close to the posterior papillary muscle. This muscle was resected, placed in a tissue bath where it was superfused with oxygenated Tyrode's solution and stimulated at a cycle length of 800 msec. A diagram of the isolated preparation is shown at the left in Figure 4.66. The site of stimulation was at the location of the upper pin. Unipolar electrograms were recorded at the sites marked by the black dots. These unipolar recordings, at the right, show two different complexes separated by an isoelectric interval that is longest at site A, shortens as site E is approached, and disappears at F. The sequence of activation of the first complex at each site shows activation moving from A to F; the sequence of activation of the second complex shows activation moving back from F to A. Figure 4.67, at the left, shows schematic drawings of the architecture in the region where some of the electrograms were recorded. The surviving muscle in the healed infarct is black and the fibrous tissue of the scar is white. At levels B, D, and E, the rim of surviving subendocardial myocardium is interrupted by connective tissue in

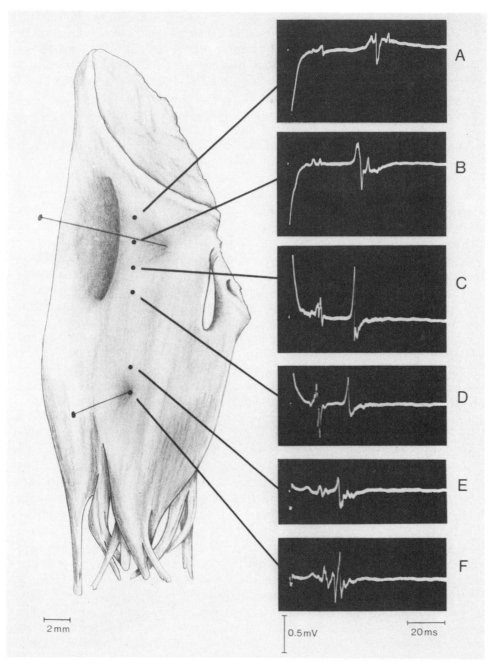

Figure 4.66: At the left is a schematic drawing of an infarcted human papillary muscle from which the extracellular electrograms shown at the right were recorded in a tissue bath. The preparation was stimulated at the site of the upper pin. Black dots indicate the recording sites. Note the presence of the two components in electrograms A-E, with the isoelectric interval becoming progressively shorter. (Reproduced from De Bakker et al. (1990) with permission.)

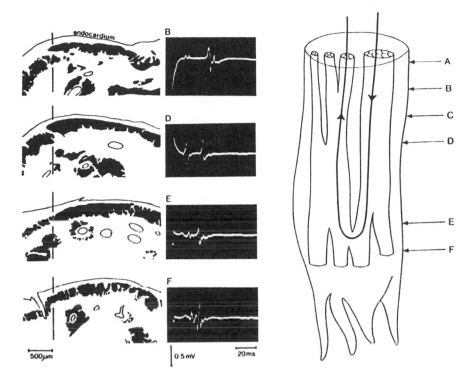

Figure 4.67: The left panel shows schematic drawings of histologic sections taken through recording sites B, D, E, and F of the infarcted papillary muscle shown in Figure 4.66. Surviving muscle is indicated by the black regions, scar indicated by the white. Note that at the level of the vertical dashed line (at the left), two areas of surviving muscle are separated by fibrous tissue at levels B, D, E, but these areas merge at level F. At the far right is a schematic drawing of the proposed "zigzag" pathway of conduction in the papillary muscle giving rise to the fractionated electrograms indicated by the large arrow. Arrows and letters at the far right indicate the recording sites in Figure 4.66. (Reproduced from De Bakker et al. (1990) with permission.)

the region where there is a vertical line drawn through the section. At site F, the muscle fibers merge as indicated by the lack of a gap between bundles at the vertical line. The diagram at the right shows the probable pathway of activation of the papillary muscle, compatible with the histologic data, leading to the occurrence of the fractionated electrograms. Activation appears to have occurred through one myocardial bundle from site A to F and then back to A through the other bundle. At each site the electrode picked up the activity in each of the bundles. Since the total distance that was traversed by the conducting impulse (from A to F to A) was about 2 cm, conduction velocity was about 45 cm/sec, a value close to normal and compatible with the presence of normal transmembrane potentials. However, the circuitous conduction pathway caused the region to be activated slowly. Therefore, in healed human infarcts, large activation delays can also occur over short distances even when conduction velocity is normal because of long, "zigzag" pathways, and these regions are characterized by the occurrence of fractionated electrograms.

In summary, the experimental studies on both canine and human infarcts *in vitro* have shown that fractionated electrograms are an indicator of slow and inhomogeneous activation of the regions in which they are recorded. The duration of the electrogram is a measurement of the amount of time required for the region around the recording electrode to be activated, the individual components of the electrogram reflect activity coming from different fiber bundles activated with delay, one from the other. Therefore, the characteristics of the electrograms can be useful indicators of conduction properties.

The characteristics of the electrograms recorded in human infarcts *in situ* have also provided invaluable information about conduction properties. In general, these electrograms indicate that conduction properties in healed human infarcts are similar to the properties defined in experimental animal models or in isolated preparations studied *in vitro*. The electrograms recorded from the endocardial regions of healed human infarcts during sinus rhythm mapping are often abnormal. Many of the electrograms have a lower amplitude than those recorded from normal regions and a longer duration (Cassidy et al. 1984a; 1984b). Some subendocardial electrograms consist of multiple components and have a fractionated appearance, consistent with slow, inhomogeneous activation of the muscle bundles trapped in the connective tissue scar. Activation of regions of the infarct where the abnormal electrograms are recorded, is often delayed (Vassallo et al. 1986; 1988). The delayed endocardial activation is the result of slow activation in the endocardial border zone reflected in the electrogram characteristics. Stimulation at sites of fractionated activity may also be followed by a long delay before inscription of the QRS, the long delay probably being caused by slow conduction out of the region with the fractionated electrograms (Stevenson et al. 1989a). Fractionated electrograms have also been recorded from the epicardial border zone of human infarcts in regions in which activation is slow and inhomogeneous (Josephson et al. 1982b; Svenson et al. 1990).

Examples of electrograms recorded during sinus rhythm with a catheter electrode from the endocardial surface of a healed human infarct are shown in Figure 4.68. The top three traces are surface electrocardiographic recordings, below which are the endocardial electrograms. The normal electrogram consists of a single biphasic deflection that has an amplitude of about 5 mV and a duration of 30 msec. The abnormal electrogram has a lower amplitude and longer duration while the fractionated and late electrogram has a still lower amplitude (less than 0.5 mV), longer duration, and consists of multiple deflections. The longer duration of both the normal and the abnormal electrograms, compared to those recorded from the isolated infarct tissue in Figure 4.64 is a result of the wider spacing (0.5 cm) between the poles of the bipolar catheter electrode, compared to the 1-mm spacing of the electrode used in the experimental study. Similar abnormal and fractionated electrograms have also been recorded during sinus rhythm from subendocardial regions of healed infarcts during surgery with closer bipolar electrodes than the catheter electrode (Klein

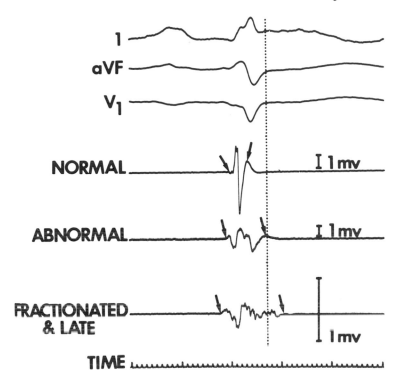

I

aVF

V₁

NORMAL

I 1 mv

ABNORMAL

I 1 mv

FRACTIONATED & LATE

I 1 mv

TIME

Figure 4.68: Three surface electrocardiographic recordings (I, aVF, and V₁) accompanied by three local bipolar electrograms (normal, abnormal, and fractionated and late) recorded from different left ventricular endocardial sites with a catheter electrode in a patient with a myocardial infarct. The dashed vertical line denotes the end of surface QRS activity. The arrows show the onset and end of local electrical activity. Each electrogram is accompanied by a 1 mV calibration signal. (Reproduced from Cassidy et al. (1984a) with permission.)

et al. 1982; Wiener et al. 1982; Kienzle et al. 1983; Weiner et al. 1984). Wiener et al. (1984) found that fractionated electrograms were more numerous, and had longer durations in patients with healed infarcts, aneurysms and ventricular tachycardia than in patients with healed infarcts and aneurysms but without tachycardia. These data might be interpreted to mean that a critical amount or area of slow, heterogeneous conduction is necessary for reentry to occur. Ventricular tachycardia often originates at sites at which abnormal or fractionated electrograms are recorded during sinus rhythm. However, normal electrograms are sometimes found at the site of origin of ventricular tachycardia (Cassidy et al. 1984a). As described above, regions within healed infarcts that have normal electrograms probably have a relatively large amount of surviving muscle bundles that are still normally arranged in parallel bundles. The lack of slow activation at some sites of origin, as indicated by normal electrograms, might mean that these sites are actually exit routes from the circuits and not the circuits themselves. Fractionated electrograms are also found during sinus rhythm at sites other than those of arrhythmia origin. Therefore, there are abnormal regions that are not responsible for the tachycardia as well as those that are (Josephson and Wit 1984; Wit and Josephson 1985).

Fractionated electrograms may be recorded during sinus rhythm at the site of origin of a ventricular tachycardia. During tachycardia the duration and fractionation of the electrogram may increase to span the entire diastolic interval indicating slow and inhomogeneous activation in the reentrant circuit (Josephson et al. 1978c). Electrograms recorded at the site of origin that may not have been fractionated during sinus rhythm sometimes fractionate during tachycardia, reflecting slow and inhomogeneous conduction in the reentrant circuit that was not present in the absence of tachycardia.

Slow activation in reentrant circuits in healed human infarcts is also indicated by other kinds of observations. One line of evidence is the large delay (100–400 msec) between stimulus artifact and resulting QRS complex when stimulating from some regions of tachycardia origin to reset or entrain the tachycardia that we discussed earlier. This delay most likely results from slow conduction of the stimulated impulse in the reentrant circuit before it emerges to cause the QRS complex (Morady et al. 1988; Stevenson et al. 1988; 1989b; Kay et al. 1990). During entrainment of tachycardia from stimulation sites outside the reentrant circuit, there may also be a long delay between pacing artifact and the time of occurrence of electrograms that are believed to be recorded from the reentrant circuit. This is also indicative of slow activation by the stimulated impulse of regions in the reentrant circuit between the site of stimulation and the electrograms (Okumura et al. 1987). Since pacing during sinus rhythm does not usually result in as long a delay between stimulus artifact and electrogram, it is likely that slow conduction increases once a presumably functional reentrant circuit is formed (Okumura et al. 1987).

Refractory Periods of Healing and Healed Infarcts

Prolonged effective and relative refractory periods have been measured in the epicardial border zone of healing infarcts caused by permanent left anterior descending coronary artery occlusion using fixed current premature stimuli applied at multiple sites (Hope et al. 1980; Gough et al. 1985; Restivo et al. 1990). The prolongation of refractory periods in the face of the shortened action potential duration during healing suggests an increase in postrepolarization refractoriness as has also been shown to occur in acute ischemia (Hope et al. 1980). We have already described the possible role of the prolongation of the refractory period in causing block of premature impulses that initiate reentry. Refractoriness of surviving muscle in epicardial border zone of healed infarcts has not been evaluated. In reperfused infarcts subepicardial, midmyocardial, and intramural sites within the infarcted region have prolonged refractory periods in addition to increased current requirements for effective stimulation (decreased excitability) (Michelson et al. 1981b). There is also a marked dispersion of excitability and refractoriness from site to site within the infarcted region. Dispersion of refractoriness may contribute to initiation of reentry. The studies determining local refractory periods are complicated by anatomical factors that may influence current flow. In reperfused infarcts the relative amount of necrotic and viable myocardium at each stimulus site differs, undoubtedly contributing to the variability in excitability. In permanent occlusion infarcts the number of cell layers in the epicardial border zone at different sites also differs and may affect excitability as well as the ability of a premature impulse to propagate.

Very little is known about refractory properties of the myocardium in healing or healed human infarcts. Vassallo et al. (1988) have measured effective refractory periods in the endocardial border zone of healed infarcts at multiple sites by applying premature stimuli through a catheter and found no difference from normal—there was no difference in dispersion of refractoriness. However, they emphasized that there was a marked increase in the dispersion of total recovery time. That is, because of the marked abnormalities in conduction in the endocardial border zone, some sites are activated long after other sites. Therefore, these sites recover excitability long after the sites that are activated early, even though the different regions may have similar refractory periods (Vassallo et al. 1988). The dispersion in recovery time that results from inhomogeneous activation could lead to conduction block of premature impulses in some regions and not others, initiating reentry.

Mechanisms Causing Reentry in Healing and Healed Infarcts

As described in Chapter I, mechanisms for reentry include anatomical reentry and functional reentry. In anatomical reentry, the reentrant pathway is formed by anatomical structures such as a loop of Purkinje fiber bundles and is therefore fixed in its size and location. Another important feature is that the reentrant circuit is around an anatomical obstacle that is the cause of the central region of block, the block that prevents the impulse from "short circuiting" the reentrant pathway and thus terminating reentry. In functional reentry, the reentrant pathway is formed because of the special electrophysiological properties of the cardiac fibers and there is no anatomical pathway or central obstacle. A central region of block that forms the obstacle still occurs, but is functional in nature. For example, in the leading circle mechanism for functional reentry, the central obstacle is caused by collision of centripetally conducting impulses (Allessie et al. 1977). In theory, a functional circuit is not fixed in size and location, but might move. This is exemplified in the excitation maps of atrial fibrillation in dogs published by Allessie et al. (1985). The reentrant excitation that causes the acute ischemic arrhythmias (see Chapter II) often is functional in nature. The functional heterogeneities in the electrophysiological properties that are required for reentry, for example refractoriness, result from the uneven effect of the ischemia on the cardiac cells. Eventually however, anatomical circuits might form when some regions become inexcitable because of cell death; then they become fixed regions of block around which reentrant excitation waves propagate. Reentrant circuits in healing or healed infarcts may also be either functional or anatomical. The kind of circuit that is formed is dependent on the extent of ischemic damage to the heart and the resultant infarct anatomy.

Again, we will begin with a description of the mechanisms causing reentrant circuits in the epicardial border zone of healing canine infarcts because studies on this experimental model have provided the most detailed activation maps of the circuits and the most detailed information on the electrophysiological and anatomical properties of the myocardium in which they occur (El-Sherif et al. 1981; Wit et al. 1982a; Mehra et al. 1983; Cardinal et al. 1984; El-Sherif 1985; Kramer et al. 1985; Cardinal et al. 1988; Dillon et al. 1988; Restivo et al. 1990; Wit et al. 1990a). Although these studies have been on healing infarcts within the first week after a coronary occlusion, some of the results may apply to healed infarcts as well. Some of the reentrant circuits in the epicardial border zone that cause nonsustained or sustained ventricular tachycardia are functional, the regions of block around which reentrant excitation circulates are not caused by any grossly visible anatomical obstacle nor are there well defined, gross anatomical pathways that form the reentrant circuit. The regions of block and the reentrant circuits are not evident in the absence of tachycardia such as during sinus beats or ventricular pacing. In Figure 4.69, an activation map of reentrant circuits in the epicardial border zone during sustained, monomorphic ventricular tachycardia is shown in panel B. In the time window that is shown, activation begins at the 10-msec isochrone, moves towards the left anterior descending coronary artery (LAD) margin (isochrones 10–60), divides into two wave fronts, one moving to the right and one to the left. Both wave fronts then move towards the lateral margin and return to the site of origin after 183 msec. This pattern of excitation is shown by the arrows. Excitation rotates around two lines of block; the lines of block are represented by the thick black vertical lines. Panel A in Figure 4.69, shows the activation map of the same region during stimulation through electrodes in the center of the epicardial border zone (at the site indicated by the pulse symbol), during sinus rhythm. Activation spreads away from the stimulus site in all directions, towards the LAD, apical, and lateral margins as indicated by the arrows. Activation spread is more rapid towards the LAD and lateral apical margins which are activated after 60–70 msec, than the base or apical margins which are activated after 80–90 msec. The direction of most rapid activation is parallel to the long axis of the myocardial fibers. The regions where the lines of apparent block were located during tachycardia did not show block during central stimulation in the absence of tachycardia. Although there is no evidence of block in the regions where block was located during tachycardia, there is slow activation transverse to the long axis of the fiber bundles in these regions. Also, during sinus rhythm, there was no evidence of the lines of block or the reentrant pathway (not shown). When sustained tachycardia was initiated by a premature impulse, the lines of block appeared and remained in the same

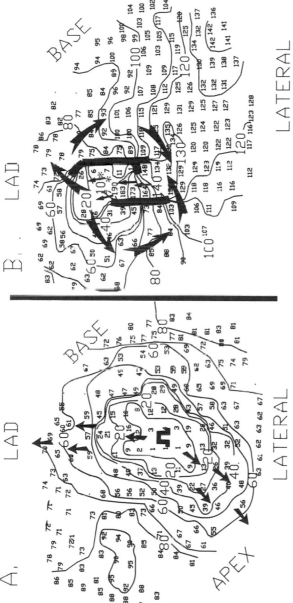

Figure 4.69: Activation map of a reentrant circuit in the epicardial border zone of a 4-day-old canine infarct during sustained ventricular tachycardia is shown in panel B. The top margin of the electrode array is adjacent to the left anterior descending coronary artery (LAD), the bottom margin of the map is toward the apical region of the lateral left ventricle. The right margin is along the base and the left margin is along the apex (see labels in panel A). On the map, the activation times at each of the recording sites indicated by the small numbers are plotted. Isochrones are drawn at 10-msec intervals and labeled with the larger numbers. Arrows indicate the sequence of isochrones and thus the direction of movement of activation. In panel A is the activation map during stimulation from the center of the epicardial border zone during sinus rhythm in the same heart. There is an elliptical pattern of activation, the arrows indicate the direction of the fast axes and the longitudinal orientation of the myocardial fibers. (Reproduced from Wit et al. (1990a) with permission.)

position throughout the duration of the tachycardia. When nonsustained tachycardia occurs or rapid tachycardias that degenerate into ventricular fibrillation, the lines of block and the circuits may shift from beat to beat. Since the lines of block and the reentrant circuits appear only during tachycardia, they may be considered to be functional.

What causes the lines of block to appear that lead to the formation of reentrant circuits similar to those shown in Figure 4.69 and what is the cause of the slow conduction around the block that enables reentry to occur? The data on action potential characteristics that we discussed earlier suggest that they might not always be depressed, and therefore, unlike in acute ischemia, reentry is not a result of depressed membrane potentials. The answers to the questions asked above are not entirely worked out, but we can formulate some possible explanations. Some insight into possible mechanisms for block and slow conduction come from a more detailed analysis of the activation maps of the reentrant circuits. Lines of conduction block in an activation map are usually indicated where closely adjacent sites are activated at sufficiently disparate times to result in a large number of interpolated isochrones. Hence, a major indication of block is the very different times of activation at the closely adjacent sites. In Figure 4.69, panel B, the thick dark black lines that are called the lines of block, appear because of the very different activation times on either side of them. By following the sequence of isochrones according to convention it seems that activation is occurring around these lines. However, the activation times and the patterns of isochrones adjacent to the lines are not easily explained if activation is spreading only around them. A portion of the activation map from Figure 4.69B is enlarged in Figure 4.70. In this map, activation times along the right side of the right-hand line of apparent block are from top to bottom: 79, 75, 84, 75, and 89 msec. In order for these recording sites to be activated at these times, which are nearly simultaneous, the reentrant wave front must have moved very slowly through what was thought to be a line of complete block, from left to right on the map as shown by the unfilled arrows. The sequence of activation times is not compatible with a wave front only moving around the upper end of the line as indicated by the solid black arrows. If this had been the case it would be expected that the activation times along the right side of the line of block would increase progressively with values compatible with the conduction velocity in cardiac muscle. Thus, the entire line might not be real block. It can be referred to as a line of apparent block. Lines of apparent block are oriented in a direction parallel to the long axis of the myocardial fibers (in the direction of the long axis of the ellipse resulting from central stimulation in Figure 4.69). Activation, if it occurred across the line from left to right in the map, occurred transverse to the long axis of the myocardial fibers. According to our discussion on anisotropy, transverse activation can be very slow even when action potentials are normal, and might account for the large differences in activation times between adjacent electrodes on different sides of the line (Dillon et al 1988).

The electrograms recorded from some regions along lines of apparent block provide further evidence that there is sometimes slow activation across them

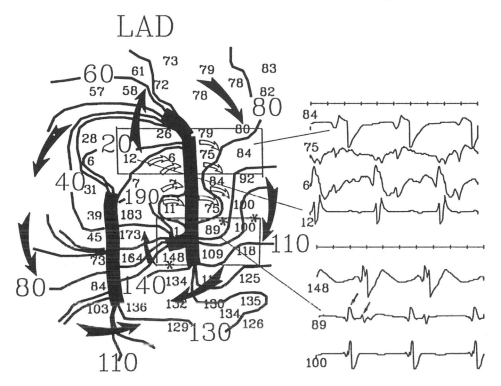

Figure 4.70: The central region of the reentrant circuit described in Figure 4.69 is enlarged in the activation map at the left. At the right are electrograms recorded at different locations in the circuit (time scale is 50 msec per division on the time line trace). The first four electrograms from the top were recorded from sites enclosed within the top rectangle. The top electrogram was recorded from the site activated at 84 msec, the next two electrograms, which are fractionated, were recorded from either side of the line of apparent block (activation times 75 and 6 msec). The fourth electrogram was recorded from the site activated at 12 msec. The next group of three electrograms was recorded from sites within the area enclosed by the lower rectangle (sites indicated by asterisks). The top electrogram was recorded from the site activated at 148 msec, the middle electrogram, which has a double component (indicated by the arrows), was assigned an activation time of 89 msec (first component), and the bottom electrogram had an activation time of 100 msec. (Reproduced from Wit et al. (1990a) with permission.)

transverse to the long axis of the muscle fibers. The electrograms may be fractionated and have long durations. These characteristics are illustrated in Figure 4.70, which, at the right, shows electrograms recorded from some sites along the right line of apparent block in the reentrant circuit. The first four electrograms (from top to bottom) were recorded from the sites within the upper rectangular box on the activation map. The first (activation time 84) and fourth (activation time 12) electrograms in this group were recorded at a distance from the line of apparent block and have only a single major deflection. However, the two electrograms between them were recorded immediately adjacent to the line of apparent block (at sites 6 and 75) and are characterized by fractionated activity. These characteristics result because there is slowly propagating activity across the line of apparent block in this region. The fractionated components are caused by asynchronous activation of adjacent fiber bundles during transverse propagation in nonuniformly anisotropic tissue (Dillon et al. 1988). The long duration and fractionated characteristics of the electrograms recorded at the lines of apparent block only occur during tachycardia and represent a dramatic change from the characteristics of these electrograms during sinus rhythm or ventricular stimulation (Dillon et al. 1988). However, there cannot be propagation across the entire line of block because a central obstacle is needed for reentry to occur. The next group of three electrograms shown at the right in Figure 4.70 was recorded at sites within the lower rectangular box. The top (activation time 148-asterisk) and the bottom (activation time 100-asterisk) electrograms in this group also have single major components. The middle electrogram recorded at the site with the 89-msec activation time has two distinct components (arrows) coinciding with the deflections at sites on either side of it. This region may be near the fulcrum of the circuit around which the reentrant wave front is revolving and the two components of the electrogram are coincident with activation on either side of the line of block (Restivo et al. 1990). This region is the location of real functional block at the center of the circuit.

The nature of the lines of block in the epicardial border zone is not always the same and for some reentrant circuits there is no evidence for slow transverse activation across the lines of block. In Figure 4.70, the activation times along the apical side of the left line of block (31, 39, 45, 73, 84 msec) provide no indication that a slowly moving transverse activation wave propagated across that line. The activation sequence and orientation of the isochrones (perpendicular to the line of block) is that which is expected if the reentrant wave front was moving around a line of real functional block. The electrograms at the line (not shown) were not fragmented but consisted of two deflections, one deflection caused by activation moving in one direction on one side of the line, and the other deflection caused by activation moving in the opposite direction on the other side of the line. Both these activation waves are moving parallel to the muscle fiber bundles. Functional conduction block, such as described for leading circle reentry, may be present along the entire length of the line of block (Cardinal et al. 1988; Restivo et al. 1990).

The characteristics of some reentrant circuits in the epicardial border zone that we just described have suggested a model for reentry in healing or healed myocardial infarcts in regions where the muscle fiber bundles have retained a parallel orientation. In these regions anisotropy is nonuniform because of the edema or connective tissue formed by the healing process. The cornerstone of the model is that the nonuniform anisotropy is a major cause of slow conduction necessary for reentry and therefore, the mechanism is that of anisotropic reentry described in Chapter I (Dillon et al. 1988). According to this model, the property of the infarct that enables reentry to occur is the parallel oriented bundles of surviving muscle fibers in which there is slow conduction transverse to the fibers and faster conduction parallel to the fibers. In the canine model of left anterior descending coronary artery occlusion, the parallel bundles are in the epicardial border zone but in other infarct models or in humans, they may sometimes be located in other regions. Figure 4.71A illustrates the characteristics of anisotropic reentry in infarcts. At the left is the figure-of-eight reentrant circuit that was previously described in Figure 4.70. However, to indicate that there is slow activation through the right line of "block", transverse to the long axis of the myocardial fibers, this line of block has been redrawn to show the individual isochrones. This region is also enlarged in the rectangle at the right. The arrows show the direction of the proposed slow activation. A central region of real block remains, around which the reentrant wave front revolves. In regions of this anisotropic circuit in which activation is occurring in the longitudinal direction of the muscle fibers, conduction is fast (approximately 0.5 m/sec), isochrones are widely separated and for the most part oriented perpendicular to the long axis of the fibers. In the regions of the circuit where activation occurs transverse to the long axis, the isochrones are bunched closely together indicating very slow activation (as slow as 0.05

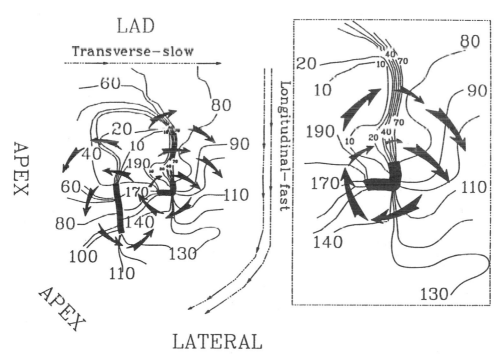

Figure 4.71A: Anisotropic reentry in the epicardial border zone of a canine infarct. The figure-of-eight reentrant circuit at the left is the one described in Figures 4.69B and 4.70. The right line of apparent block has been redrawn to show the individual isochrones resulting from slow propagation transverse to the myocardial fiber orientation. The transverse and longitudinal directions relative to the long axis of the myocardial fibers are indicated. This anisotropic reentrant circuit is enlarged in the rectangle at the right. The black arrows show the activation pattern.

m/sec) and the isochrones are oriented parallel to the fibers. It is the slow conduction transverse to the long axis of the parallel oriented muscle bundles that enables reentry to occur, not slow conduction caused by severely depressed transmembrane potentials. Therefore, despite the appearance of a long line of apparent block (shown in Figure 4.70), reentry is actually occurring around a smaller central fulcrum of block.

Another example of an anisotropic reentrant circuit is shown in Figure 4.71B. In this figure, the reentrant circuit previously described in Figure 4.42 is displayed at the left. The line of apparent block around which the reentrant wave front revolves is enlarged in the rectangle at the right. Since the 110-msec isochrone that is distal to this line is parallel to it, the reentrant impulse may be moving through the line. Therefore, the line of apparent block has been redrawn to show the individual isochrones and the unfilled arrows show propagation through this region. A region of block at the center of the circuit remains. Activation in the anisotropic circuit is slow in the direction transverse to the long axis of the myocardial fibers (isochrones are bunched closely together) and rapid in the direction of the long axis (isochrones are widely separated).

The size of the central fulcrum of block in an anisotropic reentrant circuit may vary in different circuits. In the example of the right line of block shown in Figure 4.70 and 4.71 it is probably less than 6 mm in length. However, the central region of block may also be much longer. In Figure 4.71A, the entire line of block at the left, around which a reentrant wave front rotates, may be a line of real functional block, since as we described, there is no evidence that there is slow activation across it. The slow conduction caused by anisotropy occurs at both ends of the line of block where the wave fronts turn in the direction perpendicular to the long axis of fiber bundle orientation. At these points the isochrones are bunched closely together.

The occurrence of reentry in the epicardial border zone of the canine infarcts is a result of the anatomy of the infarct. The formation of a thin "sheet" of surviving muscle forces the impulse to conduct over the epicardial surface of the heart, in a plane in which the orientation of the muscle fiber bundles can exert a significant influence on conduction velocity. Transmural activation of this region where the reentrant circuits are located is also prevented because of the underlying infarct, so the circuits are not disrupted by excitation waves coming from below. These structural features can be present in healed as well as healing infarcts. That this anatomy alone is sufficient to cause reentrant tachycardia without significant alterations in transmembrane potentials being necessary, is evident from the studies in Allessie's laboratory (Schalij 1988; Allessie et al. 1989). They mimicked the epicardial border zone in the absence of coronary occlusion by freezing the left ventricle of the Langendorff-perfused rabbit heart with a cryoprobe inserted into the ventricular cavity. The cryoprobe froze the ventricle from the endocardial surface towards the epicardial surface but a thin rim of surviving epicardial muscle was maintained by immersing the heart in warm Tyrode's solution during the freezing process. The freezing procedure did not alter the transmembrane action potentials of the

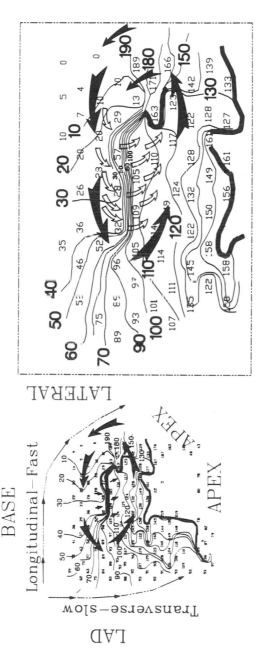

Figure 4.71B: Anisotropic reentry in the epicardial border zone of a canine infarct. The reentrant circuit at the left is the one described in Figure 4.42. The transverse and longitudinal directions relative to the long axis of the myocardial fibers are indicated. The reentrant circuit is enlarged in the rectangle at the right. The line of apparent block has been redrawn to show propagation transverse to the long axis of the myocardial fibers (unfilled arrows).

normal, surviving epicardial muscle. Whereas only fibrillation could be induced in the rabbit ventricles prior to freezing, sustained tachycardias were induced after freezing. Tachycardia was caused by reentry in the thin surviving rim of epicardial muscle. Excitation in the circuits moved around lines of block oriented parallel to the myocardial fiber bundles. Activation in the circuits was rapid in the direction parallel to the orientation of the bundles and slow perpendicular to the orientation. The slow activation resulting from the anisotropic properties caused reentry.

The events occurring at the central fulcrum of the anisotropic reentrant circuits in the epicardial border zone of the canine infarct model are unclear. High-density activation maps recorded in some experiments suggests that there might be collision of wave fronts similar to that in the leading circle model of reentry (Restivo et al. 1990). Also, the central fulcrum might sometimes be a region of anatomical block, a small region where the infarct extends all the way to the epicardial surface. The mechanism for block in the central fulcrum has been studied in the rabbit model described above since microelectrodes could be inserted into this region. (It has not been possible to do this in canine models.) The transmembrane potential recordings were reminiscent of those at the center of leading circle reentry in the atrium (Schalij 1988), with multiple depolarizations indicating collision of centripetal wave fronts in the center of the circuit. In addition, the transmembrane potential recordings in the rabbit model have shown conduction delays as the excitation waves move around the ends of the lines of block and turn from the transverse to the parallel direction. Schalij (1988) has proposed that the delay is caused by a sudden increase in the axial current load on the reentrant wave front and contributes to the occurrence of an excitable gap in anisotropic reentrant circuits. We also described in Chapter I that the changes in the wavelength of the reentrant impulse that occurs in an anisotropic circuit may also lead to an excitable gap.

Reentrant circuits in the epicardial border zone of canine infarcts that cause sustained tachycardia are stable; they are located in the same place every time tachycardia occurs in an individual heart and for each beat of the tachycardia. Why do functional circuits of this kind remain in the same location if they are not confined there by a specific anatomical pathway? We can only speculate about a possible answer to this question since there is no experimental evidence which answers it at the present time. The epicardial border zone in hearts with sustained tachycardia may have special, localized regions with the appropriate anisotropic properties that cause the necessary slow conduction that enables reentry to occur. In other regions, transverse conduction may not be slow enough and circuits attempting to settle in these regions cannot be established. Therefore, there is a heterogeneity in the anisotropic properties that may be related to the degree of fiber bundle separation by edema or connective tissue. In hearts with several different reentrant circuits causing tachycardias with different morphologies, there may be several regions with conduction properties that are appropriate for sustaining reentry. In hearts with only nonsustained tachycardia, areas with sufficiently slow conduction may not be present because of the lack of the appropriate nonuniform anisotropy. In hearts in which fibrillation occurs and is not due to hemodynamic impairment occurring during a preceding period of tachycardia, anisotropy might not cause conduction that is sufficiently slow to result in a stable reentrant circuit. Rather, the circuits may be small and unstable and resemble more the spiral waves discussed in Chapter I.

We have described that muscle bundles in some regions of healed infarcts may no longer be densely or tightly packed but are widely separated by connective tissue. The muscle bundles and fibers are also no longer oriented parallel to one another. In these regions, conduction is slow independent of the direction the wave front is moving and despite the presence of mostly normal transmembrane potentials. It would also seem that this kind of anatomical structure should provide an ideal matrix for reentrant circuits. Conduction is certainly slow enough to cause reentry. This is also a type of anisotropic reentry since the slow conduction that enables reentry to occur results from the nonuniform anisotropic properties, and not from alterations in transmembrane potentials. However, there are no data from experimental studies at present to show what such circuits look like and to characterize their properties. Conduction might be expected to be slow around the entire circuit, although probably not uniformly slow.

Studies on infarct structure also indicate that ventricular tachycardia in healing or healed infarcts can sometimes be the result of anatomical reentry. Depression of transmembrane action potentials may sometimes play a role in causing slow conduction in the circuits. In the canine model of left anterior descending coronary artery occlusion, anatomical reentry has been found in the epicardial border zones in which conduction velocities were depressed and in which there were regions of block evident during sinus rhythm or ventricular stimulation. Block occurred that was formed in regions where there were no surviving epicardial muscle bundles (Saltman et al. 1987; Saltman 1990). Reentrant excitation causing tachycardia revolved around this anatomical obstacle. In Figure 4.63, we described an activation map, during ventricular stimulation, of an epicardial border zone of a healing infarct with a region of anatomical block. The activation map of this same epicardial border zone during sustained ventricular tachycardia is shown in Figure 4.72. There are two reentrant excitation waves, each traveling in a circle around a region of conduction block, indicated by the thick black lines. Activation of the circuit at the left begins within the 10-msec isochrone (asterisk towards the apex) and moves around the area of anatomical block that was evident during ventricular pacing as indicated by the arrows. Activation of the circuit at the right begins within the 10-msec isochrone towards the lateral margin (asterisk) and moves around a region of functional block that only occurred during tachycardia. Lines of anatomical block need not be parallel to the myocardial fiber long axis (as is functional block in anisotropic reentry) although in this example part of the anatomical block is in that direction. Conduction velocities in the circuit in Figure 4.72 were slow both parallel and perpendicular to the long axis of the muscle bundles, unlike anisotropic reentry because transmembrane potentials were probably depressed. However, the circulating reentrant wave front still moves both parallel and transverse to the orientation of the myocardial fiber bundles as it travels around the areas of block and, therefore conduction veloc-

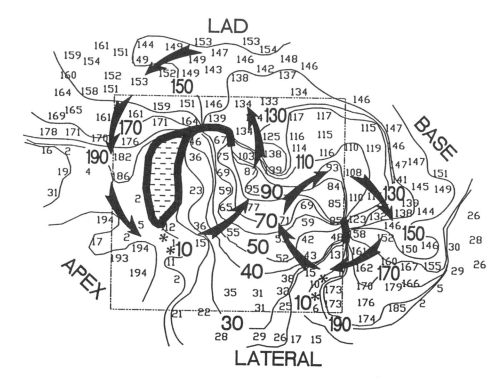

Figure 4.72: Activation map of a reentrant circuit in the epicardial border zone of a 4-day-old canine infarct during sustained ventricular tachycardia. The margins of the electrode array adjacent to the left anterior descending coronary artery (LAD), apex, lateral left ventricle and base are labeled. The small numbers are activation times at each of the recording sites. Isochrones are drawn at 10-msec intervals and are labeled with large numbers. The asterisk indicates the beginning of activation in this time window, the arrows point out the sequence of activation. The region of dashed lines is a region of conduction block. (Unpublished results of A.E. Saltman, J. Coromilas, and A.L. Wit.)

ity in regions where the wave fronts move parallel to the long axis of the fiber orientation are usually faster than conduction velocities in directions perpendicular to this orientation. The revolution time around anatomical circuits is longer than around the functional anisotropic circuits because of the larger regions of central block and the slower all-around conduction velocities caused by the depressed transmembrane potentials, leading to a longer tachycardia cycle length (Saltman 1990). Although anisotropic circuits have an excitable gap, the excitable gap of anatomical circuits is generally larger because of the short wavelength caused by slow conduction around the entire circuit and the longer path length resulting from a large anatomical obstacle. Therefore, in this experimental model of the epicardial border zone, the kind of circuit (functional or anatomical) and the cause of slow conduction in the circuit (anisotropy or depressed action potentials), can have significant effects on the properties of the tachycardia.

Other kinds of anatomical circuits in canine infarcts may involve intramural pathways of surviving bundles as was shown in Figure 4.45. As we discussed, such intramural pathways may occur after coronary occlusions that are distal along the artery or after reperfusion. Slow conduction in these circuits might still be caused by anisotropy: activation transverse to the long axis of parallel oriented muscle fibers, or slow activation in regions of fiber disarray. Slow conduction might also be the result of depressed transmembrane potentials. There are no data available to identify the cause of the slow conduction in intramural pathways at this time. The size of the anatomical circuits involving intramural pathways appears to be larger than functional circuits in the epicardial border zone and, therefore might cause tachycardias with longer cycle lengths.

Therefore, to briefly summarize, studies on reentry in experimental healing canine infarcts have shown that it may be either functional or anatomical. The exact mechanism for the functional block has not been directly proven but might sometimes be analogous to the leading circle mechanism. The anatomical block probably results from damage that is incurred during the prolonged ischemia that leads to infarction. Slow conduction in the reentrant circuits may have more than one mechanism. In some instances it may be caused by anisotropic properties of the surviving muscle that forms the reentrant circuit, while in others it may result from depression of the transmembrane action potentials. The different properties of reentrant circuits in different hearts are manifested as different properties of the tachycardia. Tachycardias caused by reentry in a circuit with anatomical block and depressed conduction have slower rates and larger excitable gaps than tachycardias caused by reentry in functional circuits with slow conduction caused only by anisotropy.

How do these data on mechanisms of reentry in experimental infarction apply to clinical tachycardia? We will make some suggestions, recognizing that there are no clinical mapping data from patients with healing infarcts, the kind of infarcts in which most of the circuits have been mapped in experimental models. The reentrant circuits we described from the clinical studies were in patients with healed infarcts, some of which were also characterized by the presence of aneurysms. The clinical mapping studies also suggest that the reentrant circuits are often in the endocardial border zone while the reentrant circuits we have emphasized in the experimental models are often in the epicardial border zone. It therefore might seem impossible to relate the experimental arrhythmias to the clinical ones. However, the mechanisms for reentry in the experimental models may not be dependent on an epicardial location of the circuits, or the fact that the infarcts are healing, rather than healed. The same mechanisms might occur in intramural circuits or subendocardial circuits in healing or healed infarcts when and where there are surviving parallel bundles of muscle fibers. In looking at both the epicardial and endocardial activation maps during clinical reentrant tachycardia, many of the features of the reentrant circuits which were described for the canine epicardial border zone are also apparent. For example, the lines of block seem to appear only during reentrant tachycardia and not during sinus rhythm or pacing, suggesting that the circuits sometimes are functional. Evidence for functional circuits not only comes from mapping studies, but also from some of the studies in which the site of tachycardia origin was stimulated both during sinus rhythm and during tachycardia. Activation maps of the reentrant circuits in human hearts also may show the "figure-of-eight" pattern that often occurs in the experimental models. The double reentrant loops with the common central conducting pathway that constitute this pattern can be a result of anisotropic reentry. Unfortunately it is not possible to determine the orientation of the myocardial fiber bundles in the published clinical maps to decipher whether slow conduction in the circuit is primarily a result of activation transverse to the long axis of the fiber bundles. Alternatively there may not be parallel oriented bundles in circuits where there is slow activation in all directions around the circuit. Similar kinds of reentrant circuits might also occur in regions where mapping studies suggested a focal site of origin. The circuits may be too small to delineate with the electrode arrays that have been used and that have a relatively low spatial resolution because of widely separated electrode contacts. The occurrence of fractionated electrograms expected to be found in regions of slow conduction in anisotropic reentrant circuits also occurs in reentrant circuits in human infarcts.

The presence of anatomical reentrant circuits has also been suggested by some of the clinical activation maps that have been discussed in previous sections. Reentry around the peripheral edges of an aneurysm constitutes anatomical reentry and the aneurysm represents the central anatomical obstacle. The activation maps shown in Figure 4.49 can be interpreted to result from reentrant circuits that are at least partly made up of narrow, intramural fiber bundles that provide long anatomical pathways for reentry. Activation through these pathways might be slow either because the transmembrane potentials of the muscle fibers constituting them are depressed or because the muscle fibers are poorly coupled to one another. Some of these circuits might also have functional components, as well as the discrete anatomical pathways, and be a combination of anisotropic and anatomical reentry.

Therefore, the evidence indicates that there are a number of different mechanisms for reentry causing clinical tachycardia. The mechanism depends on the anatomical organization of the infarct, which to some extent may be dependent on the stage of healing. As in the experimental models, there may be functional, anisotropic or anatomical circuits. Action potentials within the circuits may be normal and slow conduction dependent on structural changes in the muscle fibers or action potentials may be depressed causing slow conduction. The mechanism for reentry that is present in the heart undoubtedly influences characteristics of the tachycardia such as its rate or the presence of an excitable gap. The mechanism may also determine whether a tachycardia is nonsustained, sustained or degenerates into ventricular fibrillation. However, the exact relationships among the structure of reentrant circuits, the electrophysiological properties of the myocardial cells in the circuit, and the nature of the arrhythmias are yet to be determined.

References

Abe, S., Y. Nagamoto, Y. Fukuchi, T. Hayakawa, and A. Kuroiwa. Relationship of alternans of monophasic action potential and conduction delay inside the ischemic border zone to serious ventricular arrhythmia during acute myocardial ischemia in dogs. *Am. Heart J.* 117: 1223–1233, 1989.

Abete, P., R. Bernabei, M. Di Gennaro, G. Iacono, F. Rengo, P. Carbonin, and M. Vassalle. Electrical and ionic mechanisms of early reperfusion arrhythmias in sheep cardiac Purkinje's fibers. *J. Electrocardiol.* 21: 199–212, 1988.

Abrahamsson, T., O. Almgren, and L. Carlsson. Ischemia-induced noradrenaline release in the isolated rat heart: Influence of perfusion substrate and duration of ischemia. *J. Mol. Cell Cardiol.* 15: 821–830, 1983.

Adamantidis, M.M., J.F Caron, and B.A. Dupuis. Triggered activity induced by combined mild hypoxia and acidosis in guinea-pig Purkinje fibers. *J. Mol. Cell Cardiol.* 18: 1287–1299, 1986.

Adgey, A.A.J. Initiation of ventricular fibrillation outside hospital. In: *Acute Phase of Ischemic Heart Disease and Myocardial Infarction,* edited by A.A.J. Adgey. Martinus Nijhoff Publishers, The Hague: 1982, pp. 67–76.

Agus, Z.S., and M. Morad. Modulation of cardiac ion channels by magnesium. *Annu. Rev. Physiol.* 53: 299–307, 1991.

Akhtar, M., A.N. Damato, W.P. Batsford, J.N. Ruskin, J.B. Ogunkelu, and G. Vargas. Demonstration of re-entry within the His-Purkinje system in man. *Circulation* 50: 1150–1162, 1974.

Akhtar, M., C. Gilbert, F.G. Wolf, and D.H. Schmidt. Reentry within the His-Purkinje system. Elucidation of reentrant circuit using right bundle branch and His bundle recordings. *Circulation* 58: 295–304, 1978.

Akhtar, M. Supraventricular tachycardias. Electrophysiologic mechanisms, diagnosis, and pharmacologic therapy. In: *Tachycardias: Mechanisms, Diagnosis, Treatment,* edited by M.E. Josephson and H.J.J. Wellens. Lea & Febiger, Philadelphia: 1984, pp. 137–169.

Aksnes, G., Ø. Ellingsen, D.L. Rutlen, and A. Ilebekk. Myocardial K^+ repletion and rise in contractility after brief ischemic periods in the pig. *J. Mol. Cell. Cardiol.* 21: 681–690, 1989a.

Aksnes, G., Ø. Ellingsen, D.L. Rutlen, and A. Ilebekk. Effects of hemodynamic variables on myocardial K^+ balance during and after shortlasting ischemia. *J. Mol. Cell. Cardiol.* 21: 1273–1284, 1989b.

Allen, D.G., and C.H. Orchard. Intracellular calcium concentration during hypoxia and metabolic inhibition in mammalian ventricular muscle. *J. Physiol.* 339: 107–122, 1983.

Allen, D.G. and C.H. Orchard. Myocardial contractile function during ischemia and hypoxia. *Circ. Res.* 60: 153–168, 1987.

Allen, J.B., and J.R. Laadt. The effect of the level of the ligature on mortality following ligation of the circumflex coronary artery in the dog. *Am. Heart J.* 39: 273–278, 1950.

Allen, J.D., and A.L. Wit. Some observations on abnormal pacemaker activity in endocardial Purkinje fibres surviving myocardial infarction. *J. Physiol.* 263: 248P-249P, 1976.

Allen, J.D., F.J. Brennan, and A.L. Wit. Actions of lidocaine on transmembrane potentials of subendocardial Purkinje fibers surviving in infarcted canine hearts. *Circ. Res.* 43: 470–481, 1978.

Allessie, M.A., F.I.M. Bonke, and F.J.G. Schopman. Circus movement in rabbit atrial muscle as a mechanism of tachycardia. *Circ. Res.* 33: 54–62, 1973.

Allessie, M.A., F.I.M. Bonke, and F.J.G. Schopman. Circus movement in rabbit atrial muscle as a mechanism of tachycardia. II. The role of nonuniform recovery of excitability in the occurrence of unidirectional block, as studied with multiple microelectrodes. *Circ. Res.* 39: 168–177, 1976.

Allessie, M.A., F.I.M. Bonke, and F.J.G. Schopman. Circus movement in rabbit atrial muscle as a mechanism of tachycardia. III. The "leading circle" concept: A new model of circus movement in cardiac tissue without the involvement of an anatomical obstacle. *Circ. Res.* 41: 9–18, 1977.

Allessie, M.A., W.J.E.P. Lammers, F.I.M. Bonke, and J. Hollen. Intra-atrial reentry as a mechanism for atrial flutter induced by acetylcholine and rapid pacing in the dog. *Circulation* 70: 123–135, 1984.

Allessie, M.A., W.J.E.P. Lammers, F.I.M. Bonke, and J. Hollen. Experimental evaluation of Moe's multiple wavelet hypothesis of atrial fibrillation. In: *Cardiac Electrophysiology and Arrhythmias*, edited by D.P. Zipes, and J. Jalife. Grune and Stratton, Orlando: 1985, pp. 265–275.

Allessie, M.A., M.J. Schalij, M.S.P. Huybers, L.V.A. Boersma. Ventricular anisotropy causes an excitable gap in reentry without an anatomic obstacle. *Circulation* 78(Suppl II): II-612, 1988.

Allessie, M.A., M.J. Schalij, C.J.H.J. Kirchhof, L. Boersma, M. Huybers, and J. Hollen. Experimental electrophysiology and arrhythmogenicity. Anisotropy and ventricular tachycardia. *Eur. Heart J.* 10(Suppl. E): 2–8, 1989.

Almendral, J.M., C. Gottlieb, F.E. Marchlinski, A.E. Buxton, J.U. Doherty, and M.E. Josephson. Entrainment of ventricular tachycardia by atrial depolarizations. *Am. J. Cardiol.* 56: 298–304, 1985.

Almendral, J.M., M.E. Rosenthal, N.J. Stamato, F.E. Marchlinski, A.E. Buxton, L.H. Frame, J.M. Miller, and M.E. Josephson. Analysis of the resetting phenomenon in sustained uniform ventricular tachycardia: incidence and relation to termination. *J. Am. Coll. Cardiol.* 8: 294–300, 1986a.

Almendral, J.M., N.J. Stamato, M.E. Rosenthal, F.E. Marchlinski, J.M. Miller, and M.E. Josephson. Resetting response patterns during sustained ventricular tachycardia: relationship to the excitable gap. *Circulation* 74: 722–730, 1986b.

Almendral, J.M., C.D. Gottlieb, M.E. Rosenthal, N.J. Stamato, A.E. Buxton, F.E. Marchlinski, J.M. Miller, and M.E. Josephson. Entrainment of ventricular tachycardia: explanation for surface electrocardiographic phenomena by analysis of electrograms recorded within the tachycardia circuit. *Circulation* 77: 569–580, 1988.

Anderson, K.P., C.D. Swerdlow, and J.W. Mason. Entrainment of ventricular tachycardia. *Am. J. Cardiol.* 53: 335–340, 1984.

Antzelevitch, C., J. Jalife, and G.K. Moe. Characteristics of reflection as a mechanism of reentrant arrhythmias and its relationship to parasystole. *Circulation* 61: 182–191, 1980.

Antzelevitch, C., and G.K. Moe. Electrotonically mediated delayed conduction and reentry in relation to "slow responses" in mammalian ventricular conducting tissue. *Circ. Res.* 49: 1129–1139, 1981.

Aomine, M., S. Nobe and M. Arita. Electrophysiologic effects of a short-chain acyl carnitine, L-propionylcarnitine, on isolated canine Purkinje fibers. *J. Cardiovasc. Pharmacol.* 13: 494–501, 1989.

Araki, H., Y. Koiwaya, O. Nakagaki, and M. Nakamura. Diurnal distribution of ST-segment elevation and related arrhythmias in patients with variant angina: a study by ambulatory ECG monitoring. *Circulation* 67: 995–1000, 1983.

Argentieri, T.M., L.H. Frame, and T.J. Colatsky. Electrical properties of canine subendocardial Purkinje fibers surviving in 1-day-old experimental myocardial infarction. *Circ. Res.* 66: 123–134, 1990.

Arita, M., and T. Kiyosue. Modification of "depressed fast channel dependent slow conduction" by lidocaine and verapamil in the presence or absence of catecholamines. Evidence for alteration of preferential ionic channels for slow conduction. *Jpn. Circ. J.* 47: 68–81, 1983.

Arlock, P., and B.G. Katzung. Effects of sodium substitutes on transient inward current and tension in guinea-pig and ferret papillary muscle. *J. Physiol.* 360: 105–120, 1985.

Armour, J.A., G.R. Hageman, and W.C. Randall. Arrhythmias induced by local cardiac nerve stimulation. *Am. J. Physiol.* 223: 1068–1075, 1972.

Arnsdorf, M.F., and G.J. Sawicki. The effects of lysophosphatidylcholine, a toxic metabolite of ischemia, on the components of cardiac excitability in sheep Purkinje fibers. *Circ. Res.* 49: 16–30, 1981.

Aronson, R.S., J.M. Gelles, and B.F. Hoffman. Effect of ouabain on the current underlying spontaneous diastolic depolarization in cardiac Purkinje fibres. *Nature New Biol.* 245: 118–120, 1973.

Aronson, R.S., and P.F. Cranefield. The effect of resting potential on the electrical activity of canine cardiac Purkinje fibers exposed to Na-free solution or to ouabain. *Pflügers Arch.* 347: 101–116, 1974.

Aronson, R.S., and J.M. Gelles. The effect of ouabain, dinitrophenol, and lithium on the pacemaker current in sheep cardiac Purkinje fibers. *Circ. Res.* 40: 517–524, 1977.

Aronson, R.S. Characteristics of action potentials of hypertrophied myocardium from rats with renal hypertension. *Circ. Res.* 47: 443–454, 1980.

Aronson, R.S. Afterpotentials and triggered activity in hypertrophied myocardium from rats with renal hypertension. *Circ. Res.* 48: 720–727, 1981.

Aronson, R.S., P.F. Cranefield, and A.L. Wit. The effects of caffeine and ryanodine on the electrical activity of the canine coronary sinus. *J. Physiol.* 368: 593–610, 1985.

Assadi, M., M. Restivo, W.B. Gough, and N. El-Sherif. Reentrant ventricular arrhythmias in the late myocardial infarction period: 17. Correlation of activation patterns of sinus and reentrant ventricular tachycardia. *Am. Heart J.* 119: 1014–1024, 1990.

Attwell, D., I. Cohen, D. Eisner, M. Ohba, and C. Ojeda. The steady state TTX-sensitive ("window") sodium current in cardiac Purkinje fibres. *Pflügers Arch.* 379: 137–142, 1979.

Bache, R.J. Can drugs really limit infarct size? In: *Therapeutic Approaches to Infarct Size Limitation,* edited by D.J. Hearse and D.M. Yellon. Raven Press, New York: 1984, pp. 185–208.

Bagdonas, A.A., J.H. Stuckey, J. Piera, N.S. Amer, and B.F. Hoffman. Effects of ischemia and hypoxia on the specialized conducting system of the canine heart. *Am. Heart J.* 61: 206–218, 1961.

Bailey, J.C., K. Greenspan, M.V. Elizari, G.J. Anderson, and C. Fisch. Effects of acetylcholine on automaticity and conduction in the proximal portion of the His-Purkinje specialized conduction system of the dog. *Circ. Res.* 30: 210–216, 1972.

Bailey, J.C., A.M. Watanabe, H.R. Besch Jr., and D.A. Lathrop. Acetylcholine antagonism of the electrophysiological effects of isoproterenol on canine cardiac Purkinje fibers. *Circ. Res.* 44: 378–383, 1979.

Bailie, D.S., H. Inoue, S. Kaseda, J. Ben-David, and D.P. Zipes. Magnesium suppression of early afterdepolarizations and ventricular tachyarrhythmias induced by cesium in dogs. *Circulation* 77: 1395–1402, 1988.

Baker, P.F., M.P. Blaustein, A.L. Hodgkin, and R.A. Steinhardt. The influence of calcium on sodium efflux in squid axons. *J. Physiol.* 200: 431–458, 1969.

Balke, C.W., E. Kaplinsky, E.L. Michelson, M. Naito, and L.S. Dreifus. Reperfusion ventricular tachyarrhythmias: Correlation with antecedent coronary artery occlusion tachyarrhythmias and duration of myocardial ischemia. *Am. Heart J.* 101: 449–456, 1981.

Balke, C.W., M.D. Lesh, J.F. Spear, A. Kadish, J.H. Levine, and E.N. Moore. Effects of cellular uncoupling on conduction in anisotropic canine ventricular myocardium. *Circ. Res.* 63: 879–892, 1988.

Balschi, J.A., J.C. Frazer, J.K. Fetters, K. Clarke, C.S. Springer, T.W. Smith, and J.S. Ingwall. Shift reagent and Na-23 nuclear magnetic resonance discriminates between extra and intra cellular sodium pools in ischemic heart. (abstract) *Circulation* 72(Suppl. III): III-355, 1985.

Barber, M.J., T.M. Mueller, D.P. Henry, S.Y. Felten, and D.P. Zipes. Transmural myocardial infarction in the dog produces sympathectomy in noninfarcted myocardium. *Circulation* 67: 787–796, 1983.

Barber, M.J., T.M. Mueller, B.G. Davies, and D.P. Zipes. Phenol topically applied to canine left ventricular epicardium interrupts sympathetic but not vagal afferents. *Circ. Res.* 55: 532–544, 1984.

Barber, M.J., T.M. Mueller, B.G. Davies, R.M. Gill, and D.P. Zipes. Interruption of sympathetic and vagal-mediated afferent responses by transmural myocardial infarction. *Circulation* 72: 623–631, 1985.

Bardaji, A., J. Cinca, F. Worner, and A. Schoenenberger. Effects of anaesthesia on acute ischaemic arrhythmias and epicardial electrograms in the pig heart in situ. *Cardiovasc. Res.* 24: 227–231, 1990.

Bardy, G.H., W.M. Smith, R.M. Ungerleider, J.L. Cox, J.J. Gallagher, and R.E. Ideker. Identification of reproducible ventricular tachycardia in a canine model. *Am. J. Cardiol.* 53: 619–625, 1984.

Barr, R.C., and M.S. Spach. Sampling rates required for digital recording of intracellular and extracellular cardiac potentials. *Circulation* 55: 40–48, 1977.

Bassett, A.L., J.J. Fenoglio Jr., A.L. Wit, R.J. Myerburg, and H. Gelband. Electrophysiologic and ultrastuctural characteristics of the canine tricuspid valve. *Am. J. Physiol.* 230: 1366–1373, 1976.

Bassett, A.L., H. Gelband, K. Nilsson, A.R. Morales, and R.J. Myerburg. Electrophysiology following healed experimental myocardial infarction. In: *Reentrant Arrhythmias: Mechanisms and Treatment*, edited by H.E. Kulbertus. University Park Press, Baltimore: 1977, pp. 242–255.

Bassingthwaighte, J.B., C.H. Fry, and J.A.S. McGuigan. Relationship between internal calcium and outward current in mammalian ventricular muscle; A mechanism for the control of the action potential duration? *J. Physiol.* 262: 15–37, 1976.

Batsford, W.P., D.S. Cannom, and B.L. Zaret. Relationship between ventricular refractoriness and regional myocardial blood flow after acute coronary occlusion. *Am. J. Cardiol.* 41: 1083–1088, 1978.

Battle, W.E., S. Naimi, B. Avitall, A.H. Brilla, J.S. Banas, J.M. Bete, and H.J. Levine. Distinctive time course of ventricular vulnerability to fibrillation during and after release of coronary ligation. *Am. J. Cardiol.* 34: 42–47, 1974.

Baumgarten, C.M., C.J. Cohen, and T.F. McDonald. Heterogeneity of intracellular potassium activity and membrane potential in hypoxic guinea pig ventricle. *Circ. Res.* 49: 1181–1189, 1981.

Baumgarten, C.M., and H.A. Fozzard. The resting and pacemaker potentials. In: *The Heart and Cardiovascular System,* edited by H.A. Fozzard, E. Haber, R.B. Jennings, A.M. Katz, and H.E. Morgan. Raven Press, New York: 1986, pp. 601–626.

Bayés de Luna, A., P. Torner, J. Guindo, M. Soler, and F. Oca. Holler. ECG study of ambulatory sudden death. Review of 158 published cases. *New Trends in Arrhythmias* 1: 293–297, 1985.

Bayés de Luna, A., P. Coumel, and J.F. Leclercq. Ambulatory sudden cardiac death: mechanisms of production of fatal arrhythmia on the basis of data from 157 cases. *Am. Heart J.* 117: 151–159, 1989.

Bean, B.P. Two kinds of calcium channels in canine atrial cells. Differences in kinetics, selectivity and pharmacology. *J. Gen. Physiol.* 86: 1–30, 1985.

Becker, L.C., R. Ferreira, and M. Thomas. Mapping of left ventricular blood flow with radioactive microspheres in experimental coronary artery occlusion. *Cardiovasc. Res.* 7: 391–400, 1973.

Beeler, G.W. Jr., and H. Reuter. Voltage clamp experiments on ventricular myocardial fibers. *J. Physiol.* 207: 165–190, 1970.

Begold, A. Von den Vernderungen des Herzschlages nach Verschliessung der Coronararterien. *Untersuch. Physiol. Lab. Wurzb.* 2: 256–287, 1867.

Belardinelli, L., and G. Isenberg. Actions of adenosine and isoproterenol on isolated mammalian ventricular myocytes. *Circ. Res.* 53: 287–297, 1983.

Ben-David, J., and D.P. Zipes. Differential response to right and left ansae subclaviae stimulation of early afterdepolarizations and ventricular tachycardia induced by cesium in dogs. *Circulation* 78: 1241–1250, 1988.

Bennett, M.A., and B.L. Pentecost. Reversion of ventricular tachycardia by pacemaker stimulation. *Br. Heart J.* 33: 922–927, 1971.

Benzing, H., G. Gebert, and M. Strohm. Extracellular acid-base changes in the dog myocardium during hypoxia and local ischemia, measured by means of glass micro-electrodes. *Cardiology* 56: 85–88, 1971/1972.

Berger, M.D., H.L. Waxman, A.E. Buxton, F.E. Marchlinski, and M.E. Josephson. Spontaneous compared with induced onset of sustained ventricular tachycardia. *Circulation* 78: 885–892, 1988.

Bernstein, R.C., and L.H. Frame. Ventricular reentry around a fixed barrier. Resetting with advancement in an in vitro model. *Circulation* 81: 267–280, 1990.

Bersohn, M.M., K.D. Philipson, and J.Y. Fukushima. Sodium-calcium exchange and sarcolemmal enzymes in ischemic rabbit hearts. *Am. J. Physiol.* 242: C288-C295, 1982.

Bhandari, A.K., W.A. Shapiro, F. Morady, E.N. Shen, J. Mason, and M.M. Scheinman. Electrophysiologic testing in patients with the long QT syndrome. *Circulation* 71: 63–71, 1985.

Bhandari, A.K., P.K. Au, J.S. Rose, A. Kotlewski, S. Blue, and S.H. Rahimtoola. Decline in inducibility of sustained ventricular tachycardia from two to twenty weeks after acute myocardial infarction. *Am. J. Cardiol.* 59: 284–290, 1987.

Bigger, J.T. Jr., and B.N. Goldreyer. The mechanism of supraventricular tachycardia. *Circulation* 42: 673–688, 1970.

Bigger, J.T. Jr., R.J. Dresdale, R.H. Heissenbuttel, F.M. Weld, and A.L. Wit. Ventricular arrhythmias in ischemic heart disease: Mechanism, prevalence, significance, and management. *Prog. Cardiovasc. Dis.* 19: 255–300, 1977.

Bigger, J.T. Jr., F.M. Weld, and L.M. Rolnitzky. Prevalence, characteristics and significance of ventricular tachycardia (three or more complexes) detected with ambulatory electrocardiographic recording in the late hospital phase of acute myocardial infarction. *Am. J. Cardiol.* 48: 815–823, 1981.

Bigger, J.T. Jr., F.M. Weld, and L.M. Rolnitzky. Which postinfarction ventricular arrhythmias should be treated? *Am. Heart. J.* 103: 660–664, 1982.

Bigger, J.T. Jr., J.L. Fleiss, R. Kleiger, J.P. Miller, L.M. Rolnitzky, and the Multicenter Post-infarction Research Group. The relationships among ventricular arrhythmias, left ventricular dysfunction, and mortality in the 2 years after myocardial infarction. *Circulation* 69: 250–258, 1984.

Bigger, J.T. Jr., J.L. Fleiss, L.M. Rolnitzky, and the Multicenter Post-infarction Research Group. Prevalence, characteristics and significance of ventricular tachycardia detected by 24-hour continuous electrocardiographic recordings in the late hospital phase of acute myocardial infarction. *Am. J. Cardiol.* 58: 1151–1160, 1986a.

Bigger, J.T. Jr., L.M. Rolnitzky, and J. Merab. Epidemiology of ventricular arrhythmias and clinical trials with antiarrhythmic drugs. In: *The Heart and Cardiovascular System,* edited by H.A. Fozzard, E. Haber, R.B. Jennings, A.M. Katz, and H.E. Morgan. Raven Press, New York: 1986b, pp. 1405–1448.

Billman, G.E., P.J. Schwartz, and H.L. Stone. Baroreceptor reflex control of heart rate: a predictor of sudden cardiac death. *Circulation* 66: 874–880, 1982.

Binah, O., I.S. Cohen, and M.R. Rosen. The effects of adriamycin on normal and ouabain toxic canine Purkinje and ventricular muscle fibers. *Circ. Res.* 53: 655–662, 1983.

Binah, O., I. Rubinstein, B. Felzen, Y. Sweed, and S. Mager. Thyroid hormones and cardiac function. In: *Lethal Arrhythmias Resulting from Myocardial Ischemia and Infarction,* edited by M.R. Rosen, and Y. Palti. Kluwer Academic Publishers, Boston: 1989, pp. 117–128.

Bishop, S.P., F.C. White, and C.M. Bloor. Regional myocardial blood flow during acute myocardial infarction in the conscious dog. *Circ. Res.* 38: 429–438, 1976.

Blake, K., N.A. Smith, and W.T. Clusin. Rate dependence of ischaemic myocardial depolarisation: Evidence for a novel membrane current. *Cardiovasc. Res.* 20: 557–562, 1986.

Blake, K., W.T. Clusin, M.R. Franz, and N.A. Smith. Mechanism of depolarization in the ischaemic dog heart: Discrepancy between T-Q potentials and potassium accumulation. *J. Physiol.* 397: 307–330, 1988.

Blumgart, H.L., H.E. Hoff, M. Landowne, and M.J. Schlesinger. Experimental studies on the effect of temporary occlusion of coronary arteries in producing persistent electrocardiographic changes. *Am. J. Med. Sci.* 194: 493–502, 1937.

Blumgart, H.L., D.R. Gilligan, and M.J. Schlesinger. Experimental studies on the effect of temporary occlusion of coronary arteries. II. The production of myocardial infarction. *Am. Heart J.* 22: 374–389, 1941.

Boineau, J.P., and J.L. Cox. Slow ventricular activation in acute myocardial infarction. A source of re-entrant premature ventricular contraction. *Circulation* 48: 702–713, 1973.

Boineau, J.P., R.B. Schuessler, C.R. Mooney, A.C. Wylds, C.B. Miller, R.D.

Hudson, J.M. Borremans, and C.W. Brockus. Multicentric origin of the atrial depolarization wave: the pacemaker complex. Relation to dynamics of atrial conduction, P-wave changes and heart rate control. *Circulation* 58: 1036–1048, 1978.

Bolick, D.R., D.B. Hackel, K.A. Reimer, and R.E. Ideker. Quantitative analysis of myocardial infarct structure in patients with ventricular tachycardia. *Circulation* 74: 1266–1279, 1986.

Bolli, R., M.L. Myers, W.-X. Zhu, and R. Roberts. Disparity of reperfusion arrhythmias after reversible myocardial ischemia in open chest and conscious dogs. *J. Am. Coll. Cardiol.* 7: 1047–1056, 1986.

Bonke, F.I.M., L.N. Bouman, and H.E. van Rijn. Change of cardiac rhythm in the rabbit after an atrial premature beat. *Circ. Res.* 24: 533–544, 1969.

Borgers, M., F. de Clerck, J. van Reempts, R. Xhonneux, and J. Neuten. Selective blockade of cellular calcium overload by flunarizine. *Int. Angiol.* 3: 25–31, 1984.

Borggrefe, M., K. Haerten, and G. Breithardt. Electrophysiological characteristics of stimulus-induced ventricular tachycardia after myocardial infarction. (abstract) *J. Am. Coll. Cardiol.* 5: 471, 1985.

Boutjdir, M., N. El-Sherif, and W.B. Gough. Effects of caffeine and ryanodine on delayed afterdepolarizations and sustained rhythmic activity in 1-day-old myocardial infarction in the dog. *Circulation* 81: 1393–1400, 1990.

Boyden, P.A., P.F. Cranefield, and D.C. Gadsby. Noradrenaline hyperpolarizes cells of the canine coronary sinus by increasing their permeability to potassium ions. *J. Physiol.* 339: 185–206, 1983.

Boyden, P.A., L.P. Tilley, A. Albala, S.K. Liu, J.J. Fenoglio Jr., and A.L. Wit. Mechanisms for atrial arrhythmias associated with cardiomyopathy: a study of feline hearts with primary myocardial disease. *Circulation* 69: 1036–1047, 1984.

Boyden, P.A. Activation sequence during atrial flutter in dogs with surgically induced right atrial enlargement: I. Observations during sustained rhythms. *Circ. Res.* 62:596–608, 1988.

Boyden, P.A., P.I. Gardner, and A.L. Wit. Action potentials of cardiac muscle in healing infarcts: response to norepinephrine and caffeine. *J. Mol. Cell. Cardiol.* 20: 525–537, 1988.

Boyden, P.A., A. Albala, and K.P. Dresdner Jr. Electrophysiology and ultrastructure of canine subendocardial Purkinje cells isolated from control and 24-hour infarcted hearts. *Circ. Res.* 65: 955–970, 1989a.

Boyden, P.A., L.H. Frame, and B.F. Hoffman. Activation mapping of reentry around an anatomic barrier in the canine atrium. Observations during entrainment and termination. *Circulation* 79: 406–416, 1989b.

Boyden, P.A., and K.P. Dresdner Jr. Electrogenic N^+-K^+ pump in Purkinje myocytes isolated from control noninfarcted and infarcted hearts. *Am. J. Physiol.* 258: H766-H772, 1990.

Bozler, E. The initiation of impulses in cardiac muscle. *Am. J. Physiol.* 138: 273–282, 1943.

Brachmann, J., G. Kabell, B.J. Scherlag, L. Harrison, and R. Lazzara. Analysis of interectopic activation patterns during sustained ventricular tachycardia. *Circulation* 67: 449–456, 1983a.

Brachmann, J., B.J. Scherlag, L.V. Rosenshtraukh, and R. Lazzara. Bradycardia-dependent triggered activity: relevance to drug-induced multiform ventricular tachycardia. *Circulation* 68: 846–856, 1983b.

Breithardt, G., L. Seipel, and F. Loogen. Sinus node recovery time and calculated sinoatrial conduction time in normal subjects and patients with sinus node dysfunction. *Circulation* 56: 43–50, 1977.

Breithardt, G., M. Borggrefe, and K. Haerten. Role of programmed ventricular stimulation and noninvasive recording of ventricular late potentials for the identification of patients at risk of ventricular tachyarrhythmias after acute myocardial infarction. In: *Cardiac Electrophysiology and Arrhythmias,* edited by D.P. Zipes and J. Jalife. Grune and Stratton, Orlando: 1985, pp. 553–561.

Brennan, F.J., P.F. Cranefield, and A.L. Wit. Effects of lidocaine on slow response and depressed fast response action potentials of canine cardiac Purkinje fibers. *J. Pharmacol. Exp. Ther.* 204: 312–324, 1978.

Brennan, F.J., and J.R. Bonn. Effects of ouabain on the electrophysiological properties of subendocardial Purkinje fibers surviving in regions of acute myocardial infarction. *Am. Heart J.* 100: 201–212, 1980.

Brosnahan, G.F., R. Roberts, W.E. Shell, J. Ross Jr., and B.E. Sobel. Deleterious effects due to hemorrhage after myocardial reperfusion. *Am. J. Cardiol.* 33: 82–86, 1974.

Bril, A., A.A.A. Kinnaird, and R.Y.K. Man. Comparison of the sodium currents in normal Purkinje fibres and Purkinje fibres surviving infarction—a pharmacological study. *Br. J. Pharmacol.* 97: 999–1006, 1989.

Brooks, C.McC., B.F. Hoffman, E.E. Suckling, and O. Orias. *Excitability of the Heart.* Grune & Stratton, New York, 1955.

Brooks, C.McC., J.L. Gilbert, M.E. Greenspan, G. Lange, and H.M. Mazzella. Excitability and electrical response of ischemic heart muscle. *Am. J. Physiol.* 198: 1143–1147, 1960.

Brooks, C.McC., J.L. Gilbert, and M.J. Janse. Failure of integrated cardiac action at supernormal heart rates. *Proc. Soc. Exptl. Biol. Med.* 117: 630–634, 1964.

Brown, B.S., T. Akera, and T.M. Brody. Mechanism of grayanotoxin III-induced afterpotentials in feline cardiac Purkinje fibers. *Eur. J. Pharmacol.* 75: 271–281, 1981.

Brown, H.F., and S.J. Noble. Membrane currents underlying delayed rectification and pace-maker activity in frog atrial muscle. *J. Physiol.* 204: 717–736, 1969.

Brown, H.F., and D. DiFrancesco. Voltage-clamp investigations of membrane currents underlying pace-maker activity in rabbit sino-atrial node. *J. Physiol.* 308: 331–351, 1980.

Brown, H.F. Electrophysiology of the sinoatrial node. *Physiol. Rev.* 62: 505–530, 1982.

Brown, H.F., J. Kimura, and S. Noble. The relative contributions of various time-dependent membrane currents to pacemaker activity in the sino atrial node. In: *Cardiac Rate and Rhythm: Physiological, Morphological and Developmental Aspects,* edited by L.N. Bouman, and H.J. Jongsma. Martinus Nijhoff, The Hague: 1982, pp. 53–68.

Brown, H.F., J. Kimura, D. Noble, S.J. Noble, and A. Taupignon. The slow inward current, i_{si}, in the rabbit sino-atrial node investigated by voltage clamp and computer simulation. *Proc. R. Soc. Lond. (Biol.)* B222: 305–328, 1984.

Browning, D.J., J.S. Tiedeman, A.L. Stagg, D.G. Benditt, M.M. Scheinman, and H.C. Strauss. Aspects of rate-related hyperpolarization in feline Purkinje fibers. *Circ. Res.* 44: 612–624, 1979.

Brugada, P., H. Abdollah, B. Heddle, and H.J.J. Wellens. Results of a ventricular stimulation protocol using a maximum of 4 premature stimuli in patients without documented or suspected ventricular arrhythmias. *Am. J. Cardiol.* 52: 1214–1218, 1983.

Brugada, P., and H.J.J. Wellens. Programmed electrical stimulation of the human heart. General principles. In: *Tachycardias: Mechanisms, Diagnosis, Treatment,* edited by M.E. Josephson, and H.J.J. Wellens. Lea & Febiger, Philadelphia: 1984a, pp. 61–89.

Brugada, P., and H.J.J. Wellens. The role of triggered activity in clinical ventricular arrhythmias. *PACE* 7: 260–271, 1984b.

Brugada, P., M. Green, H. Abdollah, and H.J.J. Wellens. Significance of ventricular arrhythmias initiated by programmed ventricular stimulation: the importance of the type of ventricular arrhythmia induced and the number of premature stimuli required. *Circulation* 69: 87–92, 1984.

Brugada, P., B. Waldecker, Y. Kersschot, M. Zehender, and H.J.J. Wellens. Ventricular arrhythmias initiated by programmed stimulation in four groups of patients with healed myocardial infarction. *J. Am. Coll. Cardiol.* 8: 1035–1040, 1986.

Brugada, P., and H.J.J. Wellens (editors). *Cardiac Arrhythmias: Where To Go From Here?* Futura Publishing Company, Inc., Mt. Kisco, New York: 1987.

Brugada, J., L. Boersma, C. Kirchhof, P. Brugada, M. Havenith, H.J.J. Wellens, and M.A. Allessie. Double-wave reentry as a mechanism of acceleration of ventricular tachycardia. *Circulation* 81: 1633–1643, 1990.

Bruyneel, K.J.J. Use of moving epicardial electrodes in defining ST-segment changes after acute coronary occlusion in the baboon. Relation to primary ventricular fibrillation. *Am. Heart J.* 89: 731–741, 1975.

Burdon-Sanderson, J., and F.J.M. Page. On the time-relations of the excitatory process in the ventricle of the heart of the frog. *J. Physiol.* 2: 384–429, 1879.

Buxton, A.E., H.L. Waxman, F.E. Marchlinski, W.J. Untereker, L.E. Waspe, and M.E. Josephson. Role of triple extrastimuli during electrophysiologic study of patients with documented sustained ventricular tachyarrhythmias. *Circulation* 69: 532–540, 1984a.

Buxton, A.E., H.L. Waxman, F.E. Marchlinski, and M.E. Josephson. Electrophysiologic characterization of nonsustained ventricular tachycardia. In:

Tachycardias: Mechanisms, Diagnosis, Treatment, edited by M.E. Josephson, and H.J.J. Wellens. Lea & Febiger, Philadelphia: 1984b, pp. 353–361.

Buxton, A.E., F.E. Marchlinski, B.T. Flores, J.M. Miller, J.U. Doherty, and M.E. Josephson. Nonsustained ventricular tachycardia in patients with coronary artery disease: role of electrophysiologic study. *Circulation* 75: 1178–1185, 1987.

Caceres, J., M. Jazayeri, J. McKinnie, B. Avitall, S.T. Denker, P. Tchou, and M. Akhtar. Sustained bundle branch reentry as a mechanism of clinical tachycardia. *Circulation* 79: 256–270, 1989.

Califf, R.M., R.A. McKinnis, J.F. McNeer, F.E. Harrell Jr., K.L. Lee, D.B. Pryor, R.A. Waugh, P.J. Harris, R.A. Rosati, and G.S. Wagner. Prognostic value of ventricular arrhythmias associated with treadmill exercise testing in patients studied with cardiac catheterization for suspected ischemic heart disease. *J. Am. Coll. Cardiol.* 2: 1060–1067, 1983.

Cameron, J.S., G.H. Dersham, and J. Han. Effects of epinephrine on the electrophysiologic properties of Purkinje fibers surviving myocardial infarction. *Am. Heart J.* 104: 551–560, 1982.

Cameron, J.S., and J. Han. Effects of epinephrine on automaticity and the incidence of arrhythmias in Purkinje fibers surviving myocardial infarction. *J. Pharmacol. Exp. Ther.* 223: 573–579, 1982.

Cameron, J.S., R.J. Myerburg, S.S. Wong, M.S. Gaide, K. Epstein, R. Alvarez, H. Gelband, P.A. Guse, and A.L. Bassett. Electrophysiologic consequences of chronic experimentally induced left ventricular pressure overload. *J. Am. Coll. Cardiol.* 2: 481–487, 1983.

Cameron, J.S., and L.J. Antonik. Prevention of hypertension is associated with reduced susceptibility to histamine-induced arrhythmias in SHR. *Am. J. Hypertens.* 1: 34S–37S, 1988.

Campbell, R.W.F., A. Murray, and D.G. Julian. Ventricular arrhythmias in the first 12 hours of acute myocardial infarction. Natural history study. *Br. Heart J.* 46: 351–357, 1981.

Cannell, M.B., and W.J. Lederer. The arrhythmogenic current I_{TI} in the absence of electrogenic sodium-calcium exchange in sheep cardiac Purkinje fibres. *J. Physiol.* 374: 201–219, 1986.

Capucci, A., M.A.W. Fabius, R. Coronel, and M.J. Janse. Variability of refractory periods in acute ischemia as a possible mechanism of early arrhythmias. In: *New Frontiers of Arrhythmias,* edited by F. Furlanello, and M. Disertori. OIC Medical Press: 1984, pp. 7–17.

Cardinal, R., and B.I. Sasyniuk. Electrophysiological effects of bretylium tosylate on subendocardial Purkinje fibers from infarcted canine hearts. *J. Pharmacol. Exp. Ther.* 204: 159–174, 1978.

Cardinal, R., M.J. Janse, I. Van Eeden, G. Werner, C.N. Naumann d'Alnoncourt, and D. Durrer. The effects of lidocaine on intracellular and extracellular potentials, activation, and ventricular arrhythmias during acute regional ischemia in the isolated porcine heart. *Circ. Res.* 49: 792–806, 1981.

Cardinal, R., P. Savard, D.L. Carson, J.-B. Perry, and P. Pagé. Mapping of ventricular tachycardia induced by programmed stimulation in canine preparations of myocardial infarction. *Circulation* 70: 136–148, 1984.

Cardinal, R., P. Savard, J.A. Armour, R. Nadeau, D.L. Carson, and A.R. LeBlanc. Mapping of ventricular tachycardia induced by thoracic neural stimulation in dogs. *Can. J. Physiol. Pharmacol.* 64: 411–418, 1986.

Cardinal, R., M. Vermeulen, M. Shenasa, F. Roberge, P. Pagé, F. Hélie, and P. Savard. Anisotropic conduction and functional dissociation of ischemic tissue during reentrant ventricular tachycardia in canine myocardial infarction. *Circulation* 77: 1162–1176, 1988.

Carlsson, L. Mechanisms of local noradrenaline release in acute myocardial ischemia. *Acta Physiol. Scand.* 129(Suppl. 559): 7–85, 1987.

Carmeliet, E., and J. Vereecke. Adrenaline and the plateau phase of the cardiac action potential. Importance of Ca^{2+}, Na^+ and K^+ conductance. *Pflügers Arch.* 313: 300–315, 1969.

Carmeliet, E. Cardiac transmembrane potentials and metabolism. *Circ. Res.* 42: 577–587, 1978.

Carmeliet, E. The slow inward current: Non-voltage-clamp studies. In: *The Slow Inward Current and Cardiac Arrhythmias,* edited by D.P. Zipes, J.C. Bailey, and V. Elharrar. Martinus Nijhoff, The Hague: 1980, pp. 97–110.

Carmeliet, E. Existence of pacemaker current i_f in human atrial appendage fibres. (abstract) *J. Physiol.* 357: 125P, 1984.

Carmeliet, E. Electrophysiologic and voltage clamp analysis of the effects of sotalol on isolated cardiac muscle and Purkinje fibers. *J. Pharmacol. Exp. Ther.* 232: 817–825, 1985.

Carson, D.L., R. Cardinal, P. Savard, and M. Vermeulen. Characterisation of unipolar waveform alternation in acutely ischaemic porcine myocardium. *Cardiovasc. Res.* 20: 521–527, 1986.

Cascio, W.E., G.-X. Yan, and A.G. Kléber. Lactic acid transport inhibition and CO_2 promote cellular K^+ loss in ischemic myocardium. (abstract) *Circulation* 80(suppl): II-611, 1989.

Cascio, W.E., G.-X. Yan, and A.G. Kléber. Passive electrical properties, mechanical activity, and extracellular potassium in arterially perfused and ischemic rabbit ventricular muscle. Effects of calcium entry blockade or hypocalcemia. *Circ. Res.* 66: 1461–1473, 1990.

Case, R.B., A. Felix, and F.S. Castellana. Rate of rise of myocardial P_{CO_2} during early myocardial ischemia in the dog. *Circ. Res.* 45: 324–330, 1979.

Cassidy, D.M., J.A. Vassallo, A.E. Buxton, J.U. Doherty, F.E. Marchlinski, and M.E. Josephson. The value of catheter mapping during sinus rhythm to localize site of origin of ventricular tachycardia. *Circulation* 69: 1103–1110, 1984a.

Cassidy, D.M., J.A. Vassallo, F.E. Marchlinski, A.E. Buxton, W.J. Untereker, and M.E. Josephson. Endocardial mapping in humans in sinus rhythm with normal left ventricles: activation patterns and characteristics of electrograms. *Circulation* 70: 37–42, 1984b.

Cassidy, D.M., J.A. Vassallo, A.E. Buxton, J.U. Doherty, F.E. Marchlinski, and M.E. Josephson. Catheter mapping during sinus rhythm: relation of local electrogram duration to ventricular tachycardia cycle length. *Am. J. Cardiol.* 55: 713–716, 1985.

Castellanos, A., L. Lemberg, M.J. Centurion, and B.V. Berkovits. Concealed digitalis-induced arrhythmias unmasked by electrical stimulation of the heart. *Am. Heart J.* 73: 484–490, 1967.

Cercek, B., A.S. Lew, P. Laramee, P.K. Shah, T.C. Peter, and W. Ganz. Time course and characteristics of ventricular arrhythmias after reperfusion in acute myocardial infarction. *Am. J. Cardiol.* 60: 214–218, 1987.

Ceremużyński, L., J. Staszewska-Barczak, and K. Herbaczynska-Cedro. Cardiac rhythm disturbances and the release of catecholamines after acute coronary occlusion in dogs. *Cardiovasc. Res.* 3: 190–197, 1969.

Chadda, K.D., V.S. Banka, and R.H. Helfant. Rate dependent ventricular ectopia following acute coronary occlusion. The concept of an optimal antiarrhythmic heart rate. *Circulation* 49: 654–658, 1974.

Chen, P-S., P.D. Wolf, E.G. Dixon, N.D. Danieley, D.W. Frazier, W.M. Smith, and R.E. Ideker. Mechanism of ventricular vulnerability to single premature stimuli in open-chest dogs. *Circ. Res.* 62: 1191–1209, 1988.

Chesnais, J.M., E. Coraboeuf, M.P. Sauviat, and J.M. Vassas. Sensitivity to H, Li and Mg ions of the slow inward sodium current in frog atrial fibres. *J. Mol. Cell. Cardiol.* 7: 627–642, 1975.

Choong, C.Y., E.F. Gibbons, R.D. Hogan, T.D. Franklin, M. Nolting, D.L. Mann, and A.E. Weyman. Relationship of functional recovery to scar contraction after myocardial infarction in the canine left ventricle. *Am. Heart J.* 117: 819–829, 1989.

Chow, M.J., A.A. Piergies, D.J. Bowsher, J.J. Murphy, W. Kushner, T.I. Ruo, A. Asada, J.V. Talano, and A.J. Atkinson. Torsade de pointes induced by N-acetylprocainamide. *J. Am. Coll. Cardiol.* 4: 621–624, 1984.

Cinca, J., M.J. Janse, H. Moréna, J. Candell, V. Valle, and D. Durrer. Mechanism and time course of the early electrical changes during acute coronary artery occlusion. An attempt to correlate the early ECG changes in man to the cellular electrophysiology in the pig. *Chest* 77: 499–505, 1980.

Cinca, J., J. Figueras, G. Senador, E. García-Moreno, A. Salas, and J. Rius. Transmural DC electrograms after coronary artery occlusion and latex embolization in pigs. *Am. J. Physiol.* 246: H475–H482, 1984.

Clark, B.B., and J.R. Cummings. Arrhythmias following experimental coronary occlusion and their reponse to drugs. *Ann. N.Y. Acad. Sci.* 64: 543–551, 1956.

Clarkson, C.W., and R.E. Ten Eick. On the mechanism of lysophosphatidylcholine-induced depolarization of cat ventricular myocardium. *Circ. Res.* 52: 543–556, 1983.

Clerc, L. Directional differences of impulse spread in trabecular muscle from mammalian heart. *J. Physiol.* 255: 335–346, 1976.

Clusin, W.T., M. Buchbinder, and D.C. Harrison. Calcium overload, "injury" current, and early ischaemic cardiac arrhythmias—A direct connection. *Lancet* I: 272–273, 1983.

Clusin, W.T., M. Buchbinder, A.K. Ellis, R.S. Kernoff, J.C. Giacomini, and D.C. Harrison. Reduction of ischemic depolarization by the calcium blocker diltiazem. Correlation with improvement of ventricular conduction and early arrhythmias in the dog. *Circ. Res.* 54: 10–20, 1984.

Clusin, W.T., R. Mohabir, and H.C. Lee. Role of cytosolic calcium in the normal and ischemic heart: potential new insights from the second generation indicator, indo-1. In: *Lethal Arrhythmias Resulting from Myocardial Ischemia and Infarction,* edited by M.R. Rosen, and Y. Palti. Kluwer Academic Publishers, Boston: 1989, pp. 13–30.

Cobb, L.A., J.A. Werner, and G.B. Trobaugh. Sudden cardiac death. I. A decade's experience with out-of-hospital resuscitation. *Mod. Concepts Cardiovasc. Dis.* 49: 31–36, 1980.

Cobbe, S.M., E. Hoffman, A. Ritzenhoff, J. Brachmann, W. Kübler, and J. Senges. Action of sotalol on potential reentrant pathways and ventricular tachyarrhythmias in conscious dogs in the late postmyocardial infarction phase. *Circulation* 68: 865–871, 1983.

Cobbe, S.M., E. Hoffman, A. Ritzenhoff, J. Brachmann, W. Kübler, and J. Senges. Day-to-day variations in inducibility of ventricular tachyarrhythmias during the late post-myocardial phase in conscious dogs. *Circulation* 72: 200–204, 1985.

Coetzee, W.A., and L.H. Opie. Effects of components of ischemia and metabolic inhibition on delayed afterdepolarizations in guinea pig papillary muscle. *Circ. Res.* 61: 157–165, 1987.

Coetzee, W.A., P. Owen, S.C. Dennis, S. Saman, and L.H. Opie. Reperfusion damage: free radicals mediate delayed membrane changes rather than early ventricular arrhythmias. *Cardiovasc. Res.* 24: 156–164, 1990.

Cohen, C.J., H.A. Fozzard, and S.-S. Sheu. Increase in intracellular sodium ion activity during stimulation in mammalian cardiac muscle. *Circ. Res.* 50: 651–662, 1982.

Cohen, D., and L.A. Kaufman. Magnetic determination of the relationship between the S-T segment shift and the injury current produced by coronary artery occlusion. *Circ. Res.* 36: 414–424, 1975.

Cohen I.S., N.B. Datyner, G.A. Gintant, and R.P. Kline. Time-dependent outward currents in the heart. In: *The Heart and Cardiovascular System,* edited by H.A. Fozzard, E. Haber, R.B. Jennings, A.M. Katz, and H.E. Morgan. Raven Press, New York: 1986, pp. 637–669.

Cohen I.S., D. DiFrancesco, N. Mulrine, and P. Pennefather. Internal and external K^+ help gate the inward rectifier. *Biophys. J.* 55: 197–202, 1989.

Cohnheim J., and A.V. Schulthess-Rechberg. Über die Folgen der Kranzarterienverschliessung für das Herz. *Virchows Arch.* 85: 503–537, 1881.

Colatsky, T.J. Mechanisms of action of lidocaine and quinidine on action potential duration in rabbit cardiac Purkinje fibers. An effect on steady state sodium currents? *Circ. Res.* 50: 17–27, 1982.

Colquhoun, D., E. Neher, H. Reuter, and C.F. Stevens. Inward current channels activated by intracellular Ca in cultured cardiac cells. *Nature* 294: 752–754, 1981.

Conrad, L.L., T.E. Cuddy, and R.H. Bayley. Activation of the ischemic ventricle and acute peri-infarction block in experimental coronary occlusion. *Circ. Res.* 7: 555–564, 1959.

Constantin, L., and J.B. Martins. Autonomic control of ventricular tachycardia: direct effects of beta-adrenergic blockade in 24 hour old canine myocardial infarction. *J. Am. Coll. Cardiol.* 9: 366–373, 1987.

Constantini, C., E. Corday, T.-W. Lang, S. Meerbaum, J. Brasch, L. Kaplan, S. Rubins, H. Gold, and J. Osher. Revascularization after 3 hours of coronary arterial occlusion: Effects on regional cardiac metabolic function and infarct size. *Am. J. Cardiol.* 36: 368–384, 1975.

Coraboeuf, E., and J. Boistel. L'action des taux élevés de gaz carbonique sur le tissu cardiaque, étudiée à l'aide de microélectrodes intracellulaires. *C.R. de la Soc. de Biol.* 147: 654–658, 1953.

Coraboeuf, E., E. Deroubaix, and J. Hoerter. Control of ionic permeabilities in normal and ischemic heart. *Circ. Res.* 38(Supp I): I92-I98, 1976.

Coraboeuf, E., E. Deroubaix, and A. Coulombe. Effect of tetrodotoxin on action potentials of the conducting system in the dog heart. *Am. J. Physiol.* 236: H561-H567, 1979.

Coraboeuf, E. Voltage clamp studies of the slow inward current. In: *The Slow Inward Current and Cardiac Arrhythmias,* edited by D.P. Zipes, J.C. Bailey, and V. Elharrar. Martinus Nijhoff, The Hague: 1980, pp. 25–95.

Coraboeuf, E., E. Deroubaix, and A. Coulombe. Acidosis-induced abnormal repolarization and repetitive activity in isolated dog Purkinje fibers. *J. Physiol. (Paris)* 76: 97–106, 1980.

Corbalan, R., R.L. Verrier, and B. Lown. Differing mechanisms for ventricular vulnerability during coronary artery occlusion and release. *Am. Heart J.* 92: 223–230, 1976.

Corbin, L.V., III, and A.M. Scher. The canine heart as an electrocardiographic generator. Dependence on cardiac cell orientation. *Circ. Res.* 41: 58–67, 1977.

Coromilas, J., J.T. Bigger Jr., E.S. Gang, and J.M. Zimmerman. Relationship between infarct size and ventricular arrhythmias. In: *Cardiac Electrophysiology and Arrhythmias*, edited by D.P. Zipes, and J. Jalife. Grune & Stratton, Orlando: 1985, pp. 523–530.

Coromilas, J., A.E. Saltman, B. Waldecker, S.M. Dillon, and A.L. Wit. Arrhythmogenic effects of flecainide in a canine model. *Circulation* (in press) 1993.

Coronel, R., J.W.T. Fiolet, F.J.G. Wilms-Schopman, A.F.M. Schaapherder, T.A. Johnson, L.S. Gettes, and M.J. Janse. Distribution of extracellular potassium and its relation to electrophysiologic changes during acute myocardial ischemia in the isolated perfused porcine heart. *Circulation* 77: 1125–1138, 1988.

Coronel, R. Distribution of extracellular potassium during acute myocardial ischemia (Doctoral Thesis). University of Amsterdam; ICG Printing, Dordrecht, 1988.

Coronel, R., J.W.T. Fiolet, F.J.G. Wilms-Schopman, T. Opthof, A.F.M. Schaapherder, and M.J. Janse. Distribution of extracellular potassium and electrophysiologic changes during two-stage coronary ligation in the isolated, perfused canine heart. *Circulation* 80: 165–177, 1989.

Coronel, R., F.J.G. Wilms-Schopman, T. Opthof, F.J.L. van Capelle,and M.J. Janse. Injury current and gradients of diastolic stimulation threshold, TQ potential, and extracellular potassium concentration during acute regional ischemia in the isolated perfused pig heart. *Circ. Res.* 68: 1241–1249, 1991.

Coronel, R., F.J.G. Wilms-Schopman, T. Opthof, J. Cinca, F. Worner, J.W.T. Fiolet, and M.J. Janse. Reperfusion induced ventricular arrhythmias following regional ischemia in isolated perfused pig hearts: distribution of extracellular potassium and electrophysiological changes. 1992, submitted to Circ Res.

Corr P.B., M.E. Cain, F.X. Witkowski, D.A. Price, and B.E. Sobel. Potential arrhythmogenic electrophysiological derangements in canine Purkinje fibers induced by lysophosphoglycerides. *Circ. Res.* 44: 822–832, 1979.

Corr, P.B., D.W. Snyder, M.E. Cain, W.A. Crafford Jr., R.W. Gross, and B.E. Sobel. Electrophysiological effects of amphiphiles on canine Purkinje fibers. Implications for dysrhythmia secondary to ischemia. *Circ. Res.* 49: 354–363, 1981a.

Corr, P.B., J.A. Shayman, J.B. Kramer, and R.J. Kipnis. Increased α-adrenergic receptors in ischemic cat myocardium. A potential mediator of electrophysiological derangements. *J. Clin. Invest.* 67: 1232–1236, 1981b.

Corr, P.B., and B.E. Sobel. Amphiphilic lipid metabolism and ventricular arrhythmias. In: *Early Arrhythmias Resulting from Myocardial Ischaemia,* edited by J.R. Parratt. Oxford University Press, New York: 1982, pp. 199–218.

Corr, P.B., R.W. Gross, and B.E. Sobel. Arrhythmogenic amphiphilic lipids and the myocardial cell membrane. *J. Mol. Cell. Cardiol.* 14: 619–626, 1982.

Corr, P.B., and F.X. Witkowski. Potential electrophysiologic mechanisms responsible for dysrhythmias associated with reperfusion of ischemic myocardium. *Circulation* 68(Suppl. I): I-16–I-24, 1983.

Corr, P.B., K.A. Yamada, and F.X. Witkowski. Mechanisms controlling cardiac autonomic function and their relation to arrhythmogenesis. In: *The Heart and Cardiovascular System,* edited by H.A. Fozzard, E. Haber, R.B. Jennings, A.M. Katz, and H.E. Morgan. Raven Press, New York: 1986, pp. 1343–1404.

Corr, P.B., K.A. Yamada, M.H. Creer, A.D. Sharma and B.E. Sobel. Lysophosphoglycerides and ventricular fibrillation early after onset of ischemia. *J. Mol. Cell. Cardiol.* 19(Suppl. V): 45–53, 1987.

Corr, P.B., M.H. Creer, K.A. Yamada, J.E. Saffitz, and B.E. Sobel. Prophylaxis of early ventricular fibrillation by inhibition of acylcarnitine accumulation. *J. Clin. Invest.* 83: 927–936, 1989.

Coulombe, A., E. Coraboeuf, and E. Deroubaix. Computer simulation of acidosis-induced abnormal repolarization and repetitive activity in dog Purkinje fibers. *J. Physiol. (Paris)* 76: 107–112, 1980.

Coulombe, A., E. Coraboeuf, C. Malecot, and E. Deroubaix. Role of the 'Na window' current and other ionic currents in triggering early afterdepolarizations and resulting re-excitations in Purkinje fibers. In: *Cardiac Electrophysiology and Arrhythmias*, edited by D.P. Zipes, and J. Jalife. Grune and Stratton, Orlando: 1985, pp. 43–50.

Coumel, P., C. Cabrol, A. Fabiato, R. Gourgon, and R. Slama. Tachycardie permanente par rythme réciproque. I. Preuves du diagnostic par stimulation auriculaire et ventriculaire. II. Traitement par l'implantation intracorporelle d'un stimulateur cardiaque avec entraînement simultané de l'oreillette et du ventricule. *Arch. Mal. Coeur* 60: 1830–1864, 1967.

Coumel, P., P. Attuel, J. Lavallée, D. Flammang, J.F. Leclercq, and R. Slama. Syndrome d'arythmie auriculaire d'origine vagale. *Arch. Mal. Coeur* 71: 645–656, 1978.

Coumel, P., J.-F. Leclercq, and F. Dessertenne. Torsades de pointes. In: *Tachycardias: Mechanisms, Diagnosis, Treatment*, edited by M.E. Josephson and H.J.J. Wellens. Lea & Febiger, Philadelphia: 1984, pp. 325–351.

Coumel, P., J.-F. Leclercq, and R. Slama. Repetitive monomorphic idiopathic ventricular tachycardia. In: *Cardiac Electrophysiology and Arrhythmias*, edited by D.P. Zipes, and J. Jalife. Grune and Stratton, Orlando: 1985, pp 457–468.

Coumel, P. The management of clinical arrhythmias. An overview on invasive versus non-invasive electrophysiology. *Eur. Heart J.* 8: 92–99, 1987.

Courtemanche, M., and A.T. Winfree. Re-entrant rotating waves in a Beeler-Reuter based model of two-dimensional cardiac electrical activity. *Int J. Bifurcation and Chaos* 1: 431–444, 1991.

Covell, J.W., M.J. Lab, and R. Pavelec. Mechanical induction of paired action potentials in intact heart in situ. *J. Physiol.* 320: 34P, 1981.

Cox, J.L., T.M. Daniel, and J.P. Boineau. The electrophysiologic time-course of acute myocardial ischemia and the effects of early coronary artery reperfusion. *Circulation* 48: 971–983, 1973.

Cox, J.L., H.I. Pass, A.S. Wechsler, H.N. Oldham, and D.C. Sabiston Jr. Coronary collateral blood flow in acute myocardial infarction. *J. Thorac. Cardiovasc. Surg.* 69: 117–125, 1975.

Cox, W.V., and H.F. Robertson. The effect of stellate ganglionectomy on the cardiac function of intact dogs. And its effect on the extent of myocardial infarction and on cardiac function following coronary artery occlusion. *Am. Heart J.* 12: 285–300, 1936.

Cramer, M., M. Siegal, J.T. Bigger Jr., and B.F. Hoffman. Characteristics of extracellular potentials recorded from the sinoatrial pacemaker of the rabbit. *Circ. Res.* 41: 292–300, 1977.

Cranefield, P.F., B.F. Hoffman, and A.A. Siebens. Anodal excitation of cardiac muscle. *Am. J. Physiol.* 190: 383–390, 1957.

Cranefield, P.F., and K. Greenspan. The rate of oxygen uptake of quiescent cardiac muscle. *J. Gen. Physiol.* 44: 235–249, 1960.

Cranefield, P.F., and B.F. Hoffman. Reentry: Slow conduction, summation and inhibition. *Circulation* 44: 309–311, 1971.

Cranefield, P.F., H.O. Klein, and B.F. Hoffman. Conduction of the cardiac impulse. I. Delay, block and one-way block in depressed Purkinje fibers. *Circ. Res.* 28: 199–219, 1971.

Cranefield, P.F., A.L. Wit, and B.F. Hoffman. Conduction of the cardiac impulse. III. Characteristics of very slow conduction. *J. Gen. Physiol.* 59: 227–246, 1972.

Cranefield, P.F., A.L. Wit, and B.F. Hoffman. Genesis of cardiac arrhythmias. *Circulation* 47: 190–204, 1973.

Cranefield, P.F., and R.S. Aronson. Initiation of sustained rhythmic activity by single propagated action potentials in canine cardiac Purkinje fibers exposed to sodium-free solution or to ouabain. *Circ. Res.* 34: 477–481, 1974.

Cranefield, P.F. *The Conduction of the Cardiac Impulse: The Slow Response and Cardiac Arrhythmias.* Futura Publishing Company, Mt. Kisco, New York: 1975.

Cranefield, P.F. Action potentials, afterpotentials and arrhythmias. *Circ. Res.* 41: 415–423, 1977.

Cranefield, P.F., and F.A. Dodge. Slow conduction in the heart. In: *The Slow Inward Current and Cardiac Arrhythmias*, edited by D.P. Zipes, J.C. Bailey, and V. Elharrar. Martinus Nijhoff, The Hague: 1980, pp. 149–171.

Cranefield, P.F., and R.S. Aronson. *Cardiac Arrhythmias: The Role of Triggered Activity and Other Mechanisms.* Futura Publishing Company, Mt. Kisco, New York: 1988.

Curtis, M.J., B.A. MacLeod, and M.J.A. Walker. Models for the study of arrhythmias in myocardial ischaemia and infarction: the use of the rat. *J. Mol. Cell. Cardiol.* 19: 399–419, 1987.

Czarnecka, M., B. Lewartowski, and A. Prokopczk. Intracellular recordings from the in situ working heart in physiological conditions and during acute ischemia and fibrillation. *Acta Physiol. Pol.* 24: 331–337, 1973.

Dahl, G., and G. Isenberg. Decoupling of heart muscle cells: correlation with increased cytoplasmic calcium activity and with changes of nexus ultrastructure. *J. Membr. Biol.* 53: 63–75, 1980.

Damiano, B.P., and M.R. Rosen. Effects of pacing on triggered activity induced by early afterdepolarizations. *Circulation* 69: 1013–1025, 1984.

Damiano, R.J., P.K. Smith, H.F. Tripp Jr., T. Asano, K.W. Small, J.E.Lowe, R.E. Ideker, and J.L. Cox. The effect of chemical ablation of the endocardium on ventricular fibrillation threshold. *Circulation* 74: 645–652, 1986.

Dangman, K.H., H.H. Wang, and A.L. Wit. Electrophysiology of isolated canine hearts with acute and chronic myocardial infarction. (abstract) *Fed. Proc.* 36: 415, 1977.

Dangman, K.H., H.H. Wang, and A.L. Wit. Effects of intracoronary potassium chloride on electrograms of canine Purkinje fibers in six-hour- to four-week-old myocardial infarcts. An indication of time-dependent changes in collateral blood flow. *Circ. Res.* 44: 392–405, 1979.

Dangman, K.H., and B.F. Hoffman. Effects of nifedipine on electrical activity of cardiac cells. *Am. J. Cardiol.* 46: 1059–1067, 1980.

Dangman, K.H., and B.F. Hoffman. *In vivo* and *in vitro* antiarrhythmic and arrhythmogenic effects of N-acetyl procainamide. *J. Pharmacol. Exp. Ther.* 217: 851–862, 1981.

Dangman, K.H., and B.F. Hoffman. Studies on overdrive stimulation of canine cardiac Purkinje fibers: Maximal diastolic potential as a determinant of the response. *J. Am. Coll. Cardiol.* 2: 1183–1190, 1983.

Dangman, K.H., and B.F. Hoffman. The effects of single premature stimuli on automatic and triggered rhythms in isolated canine Purkinje fibers. *Circulation* 71: 813–822, 1985.

Dangman, K.H., K.P. Dresdner Jr., and S. Zaim. Automatic and triggered impulse initiation in canine subepicardial muscle cells from border zones of 24-hour transmural infarcts. New mechanisms for malignant cardiac arrhythmias? *Circulation* 78: 1020–1030, 1988.

Daniel, T.M., J.P. Boineau, and D.C. Sabiston. Comparison of human ventricular activation with a canine model in chronic myocardial infarction. *Circulation* 44: 74–89, 1971.

Daniel, W.G., R.H. Svenson, T.N. Masters, and F. Roblesek. Electrophysiologic effects of partial coronary flow reduction in the exposed canine heart. Effects of ischemia and ischemic-induced regional hypothermia on refractoriness and conduction delay. *Circulation* 58: 670–678, 1978.

Danilo, P. Jr., M.R. Rosen, and A.J. Hordof. Effects of acetylcholine on the ventricular specialized conducting system of neonatal and adult dogs. *Circ. Res.* 43: 777–784, 1978.

Dart, A.M., A. Schömig, R. Dietz, E. Mayer, and W. Kübler. Release of endogenous catecholamines in the ischemic myocardium of the rat. Part B: Effect of sympathetic nerve stimulation. *Circ. Res.* 55: 702–706, 1984.

Davidenko, J.M., L. Cohen, R. Goodrow, and C. Antzelevitch. Quinidine-induced action potential prolongation, early afterdepolarizations, and triggered activity in canine Purkinje fibers. Effects of stimulation rate, potassium, and magnesium. *Circulation* 79: 674–686, 1989.

Davidenko, J.M., P.F. Kent, D.R. Chialvo, D.C. Michaels, and J. Jalife. Sustained vortex-like waves in normal isolated ventricular muscle. *Proc. Natl. Acad. Sci. USA* 87: 8785–8789, 1990.

Davies, M.J. Pathological view of sudden cardiac death. *Br. Heart J.* 45: 88–96, 1981.

Davies, M.J., and A. Thomas. Thrombosis and acute coronary-artery lesions in sudden cardiac ischemic death. *N. Engl. J. Med.* 310: 1137–1140, 1984.

Davis, J., R. Glassman, and A.L. Wit. Method for evaluating the effects of antiarrhythmic drugs on ventricular tachycardias with different electrophysiologic characteristics and different mechanisms in the infarcted canine heart. *Am. J. Cardiol.* 49: 1176–1184, 1982.

Davis, L.D. Effect of changes in cycle length on diastolic depolarization produced by ouabain in canine Purkinje fibers. *Circ. Res.* 32: 206–214, 1973.

Davis, L.D. Effects of autonomic neurohumors on transmembrane potentials of atrial plateau fibers. *Am. J. Physiol.* 229: 1351–1356, 1975.

Dawson, A.K., A.S. Leon, and H.L. Taylor. Effects of pentobarbital anesthesia on vulnerability to ventricular fibrillation. *Am. J. Physiol.* 239: H427-H431, 1980.

De Bakker, J.M.T., M.J. Janse, F.J.L. van Capelle, and D. Durrer. An interactive computer system for guiding the surgical treatment of life-threatening ventricular tachycardias. *IEEE Trans. Biomed. Eng.* BME-31: 362–368, 1984.

De Bakker, J.M.T. Intraoperative mapping of endocardial electrical activity: a guide for surgical treatment of ventricular tachycardias. (Doctoral Thesis) University of Utrecht. Rodopi, Amsterdam, 1985.

De Bakker, J.M.T., F.J.L. van Capelle, and M.J. Janse. Localization of the site of origin of ventricular tachycardia in the chronic phase of myocardial infarction. In: *Nonpharmacological Therapy of Tachyarrhythmias*, edited by G. Breithardt, M. Borggrefe and D.P. Zipes. Futura Publishing Company, Mt. Kisco, New York: 1987, pp. 33–49.

De Bakker, J.M.T., F.J.L. van Capelle, M.J. Janse, A.A.M. Wilde, R. Coronel, A.E. Becker, K.P. Dingemans, N.M. van Hemel, and R.N.W. Hauer. Reentry as a cause of ventricular tachycardia in patients with chronic ischemic heart disease: electrophysiologic and anatomic correlation. *Circulation* 77: 589–606, 1988.

De Bakker, J.M.T., R. Coronel, S. Tasseron, A.A.M. Wilde, T. Opthof, M.J. Janse, F.J.L. van Capelle, A.E. Becker and G. Jambroes. Ventricular tachycardia in the infarcted, Langendorff-perfused human heart: role of the arrangement of surviving cardiac fibers. *J. Am. Coll. Cardiol.* 15: 1594–1607, 1990.

De Boer, S. *De pathologische physiologie en pharmacologie van den onregelmatige hartslag.* Groningen, Wolters, Batavia: 1935, pp. 346.

Deck, K.A. Änderungen des Ruhepotentials und der Kabeleigenschaften von Purkinje-Fäden bei der Dehnung. *Pflügers Arch* 280: 131–140, 1964.

De Hemptinne, A. Intracellular pH and surface pH in skeletal and cardiac muscle measured with a double-barrelled pH microelectrode. *Pflügers Arch.* 386: 121–126, 1980.

De Hemptinne, A., and F. Huguenin. The influence of muscle respiration and glycolysis on surface and intracellular pH in fibres of the rat soleus. *J. Physiol.* 347: 581–592, 1984.

Deitmer, J.W., and D. Ellis. The intracellular sodium activity of cardiac Purkinje fibres during inhibition and re-activation of the Na-K pump. *J. Physiol.* 284: 241–259, 1978.

Dekker, E. Direct current make and break thresholds for pacemaker electrodes on the canine ventricle. *Circ. Res.* 27: 811–823, 1970.

Délèze, J. The recovery of resting potential and input resistance in sheep heart injured by knife or laser. *J. Physiol.* 208: 547–562, 1970.

Delgado, C., B. Steinhaus, M. Delmar, D.R. Chialvo, and J. Jalife. Directional differences in excitability and margin of safety for propagation in sheep ventricular epicardial muscle. *Circ. Res.* 67: 97–110, 1990.

Delmar, M., D.C. Michaels, T. Johnson, and J. Jalife. Effects of increasing intercellular resistance on transverse and longitudinal propagation in sheep epicardial muscle. *Circ. Res.* 60: 780–785, 1987.

Dellsperger, K.C., J.L. Clothier, J.A. Hartnett, L.M. Haun, and M.L. Marcus. Acceleration of the wavefront of myocardial necrosis by chronic hypertension and left ventricular hypertrophy in dogs. *Circ. Res.* 63: 87–96, 1988.

DeMello, W.C. Effect of intracellular injection of calcium and strontium on cell communication in heart. *J. Physiol.* 250: 231–245, 1975.

Denniss, A.R., H. Baaijens, D.V. Cody, D.A. Richards, P.A. Russell, A.A. Young, D.L. Ross, and J.B. Uther. Value of programmed stimulation and exercise testing in predicting one-year mortality after acute myocardial infarction. *Am. J. Cardiol.* 56: 213–220, 1985.

Denniss, A.R., D.A. Richards, J.A. Waywood, T. Yung, C.A. Kam, D.L. Ross, and J.B. Uther. Electrophysiological and anatomic differences between canine hearts with inducible ventricular tachycardia and fibrillation associated with chronic myocardial infarction. *Circ. Res.* 64: 155–166, 1989.

Désilets, M., and C.M. Baumgarten. Isoproterenol directly stimulates the Na^+-K^+ pump in isolated cardiac myocytes. *Am. J. Physiol.* 251: H218-H225, 1986.

de Soyza, N., J.K. Bissett, J.J. Kane, M.L. Murphy, and J.E. Doherty. Association of accelerated idioventricular rhythm and paroxysmal ventricular tachycardia in acute myocardial infarction. *Am. J. Cardiol.* 34: 667–670, 1974.

De Waart, A., C.J. Storm, and A.K.J. Koumans. Ligation of the coronary arteries in Javanese monkeys. III. Further theoretical considerations of the changes in the ventricular electrocardiogram, with illustrative experiments. *Am. Heart J.* 12: 184–205, 1936.

DeWood, M.A., J. Spores, R. Notske, L.T. Mouser, R. Burroughs, M.S. Golden, and H.T. Lang. Prevalence of total coronary occlusion during the early hours of transmural myocardial infarction. *N. Engl. J. Med.* 303: 897–902, 1980.

Dialog Database, Los Angeles.

DiFrancesco, D., and C. Ojeda. Properties of the current i_f in the sino-atrial node of the rabbit compared with those of the current i_{k2} in Purkinje fibres. *J. Physiol.* 308: 353–367, 1980.

DiFrancesco, D. A new interpretation of the pace-maker current in calf Purkinje fibres. *J. Physiol.* 314: 359–376, 1981a.

DiFrancesco, D. A study of the ionic nature of the pace-maker current in calf Purkinje fibres. *J. Physiol.* 314: 377–393, 1981b.

DiFrancesco, D., A. Feroni, and S. Visentin. Barium-induced blockade of the inward rectifier in calf Purkinje fibres. *Pflügers Arch.* 402: 446–453, 1984.

DiFrancesco, D. The cardiac hyperpolarizing-activated current, i_f. Origins and developments. *Prog. Biophys. Mol. Biol.* 46: 163–183, 1985.

DiFrancesco, D., and D. Noble. A model of cardiac electrical activity incorporating ionic pumps and concentration changes. *Phil. Trans. R. Soc. Lond. B.* 307: 353–398, 1985.

DiFrancesco, D. Characterization of single pacemaker channels in cardiac sino-atrial node cells. *Nature* 324: 470–473, 1986.

DiFrancesco, D., A. Ferroni, M. Mazzanti, and C. Tromba. Properties of the hyperpolarizing-activated current (i_f) in cells isolated from the rabbit sino-atrial node. *J. Physiol.* 377: 61–88, 1986.

DiFrancesco D., and C. Tromba. Inhibition of the hyperpolarization-activated current (i_f) induced by acetylcholine in rabbit sino-atrial node myocytes. *J. Physiol.* 405: 477–491, 1988.

DiFrancesco, D. The hyperpolarization-activated current, i_f, and cardiac pacemaking. In: *Cardiac Electrophysiology: A Textbook*, edited by M.R. Rosen, M.J. Janse, and A.L. Wit. Futura Publishing Company, Mt. Kisco, New York: 1990, pp. 117–132.

Dillon, S.M., M.A. Allessie, P.C. Ursell, and A.L. Wit. Influence of anisotropic tissue structure on reentrant circuits in the epicardial border zone of sub-acute canine infarcts. *Circ. Res.* 63: 182–206, 1988.

Dillon, S.M. Optical recordings in the rabbit heart show that defibrillation strength shocks prolong the duration of depolarization and the refractory period. *Circ. Res.* 69: 842–856, 1991.

Dilly, S.G., and M.J. Lab. Electrophysiological alternans and restitution during acute regional ischaemia in myocardium of anesthetized pig. *J. Physiol.* 402: 315–333, 1988.

Dodge, F.A., and P.F. Cranefield. Nonuniform conduction in cardiac Purkinje fibers. In: *Normal and Abnormal Conduction in the Heart*, edited by A.P. Carvalho, B.F. Hoffman, and M. Lieberman. Futura Publishing Company, Mt. Kisco, New York: 1982, pp. 379–395.

Doerr, T., R. Denger and W. Trautwein. Calcium currents in single SA nodal cells of the rabbit heart studied with action potential clamp. *Pflügers Arch.* 413: 599–603, 1989.

Dominguez, G., and H.A. Fozzard. Influence of extracellular K^+ concentration on cable properties and excitability of sheep cardiac Purkinje fibers. *Circ. Res.* 26: 565–574, 1970.

Donaldson, R.M., F.S. Nashat, D. Noble, and P. Taggart. Differential effects of ischaemia and hyperkalaemia on myocardial repolarization and conduction times in the dog. *J. Physiol.* 353: 393–403, 1984.

Downar, E., and M.B. Waxman. Depressed conduction and unidirectional block in Purkinje fibres. In: *The Conduction System of the Heart*, edited by H.J.J. Wellens, K.I. Lie, and M.J. Janse. Lea & Febiger, Philadelphia: 1976, pp. 393–409.

Downar, E., M.J. Janse, and D. Durrer. The effect of acute coronary artery occlusion on subepicardial transmembrane potentials in the intact porcine heart. *Circulation* 56: 217–224, 1977a.

Downar, E., M.J. Janse, and D. Durrer. The effect of "ischemic" blood on transmembrane potentials of normal porcine ventricular myocardium. *Circulation* 55: 455–462, 1977b.

Downar, E., and I. Parson. Mechanisms underlying ventricular arrhythmias of acute myocardial ischemia and reperfusion. (abstract) *Circulation* 64: (Suppl. IV) IV-216, 1981.

Downar, E., I.D. Parson, L.L. Mickleborough, D.A. Cameron, L.C. Yao, and M.B. Waxman. On-line epicardial mapping of intraoperative ventricular arrhythmias: initial clinical experience. *J. Am. Coll. Cardiol.* 4: 703–714, 1984.

Downar, E., L. Harris, L.L. Mickleborough, N. Shaikh, and I.D. Parson. Endocardial mapping of ventricular tachycardia in the intact human ventricle: evidence for reentrant mechanisms. *J. Am. Coll. Cardiol.* 11: 783–791, 1988.

Dresdner, K.P., R.P. Kline, and A.L. Wit. Cytoplasmic K^+ and Na^+ activity in subendocardial canine Purkinje fibers from one day old infarcts using double-barrel ion selective electrodes: comparison with maximum diastolic potential. (abstract) *Biophys. J.* 47: 463a, 1985.

Dresdner, K.P., R.P. Kline, and A.L. Wit. Intracellular K^+ activity, intracellular Na^+ activity and maximum diastolic potential of canine subendocardial Purkinje cells from one-day-old infarcts. *Circ. Res.* 60: 122–132, 1987.

Dresdner, K.P. Jr., M.S. Hanna, R.P. Kline, and A.L. Wit. Na^+/K^+ pump failure in canine cardiac Purkinje fibers surviving in infarcts. *Circulation* 78(Suppl. II): II-637, 1988.

Dresdner, K.P. Jr., R.P. Kline, and A.L. Wit. Intracellular pH of canine subendocardial Purkinje cells surviving in 1-day-old myocardial infarcts. *Circ. Res.* 65: 554–565, 1989.

Dudel, J., and W. Trautwein. Das Aktionspotential und Mechanogramm des Herzmuskels unter dem Einfluss der Dehnung. *Cardiologia* 25: 344–362, 1954.

Dudel, J., K. Peper, R. Rüdel, and W. Trautwein. The effect of tetrodotoxin on the membrane current in cardiac muscle (Purkinje fibers). *Pflügers Arch.* 295: 213–226, 1967a.

Dudel, J., K. Peper, R. Rüdel, and W. Trautwein. The potassium component of membrane current in Purkinje fibers. *Pflügers Arch.* 296: 308–327, 1967b.

Duff, H.J., J.M.E. Martin, and M. Rahmberg. Time-dependent change in electrophysiologic milieu after myocardial infarction in conscious dogs. *Circulation* 77: 209–220, 1988.

Dunn, R.B., and D.M. Griggs Jr. Transmural gradients in ventricular tissue metabolites produced by stopping coronary blood flow in the dog. *Circ. Res.* 37: 438–445, 1975.

Durrer, D., and L.H. van der Tweel. Spread of activation in the left ventricular wall of the dog. I. *Am. Heart J.* 46: 683–691, 1953.

Durrer, D., P. Formijne, R.Th. Van Dam, J. Büller, A.A.W. Van Lier, and F.L. Meyler. The electrocardiogram in normal and some abnormal conditions. In revived human fetal heart and in acute and chronic coronary occlusion. *Am. Heart J.* 61: 303–314, 1961.

Durrer, D., A.A.W. Van Lier, and J. Büller. Epicardial and intramural excitation in chronic myocardial infarction. *Am. Heart J.* 68: 765–776, 1964.

Durrer, D., L. Schoo, R.M. Schuilenburg, and H.J.J. Wellens. The role of premature beats in the initiation and the termination of supraventricular tachycardia in the Wolff-Parkinson-White syndrome. *Circulation* 36: 644–662, 1967.

Durrer, D., R.Th. Van Dam, G.E. Freud, M.J. Janse, F.L. Meijler, and R.C. Arzbaecher. Total excitation of the isolated human heart. *Circulation* 41: 899–912, 1970.

Durrer, D., R.Th. Van Dam, G.E. Freud, and M.J. Janse. Reentry and ventricular arrhythmias in local ischemia and infarction of the intact dog heart. *Proc. Kon. Ned. Akad. Wetenschappen: Series* C74: 321–334, 1971.

Earm, Y.E., Y. Shimoni, and A.J. Spindler. A pace-maker-like current in the sheep atrium and its modulation by catecholamines. *J. Physiol.* 342: 569–590, 1983.

Ebert, P.A., R.B. Vanderbeek, R.J. Allgood, and D.C. Sabiston Jr. Effect of chronic cardiac denervation on arrhythmias after coronary artery ligation. *Cardiovasc. Res.* 4: 141–147, 1970.

Echt, D.S., J.C. Griffin, A.J. Ford, J.W. Knutti, R.C. Feldman, and J.W. Mason. Nature of inducible ventricular tachyarrhythmias in a canine chronic myocardial infarction model. *Am. J. Cardiol.* 52: 1127–1132, 1983.

Ehara, T., A. Noma, and K. Ono. Calcium-activated non-selective cation channel in ventricular cells isolated from adult guinea-pig hearts. *J. Physiol.* 403: 117–133, 1988.

Einthoven, W. Un nouveau galvanometre. *Arch. Neerl. Sci. Exactes Nat.* 6: 625–633, 1901.

Eisner, D.A. and W.J. Lederer. Inotropic and arrhythmogenic effects of potassium-depleted solutions on mammalian cardiac muscle. *J. Physiol.* 294: 255–277, 1979.

Eisner, D.A., and W.J. Lederer. Na-Ca exchange: stoichiometry and electrogenicity. *Am. J. Physiol.* 248: C189-C202, 1985.

Eisner, D.A. The Na-K pump in cardiac muscle. In: *The Heart and Cardiovascular System*, edited by H.A. Fozzard, E. Haber, R.B. Jennings, A.M. Katz, and H.E. Morgan. Raven Press, New York: 1986, pp. 489–507.

Elharrar, V., P.R. Foster, T.L. Jirak, W.E. Gaum, and D.P. Zipes. Alterations in canine myocardial excitability during ischemia. *Circ. Res.* 40: 98–105, 1977.

Elharrar, V., J.C. Bailey, D.A. Lathrop, and D.P. Zipes. Effects of aprindine HCl on slow channel action potentials and transient depolarizations in canine Purkinje fibers. *J. Pharmacol. Exp. Ther.* 205: 410–417, 1978.

Ellis, D. The effects of external cations and ouabain on the intracellular sodium activity of sheep heart Purkinje fibers. *J. Physiol.* 273: 211–240, 1977.

Ellis, D., and J. Noireaud. Intracellular pH in sheep Purkinje fibers and ferret papillary muscles during hypoxia and recovery. *J. Physiol.* 383: 125–141, 1987.

El-Said, G., H.S. Rosenberg, C.E. Mullins, G.L. Hallman, D.A. Cooley, and D.G.

McNamara. Dysrhythmias after Mustard's operation for transposition of the great arteries. *Am. J. Cardiol.* 30: 526–532, 1972.

El-Sherif, N., B.J. Scherlag, R. Lazzara, and P. Samet. Pathophysiology of tachycardia- and bradycardia-dependent block in the canine proximal His-Purkinje system after acute myocardial ischemia. *Am. J. Cardiol.* 33: 529-540, 1974.

El-Sherif, N., B.J. Scherlag, and R. Lazzara. Electrode catheter recordings during malignant ventricular arrhythmia following experimental acute myocardial ischemia. Evidence for re-entry due to conduction delay and block in ischemic myocardium. *Circulation* 51: 1003–1014, 1975.

El-Sherif, N., B.J. Scherlag, R. Lazzara, and R.R. Hope. Reentrant ventricular arrhythmias in the late myocardial infarction period. 1. Conduction characteristics in the infarction zone. *Circulation* 55: 686–702, 1977a.

El-Sherif, N., R.R. Hope, B.J. Scherlag, and R. Lazzara. Re-entrant ventricular arrhythmias in the late myocardial infarction period. 2. Patterns of initiation and termination of re-entry. *Circulation* 55: 702–719, 1977b.

El-Sherif, N., R. Lazzara, R.R. Hope, and B.J. Scherlag. Re-entrant ventricular arrhythmias in the late myocardial infarction period. 3. Manifest and concealed extrasystolic grouping. *Circulation* 56: 225–234, 1977c.

El-Sherif, N. Reentrant ventricular arrhythmias in the late myocardial infarction period. 6. Effect of the autonomic system. *Circulation* 58: 103–110, 1978.

El-Sherif, N., and R. Lazzara. Reentrant ventricular arrhythmias in the late myocardial infarction period. 7. Effect of verapamil and D-600 and the role of the "slow channel". *Circulation* 60: 605–615, 1979.

El-Sherif, N., R. Zeiler, and W.B. Gough. Effects of catecholamines, verapamil, and tetrodotoxin on triggered automaticity in canine ischemic Purkinje fibers. (abstract) *Circulation* 62(Suppl III): III-281, 1980.

El-Sherif, N., R.A. Smith, and K. Evans. Canine ventricular arrhythmias in the late myocardial infarction period. 8. Epicardial mapping of reentrant circuits. *Circ. Res.* 49: 255–265, 1981.

El-Sherif, N., R. Mehra, W.B. Gough, and R.H. Zeiler. Ventricular activation patterns of spontaneous and induced ventricular rhythms in canine one-day-old myocardial infarction. Evidence for focal and reentrant mechanisms. *Circ. Res.* 51: 152–166, 1982.

El-Sherif, N., R. Mehra, W.B. Gough, and R.H. Zeiler. Reentrant ventricular arrhythmias in the late myocardial infarction period. Interruption of reentrant circuits by cryothermal techniques. *Circulation* 68: 644–656, 1983a.

El-Sherif, N., W.B. Gough, R.H. Zeiler, and R. Mehra. Triggered ventricular rhythms in 1-day-old myocardial infarction in the dog. *Circ. Res.* 52: 566–579, 1983b.

El-Sherif, N, R. Mehra, W.B. Gough, and R.H. Zeiler. Reentrant ventricular arrhythmias in the late myocardial infarction period. II. Burst pacing versus multiple premature stimulation in the induction of reentry. *J. Am. Coll. Cardiol.* 4: 295–304, 1984.

El-Sherif, N. The figure 8 model of reentrant excitation in the canine postinfarction heart. In: *Cardiac Electrophysiology and Arrhythmias*, edited by D.P. Zipes, and J. Jalife. Grune & Stratton, Orlando: 1985, pp. 363–378.

El-Sherif, N., W.B. Gough, R.H. Zeiler, and R. Hariman. Reentrant ventricular arrhythmias in the late myocardial infarction period. 12. Spontaneous versus induced reentry and intramural versus epicardial circuits. *J. Am. Coll. Cardiol.* 6: 124–132, 1985.

El-Sherif, N., W.B. Gough, and M. Restivo. Reentrant ventricular arrhythmias in the late myocardial infarction period. 14. Mechanisms of resetting, entrainment, acceleration or termination of reentrant tachycardia by programmed electrical stimulation. *PACE* 10: 341–371, 1987.

Engelmann, T.W. Über die Leitung der Erregung im Herzmuskel. *Pflügers Arch.* 11: 465–480, 1875.

Engelmann, T.W. Über reciproke und irreciproke Reizleitung, mit besonderer Beziehung auf das Herz. *Pflügers Arch.* 61: 275–284, 1895.

Erichsen, J.E. On the influence of the coronary circulation on the action of the heart. *London Med. Gazette* 2: 561–565, 1841–42.

Ericsson, M., A. Granath, P. Ohlsén, T. Södermark, and U. Volpe. Arrhythmias and symptoms during treadmill testing three weeks after myocardial infarction in 100 patients. *Br. Heart J.* 35: 787–790, 1973.

Erlanger, J., and A.D. Hirschfelder. Further studies on the physiology of heartblock in mammals. *Am. J. Physiol.* 15: 153–206, 1906.

Erlanger, J., and J.R. Blackman. A study of relative rhythmicity and conductivity in various regions of the auricles of the mammalian heart. *Am. J. Physiol.* 19: 125–174, 1907.

Escande, D., E. Coraboeuf, and C. Planche. Abnormal pacemaking is modulated by sarcoplasmic reticulum in partially-depolarized myocardium from dilated right atria in humans. *J. Mol. Cell. Cardiol.* 19: 231–241, 1987.

Escher, D.J.W., and S. Furman. Emergency treatment of cardiac arrhythmias. Emphasis on use of electrical pacing. *JAMA* 214: 2028–2034, 1970.

Euler, D.E., S.B. Jones, W.P. Gunnar, J.M.Loeb, D.K. Murdock, and W.C. Randall. Cardiac arrhythmias in the conscious dog after excision of the sinoatrial node and crista terminalis. *Circulation* 59: 468–475, 1979.

Euler, D.E., C.E. Prood, J.F. Spear, and E.N. Moore. The interruption of collateral blood flow to the ischemic canine myocardium by embolization of a coronary artery with latex: Effects on conduction delay and ventricular arrhythmias. *Circ. Res.* 49: 97–108, 1981.

Euler, D.E., J.F. Spear, and E.N. Moore. Effect of coronary occlusion on arrhythmias and conduction in the ovine heart. *Am. J. Physiol.* 245: H82-H89, 1983.

Eyster, J.A.E., and W.J. Meek. The origin and conduction of the heart beat. *Physiol. Rev.* 1: 1–43, 1921.

Eyster, J.A.E., and W.J. Meek. Studies on the origin and conduction of the cardiac impulse. VIII. The permanent rhythm following destruction of the sino-auricular node. *Am. J. Physiol.* 61: 117–129, 1922.

Eyster, J.A.E., W.J. Meek, H. Goldberg, and W.E. Gilson. Potential changes in an injured region of cardiac muscle. *Am. J. Physiol.* 124: 717–728, 1938.

Fabiato, A., and F. Fabiato. Contractions induced by a calcium-triggered release of calcium from the sarcoplasmic reticulum of single skinned cardiac cells. *J. Physiol.* 249: 469–495, 1975.

Fabiato, A. Calcium-induced release of calcium from the cardiac sarcoplasmic reticulum. *Am. J. Physiol.* 245: C1-C14, 1983.

Falk, R.T., and I.S. Cohen. Membrane current following activity in canine cardiac Purkinje fibers. *J. Gen. Physiol.* 83: 771–799, 1984.

Fedida, D., D. Noble, A.C. Rankin, and A.J. Spindler. The arrhythmogenic transient inward current I_{TI} and related contraction in isolated guinea-pig ventricular myocytes. *J. Physiol.* 392: 523–542, 1987.

Fenoglio, J.J. Jr., A. Albala, F.G. Silva, P.L. Friedman, and A.L. Wit. Structural basis of ventricular arrhythmias in human myocardial infarction: A hypothesis. *Hum. Pathol.* 7: 547–563, 1976.

Fenoglio, J.J. Jr., H.S. Karagueuzian, P.L. Friedman, A. Albala, and A.L. Wit. Time course of infarct growth toward the endocardium after coronary occlusion. *Am. J. Physiol.* 236: H356-H370, 1979.

Fenoglio, J.J. Jr., T.D. Pham, A.H. Harken, L.N. Horowitz, M.E. Josephson, and A.L. Wit. Recurrent sustained ventricular tachycardia: structure and ultrastructure of subendocardial regions in which tachycardia originates. *Circulation* 68: 518–533, 1983.

Ferrer, M.I. *The Sick Sinus Syndrome.* Futura Publishing Company, Mt. Kisco, New York: 1974.

Ferrier, G.R., and G.K. Moe. Effect of calcium on acetylstrophanthidin-induced transient depolarizations in canine Purkinje tissue. *Circ. Res.* 33: 508–515, 1973.

Ferrier, G.R., J.H. Saunders, and C. Mendez. A cellular mechanism for the generation of ventricular arrhythmias by acetylstrophanthidin. *Circ. Res.* 32: 600–609, 1973.

Ferrier, G.R. Digitalis arrhythmias: Role of oscillatory afterpotentials. *Prog. Cardiovasc. Dis.* 19: 459–474, 1977.

Ferrier, G.R., and J.E. Rosenthal. Automaticity and entrance block induced by focal depolarization of mammalian ventricular tissues. *Circ. Res.* 47: 238–248, 1980.

Ferrier, G.R. Effects of transmembrane potential on oscillatory afterpotentials induced by acetylstrophanthidin in canine ventricular tissues. *J. Pharmacol. Exp. Ther.* 215: 332–341, 1980.

Ferrier, G.R., M.P. Moffat, and A. Lukas. Possible mechanisms of ventricular arrhythmias elicited by ischemia followed by reperfusion. Studies on isolated canine ventricular tissues. *Circ. Res.* 56: 184–194, 1985.

Fiolet, J.W.T., A. Baartscheer, C.A. Schumacher, R. Coronel, and H.F. ter Welle. The change of the free energy of ATP hydrolysis during global ischemia and anoxia in the rat heart. Its possible role in the regulation of transsarcolemmal sodium and potassium gradients. *J. Mol. Cell. Cardiol.* 16: 1023–1036, 1984.

Fiolet, J.W.T., A. Baartscheer, C.A. Schumacher, H.F. ter Welle, and W.J.G. Krieger. Transmural inhomogeneity of energy metabolism during acute global ischemia in the isolated rat heart: dependence on environmental conditions. *J. Mol. Cell. Cardiol.* 17: 87–92, 1985.

Fisher, J.D., R. Mehra, and S. Furman. Termination of ventricular tachycardia with bursts of rapid ventricular pacing. *Am. J. Cardiol.* 41: 94–102, 1978.

Fischmeister, R., and G. Vassort. The electrogenic Na-Ca exchange and the cardiac electrical activity. I—Simulation on Purkinje fibre action potential. *J. Physiol. (Paris)* 77: 705–709, 1981.

Fitzgerald, D.M., K.J. Friday, J.A. Yeung Lai Wah, R. Lazzara, and W.M. Jackman. Electrogram patterns predicting successful catheter ablation of ventricular tachycardia. *Circulation* 77: 806–814, 1988.

Fleet, W.F., T.A. Johnson, C.A. Graebner, and L.S. Gettes. Effect of serial brief ischemic episodes on extracellular K^+, pH, and activation in the pig. *Circulation* 72: 922–932, 1985.

Fleet, W.F., T.A. Johnson, C.A. Graebner, C.L. Engle, and L.S. Gettes. Effects of verapamil on ischemia-induced changes in extracellular K^+, pH and local activation in the pig. *Circulation* 73: 837–846, 1986.

Fontaine, G., G. Guiraudon, R. Frank, A. Gerbaux, J.P. Cousteau, A. Barrillon, J. Gay, C. Cabrol, and J. Facquet. La cartographie épicardique et le traitement chirurgical par simple ventriculotomie de certaines tachycardies ventriculaires rebelles par réentrée. *Arch. Mal. Coeur* 68: 113–124, 1975.

Fontaine, G., G. Guiraudon, R. Frank, R. Coutte, and C. Dragodanne. Epicardial mapping and surgical treatment in six cases of resistant ventricular tachycardia not related to coronary artery disease. In: *The Conduction System of the Heart*, edited by H.J.J. Wellens, K.I. Lie, and M.J. Janse. Lea & Febiger, Philadelphia: 1976, pp. 545–563.

Fontaine, G., G. Guiraudon, R. Frank, Y. Tereau, A. Pavie, C. Cabrol, G. Chomette, and Y. Grosgogeat. Management of ventricular tachycardia not related to myocardial ischemia. *Clin. Prog. Pacing Electrophysiol.* 2: 193–219, 1984.

Forbes, A., L.H. Ray, and F.R. Griffith Jr. The nature of the delay in the response to the second of two stimuli in nerve and in the nerve-muscle preparation. *Am. J. Physiol.* 66: 553–617, 1923.

Forfar, J.C., R.A. Riemersma, and M.F. Oliver. α-Adrenoceptor control of norepinephrine release from acutely ischaemic myocardium: Effects of blood flow, arrhythmias, and regional conduction delay. *J. Cardiovasc. Pharmacol.* 5: 752–759, 1983.

Forfar, J.C., R.A. Riemersma, D.C. Russell, and M.F. Oliver. Relationship of neurosympathetic responsiveness to early ventricular arrhythmias in ischaemic myocardium. *Cardiovasc. Res.* 18: 427–437, 1984.

Forfar, J.C., D.C. Russell, and R.A. Riemersma. Control of myocardial catecholamine release during acute ischemia. *J. Cardiovasc. Pharmacol.* 7(Suppl. 5): S33-S39, 1985.

Fosset, M., J.R. De Weille, R.D. Green, H. Schmid-Antomarchi, and M. Lazdunski. Antidiabetic sulfonylureas control action potential properties in heart cells via high affinity receptors that are linked to ATP-dependent K^+ channels. *J. Biol. Chem.* 263: 7933–7936, 1988.

Fozzard, H.A. Conduction of the action potential. In: *The Cardiovascular System*, edited by R.M. Berne. The American Physiological Society, Bethesda: 1979, pp. 335–356.

Fozzard, H.A., O.M. Sejersted, and J.A. Wasserstrom. Sodium activation of the Na K-pump in isolated sheep cardiac Purkinje strands. (abstract) *J. Physiol.* 381: 91P, 1986.

Fozzard, H.A. The roles of membrane potential and inward Na^+ and Ca^{2+} currents in determining conduction. In: *Cardiac Electrophysiology: A Textbook*, edited by M.R. Rosen, M.J. Janse, and A.L. Wit. Futura Publishing Company, Mt. Kisco, New York: 1990, pp. 415–425.

Frame, L.H., and B.F. Hoffman. Mechanisms of tachycardia. In: *Tachycardias*, edited by B. Surawicz, C.P. Reddy, and E.N. Prystowsky. Martinus Nijhoff, Boston: 1984, pp. 7–36.

Frame, L.H., R.L. Page, and B.F. Hoffman. Atrial reentry around an anatomic barrier with a partially excitable gap. A canine model of atrial flutter. *Circ. Res.* 58: 495–511, 1986.

Frame, L.H., R.L. Page, P.A. Boyden, J.J. Fenoglio Jr., and B.F. Hoffman. Circus movement in the canine atrium around the tricuspid ring during experimental atrial flutter and during reentry in vitro. *Circulation* 76: 1155–1175, 1987.

Frank, J., M. Dolder, M. Gertsch, U. Althaus, H.P. Gurtner. Ventrikuläre Rhythmusstörungen im akuten Stadium des experimentellen Myokardinfarktes beim Schwein; Einfluss des β-blockers Pindolol und des Calcium-Antagonisten Ro 11–1781. *Schweiz. Med. Wschr.* 108: 1740–1743, 1978.

Frank, R., J.L. Tonet, S. Kounde, G. Farenq, and G. Fontaine. Localization of the area of slow conduction during ventricular tachycardia. In: *Cardiac Arrhythmias: Where To Go From Here?*, edited by P. Brugada and H.J.J. Wellens. Futura Publishing Company, Mt. Kisco, New York: 1987, pp. 191–208.

Franz, M.R., D. Burkhoff, D.T. Yue, and K. Sagawa. Mechanically induced action potential changes and arrhythmias in isolated and in situ canine hearts. *Cardiovasc. Res.* 23: 213–223, 1989.

Freedman, R.A., C.D. Swerdlow, D.S. Echt, R.A. Winkle. V. Soderholm-Difatte, and J.W. Mason. Facilitation of ventricular tachyarrhythmia induction by isoproterenol. *Am. J. Cardiol.* 54: 765–770, 1984.

Friedman, P.L., J.R. Stewart, J.J. Fenoglio Jr., and A.L. Wit. Survival of subendocardial Purkinje fibers after extensive myocardial infarction in dogs. In vitro and in vivo correlations. *Circ. Res.* 33: 597–611, 1973a.

Friedman, P.L., J.R. Stewart, and A.L. Wit. Spontaneous and induced cardiac arrhythmias in subendocardial Purkinje fibers surviving extensive myocardial infarction in dogs. *Circ. Res.* 33: 612–626, 1973b.

Friedman, P.L., J.J. Fenoglio Jr., and A.L. Wit. Time course for reversal of electrophysiological and ultrastructural abnormalities in subendocardial Purkinje fibers surviving extensive myocardial infarction in dogs. *Circ. Res.* 36: 127–144, 1975.

Fujiwara, H., M. Ashraf, S. Sato, and R.W. Millard. Transmural cellular damage and blood flow distribution in early ischemia in pig hearts. *Circ. Res.* 51: 683–693, 1982.

Furukawa, T., S. Kimura, A. Castellanos, A.L. Bassett, and R.J. Myerburg. In vivo induction of "focal" triggered ventricular arrhythmias and responses to overdrive pacing in the canine heart. *Circulation* 82: 549–559, 1990.

Gadsby, D.C., and P.F. Cranefield. Two levels of resting potential in cardiac Purkinje fibers. *J. Gen. Physiol.* 70: 725–746, 1977.

Gadsby, D.C., A.L. Wit, and P.F. Cranefield. The effects of acetylcholine on the electrical activity of canine cardiac Purkinje fibers. *Circ. Res.* 43: 29–35, 1978.

Gadsby, D.C., and P.F. Cranefield. Electrogenic sodium extrusion in cardiac Purkinje fibers. *J. Gen. Physiol.* 73: 819–837, 1979a.

Gadsby, D.C., and P.F. Cranefield. Direct measurement of changes in sodium pump current in canine cardiac Purkinje fibers. *Proc. Natl. Acad. Sci. USA* 76: 1783- 1787, 1979b.

Gadsby, D.C., and A.L. Wit. Electrophysiologic characteristics of cardiac cells and the genesis of cardiac arrhythmias. In: *Cardiac Pharmacology*, edited by R.D. Wilkersen. Academic Press, New York: 1981, pp. 229–274.

Gadsby, D.C., and P.F. Cranefield. Effects of electrogenic sodium extrusion on the membrane potential of cardiac Purkinje fibers. In: *Normal and Abnormal Conduction in the Heart*, edited by A. Paes de Carvalho, B.F. Hoffman, and M. Lieberman. Futura Publishing Company, Mt. Kisco, New York: 1982, pp. 225–244.

Gaide, M.S., R.J. Myerburg, P.L. Kozlovskis, and A.L. Bassett. Elevated sympathetic response of epicardium proximal to healed myocardial infarction. *Am. J. Physiol.* 245: H646-H652, 1983.

Gallagher, J.D., A.J. Del Rossi, J. Fernandez, V. Maranhao, M.D. Strong, M. White, and L.J. Gessman. Cryothermal mapping of recurrent ventricular tachycardia in man. *Circulation* 71: 733–739, 1985.

Gallagher, J.J., E.L.C. Pritchett, W.C. Sealy, J. Kasell, and A.G. Wallace. The preexcitation syndromes. *Prog. Cardiovasc. Dis.* 20: 285–327, 1978.

Gambetta, M., and R.W. Childers. The initial electrophysiologic disturbance in experimental myocardial infarction. (abstract) *Ann. Intern. Med.* 70: 1076, 1969.

Gang, E.S., J.T. Bigger Jr., and F.D. Livelli Jr. A model of chronic ischemic arrhythmias: The relation between electrically inducible ventricular tachycardia, ventricular fibrillation threshold and myocardial infarct size. *Am. J. Cardiol.* 50: 469–477, 1982.

Gang, E.S., J.A. Reiffel, F.D. Livelli Jr., and J.T. Bigger Jr. Sinus node recovery times following the spontaneous termination of supraventricular tachycardia and following atrial overdrive pacing: A comparison. *Am. Heart J.* 105: 210–215, 1983.

Gang, E.S., J.T. Bigger Jr., and E.W. Uhl. Effects of timolol and propranolol on inducible sustained ventricular tachyarrhythmias in dogs with subacute myocardial infarction. *Am. J. Cardiol.* 53: 275–281, 1984.

Garan, H., J.T. Fallon, and J.N. Ruskin. Sustained ventricular tachycardia in recent canine myocardial infarction. *Circulation* 62: 980–987, 1980.

Garan, H., J.T. Fallon, and J.N. Ruskin. Nonsustained polymorphic ventricular tachycardia induced by electrical stimulation in 3 week old canine myocardial infarction. *Am. J. Cardiol.* 48: 280–286, 1981.

Garan, H., and J.N. Ruskin. Localized reentry. Mechanism of induced sustained ventricular tachycardia in canine model of recent myocardial infarction. *J. Clin. Invest.* 74: 377–392, 1984.

Garan, H., J.N. Ruskin, B. McGovern, and G. Grant. Serial analysis of electrically induced ventricular arrhythmias in a canine model of myocardial infarction. *J. Am. Coll. Cardiol.* 5: 1095–1106, 1985.

Garan, H., J.T. Fallon, S. Rosenthal, and J.N. Ruskin. Endocardial, intramural, and epicardial activation patterns during sustained monomorphic ventricular tachycardia in late canine myocardial infarction. *Circ. Res.* 60: 879–896, 1987.

Garan, H., J.M. McComb, and J.N. Ruskin. Spontaneous and electrically induced ventricular arrhythmias during acute ischemia superimposed on 2 week old canine myocardial infarction. *J. Am. Coll. Cardiol.* 11: 603–611, 1988.

Gardner, P.I., P.C. Ursell, J.J. Fenoglio Jr., M.A. Allessie, F.I.M. Bonke, and A.L. Wit. Structure of the epicardial border zone in canine infarcts is a cause of reentrant excitation. (abstract) *Circulation* 64(Suppl. IV): IV-320, 1981.

Gardner, P.I., P.C. Ursell, T.D. Pham, J.J. Fenoglio Jr., and A.L. Wit. Experimental chronic ventricular tachycardia: Anatomic and electrophysiologic substrates. In: *Tachycardias: Mechanisms, Diagnosis, Treatment*, edited by M.E. Josephson, and H.J.J. Wellens. Lea & Febiger, Philadelphia: 1984, pp. 29–60.

Gardner, P.I., P.C. Ursell, J.J. Fenoglio Jr., and A.L. Wit. Electrophysiologic and anatomic basis for fractionated electrograms recorded from healed myocardial infarcts. *Circulation* 72: 596–611, 1985.

Garrey, W.E. The nature of fibrillary contraction of the heart.—Its relation to tissue mass and form. *Am. J. Physiol.* 33: 397–414, 1914.

Garrey, W.E. Auricular fibrillation. *Physiol. Rev.* 4: 215–250, 1924.

Gaspardone, A., K.I. Shine, S.R. Seabrooke, and P.A. Poole-Wilson. Potassium loss from rabbit myocardium during hypoxia: Evidence for passive efflux linked to anion extrusion. *J. Mol. Cell. Cardiol.* 18: 389–399, 1986.

Geer, J.C., C.A. Crago, W.C. Little, L.L. Gardner, and S.P. Bishop. Subendocardial ischemic myocardial lesions associated with severe coronary atherosclerosis. *Am. J. Pathol.* 98: 663–680, 1980.

Gelband, H., and A.L. Bassett. Depressed transmembrane potentials during experimentally induced ventricular failure in cats. *Circ. Res.* 32: 625–634, 1973.

Geltman, E.M., A.A. Ehsani, M.K. Campbell, K. Schechtman, R. Roberts, and B.E. Sobel. The influence of location and extent of myocardial infarction on long-term ventricular dysrhythmia and mortality. *Circulation* 60: 805–814, 1979.

Gessman, L.J., J.B. Agarwal, and R.H. Helfant. Methyl prednisolone increases the incidence of sudden death and inducible ventricular tachycardia in dogs with myocardial infarction. (abstract) *Clin. Res.* 29: 650A, 1981.

Gessman, L.J., J.B. Agarwal, T. Endo, and R.H. Helfant. Localization and mechanism of ventricular tachycardia by ice mapping 1 week after the onset of myocardial infarction in dogs. *Circulation* 68: 657–666, 1983.

Gettes, L.S., and H. Reuter. Slow recovery from inactivation of inward currents in mammalian myocardial fibres. *J. Physiol.* 240: 703–724, 1974.

Gettes, L.S., J.W. Buchanan Jr., T. Saito, Y. Kagiyama, S. Oshita, and T. Fujino. Studies concerned with slow conduction. In: *Cardiac Electrophysiology and Arrhythmias*, edited by D.P. Zipes, and J. Jalife. Grune & Stratton, Orlando: 1985, pp. 81–87.

Gibson, J.K., and B.R. Lucchesi. Electrophysiologic actions of UM-272 (Pranolium) on reentrant ventricular arrhythmias in postinfarction canine myocardium. *J. Pharmacol. Exp. Ther.* 214: 347–353, 1980.

Giles, W., A. Van Ginneken, and E.F. Shibata. Ionic currents underlying cardiac pacemaker activity: A summary of voltage clamp data from single cells. In: *Cardiac Muscle: The Regulation of Excitation and Contraction*, edited by R. Nathan. Academic Press, New York: 1986, pp. 1–27.

Gillette, P.C. The mechanisms of supraventricular tachycardia in children. *Circulation* 54: 133–139, 1976.

Gillette, P.C., and A. Garson Jr. Electrophysiologic and pharmacologic characteristics of automatic ectopic atrial tachycardia. *Circulation* 56: 571–575, 1977.

Gillette, P.C., J.D. Kugler, A. Garson Jr., H.P. Gutgesell, D.F. Duff, and D.G. McNamara. Mechanisms of cardiac arrhythmias after the Mustard operation for transposition of the great arteries. *Am. J. Cardiol.* 45: 1225–1230, 1980.

Gilmour, R.F. Jr., and D.P. Zipes. Different electrophysiological responses of canine endocardium and epicardium to combined hyperkalemia, hypoxia and acidosis. *Circ. Res.* 46: 814–825, 1980.

Gilmour, R.F. Jr., and D.P. Zipes. Electrophysiological response of vascularized hamster cardiac transplants to ischemia. *Circ. Res.* 50: 599–609, 1982.

Gilmour, R.F. Jr., J.J. Evans, and D.P. Zipes. Purkinje-muscle coupling and endocardial response to hyperkalemia, hypoxia, and acidosis. *Am. J. Physiol.* 247: H303-H311, 1984.

Gilmour, R.F. Jr., J.J. Evans, and D.P. Zipes. Preferential interruption of impulse transmission across Purkinje-muscle junctions by interventions that depress conduction. In: *Cardiac Electrophysiology and Arrhythmias*, edited by D.P. Zipes, and J. Jalife. Grune and Stratton, Orlando: 1985, pp. 287–300.

Gilmour, R.F. Jr., and D.P. Zipes. Abnormal automaticity and related phenomena. In: *The Heart and Cardiovascular System*, edited by H.A. Fozzard, E.

Haber, R.B. Jennings, A.M. Katz, and H.E. Morgan. Raven Press, New York: 1986, pp. 1239–1257.

Gintant, G.A., and I.S. Cohen. Advances in cardiac cellular electrophysiology: Implications for automaticity and therapeutics. *Ann. Rev. Pharmacol. Toxicol.* 28: 61–81, 1988.

Gintant, G.A., I.S. Cohen, N.B. Datyner, and R.P. Kline. Time-dependent outward currents in the heart. In: *The Heart and Cardiovascular System*, edited by H.A. Fozzard, E. Haber, R.B. Jennings, A.M. Katz, and H.E. Morgan. Raven Press, New York: 1991, pp. 1121–1169.

Glitsch, H.G. Characteristics of active Na transport in intact cardiac cells. *Am. J. Physiol.* 236: H189-H199, 1979.

Goldberg, S., A.J. Greenspon, P.L. Urban, B. Muza, B. Berger, P. Walinsky, and P.R. Maroko. Reperfusion arrhythmia: A marker of restoration of antegrade flow during intracoronary thrombolysis for acute myocardial infarction. *Am. Heart J.* 105: 26–32, 1983.

Goldenberg, M., and C.J. Rothberger. Über die Wirkung von Veratrin auf den Purkinjefaden. *Pflügers Arch.* 238: 137–152, 1937.

Goldreyer, B.N., and J.T.Bigger Jr. Site of reentry in paroxysmal supraventricular tachycardia in man. *Circulation* 43: 15–26, 1971.

Goldreyer, B.N., and A.N. Damato. The essential role of atrioventricular conduction delay in the initiation of paroxysmal supraventricular tachycardia. *Circulation* 43: 679–687, 1971.

Goldreyer, B.N., J.J. Gallagher, and A.N. Damato. The electrophysiologic demonstration of atrial ectopic tachycardia in man. *Am. Heart J.* 85: 205–215, 1973.

Goldstein, S., J.R. Landis, R. Leighton, G. Ritter, C.M. Vasu, A. Lantis, and R. Serokman. Characteristics of the resuscitated out-of-hospital cardiac arrest victim with coronary heart disease. *Circulation* 64: 977–984, 1981.

Goldstein, S., S.V. Medendorp, J.R. Landis, R.A. Wolfe, R. Leighton, G. Ritter, C.M. Vasu, and A. Acheson. Analysis of cardiac symptoms preceding cardiac arrest. *Am. J. Cardiol.* 58: 1195–1198, 1986.

Goldstein, S.S., and W. Rall. Changes of action potential shape and velocity for changing core conductor geometry. *Biophys. J.* 14: 731–757, 1974.

Gomes, J.A.C., R.I. Hariman, P.S. Kang, N. El-Sherif, I. Chowdhry, and J. Lyons. Programmed electrical stimulation in patients with high-grade ventricular ectopy: electrophysiologic findings and prognosis for survival. *Circulation* 70: 43–51, 1984.

Gomes, J.A., and S.L. Winters. The origins of the sinus node pacemaker complex in man: Demonstration of dominant and subsidiary foci. *J. Am. Coll. Cardiol.* 9: 45–52, 1987.

Gorgels, A.P.M., H.D.M. Beekman, P. Brugada, W.R.M. Dassen, D.A.B. Richards, and H.J.J. Wellens. Extrastimulus-related shortening of the first postpacing interval in digitalis-induced ventricular tachycardia: observations during programmed electrical stimulation in the conscious dog. *J. Am. Coll. Cardiol.* 1: 840–857, 1983.

Gorgels, A.P.M., B. de Wit, H.D.M. Beekman, W.R.M. Dassen, and H.J.J. Wellens. Triggered activity induced by pacing during digitalis intoxication: observations during programmed electrical stimulation in the conscious dog with chronic complete atrioventricular block. *PACE* 10: 1309–1321, 1987.

Gorgels, A.P.M., M.A. Vos, I.S. Letsch, E.A. Verschuuren, F.W.H.M. Bär, J.H.A. Janssen, and H.J.J. Wellens. Usefulness of the accelerated idioventricular rhythm as a marker for myocardial necrosis and reperfusion during thrombolytic therapy in acute myocardial infarction. *Am. J. Cardiol.* 61: 231–235, 1988.

Gornick, C.C., H.G. Tobler, I.C. Tuna, and D.G. Benditt. Electrophysiological effects of left ventricular free wall traction in intact hearts. *Am. J. Physiol.* 257: H1211–H1219, 1989.

Gottlieb, C.D., M.E. Rosenthal, N.J. Stamato, L.H. Frame, M.D. Lesh, J.M. Miller, and M.E. Josephson. A quantitative evaluation of refractoriness within a reentrant circuit during ventricular tachycardia. Relation to termination. *Circulation* 82: 1289–1295, 1990.

Gough, W.B., R.H. Zeiler, and N. El-Sherif. Effects of diltiazem on triggered activity in canine 1 day old infarction. *Cardiovasc. Res.* 18: 339–343, 1984.

Gough, W.B., R. Mehra, M. Restivo, R.H. Zeiler, and N. El-Sherif. Reentrant ventricular arrhythmias in the late myocardial infarction period in the dog. 13. Correlation of activation and refractory maps. *Circ. Res.* 57: 432–442, 1985.

Gough, W.B., D. Hu, and N. El-Sherif. Effects of clofilium on ischemic subendocardial Purkinje fibers 1 day postinfarction. *J. Am. Coll. Cardiol.* 11: 431–437, 1988.

Gough, W.B., and N. El-Sherif. Dependence of delayed afterdepolarizations on diastolic potentials in ischemic Purkinje fibers. *Am. J. Physiol.* 257: H770-H777, 1989.

Gradman, A.H., P.A. Bell, and R.F. DeBusk. Sudden death during ambulatory monitoring. Clinical and electrocardiographic correlations. Report of a case. *Circulation* 55: 210–211, 1977.

Granath, A., T. Södermark, T. Winge, U. Volpe, and S. Zetterquist. Early work load tests for evaluation of long-term prognosis of acute myocardial infarction. *Br. Heart J.* 39: 758–763, 1977.

Grant, A.O., and B.G. Katzung. The effects of quinidine and verapamil on electrically induced automaticity in the ventricular myocardium of guinea pig. *J. Pharmacol. Exp. Ther.* 196: 407–419, 1976.

Grant, A.O., and C.F. Starmer. Mechanisms of closure of cardiac sodium channels in rabbit ventricular myocytes: single-channel analysis. *Circ. Res.* 60: 897–913, 1987.

Greenberg, Y.J., and M. Vassalle. On the mechanism of overdrive suppression in the guinea pig sinoatrial node. *J. Electrocardiol.* 23: 53–67, 1990.

Greene, H.L., P.R. Reid, and A.H. Schaeffer. The repetitive ventricular response in man. A predictor of sudden death. *N. Engl. J. Med.* 299: 729–734, 1978.

Guarnieri, T., and H.C. Strauss. Intracellular potassium activity in guinea pig papillary muscle during prolonged hypoxia. *J. Clin. Invest.* 69: 435–442, 1982.

Guse, P., B.J. Scherlag, G. Kabell, R.R. Hope, and R. Lazzara. Effect of methyl-prednisolone on ventricular arrhythmias, mortality and infarct size following experimental coronary artery occlusion. (abstract) *Am. J. Cardiol.* 43: 372, 1979.

Guyton, A.C. *Textbook of Medical Physiology.* W.B. Saunders Company, Philadelphia: 1986, p. 14.

Haase, M., and U. Schiller. Zur zeitlichen Parallelität zwischen der Aktivität ektopischer Schrittmacher und dem Eintritt von Kammerflimmern nach Ligatur eines Hauptkoronarastes beim Hund. *Acta Biol. Med. Germ.* 23: 413–422, 1969.

Hagiwara, N., H. Irisawa, and M. Kameyama. Contribution of two types of calcium currents to the pacemaker potentials of rabbit sino-atrial node cells. *J. Physiol.* 395: 233–253, 1988.

Halsey, R.H. A case of ventricular fibrillation. *Heart* 6: 67–76, 1915.

Hamer, A., J. Vohra, D. Hunt, and G. Sloman. Prediction of sudden death by electrophysiologic studies in high risk patients surviving acute myocardial infarction. *Am. J. Cardiol.* 50: 223–229, 1982.

Hamer, A.W., H.S. Karagueuzian, K. Sugi, C.A. Zaher, W.J. Mandel, and T. Peter. Factors related to the induction of ventricular fibrillation in the normal canine heart by programmed electrical stimulation. *J. Am. Coll. Cardiol.* 3: 751–759, 1984.

Hamlin, R.L., R.R. Burton, S.D. Leverett, and J.W. Burns. Ventricular activation process in minipigs. *J. Electrocardiol.* 8: 113–116, 1975.

Hamra, M., and M.R. Rosen. α Adrenergic receptor stimulation during simulated ischemia and reperfusion in canine cardiac Purkinje fibers. *Circulation* 78: 1495–1502, 1988.

Han, J., and G.K. Moe. Nonuniform recovery of excitability in ventricular muscle. *Circ. Res.* 14: 44–60, 1964.

Han, J., J. DeTraglia, D. Millet, and G.K. Moe. Incidence of ectopic beats as a function of basic rate in the ventricle. *Am. Heart J.* 72: 632–639, 1966.

Han, J., B.G. Goel, and C.S. Hanson. Re-entrant beats induced in the ventricle during coronary occlusion. *Am. Heart J.* 80: 778–784, 1970.

Hanich, R.F., C.D.J. De Langen, A.H. Kadish, E.L. Michelson, J.H. Levine, J.F. Spear, and E.N. Moore. Inducible sustained ventricular tachycardia 4 years after experimental canine myocardial infarction: Electrophysiologic and anatomic comparisons with early healed infarcts. *Circulation* 77: 445–456, 1988a.

Hanich, R.F., J.H. Levine, J.F. Spear, and E.N. Moore. Autonomic modulation of ventricular arrhythmia in cesium chloride-induced long QT syndrome. *Circulation* 77: 1149–1161, 1988b.

Hanna, M.S., K.P. Dresdner, R.P. Kline, and A.L. Wit. Characterization of transmembrane potential and intracellular potassium activity in the epicardial border zone 24 hours after myocardial infarction. (abstract) *Circulation* 76(Suppl. IV): IV-16, 1987.

Hansen, D.E., C.S. Craig, and L.M. Hondeghem. Stretch-induced arrhythmias in the isolated canine ventricle. Evidence for the importance of mechanoelectrical feedback. *Circulation* 81: 1094–1105, 1990.

Hariman, R.J., E. Krongrad, R.A. Boxer, F.O. Bowman Jr., J.R. Malm, and B.F. Hoffman. Methods for recording electrograms of the sinoatrial node during cardiac surgery in man. *Circulation* 61: 1024–1029, 1980.

Harris, A.S., and G.K. Moe. Idioventricular rhythms and fibrillation induced at the anode or the cathode by direct currents of long duration. *Am. J. Physiol.* 136: 318–331, 1942.

Harris, A.S., and A. Guevara Rojas. The initiation of ventricular fibrillation due to coronary occlusion. *Exp. Med. & Surg.* 1: 105–122, 1943.

Harris, A.S. Delayed development of ventricular ectopic rhythms following experimental coronary occlusion. *Circulation* 1: 1318–1328, 1950.

Harris, A.S., A. Estandia, and R.F. Tillotson. Ventricular ectopic rhythms and ventricular fibrillation following cardiac sympathectomy and coronary occlusion. *Am. J. Physiol.* 165: 505–512, 1951.

Harris, A.S., A. Bisteni, R.A. Russell, J.C. Brigham, and J.E. Firestone. Excitatory factors in ventricular tachycardia resulting from myocardial ischemia. Potassium a major excitant. *Science* 119: 200–203, 1954.

Harris, A.S., H. Otero, and A.J. Bocage. The induction of arrhythmias by sympathetic activity before and after occlusion of a coronary artery in the canine heart. *J. Electrocardiol.* 4: 34–43, 1971.

Harris, L., E. Downar, L. Mickleborough, N. Shaikh, and I. Parson. Activation sequence of ventricular tachycardia: endocardial and epicardial mapping studies in the human ventricle. *J. Am. Coll. Cardiol.* 10: 1040–1047, 1987.

Harrison, L.A., G. Kabell, J. Brachmann, B.J. Scherlag, and R. Lazzara. Ventricular arrhythmias in transmural versus subendocardial infarction. (abstract) *Circulation* 62(Suppl. III): III-197, 1980.

Hauer, R.N.W., M.T. de Zwart, J.M.T. de Bakker, J.F. Hitchcock, O.C.K.M. Penn, M. Nijsen-Karelse, and E.O. Robles de Medina. Endocardial catheter mapping: wire skeleton technique for representation of computed arrhythmogenic sites compared with intraoperative mapping. *Circulation* 74: 1346–1354, 1986.

Hauer, R.N.W. The Site of Origin of Ventricular Tachycardia. Identification, localization, and ablation using catheter techniques. (Doctoral Thesis) University of Utrecht; The Netherlands, 1987.

Hashimoto, K., and G.K. Moe. Transient depolarizations induced by acetylstrophanthidin in specialized tissue of dog atrium and ventricle. *Circ. Res.* 32: 618–624, 1973.

Hauswirth, O., D. Noble, and R.W. Tsien. The mechanism of oscillatory activity at low membrane potentials in cardiac Purkinje fibres. *J. Physiol.* 200: 255–265, 1969.

Hayashi, H., C. Ponnambalam, and T.F. McDonald. Arrhythmic activity in reoxygenated guinea pig papillary muscles and ventricular cells. *Circ. Res.* 61: 124–133, 1987.

Hearse, D.J., and D.M. Yellon (Editors). *Therapeutic Approaches to Myocardial Infarct Size Limitation.* Raven Press, New York: 1984.

Hearse, D.J. Free radicals and myocardial injury during ischemia and reperfusion: a short-lived phenomenon? In: *Lethal Arrhythmias Resulting From Myocardial Ischemia and Infarction,* edited by M.R. Rosen, and Y. Palti. Kluwer Academic Publishers, Boston: 1989, pp. 105–115.

Helfant, R.H., R. Pine, V. Kabde, and V.S. Banka. Exercise-related ventricular premature complexes in coronary heart disease. Correlations with ischemia and angiographic severity. *Ann. Intern. Med.* 80: 589–592, 1974.

Hellerstein, H.K., and I.M. Liebow. Electrical alternation in experimental coronary artery occlusion. *Am. J. Physiol.* 160: 366–374, 1950.

Henning, B., and A.L. Wit. Action potential characteristics control afterdepolarization amplitude and triggered activity in canine coronary sinus. *Circulation* 64(Suppl. IV): IV-50, 1981.

Henning, B., and A.L. Wit. The time course of action potential repolarization affects delayed afterdepolarization amplitude in atrial fibers of the canine coronary sinus. *Circ. Res.* 55: 110–115, 1984.

Henning, B., R.P. Kline, M.S. Siegal, and A.L. Wit. Triggered activity in atrial fibres of canine coronary sinus: the role of extracellular potassium accumulation and depletion. *J. Physiol.* 383: 191–211, 1987.

Herre, J.M., L. Wetstein, Y.-L. Lin, A.S. Mills, M. Dao, and M.D. Thames. Effect of transmural versus nontransmural myocardial infarction on inducibility of ventricular arrhythmias during sympathetic stimulation in dogs. *J. Am. Coll. Cardiol.* 11: 414–421, 1988.

Hess, P., and R. Weingart. Intracellular free calcium modified by pH_i in sheep cardiac Purkinje fibres. *J. Physiol.* 307: 60P-61P, 1980.

Hewett, K., L. Gessman, and M.R. Rosen. Effects of procaine amide, quinidine and ethmozin on delayed afterdepolarizations. *Eur. J. Pharmacol.* 96: 21–28, 1983.

Hewett, K.W., and M.R. Rosen. Alpha and beta adrenergic interactions with ouabain-induced delayed afterdepolarizations. *J. Pharmacol. Exp. Ther.* 229: 188–192, 1984.

Hill, J.L., and L.S. Gettes. Effects of acute coronary artery occlusion on local myocardial extracellular K^+ activity in swine. *Circulation* 61: 768–778, 1980.

Hiraoka, M. Membrane current changes induced by acetylstrophanthidin in cardiac Purkinje fibers. *Jpn. Heart J.* 18: 851–859, 1977.

Hiraoka, M., Y. Okamoto, and T. Sano. Oscillatory afterpotentials and triggered-automaticity in mammalian ventricular muscle fibres at high resting potentials. *Experientia* 35: 500–501, 1979.

Hiraoka, M., Y. Okamoto, and T. Sano. Oscillatory afterpotentials in dog ventricular muscle fibers. *Circ. Res.* 48: 510–518, 1981.

Hiraoka, M., and S. Kawano. Regulation of delayed afterdepolarizations and aftercontractions in dog ventricular muscle fibres. *J. Mol. Cell. Cardiol.* 16: 285–289, 1984.

Hirche, H.J., C. Franz, L. Bös, R. Bissig, R. Lang, and M. Schramm. Myocardial extracellular K^+ and H^+ increase and noradrenaline release as possible cause of early arrhythmias following acute coronary artery occlusion in pigs. *J. Mol. Cell. Cardiol.* 12: 579–593, 1980.

Hiromasa, S., H. Coto, Z-Y. Li, C. Maldonado, and J. Kupersmith. Dextrorotatory isomer of sotalol: electrophysiologic effects and interaction with verapamil. *Am. Heart J.* 116: 1552–1557, 1988.

Hirzel, H.O., G.R. Nelson, E.H. Sonnenblick, and E.S. Kirk. Redistribution of collateral blood flow from necrotic to surviving myocardium following coronary occlusion in the dog. *Circ. Res.* 39: 214–222, 1976.

Hodgkin, A.L., and B. Katz. The effect of sodium ions on the electrical activity of the giant axon of the squid. *J. Physiol.* 108: 37–77, 1949.

Hodgkin, A.L. and A.F. Huxley. A quantitative description of membrane current and its application to conduction and excitation in nerve. *J. Physiol.* 117: 500–544, 1952.

Hodgkin, A.L. A note on conduction velocity. *J. Physiol.* 125: 221–224, 1954.

Hoffman, A. Fibrillation of the ventricles at the end of an attack of paroxysmal tachycardia in men. *Heart* 213–217, 1911–1912.

Hoffman, B.F., E.F. Gorin, F.S. Wax, A.A. Siebens, and C.McC. Brooks. Vulnerability to fibrillation and the ventricular-excitability curve. *Am. J. Physiol.* 167: 88–94, 1951.

Hoffman, B.F., and P.F. Cranefield. *Electrophysiology of the Heart.* McGraw-Hill, New York: 1960.

Hoffman, B.F., and P.F. Cranefield. The physiological basis of cardiac arrhythmias. *Am. J. Med.* 37: 670–684, 1964.

Hoffman, B.F. The genesis of cardiac arrhythmias. *Prog. Cardiovasc. Dis.* 8: 319–329, 1966.

Hoffman, B.F., and D.H. Singer. Appraisal of the effects of catecholamines on cardiac electrical activity. In: *New Adrenergic Blocking Drugs: Their Pharmacological, Biochemical and Clinical Actions*, edited by E.M. Weyer, N.C. Moran, H. Hutchins, and M.L. McWhiney. Ann. N.Y. Acad. Sci. 139: 914–939, 1967.

Hoffman, B.F. Role of the sympathetic nervous system in arrhythmias occurring after coronary artery occlusion and myocardial infarction. In: *Neural Mechanisms in Cardiac Arrhythmias*, edited by P.J. Schwartz, A.M. Brown, A. Malliani, and A. Zanchetti. Perspectives in Cardiovascular Research, Volume 2. Raven Press, New York: 1978, pp. 155–166.

Hoffman, B.F., and M.R. Rosen. Cellular mechanisms for cardiac arrhythmias. *Circ. Res.* 49: 1–15, 1981.

Hoffman, B.F., and K.H. Dangman. Are arrhythmias caused by automatic impulse generation? In: *Normal and Abnormal Conduction in the Heart*, edited by A. Paes de Carvalho, B.F. Hoffman, and M. Lieberman. Futura Publishing Company, Mt. Kisco, New York: 1982, pp. 429–448.

Hogan, P.M., and L.D. Davis. Evidence for specialized fibers in the canine right atrium. *Circ. Res.* 23: 387–396, 1968.

Hogan, P.M., S.M. Wittenberg, and F.J. Klocke. Relationship of stimulation frequency to automaticity in the canine Purkinje fiber during ouabain administration. *Circ. Res.* 32: 377–384, 1973.

Holland, R.P., and H. Brooks. The QRS complex during myocardial ischemia. An experimental analysis in the porcine heart. *J. Clin. Invest.* 57: 541–550, 1976.

Hondeghem, L.M., and C.L. Cotner. Reproducible and uniform cardiac ischemia: Effects of antiarrhythmic drugs. *Am. J. Physiol.* 235: H574-H580, 1978.

Honjo, H., M. Hirai, T. Osaka, I. Kuodama, J. Toyama, and K. Yamada. Effects of acute ischemia on the endocardial activation sequence of canine left ventricle. *Environmental Med.* 30: 83–88, 1986.

Hope, R.R., D.O. Williams, N. El-Sherif, R. Lazzara, and B.J. Scherlag. The efficacy of antiarrhythmic agents during acute myocardial ischemia and the role of heart rate. *Circulation* 50: 507–514, 1974.

Hope, R.R., B.J. Scherlag, N. El-Sherif, and R. Lazzara. Hierarchy of ventricular pacemakers. *Circ. Res.* 39: 883–888, 1976.

Hope, R.R., B.J. Scherlag, N. El-Sherif, and R. Lazzara. Continuous concealed ventricular arrhythmias. *Am. J. Cardiol.* 40: 733–738, 1977.

Hope, R.R., B.J. Scherlag, N. El-Sherif, and R. Lazzara. Ventricular arrhythmias in healing myocardial infarction. Role of rhythm versus rate in reentrant activation. *J. Thorac. Cardiovasc. Surg.* 75. 458–400, 1978.

Hope, R.R., B.J. Scherlag, and R. Lazzara. Excitation of ischemic myocardium: Altered properties of conduction, refractoriness, and excitability. *Am. Heart J.* 99: 753–765, 1980.

Horacek, Th., M. Neumann, S. von Mutius, M. Budden, and W. Meesmann. Nonhomogeneous electrophysiological changes and the bimodal distribution of early ventricular arrhythmias during acute coronary artery occlusion. *Basic. Res. Cardiol.* 79: 649–667, 1984.

Hordof, A.J., R. Edie, J.R. Malm, B.F. Hoffman, and M.R. Rosen. Electrophysiologic properties and response to pharmacologic agents of fibers from diseased human atria. *Circulation* 54: 774–779, 1976.

Horn, E.M., N.J. Johnson, J.P. Bilezikian, and M.R. Rosen. Developmental changes in the electrophysiological properties and the β-adrenergic receptor-effector complex in atrial fibers of the canine coronary sinus. *Circ. Res.* 65: 325–333, 1989.

Horowitz, L.N., J.F. Spear, and E.N. Moore. Subendocardial origin of ventricular arrhythmias in 24-hour-old experimental myocardial infarction. *Circulation* 53: 56–63, 1976.

Horowitz, L.N., M.E. Josephson, and A.H. Harken. Epicardial and endocardial activation during sustained ventricular tachycardia in man. *Circulation* 61: 1227–1238, 1980.

Hoyt, R.H., M.L. Cohen, and J.E. Saffitz. Distribution and three-dimensional structure of intercellular junctions in canine myocardium. *Circ. Res.* 64: 563–574, 1989.

Hoyt, R.H., M.L. Cohen, P.B. Corr, and J.E. Saffitz. Alterations of intercellular junctions induced by hypoxia in canine myocardium. *Am. J. Physiol.* 258: H1439-H1448, 1990.

Hume, J., and B.G. Katzung. Physiological role of endogenous amines in the modulation of ventricular automaticity in the guinea-pig. *J. Physiol.* 309: 275–286, 1980.

Hunt, G.B., and D.L. Ross. Comparison of the effects of three anesthetic agents on induction of ventricular tachycardia in a canine model of myocardial infarction. *Circulation* 78: 221–226, 1988.

Hunt, G.B., and D.L. Ross. Influence of infarct age on reproducibility of ventricular tachycardia induction in a canine model. *J. Am. Coll. Cardiol.* 14: 765–773, 1989.

Hunt, G.B., and D.L. Ross. Effect of isoproterenol on induction of ventricular tachyarrhythmias in the normal and infarcted canine heart. *Int. J. Cardiol.* 29: 155–161, 1990.

Hunter, P.J., P.A. McNaughton, and D. Noble. Analytical models of propagation in excitable cells. *Prog. Biophys. Mol. Biol.* 30: 99–144, 1975.

Ideker, R.E., G.J. Klein, L. Harrison, W.M. Smith, J. Kasell, K.A. Reimer, A.G. Wallace, and J.J. Gallagher. The transition to ventricular fibrillation induced by reperfusion after acute ischemia in the dog: A period of organized epicardial activation. *Circulation* 63: 1371–1379, 1981.

Ikeda, K., and M. Hiraoka. Effects of hypoxia on passive electrical properties of canine ventricular muscle. *Pflügers Arch.* 393: 45–50, 1982.

Ilebekk, A., G. Aksnes, D.L. Rutlen, and Ø. Ellingsen. Myocardial potassium uptake after brief coronary artery occlusions in the pig. (abstract) *J. Mol. Cell. Cardiol.* 20(Suppl. V): S30, 1988.

Ilvento, J.P, J. Provet, P. Danilo Jr., and M.R. Rosen. Fast and slow idioventricular rhythms in the canine heart: A study of their mechanism using antiarrhythmic drugs and electrophysiologic testing. *Am. J. Cardiol.* 49: 1909–1916, 1982.

Imanishi, S. Calcium-sensitive discharges in canine Purkinje fibers. *Jpn. J. Physiol.* 21: 443–463, 1971.

Imanishi, S., and B. Surawicz. Automatic activity in depolarized guinea pig ventricular myocardium. *Circ. Res.* 39: 751–759, 1976.

Imanishi, S., R.G. McAllister Jr., and B. Surawicz. The effects of verapamil and lidocaine on the automatic depolarizations in guinea-pig ventricular myocardium. *J. Pharmacol. Exp. Ther.* 207: 294–303, 1978.

Imoto, Y., T. Ehara, and H. Matsuura. Voltage- and time-dependent block of i_{K1} underlying Ba^{2+}-induced ventricular automaticity. *Am. J. Physiol.* 252: H325-H333, 1987.

Inou, T., W.C. Lamberth Jr., S. Koyanagi, D.G. Harrison, C.L. Eastham, and M.L. Marcus. Relative importance of hypertension after coronary occlusion in chronic hypertensive dogs with LVH. *Am. J. Physiol.* 253: H1148-H1158, 1987.

Irisawa, H., and R. Sato. Intra- and extracellular actions of proton on the calcium current of isolated guinea pig ventricular cells. *Circ. Res.* 59: 348–355, 1986.

Irisawa, H. and W.R. Giles. Sinus and atrioventricular node cells: Cellular electrophysiology. In: *Cardiac Electrophysiology: From Cell to Bedside*, edited by D.P. Zipes, and J. Jalife. W.B. Saunders Company, Philadelphia: 1990, pp. 95–102.

Isenberg, G., and W. Trautwein. The effect of dihydro-ouabain and lithium-ions on the outward current in cardiac Purkinje fibers. Evidence for electrogenicity of active transport. *Pflügers Arch.* 350: 41–54, 1974.

Isenberg, G. Cardiac Purkinje fibers: cesium as a tool to block inward rectifying potassium currents. *Pflügers Arch.* 365: 99–106, 1976.

Isenberg, G. Cardiac Purkinje fibres. $[Ca^{2+}]_i$ controls steady state potassium conductance. *Pflügers Arch.* 371: 71–76, 1977.

Isenberg, G., J. Vereecke, G. van der Heyden, and E. Carmeliet. The shortening of the action potential by DNP in guinea-pig ventricular myocytes is mediated by an increase of a time-independent K conductance. *Pflügers Arch.* 397: 251–259, 1983.

Jackman, W.M., and D.P. Zipes. Low-energy synchronous cardioversion of ventricular tachycardia using a catheter electrode in a canine model of subacute myocardial infarction. *Circulation* 66: 187–195, 1982.

Jackman, W.M., M. Clark, K.J. Friday, E.M. Aliot, J. Anderson, and R. Lazzara. Ventricular tachyarrhythmias in the long QT syndromes. *Med. Clin. North Am.* 68: 1079–1109, 1984.

Jackrel, J., J.A. Miller, F.G. Schecter, S. Minkowitz, and J.H. Stuckey. Atrioventricular conduction following ligation of the anterior septal artery in the dog. An electrocardiographic, histopathologic and histochemical study. *Am. J. Cardiol.* 25: 552–561, 1970.

Jagadeesh, G., and S.D.S. Seth. Delayed development of ventricular arrhythmias following experimental coronary occlusion in pigs. *Jpn. J. Pharmacol.* 24: 479–482, 1974.

Jalife, J., and G.K. Moe. Effect of electrotonic potentials on pacemaker activity of canine Purkinje fibers in relation to parasystole. *Circ. Res.* 39: 801–808, 1976.

Jalife, J., and G.K. Moe. A biologic model of parasystole. *Am. J. Cardiol.* 43: 761–772, 1979.

Jalife, J., and G.K. Moe. Excitation, conduction, and reflection of impulses in isolated bovine and canine cardiac Purkinje fibers. *Circ. Res.* 49: 233–247, 1981.

Jalife, J., J.M. Davidenko, and D.C. Michaels. A new perspective on the mechanisms of arrhythmias and sudden cardiac death: spiral waves of excitation in heart muscle. *J. Cardiovasc. Electrophysiol.* 2:(Suppl. to #3): S133-S152, 1991.

James, T.N., J.H. Isobe, and F. Urthaler. Correlative electrophysiological and anatomical studies concerning the site of origin of escape rhythm during complete atrioventricular block in the dog. *Circ. Res.* 45: 108–119, 1979.

James, T.N. Automaticity in the atrioventricular junction. In: *Cardiac Electrophysiology: A Textbook*, edited by M.R. Rosen, M.J.J Janse, and A.L. Wit. Futura Publishing Company, Mt. Kisco, New York: 1990, pp. 191–222.

Janse, M.J., A.B.M. van der Steen, R.Th. van Dam, and D. Durrer. Refractory period of the dog's ventricular myocardium following sudden changes in frequency. *Circ. Res.* 24: 251–262, 1969.

Janse, M.J. The Effect of Changes in Heart Rate on the Refractory Period of the Heart. (Doctoral Thesis) University of Amsterdam; Mondeel-Offsetdrukkerij, Amsterdam, 1971.

Janse, M.J., F.J.L. van Capelle, G.E. Freud, and D. Durrer. Circus movement within the AV node a basis for supraventricular tachycardia as shown by multiple microelectrode recording in the isolated rabbit heart. *Circ. Res.* 28: 403–414, 1971.

Janse, M.J., F.J.L. van Capelle, R.H. Anderson, P. Touboul. and J. Billette. Electrophysiology and structure of the atrioventricular node of the isolated rabbit heart. In: *The Conduction System of the Heart*, edited by H.J.J. Wellens, K.I. Lie, and M.J. Janse. Lea & Febiger, Philadelphia: 1976, pp. 296–315.

Janse, M.J., and E. Downar. The effect of acute ischaemia on transmembrane potentials in the intact heart. The relation to reentrant mechanisms. In: *Re-Entrant Arrhythmias, Mechanisms and Treatment*, edited by H.E. Kulbertus. University Park Press, Baltimore: 1977, pp. 195–209.

Janse, M.J., A.G. Kléber, E. Downar, and D. Durrer. Changements electrophysiologiques pendant l'ischemie myocardique et mechanisme possible des troubles du rhythme ventriculaire. *Ann. Cardiol. Angeiol.* 26(Suppl): 551–554, 1977.

Janse, M.J., J. Tranum-Jensen, A.G. Kléber, and F.J.L. Van Capelle. Techniques and problems in correlating cellular electrophysiology and morphology in cardiac nodal tissues. In: *The Sinus Node. Structure, Function and Clinical Relevance*, edited by F.I.M. Bonke. Martinus Nijhoff Medical Division, The Hague: 1978, pp. 183–194.

Janse, M.J., and D. Durrer. Mechanisme en betekenis van de veranderingen in het ST-segment van het elektrocardiogram tijdens acute ischemie van de hartspier. *Ned. Tijdschr. Geneesk.* 122: 1964–1968, 1978.

Janse, M.J., J. Cinca, H. Moréna, J.W.T. Fiolet, A.G. Kléber, G.P. De Vries, A.E. Becker, and D. Durrer. The "border zone" in myocardial ischemia. An electrophysiological, metabolic and histochemical correlation in the pig heart. *Circ. Res.* 44: 576–588, 1979.

Janse, M.J., H. Moréna, J. Cinca, J.W.T. Fiolet, W.J. Krieger, and D. Durrer. Electrophysiological, metabolic and morphological aspects of acute myocardial ischemia in the isolated porcine heart. Characterization of the "border zone". *J. Physiol. (Paris)* 76: 785–790, 1980a.

Janse, M.J., H. Morsink, F.J.L. van Capelle, A.G. Kléber, F. Wilms-Schopman, and D. Durrer. Ventricular arrhythmias in the first 15 minutes of acute regional myocardial ischemia in the isolated pig heart: Possible role of injury currents. In: *Sudden Death*, edited by H.E. Kulbertus, and H.J.J. Wellens. Martinus Nijhoff Publishers, The Hague: 1980b, pp. 89–103.

Janse, M.J., F.J.L. Van Capelle, H. Morsink, A.G. Kléber, F.J.G. Wilms-Schopman, R. Cardinal, C. Naumann d'Alnoncourt, and D. Durrer. Flow of "injury" current and patterns of excitation during early ventricular arrhythmias in acute regional myocardial ischemia in isolated porcine and canine hearts. Evidence for two different arrhythmogenic mechanisms. *Circ. Res.* 47: 151–165, 1980c.

Janse, M.J., and A.G. Kléber. Electrophysiological changes and ventricular arrhythmias in the early phase of regional myocardial ischemia. *Circ. Res.* 49: 1069–1081, 1981.

Janse, M.J. Electrophysiological changes in the acute phase of myocardial ischaemia and mechanisms of ventricular arrhythmias. In: *Early Arrhythmias Resulting from Myocardial Ischaemia,* edited by J.R. Parratt. Oxford University Press, New York: 1982a, pp. 57–80.

Janse, M.J. Etiology of ventricular arrhythmias in the early phase of myocardial ischemia. Re-entry, focus and action of drugs. In: *Acute Phase of Ischemic Heart Disease and Myocardial Infarction*, edited by A.A.J. Adgey. Martinus Nijhoff Publishers, The Hague: 1982b, pp. 45–66.

Janse, M.J. Electrophysiological changes in acute myocardial ischemia. In: *What is Angina?*, edited by D.G. Julian, K.L. Lie, and L. Wilhelmsen. AB Hassle, Molndal, Sweden: 1982c, pp. 160–170.

Janse, M.J., and F.J.L. van Capelle. Electrotonic interactions across an inexcitable region as a cause of ectopic activity in acute regional myocardial ischemia. A study in intact porcine and canine hearts and computer models. *Circ. Res.* 50: 527–537, 1982a.

Janse, M.J., and F.J.L. van Capelle. Ectopic activity in the early phase of regional myocardial ischemia. In: *Cardiac Rate and Rhythm. Physiological, Morphological and Developmental Aspects,* edited by L.N. Bouman, and H.J. Jongsma. Martinus Nijhoff Publishers, The Hague: 1982b, pp. 297–320.

Janse, M.J., A. Capucci, R. Coronel, and M.A.W. Fabius. Variability of recovery of excitability in the normal canine and the ischaemic porcine heart. *Eur. Heart J.* 6(Suppl. D): 41–52, 1985a.

Janse, M.J., J.M.T. De Bakker, A.A.M. Wilde, R. Coronel, F.J.L. Van Capelle, and A.E. Becker. Conduction delay in subendocardial tissue from patients with ventricular tachycardia. (abstract) *Circulation* 72(Suppl. III): III-36, 1985b.

Janse, M.J., P.J. Schwartz, F.J.G. Wilms-Schopman, R.J.G. Peters, and D. Durrer. Effects of unilateral stellate ganglion stimulation and ablation on electrophysiologic changes induced by acute myocardial ischemia in dogs. *Circulation* 72: 585–595, 1985c.

Janse, M.J., F. Wilms-Schopman, R.J. Wilensky, and J. Tranum-Jensen. Role of the subendocardium in arrhythmogenesis during acute ischemia. In: *Cardiac Electrophysiology and Arrhythmias*, edited by D.P. Zipes, and J. Jalife. Grune and Stratton, Orlando: 1985d, pp. 353–362.

Janse, M.J. Reentry rhythms. In: *The Heart and Cardiovascular System*, edited by H.A. Fozzard, E. Haber, R.B. Jennings, A.M. Katz, and H.E. Morgan. Raven Press, New York: 1986a, pp. 1203–1238.

Janse, M.J. Electrophysiology and electrocardiology of acute myocardial ischemia. *Can. J. Cardiol.* (Suppl. A): 46A-52A, 1986b.

Janse, M.J. Electrophysiological effects of myocardial ischaemia. Relationship with early ventricular arrhythmias. *Eur. Heart J.* 7(Suppl. A): 35–43, 1986c.

Janse, M.J., A.G. Kléber, A. Capucci, R. Coronel, and F.J.G. Wilms-Schopman. Electrophysiological basis for arrhythmias caused by acute ischemia. Role of the subendocardium. *J. Mol. Cell. Cardiol.* 18: 339–355, 1986.

January, C.T., and H.A. Fozzard. The effects of membrane potential, extracellular potassium, and tetrodotoxin on the intracellular sodium ion activity in sheep cardiac muscle. *Circ. Res.* 54: 652–665, 1984.

January C.T., and H.A. Fozzard. Delayed afterdepolarizations in heart muscle: mechanisms and relevance. *Pharmacol. Rev.* 40: 219–227, 1988.

January C.T., and J.M. Riddle. Early afterdepolarizations: mechanism of induction and block. A role for L-type Ca^{2+} current. *Circ. Res.* 64: 977–990, 1989.

Jennings, R.B., H.M. Sommers, G.A. Smyth, H.A. Flack, and H. Linn. Myocardial necrosis induced by temporary occlusion of a coronary artery in the dog. *Arch. Pathol.* 70: 68–78, 1960.

Jennings, R.B., J.H. Baum, and P.B. Herdson. Fine structural changes in myocardial ischemic injury. *Arch. Pathol.* 79: 135–143, 1965.

Jennings, R.B., C.E. Ganote, and K.A. Reimer. Ischemic tissue injury. *Am. J. Pathol.* 81: 179–198, 1975.

Jennings, R.B., K.A. Reimer, M.L. Hill, and S.E. Mayer. Total ischemia in dog hearts, in vitro. 1. Comparison of high energy phosphate production, utilization, and depletion, and of adenosine nucleotide catabolism in total ischemia in vitro vs. severe ischemia in vivo. *Circ. Res.* 49: 892–900, 1981.

Johnson, E.A. First electrocardiographic sign of myocardial ischemia: An electrophysiological conjecture. *Circulation* 53(Suppl I): I-82–I-84, 1976.

Johnson, N., P. Danilo Jr., A.L. Wit, and M.R. Rosen. Characteristics of initiation and termination of catecholamine-induced triggered activity in atrial fibers of the coronary sinus. *Circulation* 74: 1168–1179, 1986.

Johnson, N.J., and M.R. Rosen. The distinction between triggered activity and other cardiac arrhythmias. In: *Cardiac Arrhythmias: Where To Go From Here?* edited by P. Brugada, and H.J.J. Wellens. Futura Publishing Company, Mt. Kisco, New York: 1987, pp. 129–145.

Johnson, T.A., R. Coronel, C.A. Graebner, J.W. Buchanan, M.J. Janse, and L.S. Gettes. Relationship between extracellular potassium accumulation and local TQ-segment potential during acute myocardial ischemia in the porcine. *J. Mol. Cell. Cardiol.* 19: 949–952, 1987.

Jones, S.B., D.E. Euler, E. Hardie, W.C. Randall, and G. Brynjolfsson. Comparison of SA nodal and subsidiary atrial pacemaker function and location in the dog. *Am. J. Physiol.* 234: H471-H476, 1978.

Jordan, J., I. Yamaguchi, W.J. Mandel, and A.E. McCullen. Comparative effects of overdrive on sinus and subsidiary pacemaker function. *Am. Heart J.* 93: 367–374, 1977.

Josephson, M.E., L.N. Horowitz, A. Farshidi, and J.A. Kastor. Recurrent sustained ventricular tachycardia. 1. Mechanisms. *Circulation* 57: 431–440, 1978a.

Josephson, M.E., L.N. Horowitz, A. Farshidi, J.F. Spear, J.A. Kastor, and E.N. Moore. Recurrent sustained ventricular tachycardia. 2. Endocardial mapping. *Circulation* 57: 440–447, 1978b.

Josephson, M.E., L.N. Horowitz, and A. Farshidi. Continuous local electrical activity. A mechanism of recurrent ventricular tachycardia. *Circulation* 57: 659–665, 1978c.

Josephson, M.E., L.N. Horowitz, A. Farshidi, S.R. Spielman, E.L. Michelson, and A.M. Greenspan. Sustained ventricular tachycardia: Evidence for protected localized reentry. *Am. J. Cardiol.* 42: 416–424, 1978d.

Josephson, M.E., A.H. Harken, and L.N. Horowitz. Endocardial excision: A new surgical technique for the treatment of recurrent ventricular tachycardia. *Circulation* 60: 1430–1439, 1979.

Josephson, M.E., and S.F. Seides. *Clinical Cardiac Electrophysiology. Techniques and Interpretations*. Lea & Febiger, Philadelphia: 1979.

Josephson, M.E., L.N. Horowitz, S.R. Spielman, A.M. Greenspan, C. VandePol, and A.II. IIarken. Comparison of endocardial catheter mapping with intraoperative mapping of ventricular tachycardia. *Circulation* 61: 395–404, 1980.

Josephson, M.E., L.N. Horowitz, H.L. Waxman, M.E. Cain, S.R. Spielman, A.M. Greenspan, F.E. Marchlinski, and M.D. Ezri. Sustained ventricular tachycardia: role of the 12-lead electrocardiogram in localizing site of origin. *Circulation* 64: 257–272, 1981.

Josephson, M.E., H.L. Waxman, M.E. Cain, M.J. Gardner, and A.E. Buxton. Ventricular activation during ventricular endocardial pacing. II. Role of pace-mapping to localize origin of ventricular tachycardia. *Am. J. Cardiol.* 50: 11–22, 1982a.

Josephson, M.E., M.B. Simson, A.H. Harken, L.N. Horowitz, and R.A. Falcone. The incidence and clinical significance of epicardial late potentials in patients with recurrent sustained ventricular tachycardia and coronary artery disease. *Circulation* 66: 1199–1204, 1982b.

Josephson, M.E., F.E. Marchlinski, A.E. Buxton, H.L. Waxman, J.U. Doherty, M.G. Kienzle, and R. Falcone. Electrophysiologic basis for sustained ventricular tachycardia—role of reentry. In: *Tachycardias: Mechanism, Diagnosis, Treatment*, edited by M.E. Josephson, and H.J.J. Wellens. Lea & Febiger, Philadelphia: 1984, pp. 305–323.

Josephson, M.E., and A.L. Wit. Fractionated electrical activity and continuous electrical activity: Fact or artifact? *Circulation* 70: 529–532, 1984.

Josephson, M.E., A.E. Buxton, F.E. Marchlinski, J.U. Doherty, D.M. Cassidy, M.G. Kienzle, J.A. Vassallo, J.M. Miller, J. Almendral, and W. Grogan. Sustained ventricular tachycardia in coronary artery disease—Evidence for reentrant mechanism. In: *Cardiac Electrophysiology and Arrhythmias*, edited by D.P. Zipes, and J. Jalife. Grune and Stratton, Orlando: 1985, pp. 409–418.

Josephson, M.E., J.M. Almendral, A.E. Buxton, and F.E. Marchlinski. Mechanisms of ventricular tachycardia. *Circulation* 75(Suppl. III): III-41–III-47, 1987.

Josephson, M.E. *Clinical Cardiac Electrophysiology*. Lea & Febiger, Philadelphia: 1992, (in press).

Joyner, R.W., R. Veenstra, D. Rawling, and A. Chorro. Propagation through electrically coupled cells. Effects of a resistive barrier. *Biophys. J.* 45: 1017–1025, 1984a.

Joyner, R.W., E.D. Overholt, B. Ramza, and R.D. Veenstra. Propagation through electrically coupled cells: two inhomogeneously coupled cardiac tissue layers. *Am. J. Physiol.* 247: H596-H609, 1984b.

Jugdutt, B.I., and R.W.M. Amy. Healing after myocardial infarction in the dog: Changes in infarct hydroxyproline and topography. *J. Am. Coll. Cardiol.* 7: 91–102, 1986.

Julian, D.G., P.A. Valentine, and G.G. Miller. Disturbances of rate, rhythm and conduction in acute myocardial infarction. A prospective study of 100 consecutive unselected patients with the aid of electrocardiographic monitoring. *Am. J. Med.* 37: 915–927, 1964.

Kabell, G., B.J. Scherlag, R.R. Hope, and R. Lazzara. Regional myocardial blood flow and ventricular arrhythmias following one-stage and two-stage coronary artery occlusion in anesthetized dogs. *Am. Heart J.* 104: 537–544, 1982.

Kabell, G., J. Brachmann, B.J. Scherlag, L. Harrison, and R. Lazzara. Mechanisms of ventricular arrhythmias in multivessel coronary disease: The effects of collateral zone ischemia. *Am. Heart J.* 108: 447–454, 1984.

Kabell, G. Modulation of conduction slowing in ischemic rabbit myocardium by calcium-channel activation and blockade. *Circulation* 77: 1385–1394, 1988.

Kagiyama, Y., J.L. Hill, and L.S. Gettes. Interaction of acidosis and increased extracellular potassium on action potential characteristics and conduction in guinea-pig ventricular muscle. *Circ. Res.* 51: 614–623, 1982.

Kakei, M., A. Noma, and T. Shibasaki. Properties of adenosine-triphosphate-regulated potassium channels in guinea-pig ventricular cells. *J. Physiol.* 363: 441–462, 1985.

Kaltenbrunner, W., R. Cardinal, M. Dubuc, M. Shenasa, R. Nadeau, G. Tremblay, M. Vermeulen, P. Savard, and P.L. Pagé. Epicardial and endocardial mapping of ventricular tachycardia in patients with myocardial infarction. Is the origin of the tachycardia always subendocardially localized? *Circulation* 84: 1058–1071, 1991.

Kammermeier, H., P. Schmidt, and E. Jüngling. Free energy change of ATP-hydrolysis: A causal factor of early hypoxic failure of the myocardium? *J. Mol. Cell. Cardiol.* 14: 267–277, 1982.

Kannel, W.B., J.T. Doyle, P.M. McNamara, P. Quickenton, and T. Gordon. Precursors of sudden coronary death. Factors related to the incidence of sudden death. *Circulation* 51: 606–613, 1975.

Kannel, W.B., and H.E. Thomas Jr. Sudden coronary death: The Framingham study. In: *Sudden Coronary Death*, edited by H.M. Greenberg and E.M.

Dwyer Jr. New York Academy of Science, New York: *Ann. N.Y. Acad. Sci.* 382: 3–20, 1982.

Kantor, P.F., W.A. Coetzee, E.E. Carmeliet, S.C. Dennis, and L.H. Opie. Reduction of ischemic K$^+$ loss and arrhythmias in rat hearts. Effect of glibenclamide, a sulfonylurea. *Circ. Res.* 66: 478–485, 1990.

Kao, C.Y., and B.F. Hoffman. Graded and decremental response in heart muscle fibers. *Am. J. Physiol.* 194: 187–196, 1958.

Kaplinsky, E., J.H. Yahini, and H.N. Neufeld. On the mechanism of sustained ventricular arrhythmias associated with acute myocardial infarction. *Cardiovasc. Res.* 6: 135–142, 1972.

Kaplinsky, E., A. Horowitz, and H.N. Neufeld. Ventricular reentry and automaticity in myocardial infarction. Effect of size of injury. *Chest* 74: 66–71, 1978.

Kaplinsky, E., S. Ogawa, C.W. Balke, and L.S. Dreifus. Two periods of early ventricular arrhythmia in the canine acute myocardial infarction model. *Circulation* 60: 397–403, 1979.

Kaplinsky, E., S. Ogawa, E.L. Michelson, and L.S. Dreifus. Instantaneous and delayed ventricular arrhythmias after reperfusion of acutely ischemic myocardium: Evidence for multiple mechanisms. *Circulation* 63: 333–340, 1981.

Karagueuzian, H.S., J.J. Fenoglio Jr., B.F. Hoffman, and A.L. Wit. Sustained ventricular tachycardia induced by electrical stimulation after myocardial infarction; Relation to infarct structure. (abstract) *Circulation* 56(Suppl. III): III-79, 1977.

Karagueuzian, H.S., J.J. Fenoglio Jr., M.B. Weiss, and A.L. Wit. Protracted ventricular tachycardia induced by premature stimulation of the canine heart after coronary artery occlusion and reperfusion. *Circ. Res.* 44: 833–846, 1979.

Karagueuzian, H.S., J.J. Fenoglio Jr., M.B. Weiss, and A.L. Wit. Coronary occlusion and reperfusion: Effects on subendocardial cardiac fibers. *Am. J. Physiol.* 238: H581-H593, 1980.

Karagueuzian, H., and B.G. Katzung. Relative inotropic and arrhythmogenic effects of five cardiac steroids in ventricular myocardium: oscillatory afterpotentials and the role of endogenous catecholamines. *J. Pharmacol. Exp. Ther.* 218: 348–356, 1981.

Karagueuzian, H.S., J.-P. Pennec, E. Deroubaix, J. de Leiris, and E. Coraboeuf. Effects of excess free fatty acids on the electrophysiological properties of ventricular specialized conducting tissue: A comparative study between the sheep and the dog. *J. Cardiovasc. Pharmacol.* 4: 462–468, 1982.

Karagueuzian, H.S., and B.G. Katzung. Voltage-clamp studies of transient inward current and mechanical oscillations induced by ouabain in ferret papillary muscle. *J. Physiol.* 327: 255–271, 1982.

Karagueuzian, H.S., K. Sugi, M. Ohta, M.C. Fishbein, W.J. Mandel, and T. Peter. Inducible sustained ventricular tachycardia and ventricular fibrillation in conscious dogs with isolated right ventricular infarction: Relation to infarct structure. *J. Am. Coll. Cardiol.* 7: 850–858, 1986a.

Karagueuzian, H.S., K. Sugi, M. Ohta, W.J. Mandel, and T. Peter. The efficacy of lidocaine and verapamil alone and in combination on spontaneously occurring automatic ventricular tachycardia in conscious dogs one day after right coronary artery occlusion. *Am. Heart J.* 111: 438–446, 1986b.

Kardesch, M., C.E. Hogancamp, and R.J. Bing. The effect of complete ischemia on the intracellular electrical activity of the whole mammalian heart. *Circ. Res.* 6: 715–720, 1958.

Kass, R.S., W.J. Lederer, R.W. Tsien, and R. Weingart. Role of calcium ions in transient inward currents and aftercontractions induced by strophanthidin in cardiac Purkinje fibres. *J. Physiol.* 281: 187–208, 1978a.

Kass, R.S., R.W. Tsien, and R. Weingart. Ionic basis of transient inward current induced by strophanthidin in cardiac Purkinje fibers. *J. Physiol.* 281: 209–226, 1978b.

Kass, R.S., and T. Scheuer. Slow inactivation of calcium channels in the cardiac Purkinje fiber. *J. Mol. Cell. Cardiol.* 14: 615–618, 1982.

Katcher, A.H., G. Peirce, and J.J. Sayen. Effects of experimental regional ischemia and levarterenol on the RS-T segment and baseline of ventricular surface electrocardiograms obtained by direct-coupled amplification. *Circ. Res.* 8: 29–43, 1960.

Katz, A.M., and F.C. Messineo. Lipid-membrane interactions and the pathogenesis of ischemic damage in the myocardium. *Circ. Res.* 48: 1–16, 1981.

Katz, A.M. Membrane-derived lipids and the pathogenesis of ischemic myocardial damage. *J. Mol. Cell. Cardiol.* 14: 627–632, 1982.

Katz, L.N., and A. Pick. *Clinical Electrocardiography. The Arrhythmias.* Lea & Febiger, Philadelphia: 1956.

Katzung, B.G., L.M. Hondeghem, and A.O. Grant. Cardiac ventricular automaticity induced by current of injury. *Pflügers Arch.* 360: 193–197, 1975.

Katzung, B.G., and J.A. Morgenstern. Effects of extracellular potassium on ventricular automaticity and evidence for a pacemaker current in mammalian ventricular myocardium. *Circ. Res.* 40: 105–111, 1977.

Kaufmann, R., and U. Theophile. Automatie fördernde Dehnungseffekte an Purkinje-Fäden, Papillarmuskeln und Vorhoftrabekeln von Rhesus-Affen. *Pflügers Arch.* 297: 174–189, 1967.

Kaufmann, R.L., M.J. Lab, R. Hennekes, and H. Krause. Feedback interaction of mechanical and electrical events in the isolated mammalian ventricular myocardium (cat papillary muscle). *Pflügers Arch.* 324: 100–123, 1971.

Kay, G.N., V.J. Plumb, J.G. Arciniegas, R.W. Henthorn, and A.L. Waldo. Torsade de pointes: The long-short initiating sequence and other clinical features: Observations in 32 patients. *J. Am. Coll. Cardiol.* 2: 806–817, 1983.

Kay, G.N., A.E. Epstein, and V.J. Plumb. Incidence of reentry with an excitable gap in ventricular tachycardia: A prospective evaluation utilizing transient entrainment. *J. Am. Coll. Cardiol.* 11: 530–538, 1988.

Kay, G.N., A.E. Epstein, and V.J. Plumb. Resetting of ventricular tachycardia by single extrastimuli. Relation to slow conduction within the reentrant circuit. *Circulation* 81: 1507–1519, 1990.

Kent, K.M., E.R. Smith, D.R. Redwood, and S.E. Epstein. Electrical stability of acutely ischemic myocardium. Influences of heart rate and vagal stimulation. *Circulation* 47: 291–298, 1973.

Kersschot, I.E., P. Brugada, M. Ramentol, M. Zehender, B. Waldecker, W.G. Stevenson, A. Geibel, C. De Zwaan, and H.J.J. Wellens. Effects of early reperfusion in acute myocardial infarction on arrhythmias induced by programmed stimulation: A prospective, randomized study. *J. Am. Coll. Cardiol.* 7: 1234–1242, 1986.

Kerzner, J., M. Wolf, B.D. Kosowsky, and B. Lown. Ventricular ectopic rhythms following vagal stimulation in dogs with acute myocardial infarction. *Circulation* 47: 44–50, 1973.

Kienzle, M.G., R.A. Falcone, F.C. Kempf, J.M. Miller, A.H. Harken, and M.E. Josephson. Intraoperative endocardial mapping: relation of fractionated electrograms in sinus rhythm to endocardial activation in ventricular tachycardia—surgical implications. (abstract) *J. Am. Coll. Cardiol.* 1: 582, 1983.

Kienzle, M.G., R.C. Tan, B.M. Ramza, M.-L. Young, and R.W. Joyner. Alterations in endocardial activation of the canine papillary muscle early and late after myocardial infarction. *Circulation* 76: 860–874, 1987.

Kieval, R.S., V.P. Butler Jr., F. Derguini, R.C. Bruening, and M.R. Rosen. Cellular electrophysiologic effects of vertebrate digitalis-like substances. *J. Am. Coll. Cardiol.* 11: 637–643, 1988.

Kimura, S., H. Nakaya, and M. Kanno. Effects of verapamil and lidocaine on changes in action potential characteristics and conduction time induced by combined hypoxia, hyperkalemia, and acidosis in canine ventricular myocardium. *J. Cardiovasc. Pharmacol.* 4: 658–667, 1982.

Kimura, S., J.S. Cameron, P.L. Kozlovskis, A.L. Bassett, and R.J. Myerburg. Delayed afterdepolarizations and triggered activity induced in feline Purkinje fibers by α-adrenergic stimulation in the presence of elevated calcium levels. *Circulation* 70: 1074–1082, 1984.

Kimura, S., A.L. Bassett, M.S. Gaide, P.L. Kozlovskis, and R.J. Myerburg. Regional changes in intracellular potassium and sodium activity after healing of experimental myocardial infarction in cats. *Circ. Res.* 58: 202–208, 1986a.

Kimura, S., A.L. Bassett, T. Kohya, P.L. Kozlovskis, and R.J. Myerburg. Simultaneous recording of action potentials from endocardium and epicardium during ischemia in the isolated cat ventricle: Relation of temporal electrophysiologic heterogeneities to arrhythmias. *Circulation* 74: 401–409, 1986b.

Kimura, S., A.L. Bassett, T. Furukawa, J. Cuevas, and R.J. Myerburg. Electrophysiological properties and responses to simulated ischemia in cat ventricular myocytes of endocardial and epicardial origin. *Circ. Res.* 66: 469–477, 1990.

Kimura, T., S. Imanishi, M. Arita, T. Hadama, and J. Shirabe. Two differential mechanisms of automaticity in diseased human atrial fibers. *Jpn. J. Physiol.* 38: 851–867, 1988.

King B.G. The effect of electric shock on heart action with special reference to varying susceptibility in different parts of the cardiac cycle. (Doctoral Thesis) Columbia University, New York. Aberdeen Press: 1934.

Kirchhof, C.J.H.J., F.I.M. Bonke, and M.A. Allessie. Evidence for the presence of electrotonic depression of pacemakers in the rabbit atrioventricular node. The effects of uncoupling from the surrounding myocardium. *Basic Res. Cardiol.* 83: 190–201, 1988.

Kirchhof, C.J.H.J. The Sinus Node and Atrial Fibrillation. (Doctoral Thesis) The University of Limburg, Maastricht, The Netherlands: 1989.

Kirkels, J.H., C.J.A. van Echteld, and T.J.C. Ruigrok. Intracellular magnesium during myocardial ischemia and reperfusion: possible consequences for postischemic recovery. *J. Mol. Cell. Cardiol.* 21: 1209–1218, 1989.

Kiyosue, T., and M. Arita. Effects of lysophosphatidylcholine on resting potassium conductance of isolated guinea pig ventricular cells. *Pflügers Arch.* 406: 296–302, 1986.

Kléber, A.G., M.J. Janse, E. Downar, and D. Durrer. Die Veränderung der TQ- und ST/T-Segmente im Elektrokardiogramm und deren Beziehung zu den ventrikulären Rhythmusstörungen während der akuten transmuralen Ischämie. *Schweiz. Med. Wochenschr.* 107: 1700–1705, 1977.

Kléber, A.G., M.J. Janse, F.J.L. Van Capelle, and D. Durrer. Mechanism and time course of S-T and T-Q segment changes during acute regional myocardial ischemia in the pig heart determined by extracellular and intracellular recordings. *Circ. Res.* 42: 603–613, 1978.

Kléber, A.G. Resting membrane potential, extracellular potassium activity, and intracellular sodium activity during acute global ischemia in isolated perfused guinea pig hearts. *Circ. Res.* 52: 442–450, 1983.

Kléber, A.G. Extracellular potassium accumulation in acute myocardial ischemia. *J. Mol. Cell. Cardiol.* 16: 389–394, 1984.

Kléber, A.G., M.J. Janse, F.J.G. Wilms-Schopman, A.A.M. Wilde, and R. Coronel. Changes in conduction velocity during acute ischemia in ventricular myocardium of the isolated porcine heart. *Circulation* 73: 189–198, 1986.

Kléber, A.G., and A.A.M. Wilde. Regulation of intracellular sodium ions in acute reversible myocardial ischemia—A perspective. *J. Mol. Cell. Cardiol.* 18(Suppl 4): 27–30, 1986.

Kléber, A.G., and C.B. Riegger. Electrical constants of arterially perfused rabbit papillary muscle. *J. Physiol.* 385: 307–324, 1987.

Kléber, A.G., C.B. Riegger, and M.J. Janse. Electrical uncoupling and increase of extracellular resistance after induction of ischemia in isolated, arterially perfused rabbit papillary muscle. *Circ. Res.* 61: 271–279, 1987a.

Kléber, A.G., C.B. Riegger, and M.J. Janse. Extracellular K^+ and H^+ shifts in early ischemia: Mechanisms and relation to changes in impulse propagation. *J. Mol. Cell. Cardiol.* 19(Suppl. V): 35–44, 1987b.

Kléber, A.G., and W.E. Cascio. Ischemia and Na^+/K^+ pump function. In: *Lethal Arrhythmias Resulting from Myocardial Ischemia and Infarction*, edited by M.R. Rosen, and Y. Palti. Kluwer Academic Publishers, Boston: 1989, pp. 77–90.

Kleiger, R.E., J.P. Miller, S. Thanavaro, M.A. Province, T.F. Martin, and G.C.

Oliver. Relationship between clinical features of acute myocardial infarction and ventricular runs 2 weeks to 1 year after infarction. *Circulation* 63: 64–70, 1981.

Klein, G.J., R.E. Ideker, W.M. Smith, L.A. Harrison, J. Kasell, A.G. Wallace, and J.J. Gallagher. Epicardial mapping of the onset of ventricular tachycardia initiated by programmed stimulation in the canine heart with chronic infarction. *Circulation* 60: 1375–1384, 1979.

Klein, H., R.B. Karp, N.T. Kouchoukos, G.L. Zorn Jr., T.N. James, and A.L. Waldo. Intraoperative electrophysiologic mapping of the ventricles during sinus rhythm in patients with a previous myocardial infarction. Identification of the electrophysiologic substrate of ventricular arrhythmias. *Circulation* 66: 847–853, 1982.

Klein, H.O., P.F. Cranefield, and B.F. Hoffman. Effect of extrasystoles on idioventricular rhythm. *Circ. Res.* 30: 651–665, 1972.

Klein, H.O., R. Lebson, P.F. Cranefield, and B.F. Hoffman. Effect of extrasystoles on idioventricular rhythm. Clinical and electrophysiologic correlation. *Circulation* 47: 758–764, 1973a.

Klein, H.O., D.H. Singer, and B.F. Hoffman. Effects of atrial premature systoles on sinus rhythm in the rabbit. *Circ. Res.* 32: 480–491, 1973b.

Klein, R.C., and C. Machell. Use of electrophysiologic testing in patients with nonsustained ventricular tachycardia: prognostic and therapeutic implications. *J. Am. Coll. Cardiol.* 14: 155–161, 1989.

Kleinfeld, M.J., and J.J. Rozanski. Alternans of the ST segment in Prinzmetal's angina. *Circulation* 55: 574–577, 1977.

Kline, R.P. and J. Kupersmith. Effects of extracellular potassium accumulation and sodium pump activation on automatic canine Purkinje fibres. *J. Physiol.* 324: 507–533, 1982.

Kline, R.P. Ion accumulation and modulation of currents. In: *Cardiac Electrophysiology: A Textbook*, edited by M.R. Rosen, M.J. Janse, and A.L. Wit. Futura Publishing Company, Mt. Kisco, New York: 1990, pp. 133–156.

Kline, R.P., M.S. Hanna, K.P. Dresdner Jr., and A.L. Wit. Time course of changes in intracellular K^+, Na^+, and pH of subendocardial Purkinje cells during the first 24 hours after coronary occlusion. *Circ. Res.* 70: 566–575, 1992.

Knabb, M.T., J.E. Saffitz, P.B. Corr, and B.E. Sobel. The dependence of electrophysiological derangements on accumulation of endogenous long-chain acyl carnitine in hypoxic neonatal rat myocytes. *Circ. Res.* 58: 230–240, 1986.

Kodama, I., J. Goto, S. Ando, J. Toyama, and K. Yamada. Effects of rapid stimulation on the transmembrane action potentials of rabbit sinus node pacemaker cells. *Circ. Res.* 46: 90–99, 1980.

Kodama, I., A.A.M. Wilde, M.J. Janse, D. Durrer, and K. Yamada. Combined effects of hypoxia, hyperkalemia and acidosis on membrane action potential and excitability of guinea-pig ventricular muscle. *J. Mol. Cell. Cardiol.* 16: 247–259, 1984.

Kohlhardt, M., K. Haap, and H.R. Figulla. Influence of low extracellular pH upon the Ca inward current and isometric contractile force in mammalian ventricular myocardium. *Pflügers Arch.* 366: 31–38, 1976.

Kokubun, S., M. Nishimura, A. Noma, and H. Irisawa. The spontaneous action potential of rabbit atrioventricular node cells. *Jpn. J. Physiol.* 30: 529–540, 1980.

Kokubun, S., M. Nishimura, A. Noma, and H. Irisawa. Membrane currents in the rabbit atrioventricular node cell. *Pflügers Arch.* 393: 15–22 1982.

Kotler, M.N., B. Tabatznik, M.M. Mower, and S. Tominaga. Prognostic significance of ventricular ectopic beats with respect to sudden death in the late postinfarction period. *Circulation* 47: 959–966, 1973.

Koyanagi, S., C. Eastham, and M.L. Marcus. Effects of chronic hypertension and left ventricular hypertrophy on the incidence of sudden cardiac death after coronary artery occlusion in conscious dogs. *Circulation* 65: 1192–1197, 1982a.

Koyanagi, S., C.L. Eastham, D.G. Harrison, and M.L. Marcus. Increased size of myocardial infarction in dogs with chronic hypertension and left ventricular hypertrophy. *Circ. Res.* 50: 55–62, 1982b.

Kozlovskis, P.L., L.A. Fieber, A.L. Bassett, J.S. Cameron, S. Kimura, and R.J. Myerburg. Regional reduction in ventricular norepinephrine after healing of experimental myocardial infarction in cats. *J. Mol. Cell. Cardiol.* 18: 413- 422, 1986.

Kramer, J.B., J.E. Saffitz, F.X. Witkowski, and P.B. Corr. Intramural reentry as a mechanism of ventricular tachycardia during evolving canine myocardial infarction. *Circ. Res.* 56: 736–754, 1985.

Krayer, O., J.J. Mandoki, and C. Mendez. Studies on veratrum alkaloids. XVI. The action of epinephrine and of veratramine on the functional refractory period of the auriculo-ventricular transmission in the heart-lung preparation of the dog. *J. Pharmacol. Exp. Ther.* 103: 412–419, 1951.

Kuchar, D.L., J.N. Ruskin, and H. Garan. Electrocardiographic localization of the site of origin of ventricular tachycardia in patients with prior myocardial infarction. *J. Am. Coll. Cardiol.* 13: 893–900, 1989.

Kuck, K.H., K.P. Kunze, N. Roewer, and W. Bleifeld. Sotalol-induced torsade de pointes. *Am. Heart J.* 107: 179–180, 1984.

Kuck, K-H., A. Costard, M. Schlüter, and K.-P. Kunze. Significance of timing programmed electrical stimulation after acute myocardial infarction. *J. Am. Coll. Cardiol.* 8: 1279–1288, 1986.

Kudenchuk, P.J., J. Kron, C.G. Walance, E.S. Murphy, C.D. Morris, K.K. Griffith, and J.H. McAnulty. Reproducibility of arrhythmia induction with intracardiac electrophysiologic testing: patients with clinical sustained ventricular tachyarrhythmias. *J. Am. Coll. Cardiol.* 7: 819–828, 1986.

Kunze, D.L. Rate-dependent changes in extracellular potassium in the rabbit atrium. *Circ. Res.* 41: 122–127, 1977.

Kuo, C.-S., K. Munakata, C.P. Reddy, and B. Surawicz. Characteristics and possible mechanism of ventricular arrhythmia dependent on the dispersion of action potential durations. *Circulation* 67: 1356–1367, 1983.

Kupersmith, J., E.M. Antman, and B.F. Hoffman. In vivo electrophysiological effects of lidocaine in canine acute myocardial infarction. *Circ. Res.* 36: 84–91, 1975.

Kupersmith, J., and P. Hoff. Occurrence and transmission of localized repolarization abnormalities in vitro. *J. Am. Coll. Cardiol.* 6: 152–160, 1985.

Kupersmith, J., P. Hoff, and G.S. Duo. In vitro characteristics of repolarization abnormality—a possible cause of arrhythmias. *J. Electrocardiol.* 19: 361–369, 1986.

Kurien, V.A., and M.F. Oliver. A metabolic cause for arrhythmias during acute myocardial hypoxia. *Lancet* 1: 813–815, 1970.

Lab, M.J. Mechanically dependent changes in action potentials recorded from the intact frog heart. *Circ. Res.* 42: 519–528, 1978.

Lab, M.J. Stress-strain-related depolarisation in the myocardium and arrhythmogenesis in early ischaemia. In: *Early Arrhythmias Resulting from Myocardial Ischaemia*, edited by J.R. Parratt. Oxford University Press, New York: 1982, pp. 81–91.

Lab, M.J., D.G. Allen, and C.H. Orchard. The effects of shortening on myoplasmic calcium concentration and on the action potential in mammalian ventricular muscle. *Circ. Res.* 55: 825–829, 1984.

Lab, M.J. Mechano-electric coupling in myocardium and its possible role in ischaemic arrhythmia. In: *Activation, Metabolism and Perfusion of the Heart*, edited by S. Sideman and R. Beyar. Martinus Nijhoff Publishers, Dordrecht: 1987, pp. 227–238.

Lado, M.G., S-S. Sheu, and H.A. Fozzard. Changes in intracellular Ca^{2+} activity with stimulation in sheep cardiac Purkinje strands. *Am. J. Physiol.* 243: H133-H137, 1982.

Lamers, J.M.J., and W.C. Hulsmann. Inhibition of $(Na^+ + K^+)$-stimulated ATPase of heart by fatty acids. *J. Mol. Cell. Cardiol.* 9: 343–346, 1977.

Lamers, J.M.J., H.T. Stinis, A. Montfoort, and W.C. Hülsmann. The effect of lipid intermediates on Ca^{2+} and Na^+ permeability and $(Na^+ + K^+)$-ATPase of cardiac sarcolemma. *Biochim. Biophys. Acta* 774: 127–137, 1984.

Lammers, W.J.E.P., M.A. Allessie, P.L. Rensma, and M.J. Schalij. The use of fibrillation cycle length to determine spatial dispersion in electrophysiological properties used to characterize the underlying mechanism of fibrillation. *New Trends in Arrhythmias* 2: 109–112, 1986.

Lammers, W.J.E.P., A.L. Wit, and M.A. Allessie. Effects of anisotropy on functional reentrant circuits: preliminary results of computer simulation studies. In: *Activation, Metabolism, and Perfusion of the Heart*, edited by S. Sideman, and R. Beyar. Martinus Nijhoff, Dordrecht: 1987, pp 133–150.

Lange, G. Action of driving stimuli from intrinsic and extrinsic sources on in situ cardiac pacemaker tissues. *Circ. Res.* 17: 449–459, 1965.

La Rovere, M.T., G. Specchia, A. Mortara, and P.J. Schwartz. Baroreflex sensitivity, clinical correlates, and cardiovascular mortality among patients with a first myocardial infarction. A prospective study. *Circulation* 78: 816–824, 1988.

Lauer, M.R., B.F. Rusy, and L.D. Davis. H^+-induced membrane depolarization in canine cardiac Purkinje fibers. *Am. J. Physiol.* 247: H312-H321, 1984.

Lazdunski, M., C. Frelin, and P. Vigne. The sodium/hydrogen exchange system in cardiac cells: its biochemical and pharmacological properties and its role in regulating internal concentrations of sodium and internal pH. *J. Mol. Cell. Cardiol.* 17: 1029–1042, 1985.

Lazzara, R., N. El-Sherif, and B.J. Scherlag. Electrophysiological properties of canine Purkinje cells in one-day-old myocardial infarction. *Circ. Res.* 33: 722–734, 1973.

Lazzara, R., N. El-Sherif, and B.J. Scherlag. Early and late effects of coronary artery occlusion on canine Purkinje fibers. *Circ. Res.* 35: 391–399, 1974.

Lazzara, R., N. El-Sherif, R.R. Hope, and B.J. Scherlag. Ventricular arrhythmias and electrophysiological consequences of myocardial ischemia and infarction. *Circ. Res.* 42: 740–749, 1978a.

Lazzara, R., R.R. Hope, N. El-Sherif, and B.J. Scherlag. Effects of lidocaine on hypoxic and ischemic cardiac cells. *Am. J. Cardiol.* 41: 872–879, 1978b.

Lazzara, R., and B.J. Scherlag. Role of the slow current in the generation of arrhythmias in ischemic myocardium. In: *The Slow Inward Current and Cardiac Arrhythmias*, edited by D.P. Zipes, J.C. Bailey, and V. Elharrar. Martinus Nijhoff, The Hague: 1980, pp. 399–416.

Lazzara, R., and S. Marchi. Electrophysiologic mechanisms for the generation of arrhythmias with adrenergic stimulation. In: *Adrenergic System and Ventricular Arrhythmias in Myocardial Infarction*, edited by J. Brachmann, and A. Schömig. Springer-Verlag, Berlin: 1989, pp. 231–238.

Leclercq, J.F., P. Coumel, P. Maison-Blanche, B. Cauchemez, M. Zimmermann, F. Chouty, and R. Slama. Mise en évidence des mécanismes déterminants de la mort subite. Enquête coopérative portant sur 69 cas enregistrés par la méthode de Holter. *Arch. Mal. Coeur* 79: 1024–1033, 1986.

Leclercq, J.F., P. Maison-Blanche, B. Cauchemez, and P. Coumel. Respective role of sympathetic tone and of cardiac pauses in the genesis of 62 cases of ventricular fibrillation recorded during Holter monitoring. *Eur. Heart J.* 9: 1276–1283, 1988.

Lederer, W.J., and R.W. Tsien. Transient inward current underlying arrhythmogenic effects of cardiotonic steroids in Purkinje fibres. *J. Physiol.* 263: 73–100, 1976.

Lee, C.O., and M. Dagostino. Effect of strophanthidin on intracellular Na ion activity and twitch tension of constantly driven canine cardiac Purkinje fibers. *Biophys. J.* 40: 185–198, 1982.

Lee, J.T., Ideker, R.E., and K.A. Reimer. Myocardial infarct size and location in relation to the coronary vascular bed at risk in man. *Circulation* 64: 526–534, 1981.

Le Marec, H., K.H. Dangman, P. Danilo Jr., and M.R. Rosen. An evaluation of automaticity and triggered activity in the canine heart one to four days after myocardial infarction. *Circulation* 71: 1224–1236, 1985.

Le Marec, H., W. Spinelli, and M.R. Rosen. The effects of doxorubicin on ventricular tachycardia. *Circulation* 74: 881–889, 1986.

Lerman, B.B., L. Belardinelli, A. West, R.M. Berne, and J.P. DiMarco. Adenosine-sensitive ventricular tachycardia: evidence suggesting cyclic AMP-mediated triggered activity. *Circulation* 74: 270–280, 1986.

Lerman, B.B. Ventricular tachycardia unassociated with coronary artery disease. *Prog. Cardiol.* 1: 255–279, 1988.

Levi, R., J.R. Malm, F.O. Bowman, and M.R. Rosen. The arrhythmogenic actions of histamine on human atrial fibers. *Circ. Res.* 49: 545–550, 1981.

Levine, J.H., J.F. Spear, T. Guarnieri, M.L. Weisfeldt, C.D.J. de Langen, L.C. Becker, and E.N. Moore. Cesium chloride-induced long QT syndrome: demonstration of afterdepolarizations and triggered activity in vivo. *Circulation* 72: 1092–1103, 1985.

Levine, J.H., T. Guarnieri, A.H. Kadish, R.I. White, H. Calkins, and J.S. Kan. Changes in myocardial repolarization in patients undergoing balloon valvuloplasty for congenital pulmonary stenosis: evidence for contraction-excitation feedback in humans. *Circulation* 77: 70–77, 1988.

Levine, J.H., J. Morganroth, and A.H. Kadish. Mechanisms and risk factors for proarrhythmia with type Ia compared with Ic antiarrhythmic drug therapy. *Circulation* 80: 1063–1069, 1989.

Levites, R., V.S. Banka, and R.H. Helfant. Electrophysiologic effects of coronary occlusion and reperfusion. Observations of dispersion of refractoriness and ventricular automaticity. *Circulation* 52: 760–765, 1975.

Levites, R., J.I. Haft, J. Calderon, and Venkatachalapathy. Effects of procain amide on the dispersion of recovery of excitability during coronary occlusion. *Circulation* 53: 982–984, 1976.

Levy, M.N. Sympathetic-parasympathetic interactions in the heart. *Circ. Res.* 29: 437–445, 1971.

Levy, M.N., and B. Blattberg. Effect of vagal stimulation on the overflow of norepinephrine into the coronary sinus during cardiac sympathetic nerve stimulation in the dog. *Circ. Res.* 38: 81–85, 1976.

Lewis, T. The experimental production of paroxysmal tachycardia and the effects of ligation of the coronary arteries. *Heart* 1: 98–137, 1909.

Lewis, T., B.S. Oppenheimer, and A. Oppenheimer. The site of origin of the mammalian heart-beat; the pacemaker in the dog. *Heart* 2: 147–169, 1910.

Lewis, T. Observations upon flutter and fibrillation. Part I. The regularity of clinical auricular flutter. *Heart* 7: 127–130, 1920.

Lewis, T., H.S. Feil, and W.D. Stroud. Observations upon flutter and fibrillation. Part II. The nature of auricular flutter. *Heart* 7: 191–245, 1920.

Liberthson, R.R., E.L. Nagel, J.C. Hirschman, S.R. Nussenfeld, B.D. Blackbourne, and J.H. Davis. Pathophysiologic observations in prehospital ventricular fibrillation and sudden cardiac death. *Circulation* 49: 790–798, 1974.

Liberthson, R.R., E.L. Nagel, and J.N. Ruskin. Pathophysiology, clinical course, and management of prehospital ventricular fibrillation and sudden cardiac death. In: *Acute Phase of Ischemic Heart Disease and Myocardial Infarction*, edited by A.A.J. Adgey. Martinus Nijhoff, The Hague: 1982, pp. 165–182.

Lichstein, E., C. Ribas-Meneclier, P.K. Gupta, and K.D. Chadda. Incidence and description of accelerated ventricular rhythm complicating acute myocardial infarction. *Am. J. Med.* 58: 192–198, 1975.

Lie, K.I., H.J.J. Wellens, R.M. Schuilenburg, and D. Durrer. Mechanism and significance of widened QRS complexes during complete atrioventricular block in acute inferior myocardial infarction. *Am. J. Cardiol.* 33: 833–839, 1974.

Lie, K.I., H.J.J. Wellens, E. Downar, and D. Durrer. Observations on patients with primary ventricular fibrillation complicating acute myocardial infarction. *Circulation* 52: 755–759, 1975.

Lie, K.I., K.L. Liem, R.M. Schuilenburg, G.K. David, and D. Durrer. Early identification of patients developing late in-hospital ventricular fibrillation after discharge from the coronary care unit. A 5 1/2 year retrospective and prospective study of 1,897 patients. *Am. J. Cardiol.* 41: 674–677, 1978.

Lipp, P., and L. Pott. Transient inward current in guinea-pig atrial myocytes reflects a change of sodium-calcium exchange current. *J. Physiol.* 397: 601–630, 1988.

Lipsius, S.L., and W.R. Gibbons. Membrane currents, contractions, and after-contractions in cardiac Purkinje fibers. *Am. J. Physiol.* 243: H77-H86, 1982.

Littmann, L., R.H. Svenson, J.J. Gallagher, J.G. Selle, S.H. Zimmern, J.M. Fedor, and P.G. Colavita. Functional role of the epicardium in postinfarction ventricular tachycardia. Observations derived from computerized epicardial activation mapping, entrainment, and epicardial laser photoablation. *Circulation* 83: 1577–1591, 1991.

Livelli, F.D., J.T. Bigger Jr., J.A. Reiffel, E.S. Gang, J.N. Patton, P.M. Noethling, L.M. Rolnitzky, and J.I. Gliklich. Response to programmed ventricular stimulation: sensitivity, specificity and relation to heart disease. *Am. J. Cardiol.* 50: 452–458, 1982.

Loeb, J.M., D.E. Euler, W.C. Randall, J.F. Moran, and G. Brynjolfsson. Cardiac arrhythmias after chronic embolization of the sinus node artery: alterations in parasympathetic pacemaker control. *Circulation* 61: 192–198, 1980.

Logic, J.R., D.H. Morrow, and R.N. Gatz. Idioventricular tachycardia complicating experimental myocardial infarction. *Dis. Chest* 56: 477–480, 1969.

Loiselle, D.S. The rate of resting heat production of rat papillary muscle. *Pflügers Arch.* 405: 155–162, 1985.

Lowe, J.E., R.G. Cummings, D.H. Adams, and E.A. Hull-Ryde. Evidence that ischemic cell death begins in the subendocardium independent of variations in collateral flow or wall tension. *Circulation* 68: 190–202, 1983.

Lown, B., R. Amarasingham, and J. Neuman. New method for terminating cardiac arrhythmias. Use of synchronized capacitor discharge. *JAMA* 182: 548–555, 1962.

Lown, B., A.M. Fakhro, W.B. Hood, and G.W. Thorn. The coronary care unit. New perspectives and directions. *JAMA* 199: 188–198, 1967a.

Lown, B., R.L. Cannon, III, and M.A. Rossi. Electrical stimulation and digitalis drugs: repetitive response in diastole. *Proc. Soc. Exptl. Biol. & Med.* 126: 698–701, 1967b.

Lown, B,. Electrical stimulation to estimate the degree of digitalization. II. Experimental studies. *Am. J. Cardiol.* 22: 251–259, 1968.

Lown, B., and M. Wolf. Approaches to sudden death from coronary heart disease. *Circulation* 44: 130–142, 1971.

Lown, B., A.F. Calvert, R. Armington, and M. Ryan. Monitoring for serious arrhythmias and high risk of sudden death. *Circulation* 52(Suppl. III): III-189–198, 1975.

Lown, B. Sudden cardiac death: The major challenge confronting contemporary cardiology. *Am. J. Cardiol.* 43: 313–329, 1979a.

Lown, B. Sudden cardiac death—1978. *Circulation* 60: 1593–1599, 1979b.

Lue, W.-M., and P.A. Boyden. Electrophysiologic properties of myocytes from normal canine epicardium and the epicardial border zone in the infarcted heart. (abstract) *Circulation* 80(Suppl. II): II-500, 1989.

Lurie, K.G., T.M. Argentieri, J. Sheldon, L.H. Frame, and F.M. Matschinsky. Metabolism and electrophysiology in subendocardial Purkinje fibers after infarction. *Am. J. Physiol.* 253: H662-H670, 1987.

Lynch, J.J., and B.R. Lucchesi. How are animal models best used for the study of antiarrhythmic drugs? In: *Life-Threatening Arrhythmias During Ischemia and Infarction*, edited by D.J. Hearse, A.S. Manning, and M.J. Janse. Raven Press, New York: 1987, pp. 169–196.

Lyons, C.J., and M.J. Burgess. Demonstration of reentry within the canine specialized conduction system. *Am. Heart J.* 98: 595–603, 1979.

MacKenzie, J. *Diseases of the Heart*. Oxford: 1918, pp. 178–254.

MacLean, W.A.H., V.J. Plumb, and A.L. Waldo. Transient entrainment and interruption of ventricular tachycardia. *PACE* 4: 358–366, 1981.

MacWilliam, J.A. Some applications of physiology to medicine. II. Ventricular fibrillation and sudden death. *Br. Med. J.* August 11 and 18, 7–43, 1923.

Mainwood, G.W., and G.E. Lucier. Fatigue and recovery in isolated frog sartorius muscles: The effects of bicarbonate concentration and associated potassium loss. *Can. J. Physiol. Pharmacol.* 50: 132–142, 1972.

Malfatto, G., T.S. Rosen, and M.R. Rosen. The response to overdrive pacing of triggered atrial and ventricular arrhythmias in the canine heart. *Circulation* 77: 1139–1148, 1988.

Maling, H.M., V.H. Cohn Jr., and B. Highman. The effects of coronary occlusion in dogs treated with reserpine and in dogs treated with phenoxybenzamine. *J. Pharmacol. Exp. Ther.* 127: 229–235, 1959.

Mann, D.E., G.M. Lawrie, J.C. Luck, J.C. Griffin, S.A. Magro, and C.R.C. Wyndham. Importance of pacing site in entrainment of ventricular tachycardia. *J. Am. Coll. Cardiol.* 5: 781–787, 1985.

Manning, A.S., and D.J. Hearse. Reperfusion-induced arrhythmias: Mechanisms and prevention. *J. Mol. Cell. Cardiol.* 16: 497–518, 1984.

Manning, G.W., C.G. McEachern, and G.E. Hall. Reflex coronary artery spasm following sudden occlusion of other coronary branches. *Arch. Intern. Med.* 64: 661–674, 1939.

Marban, E., and W.G. Wier. Ryanodine as a tool to determine the contributions of calcium entry and calcium release to the calcium transient and contraction of cardiac Purkinje fibers. *Circ. Res.* 56: 133–138, 1985.

Marban, E., S.W. Robinson, and W.G. Wier. Mechanisms of arrhythmogenic delayed and early afterdepolarizations in ferret ventricular muscle. *J. Clin. Invest.* 78: 1185–1192, 1986.

Marban, E., M. Kitakaze, H. Kusuoka, J.K. Porterfield, D.T. Yue, and V.P. Chacko. Intracellular free calcium concentration measured with ^{19}F NMR spectroscopy in intact ferret hearts. *Proc. Natl. Acad. Sci. USA* 84: 6005–6009, 1987.

Marchlinski, F.E., H.L. Waxman, A.E. Buxton, and M.E. Josephson. Sustained ventricular tachyarrhythmias during the early postinfarction period: Electrophysiologic findings and prognosis for survival. *J. Am. Coll. Cardiol.* 2: 240–250, 1983.

Marchlinski, F.E. Ventricular tachycardia associated with coronary artery disease. *Prog. Cardiol.* 1: 231–253, 1988.

Maroko, P.R., P. Libby, W.R. Ginks, C.M. Bloor, W.E. Shell,. B.E. Sobel, and J. Ross Jr. Coronary artery reperfusion. I. Early effects on local myocardial function and the extent of myocardial necrosis. *J. Clin. Invest.* 51: 2710–2716, 1972.

Marshall, R.J., and J.R. Parratt. The early consequences of myocardial ischaemia and their modification. *J. Physiol. (Paris)* 76: 699–715, 1980.

Martins, J.B., and D.P. Zipes. Epicardial phenol interrupts refractory period responses to sympathetic but not vagal stimulation in canine left ventricular epicardium and endocardium. *Circ. Res.* 47: 33–40, 1980.

Martins, J.B. Autonomic control of ventricular tachycardia: sympathetic neural influence on spontaneous tachycardia 24 hours after coronary occlusion. *Circulation* 72: 933–942, 1985.

Martins, J.B., R. Lewis, D. Wendt, D.D. Lund, and P.G. Schmid. Subendocardial infarction produces epicardial parasympathetic denervation in canine left ventricle. *Am. J. Physiol.* 256: H859-H866, 1989.

Mary-Rabine, L., A.J. Hordof, P. Danilo Jr., J.R. Malm, and M.R. Rosen. Mechanisms for impulse initiation in isolated human atrial fibers. *Circ. Res.* 47: 267–277, 1980.

Mascher, D. Electrical and mechanical responses from ventricular muscle fibers after inactivation of the sodium carrying system. *Pflügers Arch.* 317: 359–372, 1970.

Maseri, A., S. Severi, and P. Marzullo. Role of coronary arterial spasm in sudden coronary ischemic death. In: *Sudden Coronary Death*, edited by H.M. Greenberg, and E.M. Dwyer Jr. New York Academy of Sciences, New York: *Ann. N.Y. Acad. Sci.* 382: 204–216, 1982.

Mason, J.W., E.B. Stinson, R.A. Winkle, J.C. Griffen, P.E. Oyer, D.L. Ross, and G. Derby. Surgery for ventricular tachycardia: efficacy of left ventricular aneurysm resection compared with operation guided by electrical activation mapping. *Circulation* 65: 1148–1155, 1982.

Mathur, P.P., and R.B. Case. Phosphate loss during reversible myocardial ischemia. *J. Mol. Cell. Cardiol.* 5: 375–393, 1973.

Mathur, V.S., G.A. Guinn, and W.H. Burris, III. Maximal revascularization (reperfusion) in intact conscious dogs after 2 to 5 hours of coronary occlusion. *Am. J. Cardiol.* 36: 252–261, 1975.

Matsuda, K., B.F. Hoffman, C.N. Ellner, M. Katz, and C.M. Brooks. Veratridine-induced prolongation of repolarization in the mammalian heart. In: *Nineteenth International Physiological Congress.* American Physiological Society: 1953, pp. 596–597.

Matsuda, K., T. Hoshi, and S. Kameyama. Effects of aconitine on the cardiac membrane potential of the dog. *Jpn. J. Physiol.* 9: 419–429, 1959.

Matta, R.J., R.L. Verrier, and B. Lown. Repetitive extrasystole as an index of vulnerability to ventricular fibrillation. *Am. J. Physiol.* 230: 1469–1473, 1976.

Mayer, A.G. Rhythmic pulsation in scyphomedusa. Publication 47 of the Carnegie Institution. Carnegie Institution, Washington, 1906, pp. 1–62.

McAllister, R.E., and D. Noble. The time and voltage dependence of the slow outward current in cardiac Purkinje fibres. *J. Physiol.* 186: 632–662, 1966.

McCallister, L.P., S. Trapukdi, and J.R. Neely. Morphometric observations on the effects of ischemia in the isolated perfused rat heart. *J. Mol. Cell. Cardiol.* 11: 619–630, 1979.

McDonald, T.F., and D.P. MacLeod. Metabolism and the electrical activity of anoxic ventricular muscle. *J. Physiol.* 229: 559–582, 1973.

McEachern, C.G., G.W. Manning, and G.E. Hall. Sudden occlusion of coronary arteries following removal of cardiosensory pathways. An experimental study. *Arch. Intern. Med.* 65: 661–670, 1940.

McGrath, B.P., S.P. Lim, L. Leversha, and A. Shanahan. Myocardial and peripheral catecholamine responses to acute coronary artery constriction before and after propranolol treatment in the anaesthetised dog. *Cardiovasc. Res.* 15: 28–34, 1981.

McWilliam, J.A. Fibrillar contraction of the heart. *J. Physiol.* 8: 296–310, 1887.

McWilliam, J.A. Cardiac failure and sudden death. *Br. Med. J.* 1: 6–8, 1889.

Meesmann, W., F.W. Schulz, G. Schley, and P. Adolphsen. Überlebensquote nach akutem experimentellem Coronarverschluss in Abhängigkeit von Spontankollateralen des Herzens. *Z. Ges. Exp. Med.* 153: 246–264, 1970.

Meesmann, W. Early arrhythmias and primary ventricular fibrillation after acute myocardial ischemia in relation to preexisting coronary collaterals. In: *Early Arrhythmias Resulting from Myocardial Ischaemia*, edited by J.R. Parratt. Oxford University Press, New York: 1982, pp. 93–112.

Mehra, R., R.H. Zeiler, W.B. Gough, and N. El-Sherif. Reentrant ventricular arrhythmias in the late myocardial infarction period. 9. Electrophysiologic-anatomic correlation of reentrant circuits. *Circulation* 67: 11–24, 1983.

Melville, K.I., H.E. Shister, and S. Huq. Iproveratril: Experimental data on coronary dilatation and antiarrhythmic action. *Can. Med. Assoc. J.* 90: 761–770, 1964.

Mendez, C., W.J. Mueller, J. Merideth, and G.K. Moe. Interaction of transmembrane potentials in canine Purkinje fibers and at Purkinje fiber-muscle junctions. *Circ. Res.* 24: 361–372, 1969.

Méndez, C., and M. Delmar. Triggered activity: its possible role in cardiac arrhythmias. In: *Cardiac Electrophysiology and Arrhythmias*, edited by D.P. Zipes, and J. Jalife. Grune and Stratton, Orlando: 1985, pp. 311–313.

Michelson, E.L., J.F. Spear, and E.N. Moore. Electrophysiologic and anatomic correlates of sustained ventricular tachyarrhythmias in a model of chronic myocardial infarction. *Am. J. Cardiol.* 45: 583–590, 1980.

Michelson, E.L., J.F. Spear, and E.N. Moore. Description of chronic canine myocardial infarction models suitable for the electropharmacologic evaluation of new antiarrhythmic drugs. In: *The Evaluation of New Antiarrhythmic Drugs*, edited by J. Morganroth, E.N. Moore, L.S. Dreifus, and E.L. Michelson. Martinus Nijhoff, The Hague: 1981a, pp. 33–46.

Michelson, E.L., J.F. Spear, and E.N. Moore. Effects of procainamide on strength-interval relations in normal and chronically infarcted canine myocardium. *Am. J. Cardiol.* 47: 1223–1232, 1981b.

Michelson, E.L., J.F. Spear, and E.N. Moore. Further electrophysiologic and anatomic correlates in a canine model of chronic myocardial infarction susceptible to the initiation of sustained ventricular tachyarrhythmias. *Anat. Rec.* 201: 55–65, 1981c.

Michelson, E.L., J.F. Spear, and E.N. Moore. Initiation of sustained ventricular tachyarrhythmias in a canine model of chronic myocardial infarction: Importance of the site of stimulation. *Circulation* 63: 776–784, 1981d.

Millar, K., R.L. Lux, and R.F. Wyatt. Ischemia induced ventricular conduction delay: Reversal by cardiac nerve stimulation. (abstract) *Circulation* 54(Suppl. II): II-131, 1976.

Miller, J.M., A.H. Harken, W.C. Hargrove, and M.E. Josephson. Pattern of endocardial activation during sustained ventricular tachycardia. *J. Am. Coll. Cardiol.* 6: 1280–1287, 1985.

Miller, J.M., F.E. Marchlinski, A.E. Buxton, and M.E. Josephson. Relationship between the 12-lead electrocardiogram during ventricular tachycardia and endocardial site of origin in patients with coronary artery disease. *Circulation* 77: 759–766, 1988.

Mines, G.R. On dynamic equilibrium in the heart. *J. Physiol.* 46: 349–383, 1913.

Mines, G.R. On circulating excitations in heart muscles and their possible relation to tachycardia and fibrillation. *Trans. R. Soc. Can.* IV: 43–52, 1914.

Miura, D.S., B.F. Hoffman, and M.R. Rosen. The effect of extracellular potassium on the intracellular potassium ion activity and transmembrane potentials of beating canine cardiac Purkinje fibers. *J. Gen. Physiol.* 69: 463–474, 1977.

Moak, J.P., and M.R. Rosen. Induction and termination of triggered activity by pacing in isolated canine Purkinje fibers. *Circulation* 69: 149–162, 1984.

Moe, G.K., A.S. Harris, and C.J. Wiggers. Analysis of the initiation of fibrillation by electrographic studies. *Am. J. Physiol.* 134: 473–492, 1941.

Moe, G.K., J.B. Preston, and H. Burlington. Physiologic evidence for a dual A-V transmission system. *Circ. Res.* 4: 357–375, 1956.

Moe, G.K. On the multiple wavelet hypothesis of atrial fibrillation. *Arch. Int. Pharmacodyn. Ther.* 140: 183–188, 1962.

Moe, G.K., W. Cohen, and R.L. Vick. Experimentally induced paroxysmal A-V nodal tachycardia in the dog. A "case report". *Am. Heart J.* 65: 87–92, 1963.

Moe, G.K., W.C. Rheinboldt, and J.A. Abildskov. A computer model of atrial fibrillation. *Am. Heart J.* 67: 200–220, 1964.

Moe, G.K., C. Mendez, and J. Han. Aberrant A-V impulse propagation in the dog heart: a study of functional bundle branch block. *Circ. Res.* 16: 261–286, 1965.

Moe, G.K. Evidence for reentry as a mechanism of cardiac arrhythmias. *Rev. Physiol. Biochem. Pharmacol.* 72: 55–81, 1975.

Moe, G.K., J. Jalife, W.J. Mueller, and B. Moe. A mathematical model of parasystole and its application to clinical arrhythmias. *Circulation* 56: 968–979, 1977.

Moir, T.W. Study of luminal coronary collateral circulation in the beating canine heart. *Circ. Res.* 24: 735–744, 1969.

Moore, E.N., and J.F. Spear. Ventricular fibrillation threshold. Its physiological and pharmacological importance. *Arch. Intern. Med.* 135: 446–453, 1975.

Moore, E.N., J.F. Spear, L.N. Horowitz, and M.E. Josephson. Electrophysiological mechanisms causing ventricular tachyarrhythmias. In: *Management of Ventricular Tachycardia—Role of Mexiletine*, edited by E. Sandøe, D.G. Julian, and J.W. Bell. Excerpta Medica, Amsterdam: 1978, pp. 3–15.

Moore, E.N., J.F. Spear, E.L. Michelson, and D.E. Euler. What is the optimal pulse duration for programmed electrical stimulation? (abstract) *Circulation* 62(Suppl. III): III-172, 1980.

Morad, M., and E.L. Rolett. Relaxing effects of catecholamines on mammalian heart. *J. Physiol.* 224: 537–558, 1972.

Morady, F., L. DiCarlo, S. Winston, J.C. Davis, and M.M. Scheinman. A prospective comparison of triple extrastimuli and left ventricular stimulation in studies of ventricular tachycardia induction. *Circulation* 70: 52–57, 1984a.

Morady, F., W. Shapiro, E. Shen, R.J. Sung, and M.M. Scheinman. Programmed ventricular stimulation in patients without spontaneous ventricular tachycardia. *Am. Heart J.* 107: 875–882, 1984b.

Morady, F., M.M. Scheinman, L.A. DiCarlo, J.C. Davis, J.M. Herre, J.C. Griffin, S.A. Winston, M. De Buitleir, C.B. Hantler, J.A. Wahr, W.H. Kou, and S.D. Nelson. Catheter ablation of ventricular tachycardia with intracardiac shocks: results in 33 patients. *Circulation* 75: 1037–1049, 1987.

Morady, F., R. Frank, W.H. Kou, J.L. Tonet, S.D. Nelson, S. Kounde, M. De Buitleir, and G. Fontaine. Identification and catheter ablation of a zone of slow conduction in the reentrant circuit of ventricular tachycardia in humans. *J. Am. Coll. Cardiol.* 11: 775–782, 1988.

Morady, F., W.H. Kou, A.H. Kadish, S. Schmaltz, D.O. Summitt, and S. Rosenheck. Effect of basic drive train cycle length on induction of ventricular tachycardia by a single extrastimulus. *J. Electrocardiol.* 3: 111–116, 1989.

Moréna, H., M.J. Janse, J.W.T. Fiolet, W.J.G. Krieger, H. Crijns, and D. Durrer. Comparison of the effects of regional ischemia, hypoxia, hyperkalemia and acidosis on intracellular and extracellular potentials and metabolism in the isolated porcine heart. *Circ. Res.* 46: 634–646, 1980.

Morgan, J.P., and K.G. Morgan. Calcium and cardiovascular function. Intracellular calcium levels during contraction and relaxation of mammalian cardiac and vascular smooth muscle as detected with aequorin. *Am. J. Med.* 77(5A): 33–46, 1984.

Moss, A.J., R. Schnitzler, R. Green, and J. DeCamilla. Ventricular arrhythmias 3 weeks after acute myocardial infarction. *Ann. Int. Med.* 75: 837–841, 1971.

Moss, A.J., J. DeCamilla, H. Davis, L. Bayer, and S. Goldstein. Use and limitations of ventricular premature beats as prognostic indicators of the posthospital course of myocardial infarction. (abstract) *Am. J. Cardiol.* 37: 158, 1976.

Moss, A.J., J. DeCamilla, and H. Davis. Cardiac death in the first 6 months after myocardial infarction: Potential for mortality reduction in the early posthospital period. *Am. J. Cardiol.* 39: 816–820, 1977.

Moss, A.J., H.T. Davis, J. DeCamilla, and L.W. Bayer. Ventricular ectopic beats and their relation to sudden and nonsudden cardiac death after myocardial infarction. *Circulation* 60: 998–1003, 1979.

Mukharji, J., R.E. Rude, W.K. Poole, N. Gustafson, L.J. Thomas Jr., H.W. Strauss, A.S. Jaffe, J.E. Muller, R. Roberts, D.S. Raabe Jr., C.H. Croft, E. Passamani, E. Braunwald, J.T. Willerson and the MILIS Study Group. Risk factors for sudden death after acute myocardial infarction: two-year follow-up. *Am. J. Cardiol.* 54: 31–36, 1984.

Mulder, B.J.M. Damage-induced propagated contractions in cardiac muscle: implications for cardiac arrhythmias. (Doctoral Thesis) University of Amsterdam. Rodopi, Amsterdam, 1989.

Mulder, B.J.M., P.D. de Tombe, and H.E.D.J. ter Keurs. Spontaneous and propagated contractions in rat cardiac trabeculae. *J. Gen. Physiol.* 93: 943–961, 1989.

Muller, J.E., P.H. Stone, Z.G. Turi, J.D. Rutherford, C.A. Czeisler, C. Parker, W.K. Poole, E. Passamani, R. Roberts, T. Robertson, B.E. Sobel, J.T. Willerson, E. Braunwald, and the MILIS Study Group. Circadian variation in the frequency of onset of acute myocardial infarction. *N. Engl. J. Med.* 313: 1315–1322, 1985.

Muller, J.E., P.L. Ludmer, S.N. Willich, G.H. Tofler, G. Aylmer, I. Klangos, and P.H. Stone. Circadian variation in the frequency of sudden cardiac death. *Circulation* 75: 131–138, 1987.

Mullins, L.J. The generation of electric currents in cardiac fibers by Na/Ca exchange. *Am. J. Physiol.* 236: C103-C110, 1979.

Mullins, L.J. *Ion Transport in Heart*. Raven Press, New York: 1981.

Murdock, D.K., J.M. Loeb, D.E. Euler, and W.C. Randall. Electrophysiology of coronary reperfusion. A mechanism for reperfusion arrhythmias. *Circulation* 61: 175–182, 1980.

Murphy, E., C. Steenbergen, L.A. Levy, B. Raju, and R.E. London. Cytosolic free magnesium levels in ischemic rat heart. *J. Biol. Chem.* 264: 5622–5627, 1989.

Musso, E., and M. Vassalle. The role of calcium in overdrive suppression of canine cardiac Purkinje fibers. *Circ. Res.* 51: 167–180, 1982.

Myerburg, R.J., J.W. Stewart, and B.F. Hoffman. Electrophysiological properties of the canine peripheral A-V conducting system. *Circ. Res.* 26: 361–378, 1970.

Myerburg, R.J., H. Gelband, K. Nilsson, R.J. Sung, R.J. Thurer, A.R. Morales, and A.L. Bassett. Long-term electrophysiological abnormalities resulting from experimental myocardial infarction in cats. *Circ. Res.* 41: 73–84, 1977.

Myerburg, R.J., C.A. Conde, R.J. Sung, A. Mayorga-Cortes, S.M. Mallon, D.S. Sheps, R.A. Appel, and A. Castellanos. Clinical, electrophysiologic and hemodynamic profile of patients resuscitated from prehospital cardiac arrest. *Am. J. Med.* 68: 568–576, 1980.

Myerburg, R.J., A.L. Bassett, K. Epstein, M.S. Gaide, P. Kozlovskis, S.S. Wong, A. Castellanos, and H. Gelband. Electrophysiological effects of procainamide in acute and healed experimental ischemic injury of cat myocardium. *Circ. Res.* 50: 386–393, 1982a.

Myerburg, R.J., K. Epstein, M.S. Gaide, S.S. Wong, A. Castellanos, H. Gelband, and A.L. Bassett. Electrophysiologic consequences of experimental acute ischemia superimposed on healed myocardial infarction in cats. *Am. J. Cardiol.* 49: 323–330, 1982b.

Myerburg, R.J., K. Epstein, M.S. Gaide, S.S. Wong, A. Castellanos, H. Gelband, J.S. Cameron, and A.L. Bassett. Cellular electrophysiology in acute and healed experimental myocardial infarction. In: *Sudden Coronary Death*, edited by H.M. Greenberg, and E.M. Dwyer Jr. New York Academy of Sciences, New York: *Ann. N.Y. Acad. Sci.* 382: 90–113, 1982c.

Myers, W.W., and C.R. Honig. Amount and distribution of Rb[86] transported into myocardium from ventricular lumen. *Am. J. Physiol.* 211: 739–745, 1966.

Nahum, L.H., W.F. Hamilton, and H.E. Hoff. The injury current in the electrocardiogram. *Am. J. Physiol.* 139: 202–207, 1943.

Naimi, S., B. Avitall, J. Mieszala, and H.J. Levine. Dispersion of effective refractory period during abrupt reperfusion of ischemic myocardium in dogs. *Am. J. Cardiol.* 39: 407–412, 1977.

Nakata, T., D.J. Hearse, and M.J. Curtis. Are reperfusion-induced arrhythmias caused by disinhibition of an arrhythmogenic component of ischemia? *J. Mol. Cell. Cardiol.* 22: 843–858, 1990.

Nakaya, H., S. Kimura, and M. Kanno. Intracellular K^+ and Na^+ activities under hypoxia, acidosis, and no glucose in dog hearts. *Am. J. Physiol.* 249: H1078-H1085, 1985.

Nakayama, T., Y. Kurachi, A. Noma, and H. Irisawa. Action potential and membrane currents of single pacemaker cells of the rabbit heart. *Pflügers Arch.* 402: 248–257, 1984.

Naumann d'Alnoncourt, C., R. Cardinal, and M.J. Janse. Über die arrhythmogene Wirkung von Potentialdifferenzen im Ventrikelmyokard. In: *Ventrikuläre Herzrhythmusstörungen-Pathophysiologie-Klinik-Therapie*, edited by B. Lüderitz. Springer Verlag, Berlin: 1981, pp. 70–80.

Naumann d'Alnoncourt, C., W. Zierhut, and B. Lüderitz. Effects of high potassium concentrations on impulse formation in ischemic Purkinje fibers. (abstract) *Circulation* 66(Suppl. II): II-357, 1982.

Naumann d'Alnoncourt, C., W. Zierhut, J. Nitsch, and B. Lüderitz. Effects of amiodarone on Purkinje fibers. In: *New Aspects in the Medical Treatment of Tachyarrhythmias. Role of Amiodarone*, edited by G. Breithardt, and F. Loogen. Urban & Schwarzenberg, München, Wien, Baltimore: 1983, pp. 88–90.

Nguyen-Thi, A., E. Ruiz-Ceretti, and O.F. Schanne. Electrophysiologic effects and electrolyte changes in total myocardial ischemia. *Can. J. Physiol. Pharmacol.* 59: 876–883, 1981.

Niedergerke, R., and R.K. Orkand. The dependence of the action potential of the frog's heart on the external and intracellular sodium concentration. *J. Physiol.* 184: 312–334, 1966.

Nikolic, G., R.L. Bishop, and J.B. Singh. Sudden death recorded during Holter monitoring. *Circulation* 66: 218–225, 1982.

Noble, D., and R.W. Tsien. The kinetics and rectifier properties of the slow potassium current in cardiac Purkinje fibres. *J. Physiol.* 195: 185–214, 1968.

Noble, D. The surprising heart: a review of recent progress in cardiac electrophysiology. *J. Physiol.* 353: 1–50, 1984.

Noma, A., K. Yanagihara, and H. Irisawa. Inward current of the rabbit sinoatrial node cell. *Pflügers Arch.* 372: 43–51, 1977.

Noma, A., H. Kotake, and H. Irisawa. Slow inward current and its role mediating the chronotropic effect of epinephrine in the rabbit sinoatrial node. *Pflügers Arch.* 388: 1–9, 1980.

Noma, A. ATP-regulated K^+ channels in cardiac muscle. *Nature* 305: 147–148, 1983.

Noma, A., and T. Shibasaki. Membrane current through adenosine-triphosphate-regulated potassium channels in guinea-pig ventricular cells. *J. Physiol.* 363: 463–480, 1985.

Nordin, C., E. Gilat, and R.S. Aronson. Delayed afterdepolarizations and triggered activity in ventricular muscle from rats with streptozotocin-induced diabetes. *Circ. Res.* 57: 28–34, 1985.

Nordrehaug, J.E., and G. von der Lippe. Hypokalaemia and ventricular fibrillation in acute myocardial infarction. *Br. Heart J.* 50: 525–529, 1983.

Norris, R.M., and C.J. Mercer. Significance of idioventricular rhythms in acute myocardial infarction. *Prog. Cardiovasc. Dis.* 16: 455–468, 1974.

Northover, B.J. Ventricular tachycardia during the first 72 hours after acute myocardial infarction. *Cardiology* 69: 149–156, 1982.

Norwegian Multicenter Study Group. Timolol-induced reduction in mortality and reinfarction in patients surviving acute myocardial infarction. *N. Engl. J. Med.* 304: 801–807, 1981.

Ogawa, S., Y. Nakamura, L.S. Dreifus, and E. Kaplinsky. Ventricular arrhythmias in acute coronary artery ligation in dogs: Electrophysiological mechanism and its relation to the severity of myocardial ischemia. *Jpn. Circ. J.* 45: 517–523, 1981.

Ogawa, S., K. Sakurai, T. Miyazaki, T. Sakai, M. Hosokawa, and Y. Nakamura. Induction and termination of ventricular tachycardia by programmed electrical stimulation in a 7-day-old canine myocardial infarction. *Jpn. Circ. J.* 50: 74–83, 1986.

Ohta, T., J. Toyama, M. Hirai, T. Osaka, I. Kodama, and K. Yamada. Endocardial mapping of ventricular tachycardia in one day old myocardial infarction. *Jpn. Circ. J.* 50: 84–90, 1986.

Okumura, K., R.W. Henthorn, A.E. Epstein, V.J. Plumb, and A.L. Waldo. Further observations on transient entrainment: importance of pacing site and properties of the components of the reentry circuit. *Circulation* 72: 1293–1307, 1985.

Okumura, K., B. Olshansky, R.W. Henthorn, A.E. Epstein, V.J. Plumb, and A.L. Waldo. Demonstration of the presence of slow conduction during sustained ventricular tachycardia in man: use of transient entrainment of the tachycardia. *Circulation* 75: 369–378, 1987.

Olichney, M., and W. Modell. Cardiovascular and antiarrhythmic effects of pentobarbital sodium in dogs after experimental myocardial infarction. (abstract) *Fed. Proc.* 17: 401, 1958.

Oliver, G.C., J.P. Miller, R.E. Kleiger, K.W. Clark, T.F. Martin, and J.R. Cox Jr. Ventricular arrhythmias in the early post hospital phase of myocardial infarction. (abstract) *Circulation* 52(Suppl. II): II-223, 1975.

Olshansky, B., J. Martins, and S. Hunt. N-acetyl procainamide causing torsades de pointes. *Am. J. Cardiol.* 50: 1439–1441, 1982.

Olsson, S.B., P. Blomström, C. Blomström-Lundqvist, and B. Wohlfart. Endocardial monophasic action potentials: Correlations with intracellular electrical activity. In: *Electrocardiography. Past and Future*, edited by P. Coumel, and O.B. Garfein. New York Academy of Sciences, New York: *Ann. N.Y. Acad. Sci.* Sci. 601: 119–127, 1990.

Opie, L.H., and W.A. Coetzee. Are calcium ions involved in the genesis of early ischemic ventricular arrhythmias? In: *Life-Threatening Arrhythmias During Ischemia and Infarction*, edited by D.J. Hearse, A.S. Manning, and M.J. Janse. Raven Press, New York: 1987, pp. 63–75.

Opthof, T., J.J. Duivenvoorden, A.C.G. VanGinneken, H.J. Jongsma and L.N. Bouman. Electrophysiological effects of alinidine (ST 567) on sinoatrial node fibres in the rabbit heart. *Cardiovasc. Res.* 20: 727–739, 1986.

Opthof, T., A.C.G. vanGinneken, L.N. Bouman, and H.J. Jongsma. The intrinsic cycle length in small pieces isolated from the rabbit sinoatrial node. *J. Mol. Cell. Cardiol.* 19: 923–934, 1987.

Opthof, T., A.R. Ramdat Misier, R. Coronel, J.T. Vermeulen, H.J. Verberne, R.G.J. Frank, A.C. Moulijn, F.J.L. van Capelle, and M.J. Janse. Dispersion of refractoriness in canine ventricular myocardium. Effects of sympathetic stimulation. *Circ. Res.* 68: 1204–1215, 1991.

Osaka, T., I. Kodama, N. Tsuboi, J. Toyama, and K. Yamada. Effects of activation sequence and anisotropic cellular geometry on the repolarization phase of action potential of dog ventricular muscles. *Circulation* 76: 226–236, 1987.

Overholt, E.D., R.W. Joyner, R.D. Veenstra, D. Rawling, and R. Wiedmann. Unidirectional block between Purkinje and ventricular layers of papillary muscles. *Am. J. Physiol.* 247: H584–H595, 1984.

Pagé, P.L., R. Cardinal, P. Savard, and M. Shenasa. Sinus rhythm mapping in a canine model of ventricular tachycardia. *PACE* 11: 632–644, 1988.

Pagé, P.L., R. Cardinal, M. Shenasa, W. Kaltenbrunner, R. Cossette, and R. Nadeau. Surgical treatment of ventricular tachycardia. Regional cryoablation guided by computerized epicardial and endocardial mapping. *Circulation* 80(Suppl. I): I-124 -I-134, 1989.

Palileo, E.V., W.W. Ashley, S. Swiryn, R.A. Bauernfeind, B. Strasberg, A.T. Petropoulos, and K.M. Rosen. Exercise provocable right ventricular outflow tract tachycardia. *Am. Heart J.* 104: 185–193, 1982.

Pantridge, J.F., and J.S. Geddes. A mobile intensive-care unit in the management of myocardial infarction. *Lancet* 2: 271–273, 1967.

Pantridge, J.F., S.W. Webb, A.A.J. Adgey, and J.S. Geddes. The first hour after the onset of acute myocardial infarction. In: *Progress in Cardiology (3)*, edited by P.N. Yu, and J.F. Goodwin. Lea & Febiger, Philadelphia: 1974, pp. 173–188.

Pantridge, J.F., S.W. Webb, and A.A.J. Adgey. Arrhythmias in the first hours of acute myocardial infarction. *Prog. Cardiovasc. Dis.* 23: 265–278, 1981.

Parratt, J.R. Inhibitors of the slow calcium current and early ventricular arrhythmias. In: *Early Arrhythmias Resulting from Myocardial Ischemia*, edited by J.R. Parratt. Oxford University Press, New York: 1982, pp. 329–346.

Parry, C.H. An inquiry into the symptoms and causes of the syncope anginosa, commonly called angina pectori. R. Cruttwell, Bath, 1799.

Paspa, P., and M. Vassalle. Mechanism of caffeine-induced arrhythmias in canine cardiac Purkinje fibers. *Am. J. Cardiol.* 53: 313–319, 1984.

Pasyk, S., C.M. Bloor, E.M. Khouri, and D.E. Gregg. Systemic and coronary effects of coronary artery occlusion in the unanesthetized dog. *Am. J. Physiol.* 220: 646–654, 1971.

Patterson, E., J.K. Gibson, and B.R. Lucchesi. Electrophysiologic effects of disopyramide phosphate on reentrant ventricular arrhythmia in conscious dogs after myocardial infarction. *Am. J. Cardiol.* 46: 792–799, 1980.

Patterson, E., J.K. Gibson, and B.R. Lucchesi. Postmyocardial infarction reentrant ventricular arrhythmias in conscious dogs: Suppression by Brety-lium Tosylate. *J. Pharmacol. Exp. Ther.* 216: 453–458, 1981a.

Patterson, E., J.K. Gibson, and B.R. Lucchesi. Prevention of chronic canine ventricular tachyarrhythmias with Bretylium Tosylate. *Circulation* 64: 1045–1050, 1981b.

Patterson, E., K. Holland, B.T. Eller, and B.R. Lucchesi. Ventricular fibrilla-tion resulting from ischemia at a site remote from previous myocardial infarction. A conscious canine model of sudden coronary death. *Am. J. Cardiol.* 50: 1414–1423, 1982.

Patterson, E., B.J. Scherlag, and R. Lazzara. Mechanism of prevention of sud-den death by nadolol: differential actions on arrhythmia triggers and sub-strate after myocardial infarction in the dog. *J. Am. Coll. Cardiol.* 8: 1365–1372, 1986.

Patterson, E., B.J. Scherlag, and R. Lazzara. Prevention of spontaneous sus-tained ventricular tachycardia in the postinfarction dog by left stellate ganglionectomy. *J. Cardiovasc. Electrophysiol.* 2: 238–248, 1991.

Penkoske, P.A., B.E. Sobel, and P.B. Corr. Disparate electrophysiological alter-ations accompanying dysrhythmia due to coronary occlusion and reperfu-sion in the cat. *Circulation* 58: 1023–1035, 1978.

Penny, W.J., and D.J. Sheridan. Arrhythmias and cellular electrophysiological changes during myocardial "ischaemia" and reperfusion. *Cardiovasc. Res.* 17: 363–372, 1983.

Penny, W.J. The deleterious effects of myocardial catecholamines on cellular electrophysiology and arrhythmias during ischaemia and reperfusion. *Eur. Heart J.* 5: 960–973, 1984.

Penny, W.J, W Culling, M.J. Lewis, and D.J. Sheridan. Antiarrhythmic and electrophysiological effects of alpha adrenoceptor blockade during myocar-dial ischaemia and reperfusion in isolated guinea-pig heart. *J. Mol. Cell. Cardiol.* 17: 399–409, 1985.

Peon, J., G.R. Ferrier, and G.K. Moe. The relationship of excitability to conduc-tion velocity in canine Purkinje tissue. *Circ. Res.* 43: 125–135, 1978.

Peper, K., and W. Trautwein. Über den Mechanismus der Extrasystolen des Aconitin-vergifteten Herzmuskels. (abstract) *Pflügers Arch.* 291: R16, 1966.

Perticone, F., L. Adinolfi, and D. Bonaduce. Efficacy of magnesium sulfate in the treatment of torsade de pointes. *Am. Heart J.* 112: 847–849, 1986.

Petropoulos, P.C., and N.G. Meijne. Cardiac function during perfusion of the circumflex coronary artery, with venous blood, low-molecular dextran, or Tyrode solution. *Am. Heart J.* 68: 370–382, 1964.

Pisa, Z. Sudden death: A worldwide problem. In: *Sudden Death*, edited by H.E. Kulbertus, and H.J.J. Wellens. Martinus Nijhoff, The Hague: 1980, pp. 3–10.

Pitt, B. Sudden cardiac death: role of left ventricular dysfunction. In: *Sudden Coronary Death*, edited by H.M. Greenberg, and E.M. Dwyer Jr. New York Academy of Sciences, New York: *Ann. N.Y. Acad. Sci.* 382: 218–222, 1982.

Pliam, M.B., D.J. Krellenstein, M. Vassalle, and C.McC. Brooks. The influence of norepinephrine, reserpine and propranolol on overdrive suppression. *J. Electrocardiol.* 8: 17–24, 1975.

Pogwizd, S.M., J.R. Onufer, J.B. Kramer, B.E. Sobel, and P.B. Corr. Induction of delayed afterdepolarizations and triggered activity in canine Purkinje fibers by lysophosphoglycerides. *Circ. Res.* 59: 416–426, 1986.

Pogwizd, S.M., and P.B. Corr. Electrophysiologic mechanisms underlying arrhythmias due to reperfusion of ischemic myocardium. *Circulation* 76: 404–426, 1987a.

Pogwizd, S.M., and P.B. Corr. Reentrant and nonreentrant mechanisms contribute to arrhythmogenesis during early myocardial ischemia: Results using three-dimensional mapping. *Circ. Res.* 61: 352–371, 1987b.

Pogwizd, S.M., and P.B. Corr. Mechanisms underlying the development of ventricular fibrillation during early myocardial ischemia. *Circ. Res.* 66: 672–695, 1990.

Polimeni, P.I. Extracellular space and ionic distribution in rat ventricle. *Am. J. Physiol.* 227: 676–683, 1974.

Poole-Wilson, P.A., and I.R. Cameron. Intracellular pH and K^+ of cardiac and skeletal muscle in acidosis and alkalosis. *Am. J. Physiol.* 229: 1305–1310, 1975.

Porter, W.T. On the results of ligation of the coronary arteries. *J. Physiol.* 15: 121–138, 1894.

Porter, W.T. Further researches on the closure of the coronary arteries. *J. Exp. Med.* 1: 46–70, 1896.

Poser, R.F., P.J. Podrid, F. Lombardi, and B. Lown. Aggravation of arrhythmia induced with antiarrhythmic drugs during electrophysiologic testing. *Am. Heart J.* 110: 9–16, 1985.

Previtali, M., C. Klersy, J.A. Salerno, M. Chimienti, C. Panciroli, E. Marangoni, G. Specchia, M. Comolli, and P. Bobba. Ventricular tachyarrhythmias in Prinzmetal's variant angina: Clinical significance and relation to the degree and time course of S-T segment elevation. *Am. J. Cardiol.* 52: 19–25, 1983.

Prinzmetal, M., B. Simkin, H.C. Bergman, and H.E. Kruger. Studies on the coronary circulation. II. The collateral circulation of the normal human heart by coronary perfusion with radioactive erythrocytes and glass spheres. *Am. Heart J.* 33: 420–442, 1947.

Prinzmetal, M., H. Toyoshima, A. Ekmekci, Y. Mizuno, and T. Nagaya. Myocardial ischemia. Nature of ischemic electrocardiographic patterns in the mammalian ventricles as determined by intracellular electrographic and metabolic changes. *Am. J. Cardiol.* 8: 493–503, 1961.

Priori, S.G., M. Mantica, and P.J. Schwartz. Delayed afterdepolarizations elicited in vivo by left stellate ganglion stimulation. *Circulation* 78: 178–185, 1988.

Priori, S.G., M. Mantica, C. Napolitano, and P.J. Schwartz. Early afterdepolarizations induced in vivo by reperfusion of ischemic myocardium. A possible mechanism for reperfusion arrhythmias. *Circulation* 81: 1911–1920, 1990.

Priori S.G., and P.B. Corr. Mechanisms underlying early and delayed afterdepolarizations induced by catecholamines. *Am. J. Physiol.* 258: H1796-H1805, 1990.

Puddu, P.E., R. Jouve, F. Langlet, J.C. Guillen, M. Lanti, and A. Reale. Prevention of postischemic ventricular fibrillation late after right or left stellate ganglionectomy in dogs. *Circulation* 77: 935–946, 1988.

Quain, R. On fatty diseases of the heart. *Medico-Chirurg. Transactions* 15: 121–196, 1850.

Quan, W., and Y. Rudy. Unidirectional block and reentry of cardiac excitation: a model study. *Circ. Res.* 66: 367–382, 1990.

Ramanathan, K.B., M.M. Bodenheimer, V.S. Banka, and R.H. Helfant. Electrophysiologic effects of partial coronary occlusion and reperfusion. *Am. J. Cardiol.* 40: 50–54, 1977.

Ramdat Misier, A.R., J.T. Vermeulen, R.G.J. Frank, T. Opthof, A.C. Moulijn, F.J.L. van Capelle, and M.J. Janse. Simultaneous measurements of ventricular "refractoriness" at multiple sites during sympathetic stimulation. (abstract) *Circulation* 78(Suppl. II): II-6, 1988.

Randall, D.C., and D.M. Hasson. Cardiac arrhythmias in the monkey during classically conditioned fear and excitement. *Pavlov J. Biol. Sci.* 16: 97–107, 1981.

Randall, W.C. Sympathetic control of the heart. In: *Neural Regulation of the Heart*, edited by W.C. Randall. Oxford University Press, New York: 1977, pp. 43–94.

Randall, W.C., J. Talano, M.P. Kaye, D.E. Euler, S.B. Jones, and G. Brynjolfsson. Cardiac pacemakers in absence of the SA node: Responses to exercise and autonomic blockade. *Am. J. Physiol.* 234: H465-H470, 1978.

Randall, W.C., J.M. Loeb, S.B. Jones, and D.E. Euler. Neural mechanisms in the regulation of atrial pacemaker function. In: *Physiology of Atrial Pacemakers and Conductive Tissues*, edited by R.C. Little. Futura Publishing Company, Mt, Kisco, New York: 1980, pp. 113–139.

Randall, W.C., L.E. Rinkema, S.B. Jones, J.F. Moran, and G. Brynjolfsson. Overdrive suppression of atrial pacemaker tissues in the alert, awake dog before and chronically after excision of the sinoatrial node. *Am. J. Cardiol.* 49: 1166–1175, 1982a.

Randall, W.C., L.E. Rinkema, S.B. Jones, J.F. Moran, and G. Brynjolfsson. Functional characterization of atrial pacemaker activity. *Am. J. Physiol.* 242: H98-H106, 1982b.

Randall, W.C. Selective autonomic innervation of the heart. In: *Nervous Control of Cardiovascular Function*, edited by W.C. Randall. Oxford University Press, New York: 1984, pp. 46–67.

Rau, E.E., K.I. Shine, and G.A. Langer. Potassium exchange and mechanical performance in anoxic mammalian myocardium. *Am. J. Physiol.* 232: H85-H94, 1977.

Reber, W.R., and R. Weingart. Ungulate cardiac Purkinje fibres: The influence of intracellular pH on the electrical cell-to-cell coupling. *J. Physiol.* 328: 87–104, 1982.

Reddy, C.P., and L.S. Gettes. Use of isoproterenol as an aid to electric induction of chronic recurrent ventricular tachycardia. *Am. J. Cardiol.* 44:705–713, 1979.

Reimer, K.A., J.E. Lowe, M.M. Rasmussen, and R.B. Jennings. The wavefront phenomenon of ischemic cell death. 1. Myocardial infarct size vs duration of coronary occlusion in dogs. *Circulation* 56: 786–794, 1977.

Reimer, K.A., and R.B. Jennings. The "wavefront phenomenon" of myocardial ischemic cell death. II. Transmural progression of necrosis within the framework of ischemic bed size (myocardium at risk) and collateral flow. *Lab. Invest.* 40: 633–644, 1979.

Reimer, K.A., R.B. Jennings, and M.L. Hill. Total ischemia in dog hearts in vitro. 2. High energy phosphate depletion and associated defects in energy metabolism, cell volume regulation, and sarcolemmal integrity. *Circ. Res.* 49: 901–911, 1981.

Rensma, P.L., M.A. Allessie, W.J.E.P. Lammers, F.I.M. Bonke, and M.J. Schalij. Length of excitation wave and susceptibility to reentrant atrial arrhythmias in normal conscious dogs. *Circ. Res.* 62: 395–410, 1988.

Rentrop, P., H. Blanke, K.R. Karsch, H. Kaiser, H. Köstering, and K. Leitz. Selective intracoronary thrombolysis in acute myocardial infarction and unstable angina pectoris. *Circulation* 63: 307–317, 1981.

Restivo, M., W.B. Gough, and N. El-Sherif. Ventricular arrhythmias in the subacute myocardial infarction period. High-resolution activation and refractory patterns of reentrant rhythms. *Circ. Res.* 66: 1310–1327, 1990.

Reuter, H., and H. Scholz. Über den Einfluss der extracellulären Ca-Konzentration auf Membranpotential und Kontraktion isolierter Herzpräparate bei graduierter Depolarisation. *Pflügers Arch.* 300: 87–107, 1968.

Reuter, H., and N. Seitz. The dependence of calcium efflux from cardiac muscle on temperature and external ion composition. *J. Physiol.* 195: 451–470, 1968.

Reuter, H. Localization of beta adrenergic receptors, and effects of noradrenaline and cyclic nucleotides on action potentials, ionic currents and tension in mammalian cardiac muscle. *J. Physiol.* 242: 429–451, 1974.

Reuter, H., and H. Scholz. The regulation of the calcium conductance of cardiac muscle by adrenaline. *J. Physiol.* 264: 49–62, 1977.

Reuter, H. Ion channels in cardiac cell membranes. *Annu. Rev. Physiol.* 46: 473–484, 1984.

Reynolds, E.W. Jr., C.R. Vander Ark, and F.D. Johnston. Effect of acute myocardial infarction on electrical recovery and transmural temperature gradient in left ventricular wall of dogs. *Circ. Res.* 8: 730–737, 1960.

Reynolds, R.D., G.J. Kelliher, D.M. Ritchie, J. Roberts, and A.B. Beasley. Comparison of the arrhythmogenic effect of myocardial infarction in the cat and dog. *Cardiovasc. Res.* 13: 152–159, 1979.

Ribeiro, L.G.T., T.A. Brandon, T.L. Debauche, P.R. Maroko, and R.R. Miller. Antiarrhythmic and hemodynamic effects of calcium channel blocking agents during coronary artery reperfusion. Comparative effects of verapamil and nifedipine. *Am. J. Cardiol.* 48: 69–74, 1981.

Richards, D.A., D.V. Cody, A.R. Denniss, P.A. Russell, A.A. Young, and J.B.

Uther. Ventricular electrical instability: a predictor of death after myocardial infarction. *Am. J. Cardiol.* 51: 75–80, 1983.

Richards, D.A., G.J. Blake, J.F. Spear, and E.N. Moore. Electrophysiologic substrate for ventricular tachycardia: Correlation of properties in vivo and in vitro. *Circulation* 69: 369–381, 1984.

Riegger, C.B., G. Alperovich, and A.G. Kléber. Effect of oxygen withdrawal on active and passive electrical properties of arterially perfused rabbit ventricular muscle. *Circ. Res.* 64: 532–541, 1989.

Riemersma, R.A. Myocardial catecholamine release in acute myocardial ischaemia; Relationship to cardiac arrhythmias. In: *Early Arrhythmias Resulting from Myocardial Ischaemia*, edited by J.R. Parratt. Oxford University Press, New York: 1982, pp. 125–138.

Ripley, K.L., F.M. Nolle, L.J. Thomas, and G.C. Oliver. Marked increases in frequency of premature ventricular contractions at nine months following myocardial infarction. (abstract) *Circulation* 52(Suppl. II): II-94, 1975.

Rivas, F., F.R. Cobb, R.J. Bache, and J.C. Greenfield. Relationship between blood flow to ischemic regions and extent of myocardial infarction. Serial measurement of blood flow to ischemic regions in dogs. *Circ. Res.* 38: 439–447, 1976.

Roberge, F.A., A. Vinet, and B. Victorri. Reconstruction of propagated electrical activity with a two-dimensional model of anisotropic heart muscle. *Circ. Res.* 58: 461–475, 1986.

Roberts, D.E., L.T. Hersh, and A.M. Scher. Influence of cardiac fiber orientation on wavefront voltage, conduction velocity and tissue resistivity in the dog. *Circ. Res.* 44: 701–712, 1979.

Roberts, J., R. Ito, J. Reilly, and V.J. Cairoli. Influence of reserpine and βTM 10 on digitalis-induced ventricular arrhythmia. *Circ. Res.* 13: 149–158, 1963.

Roberts, R., A. Husain, H.D. Ambos, G.C. Oliver, J.R. Cox Jr., and B.E. Sobel. Relation between infarct size and ventricular arrhythmia. *Br. Heart J.* 37: 1169–1175, 1975.

Roberts, R., V. DeMello, and B.E. Sobel. Deleterious effects of methylprednisolone in patients with myocardial infarction. *Circulation* 53(Suppl. I): I-204-I-206, 1976.

Robertson, J.F., M.E. Cain, L.N. Horowitz, S.R. Spielman, A.M. Greenspan, H.L. Waxman, and M.E. Josephson. Anatomic and electrophysiologic correlates of ventricular tachycardia requiring left ventricular stimulation. *Am. J. Cardiol.* 48: 263–268, 1981.

Robinson, G.C., and G.R. Herrmann. Paroxysmal tachycardia of ventricular origin, and its relation to coronary occlusion. *Heart* 8: 59–81, 1921.

Robinson, R.B., P.A. Boyden, B.F. Hoffman, and K.W. Hewett. Electrical restitution process in dispersed canine cardiac Purkinje and ventricular cells. *Am. J. Physiol.* 253: H1018–H1025, 1987.

Roden, D.M., and B.F. Hoffman. Action potential prolongation and induction of abnormal automaticity by low quinidine concentrations in canine Purkinje fibers. Relationship to potassium and cycle length. *Circ. Res.* 56: 857–867, 1985.

Roden, D.M., R.L. Woosley, and R.K. Primm. Incidence and clinical features of the quinidine-associated long QT syndrome: Implications for patient care. *Am. Heart J.* 111: 1088–1093, 1986.

Roelandt, J., P. Klootwijk, J. Lubsen, and M.J. Janse. Sudden death during longterm ambulatory monitoring. *Eur. Heart J.* 5: 7–20, 1984.

Rosen, M.R., H. Gelband, and B.F. Hoffman. Effects of blood perfusion on electrophysiological properties of isolated canine Purkinje fibers. *Circ. Res.* 30: 575–587, 1972.

Rosen, M.R., H. Gelband, and B.F. Hoffman. Correlation between effects of ouabain on the canine electrocardiogram and transmembrane potentials of isolated Purkinje fibers. *Circulation* 47: 65–72, 1973a.

Rosen, M.R., H. Gelband, C. Merker, and B.F. Hoffman. Mechanisms of digitalis toxicity. Effects of ouabain on phase four of canine Purkinje fiber transmembrane potentials. *Circulation* 47: 681–689, 1973b.

Rosen, M.R., and P. Danilo Jr. Effects of tetrodotoxin, lidocaine, verapamil, and AHR-2666 on ouabain-induced delayed afterdepolarizations in canine Purkinje fibers. *Circ. Res.* 46: 117–124, 1980.

Rosen, M.R., C. Fisch, B.F. Hoffman, P. Danilo Jr., D.E. Lovelace, and S.B. Knoebel. Can accelerated atrioventricular junctional escape rhythms be explained by delayed afterdepolarizations? *Am. J. Cardiol.* 45: 1272–1284, 1980.

Rosen, M.R., and R.F. Reder. Does triggered activity have a role in the genesis of cardiac arrhythmias? *Ann. Intern. Med.* 94: 794–801, 1981.

Rosen, M.R., P. Danilo Jr., and R.M. Weiss. Actions of adenosine on normal and abnormal impulse initiation in canine ventricle. *Am. J. Physiol.* 244: H715- H721, 1983.

Rosenfeld, J., M.R. Rosen, and B.F. Hoffman. Pharmacologic and behavioral effects on arrhythmias that immediately follow abrupt coronary occlusion: A canine model of sudden coronary death. *Am. J. Cardiol.* 41: 1075–1082, 1978.

Rosenthal, J.E. Contribution of depolarized foci with variable conduction impairment to arrhythmogenesis in 1 day old infarcted canine cardiac tissue: an in vitro study. *J. Am. Coll. Cardiol.* 8: 648–656, 1986.

Rosenthal, M.E., N.J. Stamato, J.M. Almendral, F.E. Marchlinski, A.E. Buxton, J.M. Miller, and M.E. Josephson. Influence of the site of stimulation on the resetting phenomenon in ventricular tachycardia. *Am. J. Cardiol.* 58: 970–976, 1986.

Rosenthal, M.E., N.J. Stamato, J.M. Almendral, C.D. Gottlieb, and M.E. Josephson. Resetting of ventricular tachycardia with electrocardiographic fusion: incidence and significance. *Circulation* 77: 581–588, 1988.

Rouet, R.H., M.M. Adamantidis, E. Honore, and B.A. Dupuis. *In vitro* abnormal repetitive responses in guinea-pig ventricular myocardium exposed to combined hypoxia, hyperkalemia and acidosis. *J. Appl. Cardiol.* 4: 19–29, 1989.

Roy, D., E. Marchand, P. Théroux, D.D. Waters, G.B. Pelletier, and M.G. Bourassa. Programmed ventricular stimulation in survivors of an acute myocardial infarction. *Circulation* 72: 487–494, 1985.

Roy, D., E. Marchand, P. Théroux, D.D. Waters, G.B. Pelletier, R. Cartier, and M.G. Bourassa. Long-term reproducibility and significance of provokable ventricular arrhythmias after myocardial infarction. *J. Am. Coll. Cardiol.* 8: 32–39, 1986.

Rozanski, G.J., S.L. Lipsius, and W.C. Randall. Functional characteristics of sinoatrial and subsidiary pacemaker activity in the canine right atrium. *Circulation* 67: 1378–1387, 1983.

Rozanski, G.J., J. Jalife, and G.K. Moe. Reflected reentry in nonhomogeneous ventricular muscle as a mechanism of cardiac arrhythmias. *Circulation* 69: 163–173, 1984a.

Rozanski, G.J., S.L. Lipsius, W.C. Randall, and S.B. Jones. Alterations in subsidiary pacemaker function after prolonged subsidiary pacemaker dominance in the canine right atrium. *J. Am. Coll. Cardiol.* 4: 535–542, 1984b.

Rozanski, G.J., and S.L. Lipsius. Electrophysiology of functional subsidiary pacemakers in canine right atrium. *Am. J. Physiol.* 249: H594-H603, 1985.

Rozanski, G.J., and J. Jalife. Automaticity in atrioventricular valve leaflets of rabbit heart. *Am. J. Physiol.* 250: H397–H406, 1986.

Rozanski, G.J. Electrophysiological properties of automatic fibers in rabbit atrioventricular valves. *Am. J. Physiol.* 253: H720-H727, 1987.

Rozanski, G.J., and R.C. Witt. Early afterdepolarizations and triggered activity in rabbit cardiac Purkinje fibers recovering from ischemic-like conditions. Role of acidosis. *Circulation* 83: 1352–1360, 1991.

Ruberman, W., E. Weinblatt, J.D. Goldberg, C.W. Frank, and S. Shapiro. Ventricular premature beats and mortality after myocardial infarction. *N. Engl. J. Med.* 297: 750–757, 1977.

Rubenstein, D.S., and S.L. Lipsius. Mechanisms of automaticity in subsidiary pacemakers from cat right atrium. *Circ. Res.* 64: 648–657, 1989.

Rudy, Y., and W. Quan. A model study of the effects of the discrete cellular structure on electrical propagation in cardiac tissue. *Circ. Res.* 61: 815–823, 1987.

Ruffy, R., D.E. Lovelace, T.M. Mueller, S.B. Knoebel, and D.P. Zipes. Relationship between changes in left ventricular bipolar electrograms and regional myocardial blood flow during acute coronary artery occlusion in the dog. *Circ. Res.* 45: 764–770, 1979.

Ruiz-Ceretti, E., P. Ragault, N. Leblanc, and A.Z. Ponce Zumino. Effects of hypoxia and altered K_o on the membrane potential of rabbit ventricle. *J. Mol. Cell. Cardiol.* 15: 845–854, 1983.

Ruskin, J.N., J.P. DiMarco, and H. Garan. Out-of-hospital cardiac arrest. Electrophysiologic observations and selection of long-term antiarrhythmic therapy. *N. Engl. J. Med.* 303: 607–613, 1980.

Russell, D.C., M.F. Oliver, and J. Wojtczak. Combined electrophysiological technique for assessment of the cellular basis of early ventricular arrhythmias. Experiments in dogs. *Lancet* 2: 686–688, 1977.

Russell, D.C., and M.F. Oliver. Ventricular refractoriness during acute myocardial ischaemia and its relationship to ventricular fibrillation. *Cardiovasc. Res.* 12: 221–227, 1978.

Russell, D.C., R.A. Riemersma, J.S. Lawrie, and M.F. Oliver. Patterns of flow and conduction during early ventricular arrhythmias following coronary arterial occlusion in the dog. *Cardiovasc. Res.* 16: 613–623, 1982.

Russell, D.C., J.S. Lawrie, R.A. Riemersma, and M.F. Oliver. Mechanisms of phase 1a and 1b early ventricular arrhythmias during acute myocardial ischemia in the dog. *Am. J. Cardiol.* 53: 307–312, 1984.

Saito, T., M. Otoguro, and T. Matsubara. Electrophysiological studies on the mechanism of electrically induced sustained rhythmic activity in the rabbit right atrium. *Circ. Res.* 42: 199–206, 1978.

Sakai, T., S. Ogawa, T. Miyazaki, M. Hosokawa, K. Sakurai, H. Yoshino, and Y. Nakamura. Electrophysiological effects of acute ischaemia on electrically stable myocardial infarction. *Cardiovasc. Res.* 23: 169–176, 1989a.

Sakai, T., S. Ogawa, M. Hosokawa, T. Miyazaki, K. Sakurai, and Y. Nakamura. Electrophysiological effects of flecainide in a canine 7 day old myocardial infarction model. *Cardiovasc. Res.* 23: 177–183, 1989b.

Sakmann, B., and G. Trube. Conductance properties of single inwardly rectifying potassium channels in ventricular cells from guinea-pig heart. *J. Physiol.* 347: 641–657, 1984.

Saltman, A.E., S.M. Dillon, P.C. Ursell, J. Coromilas, and A.L. Wit. Influence of anisotropic structure of the infarct epicardial border zone on conduction. (abstract) *Fed. Proc.* 46: 1438, 1987.

Saltman, A.E. Anisotropic conduction in the infarcted canine ventricle: conduction characteristics of stimulated and reentrant beats and the influence of the antiarrhythmic drug flecainide. (Doctoral Thesis) Columbia University, 1990.

Saltman, A.E., J. Coromilas, B. Waldecker, S.M. Dillon, and. A.L. Wit. Functional and anatomical reentrant circuits cause ventricular tachycardia in healing canine myocardial infarcts. *Circulation* 1993, (in press).

Samson, W.E., and A.M. Scher. Mechanism of S-T segment alteration during acute myocardial injury. *Circ. Res.* 8: 780–787, 1960.

Sano, T., N. Takayama, and T. Shimamoto. Directional difference of conduction velocity in the cardiac ventricular syncytium studied by microelectrodes. *Circ. Res.* 7: 262–267, 1959.

Sasyniuk, B.I., and C. Mendez. A mechanism for reentry in canine ventricular tissue. *Circ. Res.* 28: 3–15, 1971.

Sasyniuk, B.I. In vitro preparation of infarcted myocardium. *Environ. Health Perspect.* 26: 233–242, 1978.

Sato, R., A. Noma, Y. Kurachi, and H. Irisawa. Effects of intracellular acidification on membrane currents in ventricular cells of the guinea pig. *Circ. Res.* 57: 553–561, 1985.

Sawanobori, T., Y. Hirano, and M. Hiraoka. Aconitine-induced delayed afterdepolarization in frog atrium and guinea pig papillary muscles in the presence of low concentrations of Ca^{2+}. *Jpn. J. Physiol.* 37: 59–79, 1987.

Schaal, S.F., A.G. Wallace, and W.C. Sealy. Protective influence of cardiac denervation against arrhythmias of myocardial infarction. *Cardiovasc. Res.* 3: 241–244, 1969.

Schalij, M.J. Anisotropic conduction and ventricular tachycardia. (Doctoral Thesis) University of Limburg, Maastrict, The Netherlands, 1988.

Schaper, W. *The Collateral Circulation of the Heart.* Amsterdam, North-Holland Publishing Company: 1971.

Schaper, W., and S. Pasyk. Influence of collateral flow on the ischemic tolerance of the heart following acute and subacute coronary occlusion. *Circulation* 53(Suppl. I): I-57-I-62, 1976.

Schechter, E., C.C. Freeman, and R. Lazzara. Afterdepolarizations as a mechanism for the long QT syndrome: Electrophysiologic studies of a case. *J. Am. Coll. Cardiol.* 3: 1556–1561, 1984.

Scheinman, M.M., D. Basu, and M. Hollenberg. Electrophysiologic studies in patients with persistent atrial tachycardia. *Circulation* 50: 266–273, 1974.

Scher, A.M., and A.C. Young. The pathway of ventricular depolarization in the dog. *Circ. Res.* 4: 461–469, 1956.

Scherf, D. Untersuchungen über die Entstehungsweise der Extrasystolen und der extrasystolischen Allorhythmien. III. Mitteilung. Über den Einfluss der Herznerven auf die Extrareizbildung in der Kammer des mit Aconotin vorbehandelten Säugetierherzens. *Zeitschr. für die ges. exp. Medizin* 65: 198–221, 1929.

Scherf, D., L.J. Morgenbesser, E.J. Nightingale, and K.T. Schaeffeler. Mechanism of ventricular fibrillation. *Cardiologia* 16: 232–242, 1950.

Scherf, D., and A. Schott. *Extrasystoles and Allied Arrhythmias.* Heinemann Medical Books Publishers, Chicago: 1973.

Scherlag, B.J., R.H. Helfant, J.I. Haft, and A.N. Damato. Electrophysiology underlying ventricular arrhythmias due to coronary ligation. *Am. J. Physiol.* 219: 1665–1671, 1970.

Scherlag, B.J., N. El-Sherif, R.R. Hope, and R. Lazzara. Characterization and localization of ventricular arrhythmias resulting from myocardial ischemia and infarction. *Circ. Res.* 35: 372–383, 1974.

Scherlag, B.J., R.R. Hope, D.O. Williams, N. El-Sherif, and R. Lazzara. Mechanisms of ectopic rhythm formation due to myocardial ischemia: Effects of heart rate and ventricular premature beats. In: *The Conduction System of the Heart,* edited by H.J.J. Wellens, K.I. Lie, and M.J. Janse. Lea & Febiger, Philadelphia: 1976, pp. 633–649.

Scherlag, B.J., G. Kabell, J. Brachmann, L. Harrison, and R. Lazzara. Mechanisms of spontaneous and induced ventricular arrhythmias in the 24-hour infarcted dog heart. *Am. J. Cardiol.* 51: 207–213, 1983.

Scherlag, B.J., J. Brachmann, G. Kabell, L. Harrison, P. Guse, and R. Lazzara. Sustained ventricular tachycardia: Common functional properties of different anatomic substrates. In: *Cardiac Electrophysiology and Arrhythmias,* edited by D.P. Zipes, and J. Jalife. Grune and Stratton, Orlando: 1985, pp. 379–387.

Scherlag, B.J., E.S. Patterson, E.J. Berbari, and R. Lazzara. Experimental simulation of sudden cardiac death in humans: electrophysiological mechanisms and role of adrenergic influences. In: *Adrenergic System and Ventricular Arrhythmias in Myocardial Infarction*, edited by J. Brachmann and A. Schömig. Springer-Verlag, Berlin: 1989, pp. 299–312.

Schmidt, R.F. Versuche mit Aconitin zum Problem der spontanen Erregungsbildung im Herzen. *Pflügers Arch.* 271: 526–536, 1960.

Schmitt, F.O., and J. Erlanger. Directional differences in the conduction of the impulse through heart muscle and their possible relation to extrasystolic and fibrillary contractions. *Am. J. Physiol.* 87: 326–347, 1928.

Schneider, J.A., and N. Sperelakis. The demonstration of energy dependence of the isoproterenol-induced transcellular Ca^{2+} current in isolated perfused guinea-pig hearts—An explanation for mechanical failure of ischemic myocardium. *J. Surg. Res.* 16: 389–403, 1974.

Schömig, A., A.M. Dart, R. Dietz, E. Mayer, and W. Kübler. Release of endogenous catecholamines in the ischemic myocardium of the rat. Part A: Locally mediated release. *Circ. Res.* 55: 689–701, 1984.

Schoenfeld, M.H., B. McGovern, H. Garan, and J.N. Ruskin. Long-term reproducibility of responses to programmed cardiac stimulation in spontaneous ventricular tachyarrhythmias. *Am. J. Cardiol.* 54: 564–568, 1984.

Schütz, E. Elektrophysiologie des Herzens bei einphasischer Ableitung. *Ergebn. Physiol.* 38: 493–620, 1936.

Schulze, R.A., H.W. Strauss, and B. Pitt. Sudden death in the year following myocardial infarction. Relation to ventricular premature contractions in the late hospital phase and left ventricular ejection fraction. *Am. J. Med.* 62: 192–199, 1977.

Schwartz, P.J., and H.L. Stone. The role of the autonomic nervous system in sudden coronary death. In: *Sudden Coronary Death*, edited by H.M. Greenberg, and E.M. Dwyer Jr. New York Academy of Sciences, New York: *Ann. N.Y. Acad. Sci.* 382: 162–180, 1982.

Schwartz, P.J., and H.L. Stone. The analysis and modulation of autonomic reflexes in the prediction and prevention of sudden death. In: *Cardiac Electrophysiology and Arrhythmias*, edited by D.P. Zipes and J. Jalife. Grune & Stratton, Orlando: 1985, pp. 165–176.

Sclarovsky, S., B. Strasberg, G. Martonovich, and J. Agmon. Ventricular rhythms with intermediate rates in acute myocardial infarction. *Chest* 74: 180–182, 1978.

Sclarovsky, S., B. Strasberg, J. Fuchs, R.F. Lewin, A. Arditi, E. Klainman, O.H. Kracoff, and J. Agmon. Multiform accelerated idioventricular rhythm in acute myocardial infarction: electrocardiographic characteristics and response to verapamil. *Am. J. Cardiol.* 52: 43–47, 1983.

Sealy, W.C., R.J. Bache, A.V. Seaber, and S.K. Bhattacharga. The atrial pacemaking site after surgical exclusion of the sinoatrial node. *J. Thorac. Cardiovasc. Surg.* 65: 841–850, 1973.

Selzer, A., and H.W. Wray. Quinidine syncope. Paroxysmal ventricular fibrillation occurring during treatment of chronic atrial arrhythmias. *Circulation* 30: 17–26, 1964.

Senges, J., J. Brachmann, D. Pelzer, T. Mizutani, and W. Kübler. Effects of some components of ischemia on electrical activity and reentry in the canine ventricular conducting system. *Circ. Res.* 44: 864–872, 1979.

Sewell, W.H., D.R. Koth, and C.E. Huggins. Ventricular fibrillation in dogs after sudden return of flow to the coronary artery. *Surgery* 38: 1050–1053, 1955.

Shabab, L., A. Wollenberger, M. Haase, and U. Schiller. Noradrenalinabgabe aus dem Hundeherzen nach vorübergehender Okklusion einer Koronararterie. *Acta. Biol. Med. Germ.* 22: 135–143, 1969.

Shah, A.K., I.S. Cohen, and N.B. Datyner. Background K^+ current in isolated canine cardiac Purkinje myocytes. *Biophys. J.* 52: 519–525, 1987.

Shaikh, N.A., and E. Downar. Time course of changes in porcine myocardial phospholipid levels during ischemia. A reassessment of the lysolipid hypothesis. *Circ. Res.* 49: 316–325, 1981.

Sharma, A.D., J.E. Saffitz, B.I. Lee, B.E. Sobel, and P.B. Corr. Alpha adrenergic mediated accumulation of calcium in reperfused myocardium. *J. Clin. Invest.* 72: 802–818, 1983.

Sharma, B., R. Asinger, G.S. Francis, M. Hodges, and R.P. Wyeth. Demonstration of exercise-induced painless myocardial ischemia in survivors of out-of-hospital ventricular fibrillation. *Am. J. Cardiol.* 59: 740–745, 1987.

Shell, W.E., and B.E. Sobel. Deleterious effects of increased heart rate on infarct size in the conscious dog. *Am. J. Cardiol.* 31: 474–479, 1973.

Sheridan, D.J., P.A. Penkoske, B.E. Sobel, and P.B. Corr. Alpha adrenergic contributions to dysrhythmia during myocardial ischemia and reperfusion in cats. *J. Clin. Invest.* 65: 161–171, 1980.

Sheridan, D.J. Reperfusion-induced arrhythmias: An experimental observation awaiting clinical discovery? In: *Life-Threatening Arrhythmias During Ischemia and Infarction*, edited by D.J. Hearse, A.S. Manning, and M.J. Janse. Raven Press, New York: 1987, pp. 49–62.

Sheu, S.-S., M. Korth, D.A. Lathrop, and H.A. Fozzard. Intra- and extracellular K^+ and Na^+ activities and resting membrane potential in sheep cardiac Purkinje strands. *Circ. Res.* 47: 692–700, 1980.

Sheu, S.-S., and H.A. Fozzard. Transmembrane Na^+ and Ca^{2+} electrochemical gradients in cardiac muscle and their relationship to force development. *J. Gen. Physiol.* 80: 325–351, 1982.

Sheu, S.-S., and W.J. Lederer. Lidocaine's negative inotropic and antiarrhythmic actions. Dependence on shortening of action potential duration and reduction of intracellular sodium activity. *Circ. Res.* 57: 578–590, 1985.

Sheu, S.-S., and M.P. Blaustein. Sodium/calcium exchange and regulation of cell calcium and contractility in cardiac muscle, with a note about vascular smooth muscle. In: *The Heart and Cardiovascular System*, edited by H.A. Fozzard, E. Haber, R.B. Jennings, A.M. Katz, and H.E. Morgan. Raven Press, New York: 1986, pp. 509–535.

Sheu, S.-S., V.K. Sharma, and M. Korth. Voltage-dependent effects of isoproterenol on cytosolic Ca concentration in rat heart. *Am. J. Physiol.* 252: H697-H703, 1987.

Shibasaki, T. Conductance and kinetics of delayed rectifier potassium channels in nodal cells of the rabbit heart. *J. Physiol.* 387:227–250, 1987.

Shibata, N., P-S Chen, E.G. Dixon, P.D. Wolf, N.D. Danieley, W.M. Smith, and R.E. Ideker. Influence of shock strength and timing on induction of ventricular arrhythmias in dogs. *Am. J. Physiol.* 255: H891-H901, 1988.

Shiki, K. and D.J. Hearse. Preconditioning of ischemic myocardium: reperfusion-induced arrhythmias. *Am. J. Physiol.* 253: H1470-H1476, 1987.

Singer, D.H., C.M. Baumgarten, and R.E. Ten Eick. Cellular electrophysiology of ventricular and other dysrhythmias: studies on diseased and ischemic heart. *Prog. Cardiovasc. Dis.* 24: 97–156, 1981.

SippensGroenewegen, A. Body surface mapping of ventricular tachycardia. Electrocardiographic localization of the site of origin. (Doctoral Thesis) University of Amsterdam. Rodopi, Amsterdam, 1990.

SippensGroenewegen, A., H. Spekhorst, N.M. van Hemel, J.H. Kingma, R.N.W. Hauer, M.J. Janse, and A.J. Dunning. Body surface mapping of ectopic left and right ventricular activation. QRS spectrum in patients without structural heart disease. *Circulation* 82: 879–896, 1990.

Skelton, R.B., N. Gergely, G.W. Manning, and J.C. Coles. Mortality studies in experimental coronary occlusion. *J. Thorac. Cardiovasc. Surg.* 44: 90–96, 1962.

Skinner, J.E., J.T. Lie, and M.L. Entman. Modification of ventricular fibrillation latency following coronary artery occlusion in the conscious pig. The effects of psychological stress and beta-adrenergic blockade. *Circulation* 51: 656–667, 1975.

Skinner, J.E. How the head rules the heart. In: *Life-Threatening Arrhythmias During Ischemia and Infarction*, edited by D.J. Hearse, A.S. Manning, and M.J. Janse. Raven Press, New York: 1987, pp. 135–151.

Smeets, J.L.R.M., M.A. Allessie, W.J.E.P. Lammers, F.I.M. Bonke, and J. Hollen. The wavelength of the cardiac impulse and reentrant arrhythmias in isolated rabbit atrium. The role of heart rate, autonomic transmitters, temperature and potassium. *Circ. Res.* 58: 96–108, 1986.

Smith, F.M. The ligation of coronary arteries with electrocardiographic study. *Arch. Intern. Med.* 22: 8–27, 1918.

Smith, G.L., and D.G. Allen. Effects of metabolic blockade on intracellular calcium concentration in isolated ferret ventricular muscle. *Circ. Res.* 62: 1223–1236, 1988.

Smith, W.M., and J.J. Gallagher. "Les torsades de pointes": An unusual ventricular arrhythmia. *Ann. Intern. Med.* 93: 578–584, 1980.

Smith, W.M., R.E. Ideker, W.M. Smith, J. Kasell, L. Harrison, G.H. Bardy, J.J. Gallagher, and A.G. Wallace. Localization of septal pacing sites in the dog heart by epicardial mapping. *J. Am. Coll. Cardiol.* 1: 1423–1434, 1983.

Snellen, H.A. *History of Cardiology.* Donker Academic Publications, Rotterdam: 1984.

Sobel, B.E., P.B. Corr, A.K. Robison, R.A. Goldstein, F.X. Witkowski, and M.S.

Klein. Accumulation of lysophosphoglycerides with arrhythmogenic properties in ischemic myocardium. *J. Clin. Invest.* 62: 546–553, 1978.

Soeima M., and A. Noma. Mode of regulation of the ACh-sensitive K-channel by the muscarinic receptor in rabbit atrial cells. *Pflügers Arch.* 400: 424–431, 1984.

Sommer, J.R., and P.C. Dolber. Cardiac muscle: Ultrastructure of its cells and bundles. In: *Normal and Abnormal Conduction in the Heart*, edited by A. Paes de Carvalho, B.F. Hoffman, and M. Lieberman. Futura Publishing Company, Mt. Kisco, New York: 1982, pp. 1–27.

Spach, M.S., M. Lieberman, J.G. Scott, R.C. Barr, E.A. Johnson, and J.M. Kootsey. Excitation sequences of the atrial septum and the AV node in isolated hearts of the dog and rabbit. *Circ. Res.* 29: 156–172, 1971.

Spach, M.S., R.C. Barr, E.A. Johnson, and J.M. Kootsey. Cardiac extracellular potentials. Analysis of complex wave forms about the Purkinje networks in dogs. *Circ. Res.* 33: 465–473, 1973.

Spach, M.S., W.T. Miller, III, E. Miller-Jones, R.B. Warren, and R.C. Barr. Extracellular potentials related to intracellular action potentials during impulse conduction in anisotropic canine cardiac muscle. *Circ. Res.* 45: 188–204, 1979.

Spach, M.S., W.T. Miller, III, D.B. Geselowitz, R.C. Barr, J.M. Kootsey, and E.A. Johnson. The discontinuous nature of propagation in normal canine cardiac muscle. Evidence for recurrent discontinuities of intracellular resistance that affect the membrane currents. *Circ. Res.* 48: 39–54, 1981.

Spach, M.S., W.T. Miller, III, P.C. Dolber, J.M. Kootsey, J.R. Sommer, and C.E. Mosher Jr. The functional role of structural complexities in the propagation of depolarization in the atrium of the dog. Cardiac conduction disturbances due to discontinuities of effective axial resistivity. *Circ. Res.* 50: 175–191, 1982.

Spach, M.S., and P.C. Dolber. The relation between discontinuous propagation in anisotropic cardiac muscle and the "vulnerable period" of reentry. In: *Cardiac Electrophysiology and Arrhythmias*, edited by D.P. Zipes, and J. Jalife. Grune and Stratton, Orlando: 1985, pp. 241–252.

Spach, M.S., and P.C. Dolber. Relating extracellular potentials and their derivatives to anisotropic propagation at a microscopic level in human cardiac muscle. Evidence for electrical uncoupling of side-to-side fiber connections with increasing age. *Circ. Res.* 58: 356–371, 1986.

Spach, M.S., P.C. Dolber, J.F. Heidlage, J.M. Kootsey, and E.A. Johnson. Propagating depolarization in anisotropic human and canine cardiac muscle: Apparent directional differences in membrane capacitance. A simplified model for selective directional effects of modifying the sodium conductance on $\dot{V}_{max}$, τ_{foot}, and the propagation safety factor. *Circ. Res.* 60: 206–219, 1987.

Spach, M.S., P.C. Dolber, and J.F. Heidlage. Influence of the passive anisotropic properties on directional differences in propagation following modification of the sodium conductance in human atrial muscle. A model of reentry based on anisotropic discontinuous propagation. *Circ. Res.* 62: 811–832, 1988.

Spach, M.S., P.C. Dolber, and J.F. Heidlage. Interaction of inhomogeneities of repolarization with anisotropic propagation in dog atria. A mechanism for both preventing and initiating reentry. *Circ. Res.* 65: 1612–1631, 1989.

Spann, J.F. Jr., R.C. Moellering Jr., E. Haber, and E.O. Wheeler. Arrhythmias in acute myocardial infarction. A study utilizing an electrocardiographic monitor for automatic detection and recording of arrhythmias. *N. Engl. J. Med.* 271: 427–431, 1964.

Spear, J.F. and E.N. Moore. Influence of brief vagal and stellate nerve stimulation on pacemaker activity and conduction within the atrioventricular conduction system of the dog. *Circ. Res.* 32: 27–41, 1973.

Spear, J.F., E.L. Michelson, S.R. Spielman, and E.N. Moore. The origin of ventricular arrhythmias 24 hours following experimental anterior septal coronary artery occlusion. *Circulation* 55: 844–852, 1977.

Spear, J.F., L.N. Horowitz, A.B. Hodess, H. MacVaugh, III, and E.N. Moore. Cellular electrophysiology of human myocardial infarction. 1. Abnormalities of cellular activation. *Circulation* 59: 247–256, 1979.

Spear, J.F., E.L. Michelson, and E.N. Moore. The use of animal models in the study of the electrophysiology of sudden coronary death. In: *Sudden Coronary Death*, edited by H.M. Greenberg, and E.M. Dwyer Jr. New York Academy of Sciences, New York: *Ann. N.Y. Acad. Sci.* 382: 78–88, 1982.

Spear, J.F., and E.N. Moore. Mechanisms of cardiac arrhythmias. *Ann. Rev. Physiol.* 44: 485–497, 1982.

Spear, J.F., E.L. Michelson, and E.N. Moore. Cellular electrophysiologic characteristics of chronically infarcted myocardium in dogs susceptible to sustained ventricular tachyarrhythmias. *J. Am. Coll. Cardiol.* 1: 1099–1110, 1983a.

Spear, J.F., E.L. Michelson, and E.N. Moore. Reduced space constant in slowly conducting regions of chronically infarcted canine myocardium. *Circ. Res.* 53: 176–185, 1983b.

Spear, J.F., D.A. Richards, G.J. Blake, and E.N. Moore. Electrophysiologic factors associated with slow conduction in infarcted myocardium: The influence of myocardial fiber orientation. In: *Cardiac Electrophysiology and Arrhythmias*, edited by D.P. Zipes, and J. Jalife. Grune & Stratton, Orlando: 1985, pp. 337–342.

Spielman, S.R., E.L. Michelson, L.N. Horowitz, J.F. Spear, and E.N. Moore. The limitations of epicardial mapping as a guide to the surgical therapy of ventricular tachycardia. *Circulation* 57: 666–670, 1978.

Spinelli, W., B. Hoffman, and B.F. Hoffman. Antiarrhythmic drug action in the Harris dog model of ventricular tachycardia. *J. Cardiovasc. Electrophysiol.* 2: 21–33, 1991.

Spurrell R.A.J., E. Sowton, and D.C. Deuchar. Ventricular tachycardia in 4 patients evaluated by programmed electrical stimulation of heart and treated in 2 patients by surgical division of anterior radiation of left bundle-branch. *Br. Heart J.* 35: 1014–1025, 1973.

Stamato, N.J., M.E. Rosenthal, J.M. Almendral, and M.E. Josephson. The resetting response of ventricular tachycardia to single and double extrastimuli: implications for an excitable gap. *Am. J. Cardiol.* 60: 596–601, 1987.

Stanton, M.S., E.N. Prystowsky, N.S. Fineberg, W.M. Miles, D.P. Zipes, and J.J. Heger. Arrhythmogenic effects of antiarrhythmic drugs: a study of 506 patients treated for ventricular tachycardia or fibrillation. *J. Am. Coll. Cardiol.* 14: 209–215, 1989.

Steenbergen, C., E. Murphy, L. Levy, and R.E. London. Elevation in cytostolic free calcium concentration early in myocardial ischemia in perfused rat heart. *Circ. Res.* 60: 700–707, 1987.

Steenbergen, C., E. Murphy, J.A. Watts, and R.E. London. Correlation between cytosolic free calcium, contracture, ATP, and irreversible ischemic injury in perfused rat heart. *Circ. Res.* 66: 135–146, 1990.

Stephenson, S.E. Jr., R.K. Cole, T.F. Parrish, F.M. Bauer Jr., I.T. Johnson Jr., M. Kochtitzky, J.S. Anderson Jr., L.L. Hibbitt, J.E. McCarty, E.R. Young, J.R. Wilson, H.N. Meiers, C.K. Meador, C.O.T. Ball, and G.R. Meneely. Ventricular fibrillation during and after coronary artery occlusion. Incidence and protection afforded by various drugs. *Am. J. Cardiol.* 5: 77–87, 1960.

Stern, M.D., H.F. Weisman, D.G. Renlund, G. Gerstenblith, O. Hano, P.S. Blank, and E.G. Lakatta. Laser backscatter studies of intracellular Ca^{2+} oscillations in isolated hearts. *Am. J. Physiol.* 257: H665-H673, 1989.

Stevenson, W.G., P. Brugada, I. Kersschot, B. Waldecker, M. Zehender, A. Geibel and H.J.J. Wellens. Electrophysiologic characteristics of ventricular tachycardia or fibrillation in relation to age of myocardial infarction. *Am. J. Cardiol.* 57:387–391, 1986.

Stevenson, W.G., J.N. Weiss, I. Wiener, D. Wohlgelernter, L. Yeatman. Localization of slow conduction in a ventricular tachycardia circuit: implications for catheter ablation. *Am. Heart J.* 114: 1253–1258, 1987.

Stevenson, W.G., J.N. Weiss, I. Wiener, K. Nademanee, D. Wohlgelernter, L. Yeatman, M. Josephson, and T. Klitzner. Resetting of ventricular tachycardia: Implications for localizing the area of slow conduction. *J. Am. Coll. Cardiol.* 11: 522–529, 1988.

Stevenson, W.G., J.N. Weiss, I. Wiener, S.M. Rivitz, K. Nademanee, T. Klitzner, L. Yeatman, M. Josephson, and D. Wohlgelernter. Fractionated endocardial electrograms are associated with slow conduction in humans: Evidence from pace-mapping. *J. Am. Coll. Cardiol.* 13: 369–376, 1989a.

Stevenson, W.G., K. Nademanee, J.N. Weiss, I. Wiener, K. Baron, L.A. Yeatman, and C.T. Sherman. Programmed electrical stimulation at potential ventricular reentry circuit sites. Comparison of observations in humans with predictions from computer simulations. *Circulation* 80: 793–806, 1989b.

Strange, R.C., M.J. Rowe, and M.F. Oliver. Lack of relation between venous plasma total catecholamine concentrations and ventricular arrhythmias after acute myocardial infarction. *Br. Med. J.* 2: 921–922, 1978.

Stratmann, H.G., K.E. Walter, and H.L. Kennedy. Torsade de pointes associated with elevated N-acetylprocainamide levels. *Am. Heart J.* 109: 375–377, 1985.

Strauss, H.C., J.T. Bigger Jr., and B.F. Hoffman. Electrophysiological and beta-receptor blocking effects of MJ 1999 on dog and rabbit cardiac tissue. *Circ. Res.* 26: 661–678, 1970.

Strauss, H.C., and J.T. Bigger Jr. Electrophysiological properties of the rabbit sinoatrial perinodal fibers. *Circ. Res.* 31: 490–506, 1972.

Strauss, H.C., A.L. Saroff, J.T. Bigger Jr., and E.G.V. Giardina. Premature atrial stimulation as a key to the understanding of sinoatrial conduction in man. Presentation of data and critical review of the literature. *Circulation* 47: 86–93, 1973.

Strauss, H.C., R. Yee, J.A. Hill Jr., and T.L. Wenger. Mechanisms of reperfusion arrhythmias. In: *Lethal Arrhythmias Resulting from Myocardial Ischemia and Infarction*, edited by M.R. Rosen, and Y. Palti. Kluwer Academic Publishers, Boston: 1989, pp. 55–73.

Suenson, M. Interaction between ventricular cells during the early part of excitation in the ferret heart. *Acta Physiologica Scandinavica* 125: 81–90, 1985.

Sugarman, H., L.N. Katz, A. Sanders, and K. Jochim. Observations on the genesis of the electrical currents established by injury to the heart. *Am. J. Physiol.* 130: 130–143, 1940.

Sugi, K., H.S. Karagueuzian, M.C. Fishbein, A. McCullen, Y. Sato, W. Ganz, W.J. Mandel, and T. Peter. Spontaneous ventricular tachycardia associated with isolated right ventricular infarction, one day after right coronary artery occlusion in the dog: Studies on the site of origin and mechanism. *Am. Heart J.* 109: 232–244, 1985.

Summitt, J., S. Rosenheck, W.H. Kou, S. Schmaltz, A.H. Kadish, and F. Morady. Effect of basic drive cycle length on the yield of ventricular tachycardia during programmed ventricular stimulation. *Am. J. Cardiol.* 65: 49–52, 1990.

Sung, R.J., E.N. Shen, F. Morady, M.M. Scheinman, D.Hess, and E.H. Botvinick. Electrophysiologic mechanism of exercise-induced sustained ventricular tachycardia. *Am. J. Cardiol.* 51: 525–530, 1983.

Sutko, J.L., and J.L. Kenyon. Ryanodine modification of cardiac muscle responses to potassium-free solutions. Evidence for inhibition of sarcoplasmic reticulum calcium release. *J. Gen. Physiol.* 82: 385–404, 1983.

Svenson, R.H., L. Littmann, J.J. Gallagher, J.G. Selle, S.H. Zimmern, J.M. Fedor, and P.G. Colavita. Termination of ventricular tachycardia with epicardial laser photocoagulation: a clinical comparison with patients undergoing successful endocardial photocoagulation alone. *J. Am. Coll. Cardiol.* 15: 163–170, 1990.

Sweeney, R.J., R.M. Gill, M.I. Steinberg, and P.R. Reid. Ventricular refractory period extension caused by defibrillation shocks. *Circulation* 82: 965–972, 1990.

Taggart, P., P.M.I. Sutton, D.W. Spear, H.F. Drake, R.H. Swanton, and R.W. Emanuel. Simultaneous endocardial and epicardial monophasic action potential recordings during brief periods of coronary artery ligation in the dog: influence of adrenaline, beta blockade and alpha blockade. *Cardiovasc. Res.* 22: 900–909, 1988.

Tajima, T., and Y. Dohi. Histamine induced or enhanced delayed afterdepolarization and triggered activity in guinea-pig papillary muscles. A preliminary study. *Jpn. Heart J.* 26: 985–992, 1985.

Tchou, P., M. Jazayeri, S. Denker, J. Dongas, J. Caceres, and M. Akhtar. Transcatheter electrical ablation of the right bundle branch. A method of treating macroreentrant ventricular tachycardia attributed to bundle branch reentry. *Circulation* 78: 246–257, 1988.

Temte, J.V., and L.D. Davis. Effect of calcium concentration on the transmembrane potentials of Purkinje fibers. *Circ. Res.* 20: 32–44, 1967.

Ten Eick, R.E., D.H. Singer, and L.E. Solberg. Coronary occlusion. Effect on cellular electrical activity of the heart. *Med. Clin. North Am.* 60: 49–67, 1976.

Ten Eick, R.E., and D.H. Singer. Electrophysiological properties of diseased human atrium. I. Low diastolic potential and altered cellular response to potassium. *Circ. Res.* 44: 545–557, 1979.

Tennant, R., and C.J. Wiggers. The effect of coronary occlusion on myocardial contraction. *Am. J. Physiol.* 112: 351–361, 1935.

Théroux, P., D.D. Waters, C. Halphen, J.-C. Debaisieux, and H.F. Mizgala. Prognostic value of exercise testing soon after myocardial infarction. *N. Engl. J. Med.* 301: 341–345, 1979.

Thind, G.S., W.S. Blakemore, and H.F. Zinsser. Ventricular aneurysmectomy for the treatment of recurrent ventricular tachyarrhythmia. *Am. J. Cardiol.* 27: 690–694, 1971.

Thompson, P.L., and B. Lown. Sequential R/T pacing to expose electrical instability in the ischemic ventricle. (abstract) *Clin. Res.* 20: 401, 1972.

Toda, N., and T.C. West. Changes in sino-atrial node transmembrane potentials on vagal stimulation of the isolated rabbit atrium. *Nature* 205: 808–809, 1965.

Tosaki, A., M. Koltai, and P. Braquet. Effects of low extracellular sodium concentration on reperfusion induced arrhythmias: changes in the myocardial sodium, potassium and calcium contents in isolated guinea pig hearts. *Cardiovasc. Res.* 23: 993–1000, 1989.

Tranum-Jensen, J., M.J. Janse, J.W.T. Fiolet, W.J.G. Krieger, C. Naumann d'Alnoncourt, and D. Durrer. Tissue osmolality, cell swelling, and reperfusion in acute regional myocardial ischemia in the isolated porcine heart. *Circ. Res.* 49: 364–381, 1981.

Trautwein, W., U. Gottstein, and J. Dudel. Der Aktionsstrom der Myocardfaser im Sauerstoffmangel. *Pflügers Arch.* 260: 40–60, 1954.

Trautwein, W., and R.F. Schmidt. Zur Membranwirkung des Adrenalins an der Herzmuskelfaser. *Pflügers Arch.* 271: 715–726, 1960.

Trautwein, W. Mechanisms of tachyarrhythmias and extrasystoles. In: *Symposium on Cardiac Arrhythmias*, edited by E. Sandøe, E. Flensted-Jensen, and K.H. Olesen. AB Astra, Södertälje, Sweden: 1970, pp. 53–66.

Trautwein, W. Effects of acetylcholine on the S-A node of the heart. In: *Cellular Pacemakers. Vol. 1. Mechanisms of Pacemaker Generation*, edited by D.O. Carpenter. John Wiley and Sons, New York: 1982, pp. 127–160.

Tseng, G.-N., and A.L. Wit. Studies on the intracellular Ca sources for aftercontractions and delayed afterdepolarizations; a comparison with Ca sources for twitches. (abstract) *Biophys. J.* 47: 459a, 1985.

Tseng, G.-N., and A.L. Wit. Characteristics of a transient inward current that causes delayed afterdepolarizations in atrial cells of the canine coronary sinus. *J. Mol. Cell. Cardiol.* 19: 1105–1119, 1987a.

Tseng, G.-N., and A.L. Wit. Effects of reducing $[Na^+]_o$ on catecholamine-induced delayed afterdepolarizations in atrial cells. *Am. J. Physiol.* 253: H115-H125, 1987b.

Tsien, R.W. Effects of epinephrine on the pacemaker potassium current of cardiac Purkinje fibers. *J. Gen. Physiol.* 64: 293–319, 1974.

Tsien, R.W. Calcium channels in excitable cell membranes. *Annu. Rev. Physiol.* 45: 341–358, 1983.

Tsuboi, N., I. Kodama, J. Toyama, and K. Yamada. Anisotropic conduction properties of canine ventricular muscles. Influence of high extracellular K^+ concentration and stimulation frequency. *Jpn. Circ. J.* 49: 487–498, 1985.

Tsuchida, T. Experimental studies of the excitability of ventricular musculature in infarcted region. *Jpn. Heart J.* 6: 152–164, 1965.

Tzivoni, D., A. Keren, H. Granot, S. Gottlieb, J. Benhorin, and S. Stern. Ventricular fibrillation caused by myocardial reperfusion in Prinzmetal's angina. *Am. Heart J.* 105: 323–325, 1983.

Tzivoni, D., A. Keren, A.M. Cohen, H. Loebel, I. Zahavi, A. Chenzbraun, and S. Stern. Magnesium therapy for torsades de pointes. *Am. J. Cardiol.* 53: 528–530, 1984.

Uemura, N., D.R. Knight, Y.-T. Shen, J. Nejima, M.V. Cohen, J.X. Thomas Jr., and S.F. Vatner. Increased myocardial infarct size because of reduced coronary collateral blood flow in beagles. *Am. J. Physiol.* 257: H1798-H1803, 1989.

Ursell, P.C., P.I. Gardner, A. Albala, J.J. Fenoglio Jr., and A.L. Wit. Structural and electrophysiological changes in the epicardial border zone of canine myocardial infarcts during infarct healing. *Circ. Res.* 56: 436–451, 1985.

Valenzuela, F., and M. Vassalle. Interaction between overdrive excitation and overdrive suppression in canine Purkinje fibres. *Cardiovasc. Res.* 17: 608–619, 1983.

Valenzuela, F., and M. Vassalle. Overdrive excitation and cellular calcium load in canine cardiac Purkinje fibers. *J. Electrocardiol.* 18: 21–33, 1985.

Van Bogaert, P-P., J.S. Vereecke, and E.E. Carmeliet. The effect of raised pH on pacemaker activity and ionic currents in cardiac Purkinje fibers. *Pflügers Arch.* 375: 45–52, 1978.

Van Capelle, F.J.L., and M.J. Janse. Influence of geometry on the shape of the propagated action potential. In: *The Conduction System of the Heart*, edited by H.J.J. Wellens, K.I. Lie, and M.J. Janse. Lea & Febiger, Philadelphia: 1976, pp. 316–335.

Van Capelle, F.J.L., and D. Durrer. Computer simulation of arrhythmias in a network of coupled excitable elements. *Circ. Res.* 47: 454–466, 1980.

Van Capelle, F.J.L. Slow conduction and cardiac arrhythmias. (Doctoral Thesis) University of Amsterdam. The Netherlands, 1983.

Van Capelle, F.J.L, and M.A. Allessie. Computer simulation of anisotropic propagation: characteristics of action potentials during re-entrant arrhythmias. In: *Cell to Cell Signalling. From Experiments to Theoretical Models*, edited by A. Goldbeter. Academic Press Ltd., Harcourt Brace Jovanovich Publishing, London: 1989, pp. 577–588.

Van Dam, R.Th., D. Durrer, J. Strackee, and L.H. van der Tweel. The excitability cycle of the dog's left ventricle determined by anodal, cathodal and bipolar stimulation. *Circ. Res.* 4: 196–204, 1956.

Van Dam, R.Th. Experimenteel onderzoek naar het prikkelbaarheidsverloop van de hartspier. (Doctoral Thesis) University of Amsterdam. The Netherlands, 1960.

Van Durme, J.-P., and R.H. Pannier. Prognostic significance of ventricular dysrhythmias 1 year after myocardial infarction. (abstract) *Am. J. Cardiol.* 37: 178, 1976.

Vandepol, C.J., A. Farshidi, S.R. Spielman, A.M. Greenspan, L.N. Horowitz, and M.E. Josephson. Incidence and clinical significance of induced ventricular tachycardia. *Am. J. Cardiol.* 45: 725–731,1980.

Van der Vusse, G.J., T. Arts, J.F.C. Glatz, and R.S. Reneman. Transmural differences in energy metabolism of the left ventricular myocardium: fact or fiction. *J. Mol. Cell. Cardiol.* 22: 23–37, 1990.

Vanheel, B., and A. de Hemptinne. Intracellular pH in depolarized cardiac Purkinje strands. *Pflügers Arch.* 405: 118–126, 1985.

Vassalle, M. Cardiac pacemaker potentials at different extra- and intracellular K concentrations. *Am. J. Physiol.* 208: 770–775, 1965.

Vassalle, M., D.L. Caress, A.J. Slovin, and J.H. Stuckey. On the cause of ventricular asystole during vagal stimulation. *Circ. Res.* 20: 228–241, 1967.

Vassalle, M., M.J. Levine, and J.H. Stuckey. On the sympathetic control of ventricular automaticity. The effects of stellate ganglion stimulation. *Circ. Res.* 23: 249–258, 1968.

Vassalle, M. Electrogenic suppression of automaticity in sheep and dog Purkinje fibers. *Circ. Res.* 27: 361–377, 1970.

Vassalle, M., and R. Carpentier. Overdrive excitation: onset of activity following fast drive in cardiac Purkinje fibers exposed to norepinephrine. *Pflügers Arch.* 332: 198–205, 1972.

Vassalle, M., M. Cummins, C. Castro, and J.H. Stuckey. The relationship between overdrive suppression and overdrive excitation in ventricular pacemakers in dogs. *Circ. Res.* 38: 367–374, 1976.

Vassalle, M. The relationship among cardiac pacemakers. Overdrive suppression. *Circ. Res.* 41: 269–277, 1977.

Vassalle, M., and A. Mugelli. An oscillatory current in sheep cardiac Purkinje fibers. *Circ. Res.* 48: 618–631, 1981.

Vassallo, J.A., D.M. Cassidy, F.E. Marchlinski, J.M. Miller, A.E. Buxton, and M.E. Josephson. Abnormalities of endocardial activation pattern in patients with previous healed myocardial infarction and ventricular tachycardia. *Am. J. Cardiol.* 58: 479–484, 1986.

Vassallo, J.A., D.M. Cassidy, K.E. Kindwall, F.E. Marchlinski, and M.E. Josephson. Nonuniform recovery of excitability in the left ventricle. *Circulation* 78: 1365–1372, 1988.

Velebit, V., P. Podrid, B. Lown, B.H. Cohen, and T.B. Graboys. Aggravation and provocation of ventricular arrhythmias by antiarrhythmic drugs. *Circulation* 65: 886–894, 1982.

Veltri, E.P., E.V. Platia, L.S.C. Griffith, and P.R. Reid. Programmed electrical stimulation and long-term follow-up in asymptomatic, nonsustained ventricular tachycardia. *Am. J. Cardiol.* 56: 309–314, 1985.

Verrier, R.L., and B. Lown. Influence of neural activity on ventricular electrical stability during acute myocardial ischemia and infarction. In: *Management of Ventricular Tachycardia—Role of Mexiletine*, edited by E. Sandøe, D.G. Julian, and J.W. Bell. Excerpta Medica, Amsterdam: 1978, pp. 133–150.

Verrier, R.L., E.L. Hagestad, and B. Lown. Delayed myocardial ischemia induced by anger. *Circulation* 75: 249–254, 1987.

Vismara, L.A., E.A. Amsterdam, and D.T. Mason. Relation of ventricular arrhythmias in the late hospital phase of acute myocardial infarction to sudden death after hospital discharge. *Am. J. Med.* 59: 6–12, 1975.

Vleugels, A., J. Vereecke, and E. Carmeliet. Ionic currents during hypoxia in voltage-clamped cat ventricular muscle. *Circ. Res.* 47: 501–508, 1980.

Vogel, W.M., V.G. Zannoni, G.D. Abrams, and B.R. Lucchesi. Inability of methylprednisolone sodium succinate to decrease infarct size or preserve enzyme activity measured 24 hours after coronary occlusion in the dog. *Circulation* 55: 588–595, 1977.

Vos, M.A., A.P.M. Gorgels, J.D.M. Leunissen-Beekman, P. Brugada, and H.J.J. Wellens. The effect of an entrainment protocol on ouabain-induced ventricular tachycardia. *PACE* 12: 1485–1493, 1989.

Vos, M.A., A.P.M. Gorgels, J.D.M. Leunissen, and H.J.J. Wellens. Flunarizine allows differentiation between mechanisms of arrhythmias in the intact heart. *Circulation* 81: 343–349, 1990.

Wald, R.W., and M.B. Waxman. Pacing-induced automaticity in sheep Purkinje fibers. *Circ. Res.* 48: 531–538, 1981.

Waldecker, B., A.E. Saltman, J. Coromilas, S.M. Dillon, and A.L. Wit. Mechanisms for entrainment of functional reentrant circuits in the infarcted canine heart. *Circulation* 1993, (in press).

Waldo, A.L., and G.A. Kaiser. A study of ventricular arrhythmias associated with acute myocardial infarction in the canine heart. *Circulation* 47: 1222-1228, 1973.

Waldo, A.L., V.J. Plumb, J.G. Arciniegas, W.A.H. MacLean, T.B. Cooper, M.F.

Priest, and T.N. James. Transient entrainment and interruption of the atrioventricular bypass pathway type of paroxysmal atrial tachycardia. A model for understanding and identifying reentrant arrhythmias. *Circulation* 67: 73–83, 1983.

Waldo, A.L., R.W. Henthorn, V.J. Plumb, and W.A.H. MacLean. Demonstration of the mechanism of transient entrainment and interruption of ventricular tachycardia with rapid atrial pacing. *J. Am. Coll. Cardiol.* 3: 422–430, 1984.

Waldo, A.L., B. Olshansky, K. Okumura, and R.W. Henthorn. Current perspective on entrainment of tachyarrhythmias. In: *Cardiac Arrhythmias: Where To Go From Here?*, edited by P. Brugada, and H.J.J. Wellens. Futura Publishing Company, Mt. Kisco, New York: 1987, pp. 171–189.

Walker, M.J.A., M.J. Curtis, D.J. Hearse, R.W.F. Campbell, M.J. Janse, D.M. Yellon, S.M. Cobbe, S.J. Coker, J.B. Harness, D.W.G. Harron, A.J. Higgins, D.G. Julian, M.J. Lab, A.S. Manning, B.J. Northover, J.R. Parratt, R.A. Riemersma, E. Riva, D.C. Russell, D.J. Sheridan, E. Winslow, and B. Woodward. The Lambeth Conventions: guidelines for the study of arrhythmias in ischaemia, infarction, and reperfusion. *Cardiovasc. Res.* 22: 447–455, 1988.

Wallace, A.G., and R.J. Mignone. Physiologic evidence concerning the reentry hypothesis for ectopic beats. *Am. Heart J.* 72: 60–70, 1966.

Wallick, D.W., M.N. Levy, D.S. Felder, and H. Zieske. Effects of repetitive bursts of vagal activity on atrioventricular junctional rate in dogs. *Am. J. Physiol.* 237: H275–H281, 1979.

Waspe, L.E., R. Brodman, S.G. Kim, J.A. Matos, D.R. Johnston, G.M. Scavin, and J.D. Fisher. Activation mapping in patients with coronary artery disease with multiple ventricular tachycardia configurations: occurrence and therapeutic implications of widely separate apparent sites of origin. *J. Am. Coll. Cardiol.* 5: 1075–1086, 1985a.

Waspe, L.E., D. Seinfeld, A. Ferrick, S.G. Kim, J.A. Matos, and J.D. Fisher. Prediction of sudden death and spontaneous ventricular tachycardia in survivors of complicated myocardial infarction: value of the response to programmed stimulation using a maximum of three ventricular extrastimuli. *J. Am. Coll. Cardiol.* 5: 1292–1301, 1985b.

Wasserstrom, J.A., and G.R. Ferrier. Voltage dependence of digitalis afterpotentials, aftercontractions, and inotropy. *Am. J. Physiol.* 241: H646–H653, 1981.

Weaver, W.D., G.S. Lorch, H.A. Alvarez, and L.A. Cobb. Angiographic findings and prognostic indicators in patients resuscitated from sudden cardiac death. *Circulation* 54: 895–900, 1976.

Webb, S.W., A.A.J. Adgey, and J.F. Pantridge. Autonomic disturbance at onset of acute myocardial infarction. *Br. Med. J.* 3: 89–92, 1972.

Webb, W.R., and S.E. Field Jr. Effect of anesthetization of A-V node on ventricular fibrillation following acute coronary arterial occlusion. *Am. J. Physiol.* 195: 403–406, 1958.

Weidmann, S. The effect of the cardiac membrane potential on the rapid availability of the sodium-carrying system. *J. Physiol.* 127: 213–224, 1955.

Weidmann, S. *Elektrophysiologie Der Herzmuskelfaser.* Medizinischer Verlag Hans Huber, Bern Und Stuttgart, 1956.

Weingart, R. The actions of ouabain on intercellular coupling and conduction velocity in mammalian ventricular muscle. *J. Physiol.* 264: 341–365, 1977.

Weiss, J., and K.I. Shine. Extracellular potassium accumulation during myocardial ischemia: Implications for arrhythmogenesis. *J. Mol. Cell. Cardiol.* 13: 699–704, 1981.

Weiss, J., and K.I. Shine. Extracellular K^+ accumulation during myocardial ischemia in isolated rabbit heart. *Am. J. Physiol.* 242: H619-H628, 1982a.

Weiss, J., and K.I. Shine. $[K^+]_o$ accumulation and electrophysiological alterations during early myocardial ischemia. *Am. J. Physiol.* 243: H318-H327, 1982b.

Weiss, J., and K.I. Shine. Effects of heart rate on extracellular $[K^+]$ accumulation during myocardial ischemia. *Am. J. Physiol.* 250: H982-H991, 1986.

Weiss, J.N., S.T. Lamp, and K.I. Shine. Cellular K^+ loss and anion efflux during myocardial ischemia and metabolic inhibition. *Am. J. Physiol.* 256: H1165-H1175, 1989.

Weisse, A.B., K. Kearney, R.M. Narang, and T.J. Regan. Comparison of the coronary collateral circulation in dogs and baboons after coronary occlusion. *Am. Heart J.* 92: 193–200, 1976.

Weld, F.M., K-L. Chu, J.T. Bigger Jr., and L.M. Rolnitzky. Risk stratification with low-level exercise testing 2 weeks after acute myocardial infarction. *Circulation* 64: 306–314, 1981.

Wellens, H.J.J. Electrical stimulation of the heart in the study and treatment of tachycardias. (Doctoral Thesis) University of Amsterdam, The Netherlands. H.E. Stenfert Kroese N.V., Leiden: 1971.

Wellens, H.J.J., R.M. Schuilenberg, and D. Durrer. Electrical stimulation of the heart in patients with Wolff-Parkinson-White syndrome, type A. *Circulation* 43: 99–114, 1971.

Wellens, H.J.J., R.M. Schuilenburg, and D. Durrer. Electrical stimulation of the heart in patients with ventricular tachycardia. *Circulation* 46: 216–226, 1972.

Wellens, H.J.J., K.I. Lie, and D. Durrer. Further observations on ventricular tachycardia as studied by electrical stimulation of the heart. Chronic recurrent ventricular tachycardia and ventricular tachycardia during acute myocardial infarction. *Circulation* 49: 647–653, 1974.

Wellens, H.J.J., and D. Durrer. The role of an accessory atrioventricular pathway in reciprocal tachycardia. Observations in patients with and without the Wolff-Parkinson-White syndrome. *Circulation* 52: 58–72, 1975.

Wellens, H.J.J., D.R. Düren, and K.I. Lie. Observations on mechanisms of ventricular tachycardia in man. *Circulation* 54: 237–244, 1976.

Wellens, H.J.J. Value and limitations of programmed electrical stimulation of the heart in the study and treatment of tachycardias. *Circulation* 57: 845–853, 1978.

Wellens, H.J.J., P. Brugada, C. de Zwaan, P. Bendermacher, and F.W. Bär. Clinical characteristics, prognostic significance, and treatment of sustained ventricular tachycardia following acute myocardial infarction. In: *The First Year After a Myocardial Infarction*, edited by H.E. Kulbertus, and H.J.J. Wellens. Futura Publishing Company, Mt. Kisco, New York: 1983, pp. 227–237.

Wellens, H.J.J., and P. Brugada. Value of programmed stimulation of the heart in patients with the Wolff-Parkinson-White syndrome. In: *Tachycardias: Mechanisms, Diagnosis, Treatment*, edited by M.E. Josephson, and H.J.J. Wellens. Lea & Febiger, Philadelphia: 1984, pp. 199–221.

Wenckebach, K.F. Arrhythmias of the heart (translated by Thos. Snowball). Edinburgh, London: 1904.

Wenger, T.L., F.E. Harrell Jr., K.K. Brown, S. Lederman, and H.C. Strauss. Ventricular fibrillation following canine coronary artery reperfusion: different outcomes with pentobarbital and α-chloralose. *Can. J. Physiol. Pharmacol.* 62: 224–228, 1984.

Wennemark, J.R., V.J. Ruesta, and D.A. Brody. Microelectrode study of delayed conduction in the canine right bundle branch. *Circ. Res.* 23: 753–769, 1968.

West, T.C. Ultramicroelectrode recording from the cardiac pacemaker. *J. Pharmacol. Exp. Ther.* 115: 283–290, 1955.

Wetstein, L., E.L. Michelson, M.B. Simson, E.N. Moore, and A.H. Harken. Initiation of ventricular tachyarrhythmia with programmed stimulation: sensitivity and specificity in an experimental canine model. *Surgery* 92: 206–211, 1982.

Wetstein, L., E.L. Michelson, E.N. Moore, and A.H. Harken. Evaluation of arrhythmogenicity of surgically induced endocardial versus ischemic myocardial damage. *J. Thorac. Cardiovasc. Surg.* 87: 571–576, 1984.

Wetstein, L., R. Mark, G.J. Kelliher, T. Friehling, K.M. O'Connor, and P.R. Kowey. Arrhythmia inducibility and ventricular vulnerability in a chronic feline infarction model. *Am. Heart J.* 110: 955–960, 1985a.

Wetstein, L., R. Mark, E. Kaplinsky, H. Mitamura, A. Kaplan, C. Sauermelch, and E.L. Michelson. Histopathologic factors conducive to experimental ventricular tachycardia. *Surgery* 98: 532–538, 1985b.

Wiegand, V., M. Güggi, W. Meesmann, M. Kessler, and F. Greitschus. Extracellular potassium activity changes in the canine myocardium after acute coronary occlusion and the influence of beta-blockade. *Cardiovasc. Res.* 13: 297–302, 1979.

Wieland, J.M., and F.E. Marchlinski. Electrocardiographic response of digoxin-toxic fascicular tachycardia to Fab fragments: Implications for tachycardia mechanism. *PACE* 9: 727–738, 1986.

Wiener, I., B. Mindich, and R. Pitchon. Determinants of ventricular tachycardia in patients with ventricular aneurysms: Results of intraoperative epicardial and endocardial mapping. *Circulation* 65: 856–861, 1982.

Wiener, I., B. Mindich, and R. Pitchon. Fragmented endocardial electrical activity in patients with ventricular tachycardia: a new guide to surgical therapy. *Am. Heart J.* 107: 86–90, 1984.

Wiggers, C.J., and R. Wégria. Ventricular fibrillation due to single, localized induction and condenser shocks applied during the vulnerable phase of ventricular systole. *Am. J. Physiol.* 128: 500–505, 1940.

Wiggers, C.J., R. Wégria, and B. Piñera. The effects of myocardial ischemia on the fibrillation threshold—The mechanism of spontaneous ventricular fibrillation following coronary occlusion. *Am. J. Physiol.* 131: 309–316, 1940.

Wiggers, C.J. The functional importance of coronary collaterals. *Circulation* 5: 609–615, 1952.

Wilber, D.J., J.J. Lynch, D. Montgomery, and B.R. Lucchesi. Postinfarction sudden death: Significance of inducible ventricular tachycardia and infarct size in a conscious canine model. *Am. Heart J.* 109: 8–18, 1985.

Wilber, D.J., B. Olshansky, J.F. Moran, and P.J. Scanlon. Electrophysiological testing and nonsustained ventricular tachycardia. Use and limitations in patients with coronary artery disease and impaired ventricular function. *Circulation* 82: 350–358, 1990.

Wilde, A.A.M., and A.G. Kléber. The combined effects of hypoxia, high K^+, and acidosis on the intracellular sodium activity and resting potential in guinea pig papillary muscle. *Circ. Res.* 58: 249–256, 1986.

Wilde, A.A.M. Myocardial ischemia and hypoxia. Cellular ionic and electrical activity. (Doctoral Thesis) University of Amsterdam. Rodopi, Amsterdam, 1988.

Wilde, A.A.M., R.J.G. Peters, and M.J. Janse. Catecholamine release and potassium accumulation in the isolated globally ischemic rabbit heart. *J. Mol. Cell. Cardiol.* 20: 887–896, 1988.

Wilde, A.A.M., D. Escande, C.A. Schumacher, D. Thuringer, M. Mestre, and J.W.T. Fiolet. Glibenclamide inhibition of ATP-sensitive K^+ channels and ischemia-induced K^+ accumulation in the mammalian heart. *Pflügers Arch.* 414(Suppl. 1): S176, 1989.

Wilde, A.A.M., D. Escande, C.A. Schumacher, D. Thuringer, M. Mestre, J.W.T. Fiolet, and M.J. Janse. Potassium accumulation in the globally ischemic mammalian heart. A role for the ATP-sensitive potassium channel. *Circ. Res.* 67: 835–843, 1990.

Wilensky, R.L., J. Tranum-Jensen, R. Coronel, A.A.M. Wilde, J.W.T. Fiolet, and M.J. Janse. The subendocardial border zone during acute ischemia of the rabbit heart: An electrophysiologic, metabolic, and morphologic correlative study. *Circulation* 74: 1137–1146, 1986.

Willems, A.R. Ventricular tachycardia or ventricular fibrillation late after myocardial infarction. (Doctoral Thesis) University of Amsterdam. ICG Printing BV, Dordrecht, 1990.

Willems, A.R., J.G.P. Tijssen, F.J.L. van Capelle, J.H. Kingma, R.N.W. Hauer, F.E.E. Vermeulen, P. Brugada, D.C.A. van Hoogenhuyze, and M.J. Janse. On behalf of the Dutch Ventricular Tachycardia Study Group of the Interuniversity Cardiology Institute of the Netherlands. Determinants of prognosis in symptomatic ventricular tachycardia or ventricular fibrillation late after myocardial infarction. *J. Am. Coll. Cardiol.* 16: 521–530, 1990.

Williams, D.O., B.J. Scherlag, R.R. Hope, N. El-Sherif, and R. Lazzara. The pathophysiology of malignant ventricular arrhythmias during acute myocardial ischemia. *Circulation* 50: 1163–1172, 1974.

Williams, H.B., B.G. King, L.P. Ferris, and P.W. Spence. Susceptibility of heart to electric shock in different phases of the cardiac cycle. *Proc. Soc. Exptl. Biol. & Med.* 31: 873–874, 1934.

Windisch, H., and H.A. Tritthart. Isoproterenol, norepinephrine and phosphodiesterase inhibitors are blockers of the depressed fast Na^+-system in ventricular muscle fibers. *J. Mol. Cell. Cardiol.* 14: 431–434, 1982.

Winfree, A.T. Electrical instability in cardiac muscle: phase singularities and rotors. *J. Theor. Biol.* 138: 353–405, 1989.

Winfree, A.T. Stable particle-like solutions to the nonlinear wave equations of three-dimensional excitable media. *SIAM Rev* 32: 1–53, 1990a.

Winfree, A.T. Ventricular reentry in three dimensions. In: *Cardiac Electrophysiology: From Cell to Bedside*, edited by D.P. Zipes, and J. Jalife. W.B. Saunders, Philadelphia: 1990b, pp. 224–234.

Winfree, A.T. Vortex action potentials in normal ventricular muscle. In: *Mathematical Approaches to Cardiac Arrhythmias*, edited by J. Jalife. New York Academy of Sciences, New York: *Ann. N.Y. Acad. Sci.* 591:190–207, 1990c.

Wit, A.L., B.N. Goldreyer, and A.N. Damato. An in vitro model of paroxysmal supraventricular tachycardia. *Circulation* 43: 862–875, 1971.

Wit, A.L., B.F. Hoffman, and P.F. Cranefield. Slow conduction and reentry in the ventricular conducting system. I. Return extrasystole in canine Purkinje fibers. *Circ. Res.* 30: 1–10, 1972a.

Wit, A.L., P.F. Cranefield, and B.F. Hoffman. Slow conduction and reentry in the ventricular conducting system. II. Single and sustained circus movement in networks of canine and bovine Purkinje fibers. *Circ. Res.* 30: 11–22, 1972b.

Wit, A.L., J.J. Fenoglio Jr., B.M. Wagner, and A.L. Bassett. Electrophysiological properties of cardiac muscle in the anterior mitral valve leaflet and the adjacent atrium in the dog. Possible implications for the genesis of atrial dysrhythmias. *Circ. Res.* 32: 731–745, 1973.

Wit, A.L., and J.T. Bigger Jr. Possible electrophysiological mechanisms for lethal arrhythmias accompanying myocardial ischemia and infarction. *Circulation* 52(Suppl. III): III-96-III-115, 1975.

Wit, A.L., and P.L. Friedman. The basis for ventricular arrhythmias accompanying myocardial infarction: Alterations in electrical activity of ventricular muscle and Purkinje fibers after coronary artery occlusion. *Arch. Intern. Med.* 135: 459–471, 1975.

Wit, A.L., B.F. Hoffman, and M.R. Rosen. Electrophysiology and pharmacology of cardiac arrhythmias. IX. Cardiac electrophysiologic effects of beta adrenergic receptor stimulation and blockade. Part A. *Am. Heart J.* 90: 521–533, 1975.

Wit, A.L., J.R. Wiggins, and P.F. Cranefield. Some effects of electrical stimulation on impulse initiation in cardiac fibers; its relevance for the determination of the mechanisms of clinical cardiac arrhythmias. In: *The Conduction System of the Heart*, edited by H.J.J. Wellens, K.I. Lie, and M.J. Janse. Lea & Febiger, Philadelphia: 1976, pp. 163–181.

Wit, A.L., and P.F. Cranefield. Triggered activity in cardiac muscle fibers of the simian mitral valve. *Circ. Res.* 38: 85–98, 1976.

Wit, A.L., and P.F. Cranefield. Triggered and automatic activity in the canine coronary sinus. *Circ. Res.* 41: 435–445, 1977.

Wit, A.L., and P.F. Cranefield. Reentrant excitation as a cause of cardiac arrhythmias. *Am. J. Physiol.* 235: H1-H17, 1978.

Wit, A.L., P.A. Boyden, D.C. Gadsby, and P.F. Cranefield. Triggered activity as a cause of atrial arrhythmias. In: *Cardiac Arrhythmias: Electrophysiology, Diagnosis and Management*, edited by O.S. Narula. Williams and Wilkins, Baltimore: 1979, pp. 14–31.

Wit, A.L., P.F. Cranefield, and D.C. Gadsby. Triggered activity. In: *The Slow Inward Current and Cardiac Arrhythmias*, edited by D.P. Zipes, J.C. Bailey, and V. Elharrar. Martinus Nijhoff, The Hague: 1980, pp. 437–454.

Wit, A.L., M.A. Allessie, J.J. Fenoglio Jr., F.I.M. Bonke, W.J.E.P. Lammers, and J. Smeets. Significance of the endocardial and epicardial border zones in the genesis of myocardial infarction arrhythmias. In: *Cardiac Arrhythmias: A Decade of Progress*, edited by D.C. Harrison. G.K. Hall Medical Publishers, Boston: 1981a, pp. 39–68.

Wit, A.L., P.F. Cranefield, and D.C. Gadsby. Electrogenic sodium extrusion can stop triggered activity in the canine coronary sinus. *Circ. Res.* 49: 1029–1042, 1981b.

Wit, A.L., and P.F. Cranefield. Mechanisms of impulse initiation in the atrioventricular junction and the effects of acetylstrophanthidin. (abstract) *Am. J. Cardiol.* 49: 921, 1982.

Wit, A.L., M.A. Allessie, F.I.M. Bonke, W. Lammers, J. Smeets, and J.J. Fenoglio Jr. Electrophysiologic mapping to determine the mechanism of experimental ventricular tachycardia initiated by premature impulses. Experimental approach and initial results demonstrating reentrant excitation. *Am. J. Cardiol.* 49: 166–185, 1982a.

Wit, A.L., M.A. Allessie, F.I.M. Bonke, J.J. Fenoglio Jr., W. Lammers, and J. Smeets. Reentrant excitation in the infarcted canine ventricle. In: *Normal and Abnormal Conduction in the Heart*, edited by A. Paes de Carvalho, B.F. Hoffman, and M. Lieberman. Futura Publishing Company, Mt. Kisco, New York: 1982b, pp. 483–510.

Wit, A.L., and M.R. Rosen. Cellular electrophysiology of cardiac arrhythmias. In: *Tachycardias: Mechanisms, Diagnosis, Treatment*, edited by M.E. Josephson, and H.J.J. Wellens. Lea & Febiger, Philadelphia: 1984, pp. 1–27.

Wit, A.L. and M.E. Josephson. Fractionated electrograms and continuous electrical activity: fact or artifact. In: *Cardiac Electrophysiology and Arrhythmias*, edited by D.P. Zipes, and J. Jalife. Grune and Stratton, Orlando: 1985, pp. 343–351.

Wit, A.L., and M.R. Rosen. Afterdepolarizations and triggered activity. In: *The Heart and Cardiovascular System*, edited by H.A. Fozzard, E. Haber, R.B. Jennings, A.M. Katz, and H.E. Morgan. Raven Press, New York: 1986, pp. 1449–1490.

Wit, A.L., S. Dillon, and P.C. Ursell. Influences of anisotropic tissue structure on reentrant ventricular tachycardia. In: *Cardiac Arrhythmias: Where To Go From Here?*, edited by P. Brugada, and H.J.J. Wellens. Futura Publishing Company, Mt. Kisco, New York: 1987, pp. 27–50.

Wit, A.L. Anisotropic reentry: a model of arrhythmias that may necessitate a new approach to antiarrhythmic drug development. In: *Lethal Arrhythmias Resulting From Myocardial Ischemia and Infarction*, edited by M.R. Rosen, and Y. Palti. Kluwer Academic Publishers, Boston: 1989, pp. 199–213.

Wit, A.L., and M.R. Rosen. Cellular electrophysiological mechanisms of cardiac arrhythmias. In: *Comprehensive Electrocardiology. Theory and Practice in Health and Disease*. Vol. 2, edited by P.W. Macfarlane, and T.D. Veitch Lawrie. Pergamon Press, New York: 1989, pp. 801–841.

Wit, A.L., S.M. Dillon, J. Coromilas, A.E. Saltman, and R. Waldecker. Anisotropic reentry in the epicardial border zone of myocardial infarcts. In: *Mathematical Approaches to Cardiac Arrhythmias*, edited by J. Jalife. New York Academy of Sciences, New York: *Ann. N.Y. Acad. Sci.* 591: 86–108, 1990a.

WWit, A.L., G.-N. Tseng, B. Henning, and M.S. Hanna. Arrhythmogenic effects of quinidine on catecholamine-induced delayed afterdepolarizations in canine atrial fibers. *J. Cardiovasc. Elect.* 1: 15–30 1990b.

Wittenberg, S.M., Streuli, F., and F.J. Klocke. Acceleration of ventricular pacemakers by transient increases in heart rate in dogs during ouabain administration. *Circ. Res.* 26: 705–716, 1970.

Wittig, J.H., and J.P. Boineau. Surgical treatment of ventricular arrhythmias using epicardial, transmural and endocardial mapping. *Ann. Thorac. Surg.* 20: 117–125, 1975.

Wojtczak, J. Contractures and increase in internal longitudinal resistance of cow ventricular muscle induced by hypoxia. *Circ. Res.* 44: 88–95, 1979.

Wolferth, C.C. So called interpolation of extrasystoles during idio-ventricular rhythm. *Am. Heart J.* 5: 482–485, 1930.

Wolleben, C.D., M.C. Sanguinetti, and P.K.S. Siegl. Influence of ATP-sensitive potassium channel modulators on ischemia-induced fibrillation in isolated rat hearts. *J. Mol. Cell. Cardiol.* 21: 783–788, 1989.

Wong, S.S., A.L. Bassett, J.S. Cameron, K. Epstein, P. Kozlovskis, and R.J. Myerburg. Dissimilarities in the electrophysiological abnormalities of lateral border and central infarct zone cells after healing of myocardial infarction in cats. *Circ. Res.* 51: 486–493, 1982.

Worley, S.J., G.H. Bardy, W.M. Smith, and R.E. Ideker. Continuous fractionated electrical activity from the composite electrode during slow orderly epicardial depolarization. (abstract) *Am. J. Cardiol.* 49: 946, 1982.

Wüsten, B., W. Flameng, and W. Schaper. The distribution of myocardial flow:

Part I: Effects of experimental coronary occlusion. *Basic Res. Cardiol.* 69: 422–434, 1974.

Wybauw, R. Sur le point d'origine de la systole cardiaque dans l'oreillette droite. *Arch. Int. Physiol.* 10: 78–89, 1910.

Yamada, M., M.J. Curtis, and D.J. Hearse. Is reperfusion-induced ventricular fibrillation an oxygen-dependent or a flow-dependent phenomenon? (abstract) *J. Mol. Cell. Cardiol.* 20(Suppl. V): S.29, 1988.

Yamazaki, S., Y. Fujibayashi, R.E. Rajagopalan, S. Meerbaum, and E. Corday. Effects of staged versus sudden reperfusion after acute coronary occlusion in the dog. *J. Am. Coll. Cardiol.* 7: 564–572, 1986.

Yanagihara, K., and H. Irisawa. Potassium current during the pacemaker depolarization in rabbit sinoatrial node cell. *Pflügers Arch.* 388: 255–260, 1980.

Zheutlin, T.A., H. Roth, W. Chua, R. Steinman, C. Summers, M. Lesch, and R.F. Kehoe. Programmed electrical stimulation to determine the need for antiarrhythmic therapy in patients with complex ventricular ectopic activity. *Am. Heart J.* 111: 860–867, 1986.

Zimmermann, M., P. Maisonblanche, B. Cauchemez, J.-F. Leclercq, and P. Coumel. Determinants of the spontaneous ectopic activity in repetitive monomorphic idiopathic ventricular tachycardia. *J. Am. Coll. Cardiol.* 7: 1219–1227, 1986.

Zipes, D.P., and C. Mendez. Action of manganese ions and tetrodotoxin on atrioventricular nodal transmembrane potentials in isolated rabbit hearts. *Circ. Res.* 32: 447–454, 1973.

Zipes, D.P., E. Arbel, R.F. Knope, and G.K. Moe. Accelerated cardiac escape rhythms caused by ouabain intoxication. *Am. J. Cardiol.* 33: 248–253, 1974.

Zipes, D.P. Influence of myocardial ischemia and infarction on autonomic innervation of heart. *Circulation* 82: 1095–1105, 1990.

Zuanetti, G., G.M. De Ferrari, S.G. Priori, and P.J. Schwartz. Protective effect of vagal stimulation on reperfusion arrhythmias in cats. *Circ. Res.* 61: 429–435, 1987.

Index

635